Cardiac Imaging Update 2025

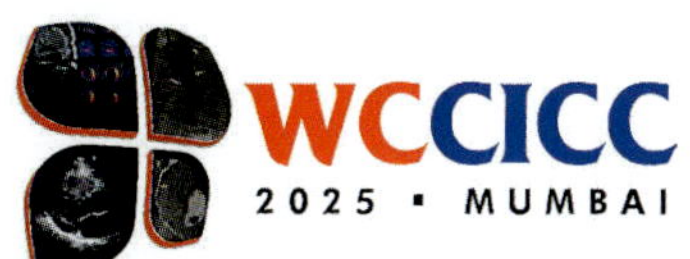

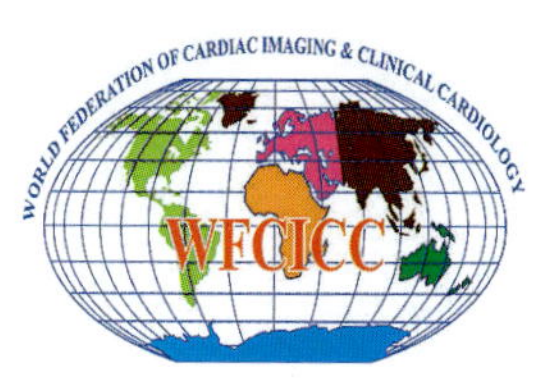

Cardiac Imaging Update 2025

Editors

GN Mahapatra
DRM DSc FRCP FCCP FICA FIAMS
Director
Department of Nuclear Medicine and PET-CT and Cardiac Imaging
Sri Aurobindo Institute of Medical Sciences
Indore, Madhya Pradesh, India
Senior Consultant and Head
Department of Nuclear Medicine, PET-CT, and SPECT
Seven Hills Hospital
Mumbai, Maharashtra, India
Director
West Coast Medical Center
Mumbai, Maharashtra, India

PC Manoria
MD DM FACC FESC FAPSC
Director
Department of Cardiology
Manoria Heart and Critical Care Hospital
Bhopal, Madhya Pradesh, India

Diwakar Jain
MD FACC FRCP MASNC FSNMMI
Professor of Medicine
New York Medical College
Director, Nuclear Cardiovascular Imaging Laboratory
Director, Cardio-Oncology Service
Department of Cardiovascular Medicine
Westchester Medical Center
Valhalla, New York, USA

Foreword

HK Chopra

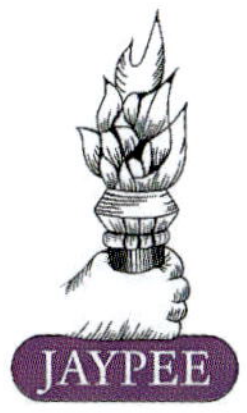

JAYPEE BROTHERS MEDICAL PUBLISHERS
The Health Sciences Publisher
New Delhi | London

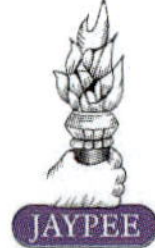

Jaypee Brothers Medical Publishers (P) Ltd

Headquarters
EMCA House, 23/23-B
Ansari Road, Daryaganj
New Delhi 110 002, India
Landline: +91-11-23272143, +91-11-23272703
+91-11-23282021, +91-11-23245672
e-mail: jaypee@jaypeebrothers.com

Corporate Office
4838/24, Ansari Road, Daryaganj
New Delhi 110 002, India
Phone: +91-11-43574357
Fax: +91-11-43574314
e-mail: jaypee@jaypeebrothers.com

Overseas Office
JP Medical Ltd.
83, Victoria Street, London
SW1H 0HW (UK)
Phone: +44-20 3170 8910
e-mail: info@jpmedpub.com

EU GPSR Authorised Representative
Logos Europe, 9 rue Nicolas Poussin
17000, La Rochelle, France
Phone: +33 (0) 6 67 93 73 78
e-mail: contact@logoseurope.eu

Website: www.jaypeebrothers.com
Website: www.jaypeedigital.com

Cardiac Imaging Update 2025

First Edition: **2026**

ISBN: 978-93-7202-540-8

Printed at: Samrat Offset Pvt. Ltd.

प्रारूप आरजी - 2
Form RG - 2

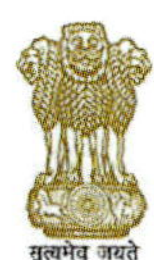

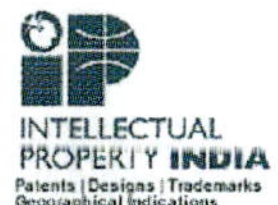

भारत सरकार
Government of India
व्यापार चिन्ह रजिस्ट्री
Trade Marks Registry

क्रमांक
No. 2442588

व्यापार चिन्ह अधिनियम, 1999
Trade Marks Act, 1999

व्यापार चिन्ह के रजिस्ट्रीकरण का प्रमाणपत्र, धारा 23 (2), नियम 56 (1)
Certificate of Registration of Trade Mark, Section 23 (2), Rule 56 (1)

व्यापार चिन्ह संख्या / **Trade Mark No.** 3436251 दिनांक /**Date** 19/12/2016 ज. संख्या /**J. No.** 1930

यह प्रमाणित किया जाता है कि जिस प्रकार चिन्ह की समाकृति इसके साथ संलग्न है, वह ....
के बारे में दिनांक ....नाम से रजिस्ट्रीकृत हो चुका है।
Certified that Trade Mark / a representation is annexed hereto, has been registered in the name(s) of :-
JAYPEE BROTHERS MEDICAL PUBLISHERS PRIVATE LIMITED, 4838/24, ANSARI ROAD, DARYAGANJ, NEW DELHI-110002, Body Incorporate, Service Provider, (Body Incorporate)

In Class 41 Under No. 3436251 as of the date 19 December 2016 in respect of

PUBLICATION SERVICES RELATING TO BOOKS, NOTE-BOOKS, MAGAZINES, BROCHURES, PAMPHLETS, MANULAS, PUBLICATION OF PRINTED MATTERS, ELECTRONIC PUBLICATON INCLUDED IN CLASS-41

JAYPEE BROTHERS MEDICAL PUBLISHERS

मेरे निर्देश पर आज .... के .... मास के .... वे दिन को इस पर मुद्रा लगायी गई
Sealed at my direction, this 07th day of August , 2020

व्यापार चिन्ह रजिस्ट्री
Trade Marks Registry MUMBAI

व्यापार चिन्ह रजिस्ट्रार
Registrar of Trademarks

रजिस्ट्रीकरण आवेदन की तारीख से १० वर्ष के लिए है और तदोपरांत वह १० वर्ष की कालावधि के लिए और प्रत्येक १० वर्ष की कालावधि के अवसान पर भी नवीनीकृत किया जा सकेगा।
Registration is for 10 years from the date of application and may then be renewed for a period of 10 years and also at the expiration of each period of 10 years.
यह प्रमाणपत्र विधि कार्यवाहियों में प्रयोग के लिए या विदेश में रजिस्ट्रीकरण अभिप्राप्त करने के लिए नहीं है
This certificate is not for use in legal proceedings or for obtaining Registration abroad.
टिप्पणी - इस व्यापार चिन्ह के स्वामित्व में कोई परिवर्तन होने पर, या कारोबार के मुख्य स्थान के पते में या भारत में तामील के लिए पते में परिवर्तन होने पर परिवर्तन के लिए आवेदन तुरंत किया जाना चाहिए.
Note: Upon any change of ownership of this Trademark, or change in address, of the principal place of business or address for service in India a request should **AT ONCE** be made to register the change.

Govt. Issued Document; Copying is an Illegal Act.

INTELLECTUAL PROPERTY **INDIA**
PATENTS | DESIGNS | TRADE MARKS
GEOGRAPHICAL INDICATIONS

सत्यमेव जयते

प्रारूप आरजी - 2
Form RG - 2
क्रमांक **No.** 3772319

व्यापार चिन्ह रजिस्ट्री, भारत सरकार Trade Marks Registry, Government Of India

व्यापार चिन्ह अधिनियम, 1999 Trade Marks Act, 1999

व्यापार चिन्ह के रजिस्ट्रीकरण का प्रमाणपत्र | Certificate of Registration of Trade Mark

(धारा 23 (2), नियम 56 (1)) | Section 23 (2), Rule 56 (1)

व्यापार चिन्ह संख्या / Trade Mark No. : 5191318
दिनांक / Date : 28-10-2021
ज. संख्या / J. No. : 2158

प्रमाणित किया जाता है कि व्यापार चिन्ह / जिसका प्रतिरूप इसके साथ संलग्न है, वह .... के नाम से .... वर्ग में .... संख्या के अधीन दिनांक .... को .... के संबंध में रजिस्ट्रीकृत किया गया है।

Certified that Trade Mark / a representation is annexed hereto, has been registered in the name(s) of :- JAYPEE BROTHERS MEDICAL PUBLISHERS PRIVATE LIMITED, 4838/24, ANSARI ROAD, DARYAGANJ, NEW DELHI-110002., Body Incorporate, (Body Incorporate)

In Class 41 Under No. 5191318 as of the date 28 October 2021 in respect of

Publication Services, Electronic Publication, Issue of Publications, Publication of Books and Textbooks, Publication of Booklets, Publication of Brochures, Publication of Journals, included Under Class-41.

Trade Mark as annexed

आज वर्ष 20.................... के .... माह के .... वें दिन को मेरे निर्देश पर मुद्रांकित किया गया

Sealed at my direction, this 19th day of October, 2024

व्यापार चिन्ह रजिस्ट्री मुंबई
Trade Marks Registry MUMBAI

उन्नत पी पंडित
व्यापार चिन्ह रजिस्ट्रार
Registrar of Trademarks

रजिस्ट्रीकरण आवेदन की तारीख से १० वर्ष के लिए है और तदोपरांत वह १० वर्ष की अवधि के लिए और प्रत्येक १० वर्ष की अवधि की समाप्ति पर भी नवीनीकृत किया जा सकेगा।
यह प्रमाणपत्र विधि कार्यवाहियों में प्रयोग के लिए या विदेश में रजिस्ट्रीकरण प्राप्त करने के लिए नहीं है
टिप्पणी : इस व्यापार चिन्ह के स्वामित्व में कोई परिवर्तन होने पर, या कारोबार के मुख्य स्थान के पते में या भारत में सेवा के लिए पते में परिवर्तन होने पर परिवर्तन को दर्ज करने के लिए एक बार अनुरोध किया जाना चाहिए.
Registration is for 10 years from the date of application and may then be renewed for a period of 10 years and also at the expiration of each period of 10 years.
This certificate is not for use in legal proceedings or for obtaining Registration abroad.
Note: Upon any change of ownership of this Trademark, or change in address, of the principal place of business or address for service in India a request should AT ONCE be made to register the change.

व्यापार चिन्ह के लिए अनुलग्नक / Annexure of Trade Mark Certificate

क्रमांक / No. **3772319**

व्यापार चिन्ह संख्या / Trade Mark No. **5191318**

दिनांक / Date **28-10-2021**

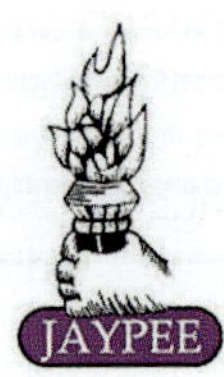

Contributors

A Muruganathan MD
Emeritus Professor
The Tamil Nadu Dr MGR Medical University
Chennai, Tamil Nadu
Senior Physician
Shristi AG Hospital
Tiruppur, Tamil Nadu, India

Aarathy Kannan
MD Dip Diab FDI FCDM MBA (HM)
Director
Sundaram Arulrhaj Hospitals
Consultant Physician and Diabetologist
Dr Aruls Diabetes, Lifestyle and Research Centre
Thoothukudi, Tamil Nadu, India

Abhishek Garg MD
Resident (DM)
Department of Cardiology
Dayanand Medical College and Hospital
Unit Hero DMC Heart Institute
Ludhiana, Punjab, India

Abhishek Kumar Tiwari MD DM
Associate Consultant
Cardiac Care
Medanta—The Medicity
Gurugram, Haryana, India

Abraham Oomman MD DM
Senior Consultant Cardiologist and HF Specialist
Department of Heart Lung Transplant
Apollo Hospitals
Chennai, Tamil Nadu, India

Ajit G Desai MD DM DNB AFACC
Additional Director
Department of Cardiology
Jaslok Hospital, Mumbai
Interventional Cardiologist
Department of Cardiology
HN Reliance Foundation Hospital
Mumbai, Maharashtra, India

AK Pancholia
MD FACC FESC FCSI FISH FIMSA MAMS
Head
Department of Medicine, Clinical and Preventive Cardiology
Arihant Hospital
Indore, Madhya Pradesh, India

Akshit Kumar MD
Senior Resident
Department of Cardiothoracic Radiology and Endovascular Interventions
All India Institute of Medical Sciences
New Delhi, India

Alok Modi
MD FISH (India) FACP (USA)
Medical Director
Alok Modi's Diabetes Centre and Kevalya Hospital
Consultant Physician and Diabetologist
Jupiter Hospital, Thane
Mumbai, Maharashtra, India

Amrish Agrawal
MD DM (Card) FACC FRCP (Glasg) FRCP (Edin) MRCP (UK) FCCP FCSI Fellow Cardiology (Australia)
Senior Consultant Cardiologist
Professor of Cardiology
Fujairah Hospital EHS
Fujairah, UAE

Anita Saxena MD DM FACC
Executive Director
Department of Cardiology
Fortis Escorts Heart Institute
New Delhi, India

Aparna Mukund Patankar
DNB (Radiology)
Consultant Radiologist
Department of Radiology
Nanavati Max Superspecialty Hospital
Mumbai, Maharashtra, India

Arindam Pande
MD (Med) DM (Cardio) FICC FESC FSCAI (USA) FACC (USA) FRCP (Glasg)
Senior Consultant Cardiologist
Department of Cardiology
Medica Superspecialty Hospital
Kolkata, West Bengal, India

Aruna Korde PhD
Radiopharmaceutical Scientist
Department of Nuclear Sciences and Applications
International Atomic Energy Agency (IAEA)
Vienna International Centre
Vienna, Austria

Asha Moorthy
MD DM FCCP FIACM FICP FIMSA FICC
Senior Consultant Cardiologist
AINU V Scans Centre, Chennai
Former Professor and Head
Department of Cardiology
SRMC and Saveetha Medical College
Chennai, Tamil Nadu, India

Ashok Das
MD FAMS FICP PhD FRCP
Dean and Medical Superintendent
Jawaharlal Institute of Postgraduate Medical Education and Research, Puducherry
Professor of Medicine
Professor and Head of Endocrinology
Pondicherry Institute of Medical Sciences
Puducherry, India

Banshi Saboo
MD PhD FACE
Chairman and Chief Diabetologist
Dia Care, Diabetes Care and Hormone Clinic
Ahmedabad, Gujarat, India

Bharat Saboo
MBBS Diploma in Diabetology PGP (Diabetology & Cardiology)
Diabetologist
Prayas Diabetes Centre
Indore, Madhya Pradesh, India

Bhargav Kiran Gaddam MD
Associate Professor
Department of General Medicine
Mahatma Gandhi Medical College and Research Institute
Sri Balaji Vidyapeeth
(Deemed to be University)
Puducherry, India

Bhavya Mody MBBS
Resident Doctor
Department of Internal Medicine
Trinity Health Hospital
Livonia, Michigan, USA

Bhukya Anji Babu MD
Senior Resident
Department of Cardiology
KIMS Hospitals
Secunderabad, Telangana, India

Blessvin Jino MD DM FNB
Consultant Interventional Cardiologist
Department of Cardiology
Meditrina Hospitals Pvt Ltd
Kollam, Kerala, India

Chris Alvis Shaji MD
Senior Resident
Internal Medicine
Medanta—The Medicity
Gurugram, Haryana, India

Cigdem Akincioglu MD
Associate Professor
Division of Molecular Imaging and Theranostics
University of Western Ontario
London, Ontario, Canada

Dayasagar Rao V
DM (Cardiology) FRCP (Canada) FRCP (Edinburgh)
Senior Consultant Interventional Cardiologist
Department of Cardiology
KIMS Hospitals
Secunderabad, Telangana, India

Debabrata Dash
MD DM FICC FAPSC FCCP FSCA
Senior Consultant and Interventional Cardiologist
Department of Cardiology
Aster Hospital
Dubai, Al Qusais, UAE

Dhinesh Kumar MD
DNB Resident
Internal Medicine
Sundaram Arulrhaj Hospitals
Tuticorin, Tamil Nadu, India

Diwakar Jain
MD FACC FRCP MASNC FSNMMI
Professor of Medicine
New York Medical College
Director, Nuclear Cardiovascular Imaging Laboratory
Director, Cardio-Oncology Service
Department of Cardiovascular Medicine
Westchester Medical Center
Valhalla, New York, USA

Geetha Priya V MD (Medicine)
Resident (DNB)
Department of Cardiology
Manipal Hospitals
Bengaluru, Karnataka, India

Girish G
DNB (Cardiology) MRCP FRCPC
Interventional Cardiologist
Department of Cardiology
Manipal Hospital
Bengaluru, Karnataka, India

GN Mahapatra
DRM DSc FRCP FCCP FICA FIAMS
Director
Department of Nuclear Medicine and PET-CT and Cardiac Imaging
Sri Aurobindo Institute of Medical Sciences
Indore, Madhya Pradesh, India
Senior Consultant and Head
Department of Nuclear Medicine, PET-CT, and SPECT
Seven Hills Hospital
Mumbai, Maharashtra, India
Director
West Coast Medical Center
Mumbai, Maharashtra, India

Gurpreet Singh Wander MD DM
Professor
Department of Cardiology
Dayanand Medical College and Hospital
Unit Hero DMC Heart Institute
Ludhiana, Punjab, India

Harsh Hirani MBBS CCGDM
Diabetologist
Life Care Centre for Diabetes
Hyderabad, Telangana, India

HK Chopra MD DM
Senior Consultant Cardiologist
Department of Cardiology
Medanta Moolchand Heart Institute
New Delhi, India

Iyengar SS
DM (Cardiology) FRCP (E)
Consultant
Department of Cardiology
Manipal Hospitals
Bengaluru, Karnataka, India

Jayanta K Panda
MD (Internal Medicine) FICP FACP FRSSDI FIMAMS
Consultant in Diabetes
Metabolic and Critical Care Medicine
Professor (PG)
Department of Medicine
SCB Medical College
Cuttack, Odisha, India

Johann Christopher
MD DNB FICI FACC
Consultant Cardiologist
Director of Cardiac Imaging
Care Hospitals
Hyderabad, Telangana, India

John LaForge MBBS
Resident
Internal Medicine
University of Alabama at Birmingham
Birmingham, Alabama, USA

Kabir Sethi MD DM FESC
Department of Structural Heart Disease
Hospital of University of Mainz
Mainz, Germany

Kamal K Sethi
MD DM FACC FHRS FCSI FISE
Director of Cardiology
Chairman and Managing Director
Delhi Heart and Lung Institute
New Delhi, India

Karthik Ananthasubramaniam
MD FACC FASE FASNC FSCCT FSCMR FRCP
Director of Echocardiography
Nuclear Cardiology/Cardiac PET
Heart and Vascular Institute
Henry Ford West Bloomfield Hospital
West Bloomfield, Michigan, USA

Madhumanti Panja
MD DNB (Cardiology)
Consultant Interventional Cardiologist
Belle Vue Clinic
AMRI Hospital
Kolkata, West Bengal, India

Manish Bansal MD DNB
Senior Director
Clinical and Preventive Cardiology
Medanta—The Medicity
Gurugram, Haryana, India

Manish Ora MD
Assistant Professor
Department of the Nuclear Medicine
Sanjay Gandhi Postgraduate Institute
of Medical Sciences
Lucknow, Uttar Pradesh, India

Manoranjan Behera MD FICP
Professor
Postgraduate Department of Medicine
SCB Medical College
Cuttack, Odisha, India

Manu Rajendran MD DM (Cardiology)
Senior Consultant and Interventional
Cardiologist
Department of Cardiology
Meditrina Hospitals Pvt Ltd
Kollam, Kerala, India

Meera Venkatesh PhD
Retiree Director
Division of Physical and
Chemical Sciences
International Atomic Energy Agency
Vienna, Austria

Mitendra Singh Yadav MD DNB
Associate Director
Department of Cardiology
Max Super Specialty Hospital
New Delhi, India

Monotosh Panja
MD FACC (USA) FCSI FICP DM (Cardiology)
Senior Consultant and Interventional
Cardiologist
Belle Vue Clinic, Kolkata
BM Birla Heart Institute, Kolkata
Former Director, ICVS
Institute of Postgraduate Medical
Education and Research
and SSKM Hospital
Kolkata, West Bengal, India

N Ramamoorthy PhD
Adjunct Professor
National Institute of Advanced Studies
Bengaluru, Karnataka, India

Narra Lavanya MD DrNB
Consultant Cardiology
Department of Cardiology
KIMS Hospital
Hyderabad, Telangana, India

Navin C Nanda MD DSc (Hon)
Distinguished Professor
Division of Cardiovascular Disease
Department of Medicine
University of Alabama at Birmingham
Birmingham, Alabama, USA

Nikesh D Jain
DNB (Med) DNB (Card) FESC FSCAI
Interventional Cardiologist
Department of Cardiology
Masina Heart Institute
Mumbai, Maharashtra, India

Nilay S Nimbalkar DMRD DNB
Director and Head for Postgraduate and
Fellowship Studies
Precision Scan and Research Centre
Nagpur, Maharashtra, India

Nitesh Raj Dulal MBBS
Research Fellow, Echocardiography
Laboratory
Cardiology Division
University of Alabama at Birmingham
Birmingham, Alabama, USA

Pankaj Manoria MD DM FACC FESC
Director
Department of Cardiology
Manoria Heart and Critical Care Hospital
Bhopal, Madhya Pradesh, India

Parneesh Arora MD DM
Director (Cardiac Sciences)
Medanta Super Speciality Hospital
Noida, Uttar Pradesh, India

Parul Samir Garde
DNB (Radiology) DMRD
Associate Director
Department of Radiology
Nanavati Max Super Specialty Hospital
Mumbai, Maharashtra, India

PC Manoria MD DM FACC FESC FAPSC
Director
Department of Cardiology
Manoria Heart and Critical Care Hospital
Bhopal, Madhya Pradesh, India

PC Rath
MD DM FESC FACC FICC FRCP (London)
FRCP (Edinburgh)
Director and Head
Department of Cardiology
Apollo Hospitals
Hyderabad, Telangana, India

Perry Gerard MD
Professor of Radiology and Medicine
New York Medical College
Director of Nuclear Medicine
Vice Chair, Department of Radiology
Westchester Medical Center
Valhalla, New York, USA

Prajakta Kirdatpatil
MD (Radiodiagnosis)
Fellowship in Cardiothoracic Imaging
Precision Scan and Research Centre
Nagpur, Maharashtra, India

Prajwal Chauhan MBBS
Junior Resident
Department of Nuclear Medicine
Sanjay Gandhi Postgraduate Institute
of Medical Sciences
Lucknow, Uttar Pradesh, India

Prashant Moorthy MD FRCR
Senior Consultant Radiologist
MGM College and Hospital
Chennai, Tamil Nadu, India

Prathap Kumar MD DM FIC
Chief Interventional Cardiologist
Department of Cardiology
Meditrina Hospital
Kollam, Kerala, India
Course Director Indo Japanese CTO Club (IJCTO)

Preeti Neve DMRD DNB (Radiodiagnosis)
Consultant and Cardiothoracic Radiologist
Star Imaging and Research Center
Department of Radiology
Pune, Maharashtra, India

Priya Jagia MD DNB
Professor and Head
Department of Cardiothoracic Radiology and Endovascular Interventions
All India Institute of Medical Sciences
New Delhi, India

Raj Wasan
College of William and Mary
Williamsburg, Virginia, USA

Rakesh Gupta
MD FASE FISCU FACC (USA) FCSI FIAE FICP FIMSA FIACTA
Director and Chief Cardiologist
JROP Institute of Echocardiography, Ultrasound, and Vascular Doppler
New Delhi, India

Ravi R Kasliwal MD DM
Chairman
Clinical and Preventive Cardiology
Medanta—The Medicity
Gurugram, Haryana, India

Ravi Ranjan Kindo
MD DM (Cardiology)
Consultant Cardiologist
Department of Cardiology
SMC Heart Institute
Raipur, Chhattisgarh, India

Ravindra Bhardwaj
MD MPH FACC FACP
Consultant Cardiologist
Department of Cardiology
Krishna Heart Care
El Dorado, Arkansas, USA

Reefa Dsouza
MD (Pharmacology CCD Diabetes)
Director
Souza Clinic
EX Goa Medical College
Bambolim, Goa, India

Richa Kothari DNB (Radiodiagnosis)
Consultant
Department of Radiology
Narayana Institute of Cardiac Sciences
Bengaluru, Karnataka, India

RM Anitha MD
Assistant Professor
Department of General Medicine
Mahatma Gandhi Medical College and Research Institute
Sri Balaji Vidyapeeth
(Deemed to be University)
Puducherry, India

Rohit Mody
MD DM FSCAI FCSI FAPSIC MES
Director and Head
Department of Cardiology
Mody Harvard Cardiac Institute and Research Centre
Krishna Super Specialty Hospital
Bathinda, Punjab India

Roxy Senior
MD DM FRCP (Lond) FACC FESC FASE (Hon)
Professor of Clinical Cardiology
Consultant Cardiologist
Director of Echocardiography
Royal Brompton Hospital (Part of GSTT)
London, UK

Runa Zaidi MD (Radiodiagnosis) EDiR
Junior Consultant
Department of Radiology
Narayana Institute of Cardiac Sciences
Bengaluru, Karnataka, India

S Arulrhaj
MD PhD DSc (Hony) FRCP (G) FRCP (L) MBA
Chairman and Chief Physician
Department of Internal Medicine
Sundaram Arulrhaj Hospital
Thoothukudi, Tamil Nadu, India

Sangeeta Dhir
MDS (Periodontology) Fellow (Implantology) Fellow (Diabetes India)
Consultant
(Dentistry and Clinical Research)
Department of Cardiology
Max Super Specialty Hospital
New Delhi, India

Sanjay Gambhir
MBBS DRM DNB
Professor and Head
Department of the Nuclear Medicine
Sanjay Gandhi Postgraduate Institute of Medical Sciences
Lucknow, Uttar Pradesh, India

Sanjay Mittal MD DM
Vice Chairman
Clinical and Preventive Cardiology
Medanta—The Medicity
Gurugram, Haryana, India

Sarita Rao
MD DM FACC FSCAI
Senior Interventional Cardiologist and Director (Cathlab)
Department of Cardiology
Apollo Hospitals
Indore, Madhya Pradesh, India

Satish Kumar Parashar
MD FACC FCSI FIAE
Director
Department of Non-invasive Cardiology
Heart Institute
Lajpat Nagar, New Delhi, India

Satyanarayan Routray
MD DM (Cardiology)
Professor and Head
Department of Cardiology
SCB Medical College and Hospital
Cuttack, Odisha, India

Saurabh Malhotra MD MPH
Director of Advanced Cardiac Imaging
Cook County Health
Associate Professor of Medicine (Cardiology)
Rush Medical College
Chicago, IL, USA

Shabbir Ali Shaik MD DM FNB FESC
Consultant Cardiologist
Department of Cardiology
AIG Hospitals
Hyderabad, Telangana, India

Shreya Ohri
MD (Cardiology) MD (Physician)
Senior Clinical Fellow
Echocardiography
Royal Brompton Hospital (Part of GSTT)
London, UK

Shruthi Kalyan DNB
Consultant and Cardiac Radiologist
Star Hospitals
Hyderabad, Telangana, India

Siddharth Sharma MD
Additional Professor
Department of the Nuclear Medicine
Sanjay Gandhi Postgraduate Institute of Medical Sciences
Lucknow, Uttar Pradesh, India

Simranpreet Singh Daid MBBS
Research Fellow
Cardiology Division
University of Alabama at Birmingham
Birmingham, AL, USA

Sradhananda Rout MD DM (Cardiology)
Senior Resident
Department of Cardiology
SMC Heart Institute
Raipur, Chhattisgarh, India

Subhajyoti Ghosh MD PhD
Metabolic Physician and Diabetologist
Apollo Clinic
Dibrugarh, Assam, India

Supraja Moorthy MD DNB FRCR
Assistant Professor
Department of Radiology
Pondicherry Institute of Medical Sciences
Puducherry, India

Supreetha Hegde A MD (Radiology)
Assistant Professor
Department of Radiodiagnosis
Kasturba Medical College
Manipal, Karnataka, India

Suraj Gowda MD DNB
Consultant Radiologist
Cardiothoracic Imaging Unit
Department of Radiology
Narayana Institute of Cardiac Sciences
Bengaluru, Karnataka, India

Sureshkumar Vellingiri MD
Assistant Professor
Department of General Medicine
Mahatma Gandhi Medical College and Research Institute
Sri Balaji Vidyapeeth
Puducherry, India

Thair Khuziem PhD (Cardiology)
Consultant Interventional Cardiologist
Department of Cardiology
Fujairah Hospital EHS
Fujairah, UAE

Tosha J Desai MD (Radiodiagnosis)
Consultant Radiologist
Department of Radiodiagnosis
Asian Heart Institute
Mumbai, Maharashtra, India

Upendra Kaul
MD DM FCSI FICC FACC FAPSIC FSCAI FAMS
Chairman (Cardiology) and
Dean (Academics and Research)
Batra Hospital and Medical Research Center
New Delhi, India

Vidit Bhatia MBBS
Student
Hamdard Institute of Medical Sciences and Research
New Delhi, India

Vijay Negalur
MD FICP FACP PGDDM FACE
Director
Renuka Hospital—Diabetes Care Centre
Dombivli
Director
Dr Negalur's Diabetes and Thyroid Specialties Center, Thane
Consulting Diabetologist
Jupiter Hospital
Thane, Maharashtra, India

Vijay Panikar MD DNB FCPS
Consultant
Department of Endocrinology and Diabetes
Lilavati Hospital and Research Centre
Director
Dr Panikar's Specialty Care Centres
Mumbai, Maharashtra India

Vineet Bhatia MD DM DNB
Director (Cardiac Sciences)
Medanta Super Speciality Hospital
Noida, Uttar Pradesh, India

Vishal Agrawal MBBS MRCP (UK)
Specialty Registrar
Department of Radiology
Mersey and West Lancashire Teaching Hospitals NHS Trust
Merseyside, UK

Viswanathan Venkatachalam
DM (Cardiology) DNB FRACP FCSANZ
Consultant Interventional Cardiologist
Heart and Beyond
Wahroonga and Norwest
New South Wales, Australia

Viveka Kumar
MD DM FSCAI FACC FECS FAPSIC FRCP (Edin)
Principal Director and Chief of Cath Labs
Cardiac Sciences
Max Super specialty Hospital
New Delhi, India

Vivekanand S Gajapati MD DM
Consultant Cardiologist
SDM Narayana Heart Centre
Dharwad, Karnataka, India

Zeeshan Sakina A Lakhani DNB (RD)
Director (Cardiac Imaging)
Aster Kerala Cluster and Meitra hospitals
Consultant and Cardiac Radiologist
MGM Healthcare, Apollo Hospitals and MMM Hospitals
Chennai, Tamil Nadu, India

Foreword

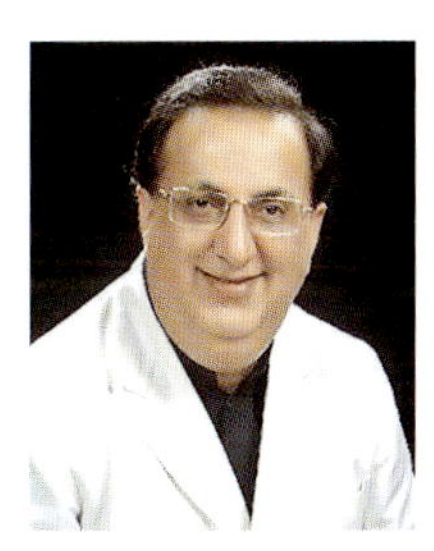

It is a great pleasure and honor indeed for me in writing the foreword for the need-based state-of-art textbook on *Cardiac Imaging Update 2025*, first of its kind, from India to the world with brainstorming, mind-boggling, and scintillating, and thought-provoking contents on every possible aspect.

It is one of the most-needed, comprehensive, illustrative, and well-structured books, published with enormous information about advances in clinical approach, imaging including echocardiography, multimodality imaging, drug, mechanical and surgical interventions for better patient care in various clinical situations.

This book comprises six sections, 49 chapters including Clinical Cardiology, Imaging Echocardiography, Nuclear Imaging and PET, Cardio-diabetology, CT and MRI, etc.

The chapters are well outlined, structured, well written, and referenced. The writing style of every chapter is vivid, concise, and practical. There are excellent graphics, tables, figures, and algorithms that present the relevant information. The printing and binding are of excellent quality. This book will represent a milestone for *Cardiac Imaging*, one of its kind from India to the world.

I congratulate the Editors, Dr GN Mahapatra, Dr PC Manoria, Dr Diwakar Jain, and all the contributors for accomplishing this prodigious achievement of great clinical relevance in Cardiology practice today for meticulous advances in *Cardiac Imaging Update 2025.*

I am sure that everyone will find this book very useful in providing comprehensive update on clinical application of all the sections mentioned above to enhance the potential, power, and promise clinical cardiology to improve the patient's care and thereby enhancing morbidity and mortality benefits.

I wish this textbook on *Cardiac Imaging Update 2025,* a great success to impact globally.

The good physician treats the disease; the great physician treats the patient who has the disease, and a super great physician prevents the disease by enhancing awareness on Clinical and Cardiac Imaging.

HK Chopra
Senior Cardiologist
Medanta Moolchand Heart Institute
Chairman CME, Moolchand Medcity, New Delhi
President, World Wellness Foundation, WHA
Country Head, AHA
Editor-in-Chief, Top 14 Focused Textbooks of Cardiology
Editor-in-Chief, 40 Handbooks in Cardiology and Medicine
National Awardee, DST, Govt of India
National Past President, CSI and IAE

Preface

Cardiac Imaging Update 2025 appears to be a valuable resource in the ever-evolving field of cardiovascular medicine, particularly given the rapid advancements in imaging technologies and their clinical applications. Here is why this book stands out:

As we stand at the precipice of a new era in cardiac care, *Cardiac Imaging Update 2025* emerges as the seminal guide to mastering today's most advanced diagnostic technologies. This meticulously curated volume represents the pinnacle of contemporary knowledge, offering unparalleled insights into the rapidly evolving landscape of cardiovascular imaging by a galaxy of experts who have excelled in their field.

The book provides current information on various imaging technologies used to evaluate the heart. It covers both common and advanced techniques such as echocardiography, computed tomography, and CT angiography, fractional flow reserve, single photon emission computed tomography, cardiac magnetic resonance positron emission tomography—CT and Intravascular Ultrasound and Optical Coherence Tomography. Besides this, the book also focused on lipidology, hypertension, cardio-diabetology, coronary artery disease, and heart failure.

We are very sure that the book will be of immense benefit to postgraduate students, physicians, and specialists of diverse fields and will immensely contribute to better patient's care.

GN Mahapatra
PC Manoria
Diwakar Jain

Contents

SECTION 1: Clinical Cardiology

SECTION 4: Cardiodiabetology

SECTION 5: Computed Tomography and Magnetic Resonance Imaging

SECTION 6: Miscellaneous

Clinical Cardiology

Coronary Artery Disease in Women: How is it Different?

Sarita Rao

INTRODUCTION

Cardiovascular disease (CVD), particularly coronary artery disease (CAD), is the leading global cause of mortality and morbidity.[1] Despite affecting both sexes, CVD in women presents unique challenges due to the interplay of biological, hormonal, and sociocultural factors that influence its prevalence, diagnosis, and outcomes. The misconception that heart disease is predominantly a "man's disease" contributes to the underdiagnosis and undertreatment of women, resulting in disproportionately higher mortality rates.[2] Globally, CAD causes over one-third of all deaths, with women accounting for 1 in 3 fatalities.[3] In India, the burden of CAD among women has reached epidemic levels, as highlighted by the INTERHEART study, which showed that women experience their first coronary event about 10 years later than men, often postmenopause. Despite this delay, mortality rates among women are rising faster than in men.[4]

Biological differences such as smaller coronary vessels, lower body surface area, and hormonal variations play a crucial role. Menopause-associated hormonal changes increase atherosclerosis risk, while elevated biomarkers like low-density lipoprotein (LDL) cholesterol, lipoprotein(a), and high-sensitivity CRP are critical predictors of cardiovascular events. Sociocultural factors further delay diagnosis and limit treatment, with gender biases and inadequate awareness compounding the issue.[5] A significant barrier to progress is the underrepresentation of women in clinical trials, resulting in limited sex-specific guidelines. The Lancet Women and Cardiovascular Disease Commission highlights that CVD in women remains understudied, under-recognized, under-diagnosed, and under-treated.[6] This chapter explores the biological, hormonal, and sociocultural factors influencing CAD in women, with a focus on the pathophysiology, diagnosis, and management of the disease in this population.

RISK FACTORS

General Risk Factors for Coronary Artery Disease in Women

Smoking is more detrimental to women than to men, raising the risk of myocardial infarction six times in women, compared to a threefold increase in men.[7] The risk of CAD in women increases with age, especially after menopause, due to the decline in estrogen's vascular protective effects. Younger women experiencing acute coronary syndromes often face higher mortality rates compared to men.[8] A family history of CAD, particularly involving first-degree relatives with early-onset myocardial infarction or sudden cardiac death, significantly elevates risk. Certain racial and ethnic groups, such as Asian Indian women, are predisposed to higher rates of premature CAD, often linked to genetic factors like elevated lipoprotein(a) levels and lifestyle changes.[9]

Hypertension is a more potent risk factor for women than men, particularly in those over 45 years of age or with obesity. Effective weight management can help to mitigate this risk. Dyslipidemia, especially low HDL cholesterol levels and elevated LDL cholesterol and triglycerides, is a strong predictor of CAD, particularly postmenopause.[10] Diabetes and metabolic syndrome further amplify CAD risk, with diabetic women facing a three- to sevenfold higher risk of CAD and an eightfold greater likelihood of heart failure compared to men. Women with diabetes often have diabetic dyslipidemia, marked by elevated triglycerides, low HDL, and small dense LDL particles, necessitating aggressive lipid management.[11]

Women-specific Risk Factors for Coronary Artery Disease

Hormonal changes in postmenopausal women increase the risk of hypertension, dyslipidemia, diabetes, and central obesity, collectively elevating the CAD risk. Estrogen promotes coronary vasodilation and reduces plaque accumulation, but its protective effect diminishes after menopause.[11] Women are more prone to plaque erosion, whereas men predominantly experience plaque rupture, influencing CAD pathophysiology. Central obesity, more common in women, is strongly associated with metabolic syndrome, hypertension, and diabetes. Tobacco use negates estrogen's protective effects, making female smokers as susceptible to CAD as males. Smoking remains a concern among Indian women, especially in rural areas.[12] Adverse pregnancy outcomes such as hypertensive disorders, preterm birth, and intrauterine growth restriction, increase the risk of CAD later in life. Preeclampsia doubles the risk of major cardiovascular events, emphasizing the need for thorough obstetrical history-taking in cardiovascular risk assessment.[13]

Polycystic ovary syndrome affecting 10–15% of reproductive-age women, is linked to higher cardiovascular risk. A Danish registry cohort study found that women with PCOS had a significantly greater risk of CVD.[14] Menopause contributes to central adiposity, insulin resistance, and a proatherogenic lipid profile, elevating CAD risk. Surgical menopause and early natural menopause further increase this risk, while vasomotor symptoms are associated with endothelial dysfunction.[14] Menopausal hormone therapy (MHT), once thought to be cardioprotective, was found in studies like the Women's Health Initiative to increase CAD risk in postmenopausal women. Current guidelines advise against using MHT for primary or secondary CVD prevention.[13] Advances in breast cancer treatment have improved survival rates, but chemotherapy and radiation can have cardiotoxic effects, increasing CAD risk. Recognizing women-specific CAD risk factors is crucial for early detection and better outcomes.[14]

TYPES OF CORONARY ARTERY DISEASE

Obstructive Coronary Artery Disease

Obstructive CAD manifests similarly in men and women, with central chest pain being the most common symptom. However, women are more likely to experience atypical symptoms, such as chest pain at rest, during sleep, or under mental stress. They may also report pain in less typical locations, including the upper back, arms, neck, or jaw, alongside other symptoms such as shortness of breath, nausea, sweating, dizziness, and weakness.[15] Women aged 55 years and younger are significantly more likely than men to present with acute coronary syndrome without chest pain, leading to delayed or missed diagnoses and increasing their risk of adverse outcomes.[16]

Ischemia with Nonobstructive Coronary Artery Disease

Ischemia with nonobstructive coronary artery disease (INOCA) results from coronary microvascular dysfunction or epicardial vascular spasm. It is particularly prevalent in women aged 45–65 years and is often underdiagnosed due to normal findings on routine noninvasive tests. Research shows that individuals with INOCA have an all-cause mortality or myocardial infarction rate of 0.98 per 100 person-years compared to 0.2 per 100 person-years in the general population. Additionally, about 50% of patients with INOCA experience recurrent episodes of ischemic chest pain, similar to those with obstructive CAD. Diagnosis requires functional coronary angiography to measure coronary flow reserve and microvascular resistance, as traditional diagnostic tools often miss this condition.[17]

Myocardial Infarction with Nonobstructive Coronary Artery Disease

Myocardial infarction with nonobstructive coronary artery disease (MINOCA) is more prevalent in women, occurring three times as often as in men. Approximately 25% of MINOCA patients experience ongoing angina, a rate comparable to those with myocardial infarction and obstructive CAD. In about one-quarter of MINOCA cases, the exact pathophysiology remains unclear. Possible causes include epicardial vessel abnormalities, coronary microvascular dysfunction, and overlaps with mild forms of Takotsubo syndrome. These mechanisms prevent adequate myocardial blood flow in response to increased oxygen demand, contributing to ischemic symptoms despite the absence of significant coronary blockages.[18]

Takotsubo Syndrome

Takotsubo syndrome, also known as stress-induced cardiomyopathy, accounts for 7.5% of acute myocardial infarction cases in women, with 90% occurring in postmenopausal women aged 50–75 years. The condition is typically triggered by emotional or physical stress, leading to heightened sympathetic activity. Patients present with symptoms and ECG changes similar to acute coronary syndrome, but angiography reveals no obstructive CAD. The hallmark feature is reversible left ventricular ballooning, although cardiac arrest occurs in 5.9% of cases. Early recognition is crucial for appropriate management and improved outcomes.[19]

Spontaneous Coronary Artery Dissection

Spontaneous coronary artery dissection (SCAD) is a significant cause of myocardial infarction in younger women, particularly those aged 60 years or younger, and accounts for at least 25% of myocardial infarction cases in this population. It is also the most common cause of pregnancy-associated myocardial infarction, primarily occurring during the third trimester or postpartum period. SCAD is typically unrelated to traditional cardiovascular risk factors or atherosclerosis, with a high recurrence risk due to an independent pathological process. Preventive strategies include avoiding hormonal therapy and subsequent pregnancies, but evidence-based treatment guidelines are currently lacking.[20]

Cardiac Syndrome X

Cardiac Syndrome X, a subset of coronary microvascular dysfunction, involves angina with normal coronary arteries on angiography. Women are disproportionately affected by this condition, which can significantly impair quality of life. The symptoms often resemble those of obstructive CAD, leading to frequent misdiagnosis or underestimation of its clinical significance. Proper recognition and management of this syndrome are essential to reduce morbidity.[21]

PATHOPHYSIOLOGY OF CORONARY ARTERY DISEASE IN WOMEN

The pathophysiology of CAD in women differs significantly from that in men, with emerging evidence highlighting more severe and unique mechanisms. Women often experience less extensive atherosclerosis, and acute events are more commonly attributed to plaque erosion rather than plaque rupture. This distinction is important as plaque erosion results in a more fibrotic type of remodeling with increased deposition of vascular smooth muscle cells (VSMCs), proteoglycans, and fibrotic tissue. While plaque erosion is more common in younger women, this trend diminishes postmenopause when plaque rupture becomes more frequent due to declining estrogen levels and associated cardiovascular changes. In women, these changes are significantly influenced by menopause.[22] The decline in estrogen levels leads to increased expression of endothelins (potent vasoconstrictors), activation of the renin-angiotensin-aldosterone system, oxidative stress, endothelial dysfunction, dyslipidemia, and arterial stiffness, all of which accelerate vascular aging, hypertension, and atherosclerosis.[23]

The distinct pathophysiological processes in women also extend to nonobstructive CAD, which is more prevalent in women and includes conditions such as coronary microvascular dysfunction, vasospasms, vasomotor abnormalities, and spontaneous coronary artery dissection.[24,25] Pregnancy introduces additional physiological changes that may contribute to CAD, such as increased blood volume, VSMC hypertrophy, and loss of vascular intercellular matrix, further complicating diagnosis and care in women. Moreover, the persistence of "Yentl syndrome," where women presenting with CAD-like symptoms are managed identically to men despite differing underlying pathology, highlights the need for heightened clinical awareness and nuanced approaches to treatment.[12]

DIAGNOSIS

Women are often under-referred for appropriate diagnostic and therapeutic procedures for CVD compared to men. This discrepancy may stem from a long-standing bias that CAD predominantly affects men, leading to an underestimation of its severity in women. Consequently, women experience lower rates of invasive testing and intervention (**Table 1**). Such biases are particularly pronounced in younger women, as CAD has a lower incidence in this group.[26]

MANAGEMENT OF CORONARY ARTERY DISEASE IN WOMEN

Lifestyle Modifications and Prevention

A comprehensive lifestyle modification is crucial in managing and preventing further complications of CAD in women. Heart-healthy diets, such as the Mediterranean diet, and routine aerobic exercise play a vital role in reducing cardiovascular risks in women. These approaches help lower blood pressure, improve lipid profiles, promote weight management, and are particularly beneficial for women with pregnancy-related complications like preeclampsia or gestational diabetes. Obesity, especially after menopause due to hormonal changes, significantly increases CAD risk in women.[27] Stress, depression, and anxiety, which are more common in women, further

TABLE 1: Various diagnostic modalities for the diagnosis of coronary artery disease (CAD) in women.

Test/procedure	*Sex-specific considerations*
Stress testing	Women have a higher rate of false-positive results due to lower pretest probability. Exercise echocardiography is preferred to avoid radiation exposure. CT coronary angiography offers superior prognostic information for women
Electrocardiography	Women show resting tachycardia and a longer QT interval. Pregnancy-related heart changes (e.g., left axis deviation, ST/T wave changes) can complicate diagnosis
Exercise testing	Reduced sensitivity/specificity in women due to lower exercise capacity, smaller coronary vessels, and nonspecific ECG changes. Female-specific normograms improve accuracy. Limited exercise capacity predicts higher 5-year mortality
Holter monitoring	Effective for identifying arrhythmias like VT, AF, or persistent arrhythmias in women with palpitations or CAD history
Coronary angiography	Women often show plaque in microvasculature rather than large epicardial vessels. Microvascular dysfunction and angina are more common in women, leading to worse outcomes
Invasive testing	Women are less likely to be referred for invasive tests despite positive stress results, leading to higher rates of MI and death. Consistent referral practices are needed

(AF: atrial fibrillation; MI: myocardial infarction; VT: ventricular tachycardia)

amplify CAD risks. The loss of estrogen's cardioprotective effects after menopause further heightens CAD risk. While HRT may help with menopausal symptoms, it is not recommended for CAD prevention, emphasizing the need for lifestyle changes and risk factor management.[28] Additionally, cardiac rehabilitation programs, including supervised exercise, dietary counseling, and emotional support, have shown significant benefits in improving physical and mental health, reducing recurrent cardiovascular events, and lowering mortality in women.

PHARMACOTHERAPY

Pharmacotherapy plays a pivotal role in managing CAD, particularly in addressing the distinct challenges women face in treatment adherence, dosing, and side effect profiles. Aspirin plays a pivotal role in cardiovascular event prevention, with its utility varying between primary and secondary prevention in women.[29] For primary prevention, its benefit in reducing MI is limited, especially in women under 65 years of age, where bleeding risks often outweigh the benefits. In secondary prevention, aspirin is well-supported, with studies like ISIS-2 showing a 16% reduction in vascular mortality postmyocardial infarction (MI).[30] Dual antiplatelet therapy is effective for recurrent events but may cause issues like heavy menstrual bleeding in younger women, requiring careful monitoring. Statins are essential for lipid-lowering therapy, with robust evidence like the PROVE IT-TIMI 22 trial highlighting their efficacy in reducing cardiovascular events, though misconceptions and side effect concerns often hinder adherence among women.[31] In anticoagulation, women face a higher bleeding risk, necessitating precise dosing and safer alternatives in high-risk cases. Nonobstructive CAD, common in women, leads to higher use of nitrates and calcium-channel blockers, with specialized care required during pregnancy to manage contraindications with standard therapies like statins and angiotensin-converting enzyme (ACE) inhibitors.[32]

INTERVENTIONAL STRATEGIES

Revascularization strategies, including percutaneous coronary intervention (PCI) and coronary artery bypass grafting (CABG), are essential in managing CAD in women. However, women face unique challenges that influence outcomes. These include smaller coronary vessels, older age at presentation, delayed symptom recognition, and higher rates of comorbidities such as diabetes, hypertension, and heart failure. Women often experience longer door-to-balloon times in acute coronary syndromes, which can delay reperfusion and worsen outcomes. Despite these barriers, advances in PCI, such as improved stent technologies and procedural techniques, have enhanced safety and efficacy, narrowing the gender gap in outcomes. However, women undergoing PCI still face higher rates of complications, including vascular injury, bleeding, and stent thrombosis. Careful vascular access site selection and use of radial access are strategies to reduce these risks.[33] CABG outcomes in women are generally less favorable than in men due to higher perioperative risks, including bleeding, infection, and prolonged recovery times. Additionally, women often present with more diffuse and advanced coronary disease at the time of surgery, which can complicate grafting procedures. Techniques such as off-pump CABG and arterial grafting, however, have improved outcomes by reducing surgical stress and enhancing graft longevity. Women also face unique postoperative challenges, including a higher likelihood of atrial fibrillation and complications related to delayed sternal healing.[33]

CONCLUSION

Coronary artery disease in women is a multifaceted condition influenced by biological, hormonal, and socio-cultural factors, leading to unique challenges in diagnosis, management, and outcomes. Despite advancements in understanding and treating CAD, significant gaps remain in awareness, research, and healthcare equity for women. These disparities, compounded by the under-representation of women in clinical trials, underscore the urgent need for sex-specific guidelines and tailored approaches to cardiovascular care. By addressing the distinct pathophysiology, risk factors, and clinical presentations of CAD in women, we can enhance diagnostic accuracy, optimize management strategies, and improve outcomes. Furthermore, increased focus on education, lifestyle modifications, and targeted prevention measures can play a pivotal role in mitigating the burden of CAD in women, ensuring that they receive the care and attention they deserve.

REFERENCES

1. Kreatsoulas C, Sloane D, Pogue J, Velianou JL, Anand SS. Referrals in acute coronary events for cardiac catheterization: The RACE CAR Trial. Can J Cardiol. 2010;8:e290-e296.
2. Bosomworth J, Khan Z. Analysis of gender-based inequality in cardiovascular health: an umbrella review. Cureus. 2023;15(8):e43482.
3. Pathak LA, Shirodkar S, Ruparelia R, Rajebahadur J. Coronary artery disease in women. Indian Heart J. 2017;69(4):532-8.
4. Yusuf S, Hawken S, Ounpuu S, Dans T, Avezum A, Lanas F, et al. Effect of potentially modifiable risk factors associated with myocardial infarction in 52 countries (the INTERHEART study): case-control study. Lancet. 2004;364:937-52.
5. Montarello N, Chan WPA. Coronary artery disease in women. Aust Prescr. 2022;45(6):193-9.
6. Vogel B, Acevedo M, Appelman Y, Bairey Merz CN, Chieffo A, Figtree GA, et al. The Lancet women and cardiovascular disease Commission: reducing the global burden by 2030. Lancet. 2021;397(10292):2385-438.
7. Njølstad I, Arnesen E, Lund-Larsen PG. Smoking, serum lipids, blood pressure, and sex differences in myocardial infarction. Circulation. 1996;93:450-6.
8. Norris CM, Yip CY, Nerenberg KA, Clavel MA, Pacheco C, Foulds HJ, et al. state of the science in women's cardiovascular disease: a canadian perspective on the influence of sex and gender. J Am Heart Assoc. 2020;9:e015634.
9. Matthews KA, Crawford SL, Chae CU, Everson-Rose S, Sowers MF, Sternfeld B, et al. Are changes in cardiovascular disease risk factors in midlife women due to chronological aging or to the menopausal transition? J Am Coll Cardiol. 2009;54:2366-73.
10. Shufelt CL, Merz CNB. Contraceptive hormone use and cardiovascular disease. J Am Coll Cardiol. 2009;53:221-31.
11. Regensteiner JG, Golden S, Huebschmann AG, Barrett-Connor E, Chang AY, Chyun D, et al. Sex differences in the cardiovascular consequences of diabetes mellitus. Circulation. 2015;132:2424-47.
12. Grandi SM, Filion KB, Yoon S, Ayele HT, Doyle CM, Hutcheon JA, et al. Cardiovascular disease-related morbidity and mortality in women with a history of pregnancy complications. Circulation. 2019;139:1069-79.
13. Dam V, Van Der Schouw YT, Onland-Moret NC, Groenwold RHH, Peters S, Burgess S, et al. Association of menopausal characteristics and risk of coronary heart disease: a pan-European case-cohort analysis. Int J Epidemiol. 2019;48:1275-85.
14. Maas AHEM, Rosano G, Cifkova R, Chieffo A, van Dijken D, Hamoda H, et al. Cardiovascular health after menopause transition, pregnancy disorders, and other gynaecologic conditions: A consensus document from European cardiologists, gynaecologists, and endocrinologists. Eur Heart J. 2021;42:967-84.
15. Mehta LS, Beckie TM, DeVon HA, Grines CL, Krumholz HM, Johnson MN, et al. Acute myocardial infarction in women: a scientific statement from the American Heart Association. Circulation. 2016;133:916-47.
16. Khan NA, Daskalopoulou SS, Karp I, Eisenberg MJ, Pelletier R, Tsadok MA, et al. Sex differences in acute coronary syndrome symptom presentation in young patients. JAMA Intern Med. 2013;173:1863-71.
17. Mehta PK, Huang J, Levit RD, Malas W, Waheed N, Bairey Merz CN. Ischemia and no obstructive coronary arteries (INOCA): A narrative review. Atherosclerosis. 2022;363:8-21.
18. Squires I, Khalil S, Patel A, Katukari N. MINOCA: Predictors and future management. Indian J Cardiovasc Dis Women. 2025;10:45-50.
19. Gili S, Cammann VL, Schlossbauer SA, Kato K, D'Ascenzo F, Di Vece D, et al. Cardiac arrest in takotsubo syndrome: results from the InterTAK Registry. Eur Heart J. 2019;40:2142-51.
20. Elkayam U, Jalnapurkar S, Barakkat MN, Khatri N, Kealey AJ, Mehra A, et al. Pregnancy-associated acute myocardial

infarction: a review of contemporary experience in 150 cases between 2006 and 2011. Circulation. 2014;129: 1695-702.
21. Geraghty L, Figtree GA, Schutte AE, Patel S, Woodward M, Arnott C. Cardiovascular disease in women: from pathophysiology to novel and emerging risk factors. Heart Lung Circ. 2020;30(1):9-17.
22. Pravda NS, Karny-Rahkovich O, Shiyovich A, Pravda MS, Rapeport N, Vaknin-Assa H, et al. Coronary artery disease in women: a comprehensive appraisal. J Clin Med. 2021;10(20):4664.
23. Reynolds H, Shaw LJ, Min K, Spertus JA, Chaitman BR, Berman DS, et al. Association of sex with severity of commary artery disease, ischemia, and symptom burden in patients with moderate or severe ischemia. JAMA Cardiol. 2020;5:773-86.
24. Sedlak TL, Guan M, Lee M, Humphries KH, Johnson BD, Pepine CJ, et al. Ischemic predictors of outcomes in women with signs and symptoms of ischemia and nonobstructive coronary artery disease. JAMA Cardiol. 2016;1(4):491-2.
25. Reis SE, Holubkov R, Lee JS, Sharaf B, Reichek N, Rogers WJ, et al. Coronary flow velocity response to adenosine characterizes coronary microvascular function in women with chest pain and no obstructive coronary disease. Results from the pilot phase of the Women's Ischemia Syndrome Evaluation (WISE) study. J Am Coll Cardiol. 1999;33(6):1469-75.
26. Vijayalakshmi IB, Nemani L, Kher M, Kumar A. The gamut of coronary artery disease in Indian women. Indian J Cardiovas Dis Women. 2023;8:43-51.
27. Rippe JM. Lifestyle strategies for risk factor reduction, prevention, and treatment of cardiovascular disease. Am J Lifestyle Med. 2018;13(2):204-12.
28. Ghodeshwar GK, Dube A, Khobragade D. Impact of lifestyle modifications on cardiovascular health: a narrative review. Cureus. 2023;15(7):e42616.
29. Augustovski FA, Cantor SB, Thach CT, Spann SJ. Aspirin for primary prevention of cardiovascular events. J Gen Intern Med. 1998;13(12):824-35.
30. Maxwell S, Waring WS. Drugs used in secondary prevention after myocardial infarction: case presentation. Br J Clin Pharmacol. 2000;50(5):405-17.
31. Virk HUH, Escobar J, Rodriguez M, Bates ER, Khalid U, Jneid H, et al. Dual antiplatelet therapy: a concise review for clinicians. life (Basel). 2023;13(7):1580.
32. Daughety MM, Zilberman-Rudenko J, Shatzel JJ, McCarty OJT, Raghunathan V, DeLoughery TG. Management of anticoagulation in pregnant women with mechanical heart valves. Obstet Gynecol Surv. 2020;75(3):190-8.
33. Gaudino M, Di Franco A, Cao D, Giustino G, Bairey Merz CN, Fremes SE, et al. Sex-related outcomes of medical, percutaneous, and surgical interventions for coronary artery disease: jacc focus seminar 3/7. J Am Coll Cardiol. 2022;79(14):1407-25.

CHAPTER 2

Cardiac Troponins in Coronary Artery Disease

Kamal K Sethi, Kabir Sethi

INTRODUCTION

What are Cardiac Troponins?

The troponin complex, located on the myofibrillar thin (actin) filament of striated (skeletal and cardiac) muscle consists of three subunits—troponin C, troponin I, and troponin T. Of these, the isoforms T and I are found in the cardiac muscle and form the cTn complex, which regulates the excitation-contraction coupling in the heart. Near about 4–5% of cTn is found in the cytosol, while the rest is found in the sarcomere.[1] Following myocyte injury, the initial release of troponin occurs from cytoplasm, followed by a slower and more continuous release from the rest of the contractile apparatus.

Ever since the European Society of Cardiology (ESC) and the American College of Cardiology jointly redefined myocardial infarction (MI) as clinical evidence of myocardial ischemia in conjunction with elevation of cardiac troponin T (cTnT) or I (cTnI), the two have emerged as preferred biochemical markers for the diagnosis of MI.[2] Because high-sensitivity cardiac troponin (hs-cTn) assays have the ability to detect minute troponin concentrations, its elevation can be noted in a number of potential diseases including pulmonary embolism, heart failure (HF), myocarditis, end-stage renal disease, and so forth. Regardless of the release mechanics, elevated cTnT and cTnI almost always imply a poor prognosis.

CHARACTERISTICS OF HIGH-SENSITIVITY CARDIAC TROPONIN ASSAYS

Enhancements in assay technology and widespread availability have made cTn the biomarker of choice for evaluating patients with suspected acute myocardial injury. Fundamental to the diagnosis of acute myocardial infarction (AMI) is a rise and/or fall of cTn with at least 1 value above the 99th percentile from a normal population.[3,4] Clinically, the most relevant point to understand is that a value above the 99th percentile of hs-cTn assay is indicative of myocardial injury.[3] Myocardial injury is considered acute if there is a rise and/or fall of cTn concentration over serial measurements and chronic if the cTn level remains elevated without significant rise or fall.[3]

Compared with standard cTn assays, hs-cTn assays have higher negative predictive value for AMI and reduce the "Troponin-blind" interval, leading to earlier detection of AMI. This results in ~4% absolute and ~20% relative increases in the detection of type 1 MI and a corresponding decrease in the diagnosis of unstable angina. High-sensitivity troponins are also associated with a twofold increase in the detection of type 2 MI. Levels of hs-cTn should be interpreted as quantitative markers of cardiomyocyte damage (i.e., the higher the level, the greater the likelihood of MI). Elevations beyond fivefold the upper reference limit have high (>90%) positive predictive value for acute type 1 MI. Elevations beyond threefold the upper reference limit have only limited (50–60%) positive predictive value for AMI and may be associated with a broad spectrum of conditions. It is common to detect circulating level of cTn in healthy individuals. Rising and/or falling cTn levels differentiate acute (as in MI) from chronic cardiomyocyte damage (the more pronounced the change, the higher the likelihood of AMI).

Patient characteristics are likely to have an influence on hs-cTn values. Men, due to increased left ventricle size and more prevalent subclinical cardiovascular disease, have higher hs-cTn concentrations than women.[5] Thus, the 99th percentile cutoff is higher for men than women. Other conditions known to be associated with increased levels of hs-cTn include older age, left ventricular hypertrophy, hypertension, chronic kidney disease (CKD), critical illness, sepsis, acute respiratory distress syndrome, and stroke[6-11] **(Box 1)**. High-sensitivity assays are recommended as their diagnostic accuracy is higher. Assays run on automated platforms in the laboratory are much more sensitive than point-of-care tests and are preferable.

BOX 1: Conditions other than type 1 myocardial infarction (MI) associated with cardiac troponin elevation.

- **Tachyarrhythmias**
- **Heart failure**
- **Hypertensive emergencies**
- **Critical illness (e.g., shock/sepsis/burns)**
- **Myocarditis***
- **Takotsubo syndrome**
- **Valvular heart disease (e.g., aortic stenosis)**
- **Aortic dissection**
- **Pulmonary embolism and pulmonary hypertension**
- **Renal dysfunction and associated cardiac disease**
- **Acute neurological event (e.g., stroke or subarachnoid hemorrhage)**
- Cardiac contusion or cardiac procedure (CABG, PCI, ablation, pacing, cardioversion, or endomyocardial biopsy)
- Hypo- and hyperthyroidism
- Infiltrative diseases (e.g., amyloidosis, hemochromatosis, sarcoidosis, and scleroderma)
- Myocardial drug toxicity or poisoning (e.g., doxorubicin, 5-fluorouracil, herceptin, and snake venoms)
- **Extreme endurance efforts**
- Rhabdomyolysis

Bold sentence: Most frequent condition
*Includes myocardial extension of endocarditis or pericarditis.
(CABG: coronary artery bypass graft(ing); PCI: percutaneous coronary intervention)
Source: Adapted from Collet JP, et al.[12]

HIGH-SENSITIVITY CARDIAC TROPONIN IN THE DIAGNOSIS OF MYOCARDIAL INFARCTION

According to the Fourth Universal Definition,[3] to diagnose MI in the presence of acute myocardial injury (elevated cTn), there must also be evidence of myocardial ischemia with at least one of the following present: (1) Symptoms of myocardial ischemia, (2) new ischemic changes on the electrocardiogram (ECG), (3) new pathological Q waves, (4) new ischemic regional wall motion abnormalities on cardiac imaging, or (5) acute coronary thrombus on coronary angiography.

Not only do the cTns allow for more sensitive diagnosis of AMI but also indicate the adverse prognostic risk associated with its elevation. Multiple randomized studies and several meta-analyses have substantiated the adverse outcome associated with elevated cTn with higher odds (3.44-fold) of death and MI at 30 days in patients with elevated cTn in comparison to those presenting with unstable angina.[13] In order to understand the characteristics of an abnormal hs-cTn better, clinicians should look at cTn as a continuous value with higher concentrations more likely linked to AMI. All efforts must be made to measure the biomarker serially, seeking a rise and/or fall in concentration. The ESC 2020 non-ST-segment elevation acute coronary syndrome (ACS) guideline favors hs-cTn testing at 0 hour and 1 hour using the ESC 0/1-hour algorithm with later sampling (e.g., at 2 or 3 hours) as reasonable alternatives.[13] Using the ESC 0/1-hour algorithm, MI may be excluded when single-sample hs-cTn concentrations are found to be below the limit of detection (LoD) (the lowest concentration the assay can reliably measure) when measured at least 3 hours after symptom onset.[14,15] In early presenters, i.e., the ones presenting within 1 hour of symptom onset, repeat sampling should be considered at 3 hours.[12]

The early absolute changes of cTn within 1 or 2 hours can provide incremental diagnostic value jointly with ECG and clinical findings. However, assay-specific cutoff values must be applied for 0/1-hour or 0/2-hour algorithms **(Table 1)**.

How to Implement the European Society of Cardiology 0/1-hour Algorithm?

It is important to understand that the ESC 0/1-hour algorithm is irrespective of the local turnaround time and the 0 hour and 1 hour refer to the point at which the blood is drawn and not to the time from the onset of symptoms. In order to maximize the safety and feasibility of the process, the nursing team should obtain samples for cTn following the 0/1-hour algorithm irrespective of other clinical details and pending results. Documentation of the 0-hour blood draw allows exact determination of the time window of the 1-hour blood draw (±10 minutes). If the 1-hour blood draw is not feasible then blood should be drawn at 2 hours and ESC 0/2-hour algorithm must be applied[12] **(Fig. 1)**.

HIGH-SENSITIVITY CARDIAC TROPONIN IN STABLE CORONARY ARTERY DISEASE

Various studies in the recent past have suggested the association of hs-cTn with the presence and severity of coronary artery disease (CAD) among stable outpatients. The PROMISE (Prospective Multicenter Imaging Study for Evaluation of Chest Pain) study, which enrolled 1,844 outpatients with suspected CAD, highlighted the association of hs-cTnI concentrations with severity of coronary artery calcium and presence of obstructive CAD (odds ratio: 1.25 per interquartile range increase; $p = 0.001$).[16] In a subsequent analysis performed in a

TABLE 1: Assay-specific cutoff levels in ng/L within the 0/1-hour and 0/2-hour algorithms.

0/1-hour algorithm	*Very low*	*Low*	*No 1 hΔ*	*High*	*1 hΔ*
hs-cTnT (Elecsys; Roche)	<5	<12	<3	≥52	≥5
hs-cTnI (Architect; Abbott)	<4	<5	<2	≥64	≥6
hs-cTnI (Centaur; Siemens)	<3	<6	<3	≥120	≥12
hs-cTnI (Access; Beckman Coulter)	<4	<5	<4	≥50	≥15
hs-cTnI (Clarity; Singulex)	<1	<2	<1	≥30	≥6
hs-cTnI (Vitros; Clinical Diagnostics)	<1	<2	<1	≥40	≥4
hs-cTnI (Pathfast; LSI Medience)	<3	<4	<3	≥90	≥20
hs-cTnI (TriageTrue; Quidel)	<4	<5	<3	≥60	≥8
0/2-hour algorithm	*Very low*	*Low*	*No 2 hΔ*	*High*	*2 hΔ*
hs-cTnT (Elecsys; Roche)	<5	<14	<4	≥52	≥10
hs-cTnI (Architect; Abbott)	<4	<6	<2	≥64	≥15
hs-cTnI (Centaur; Siemens)	<3	<8	<7	≥120	≥20
hs-cTnI (Access; Beckman Coulter)	<4	<5	<5	≥50	≥20
hs-cTnI (Clarity; Singulex)	<1	TBD	TBD	≥30	TBD
hs-cTnI (Vitros; Clinical Diagnostics)	<1	TBD	TBD	≥40	TBD
hs-cTnI (Pathfast; LSI Medience)	<3	TBD	TBD	≥90	TBD
hs-cTnI (TriageTrue; Quidel)	<4	TBD	TBD	≥60	TBD

(TBD: to be determine)
Source: Adapted from Collet JP, et al.[12]

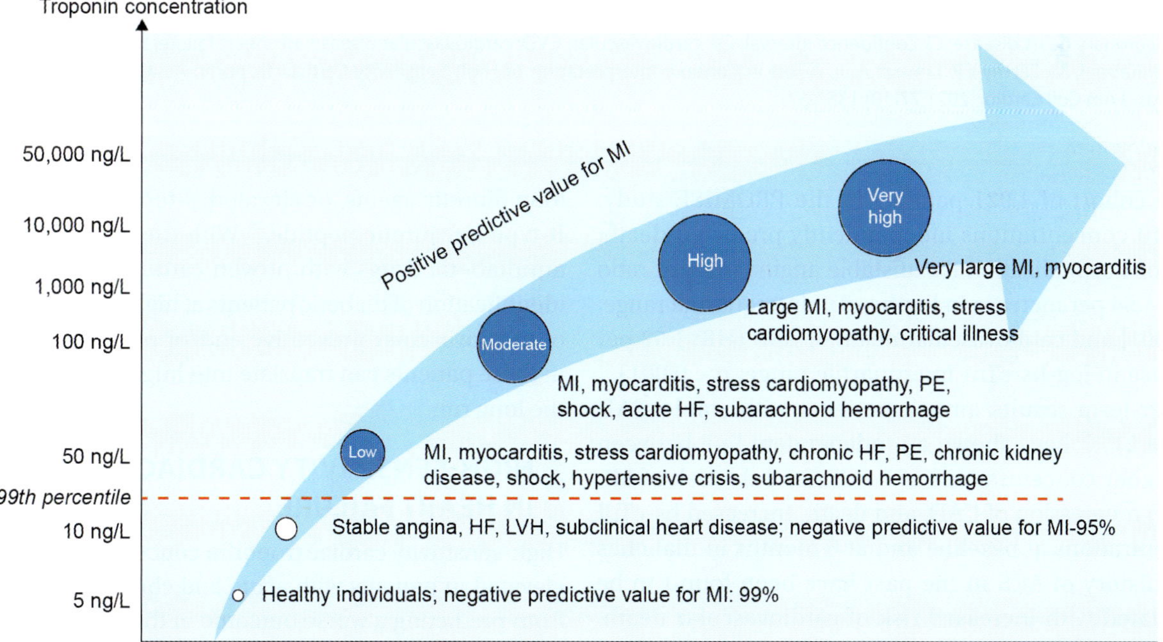

Fig. 1: Range of diagnoses across hs-cTn concentrations. (HF: heart failure; hs-cTn: high-sensitivity cardiac troponin; LVH: left ventricular hypertrophy; MI: myocardial infarction; PE: pulmonary embolism)
Source: Raber I, McCarthy CP, Januzzi JL Jr. A Test in Context: Interpretation of High-Sensitivity Cardiac Troponin Assays in Different Clinical Settings. J Am Coll Cardiol. 2021;77(10):1307-67.

TABLE 2: High-sensitivity cardiac troponin (hs-cTn) in "stable" coronary artery disease.*

First author (reference), year	*N*	*Cardiac troponin cutoff, ng/L*	*Troponin assay*	*% Individuals above troponin cutoff*	*Outcome*	*Adjusted HR (95% CI)*
deFilippi, et al. (36), 2010	4,221	hs-cTnT ≥13	Roche Elecsys	17	11.8-year incident HF	2.5 (2.0–3.0)
deFilippi, et al. (36), 2010	4,221	hs-cTnT ≥13	Roche Elecsys	17	11.8-year CV mortality	2.9 (2.4–3.6)
de Lemos, et al. (8), 2010	3,546	hs-cTnT ≥14	Roche Elecsys	2	6.4-year all-cause mortality	2.8 (1.4–5.2)
Saunders, et al. (37), 2011	9,698	hs-cTnT ≥14	Roche Elecsys	7	10-year all-cause mortality	4.0 (3.2–4.9)
Saunders, et al. (37), 2011	9,698	hs-cTnT ≥14	Roche Elecsys	7	10-year CV mortality	7.6 (3.8–15.3)
Saunders, et al. (37), 2011	9,698	hs-cTnT ≥14	Roche Elecsys	7	10-year incident HF	6.0 (4.5–7.9)
McEvoy, et al. (7), 2016	8,838	hs-cTnT ≥5	Roche Elecsys	56	14-year incident CHD	1.4 (1.2–1.6)
McEvoy, et al. (7), 2016	8,838	hs-cTnT ≥5	Roche Elecsys	56	14-year incident HF	2.0 (1.6–2.4)
McEvoy, et al. (7), 2016	8,838	hs-cTnT ≥5	Roche Elecsys	56	14-year mortality	1.5 (1.3–1.7)
Welsh, et al. (38), 2019	19,501	hs-cTnT ≥5	Roche Elecsys	Not reported	7.8-year CVD composite	1.0 (0.8–1.2)
Welsh, et al. (38), 2019	19,501	hs-cTnI ≥5	Abbott Architect	Not reported	7.8-year CVD composite	1.5 (1.2–1.9)
Yan, et al. (40), 2020	48,455	hs-cTnI ≥3.2	Abbott Architect	31	6.6-year incident HF	1.6 (1.3–2.0)
Blankenberg, et al. (39), 2016	74,738	hs-cTnI ≥6.0	Abbott Architect	Highest quintile	12.1-year all-cause mortality	1.6 (1.5–1.8)
Blankenberg, et al. (39), 2016	74,738	hs-cTnI ≥6.0	Abbott Architect	Highest quintile	13.8-year CV mortality	2.6 (2.3–2.9)

*Select rather than an entire list of studies examining high-sensitivity troponin in ambulatory populations included.
Note: The reference numbers cited in parenthesis are from the original article and do not correspond with the current references.
(CHD: coronary heart disease; CI: confidence interval; CV: cardiovascular; CVD: cardiovascular disease; HF: heart failure; HR: hazard ratio)
Source: Raber I, McCarthy CP, Januzzi JL Jr. A Test in Context: Interpretation of High-Sensitivity Cardiac Troponin Assays in Different Clinical Settings. J Am Coll Cardiol. 2021;77(10):1357-67.

larger cohort of 4,021 patients in the PROMISE study, hs-cTnI concentrations independently predicted death, AMI, or hospitalization for unstable angina [hazard ratio (HR): 1.54 per increase in log-hs-cTnI interquartile range; p <0.001] and cardiovascular death or AMI (HR: 1.52 per increase in log-hs-cTnI interquartile range; p < 0.001).[17] Longer-term results among patients with stable CAD **(Table 2)**[17-23] have shown an independent link between the higher concentrations of hs-cTn and the risk of MI, stroke, progression of CAD, and death. Increased hs-cTnI concentrations at baseline and at 6 months in diabetics with history of ACS in the past have been found to be associated with increased risk of cardiovascular death, MI, or stroke.[24] In the same cohort, hs-cTnI >16 ng/L for women and hs-cTnI >33 ng/L for men were associated with an increased risk of a composite outcome of cardiovascular death, HF hospitalization, initiation of loop diuretic agents, or elevated N-terminal prohormone B-type natriuretic peptide.[25] With the expanding role of antidiabetic drugs with proven cardiovascular benefits, identification of diabetic patients at high risk and initiation of cardiovascular preventive and/or protective strategies in these patients can translate into huge clinical benefit in the long run.

HIGH-SENSITIVITY CARDIAC TROPONIN IN HEART FAILURE

High-sensitivity cardiac troponin concentrations are often elevated in patients with acute and chronic HF, and apart from predicting a worse outcome in these patients, it may offer additional prognostic information in both settings **(Tables 3 and 4)**.[26-36]

Even though cTn measurement is recommended in patients presenting with acute HF (to rule out type 1 MI

TABLE 3: Effect of high-sensitivity cardiac troponin (hs-cTn) on prognosis in heart failure.*

First author (reference), year	*N*	*Cardiac troponin cutoff, ng/L*	*Troponin assay*	*% Individuals above troponin cutoff*	*Outcome*	*Adjusted HR (95% CI)*
Nakamura, et al. (68), 2014	444	hs-cTnT ≥28	Roche Elecsys	50	15-month CV mortality	4.0 (1.9–8.3)
Nakamura, et al. (68), 2014	444	hs-cTnT ≥28	Roche Elecsys	50	15-month all-cause mortality	2.9 (1.6–5.0)
Felker, et al. (69), 2015	1,074	Doubling in peak change in hs-cTnT	Roche Elecsys	–	180-day CV mortality	1.4 (1.2–1.6)
Diez, et al. (76), 2016	187	hs-cTnT >42	Roche Elecsys	50	90-day mortality or readmission	1.7 (0.9–3.0)
Fudim, et al. (70), 2018	139	Per doubling of baseline hs-cTnI	Beckman Coulter Access	–	Emergency room visits, readmissions, and death at day 60	1.2 (1.0–1.4)
Aimo, et al. (80), 2019	1,499	hs-cTnT ≥43	Roche Elecsys	50	All-cause mortality at 2 years	1.9 (1.3–2.8)

*Select rather than an entire list of studies examining high-sensitivity troponin in acute heart failure included.

Note: The reference numbers cited in parenthesis are from the original article and do not correspond with the current bibliography.

(CI: confidence interval; CV: cardiovascular; HR: hazard ratio)

Source: Raber I, McCarthy CP, Januzzi JL Jr. A Test in Context: Interpretation of High-Sensitivity Cardiac Troponin Assays in Different Clinical Settings. J Am Coll Cardiol. 2021;77(10):1357-67.

TABLE 4: High-sensitivity cardiac troponin (hs-cTn) and long-term risk in heart failure.

First author (reference), year	*N*	*Cardiac troponin cutoff, ng/L*	*Troponin assay*	*% Individuals above troponin cutoff*	*Outcome*	*Adjusted HR (95% CI)*
Latini, et al. (71), 2007	4,053	Per increments of hs-cTnT 10	Roche Elecsys	–	2-year all-cause mortality	1.05 (1.0–1.1)
Alehagen, et al. (72), 2010	470	hs-cTnT >18 (men) hs-cTnT >8 (women)	Roche Elecsys	37	10-year CV mortality	2.2 (1.5–3.4)
Tentzeris, et al. (73), 2011	172	hs-cTnT >14	Roche Elecsys	58	3.5-year all-cause mortality or HF hospitalization	1.9 (1.1–3.3)
Eggers, et al. (74), 2011	103	hs-cTnT >13.5	Roche Elecsys	36	2-year all-cause mortality	2.0 (1.3–3.1)
Eggers, et al. (74), 2011	103	hs-cTnI >14.4	Beckman-Coulter	48	2-year all-cause mortality	1.9 (1.2–2.8)
Masson, et al. (78), 2012	554	Per 1-U increment in hs-cTnT on log scale	Roche Elecsys	–	2-year all-cause mortality	1.6 (1.4–1.8)
Egstrup, et al. (75), 2012	416	hs-cTnT >18 (men) hs-cTnT >8 (women)	Roche Elecsys	57	4.4-year all-cause mortality	1.7 (1.2–2.5)
Aimo, et al. (60), 2018	7,382	hs-cTnT >18	Roche Elecsys	–	2.4-year CV hospitalization	1.4 (1.4–1.5)
Aimo, et al. (60), 2018	7,553	hs-cTnT >18	Roche Elecsys	–	2.4-year CV death	1.4 (1.3–1.5)
Aimo, et al. (60), 2018	9,289	hs-cTnT >18	Roche Elecsys	–	2.4-year all-cause mortality	1.5 (1.4–1.6)
Welsh, et al. (77), 2018	1,853	Per 1-SD hs-cTnT	Roche Elecsys	–	28-month all-cause mortality	1.6 (1.5–1.8)
Welsh, et al. (77), 2018	1,853	Per 1-SD hs-cTnT	Roche Elecsys	–	28-month HF hospitalization or CV death	1.6 (1.5–1.7)

Note: The reference numbers cited in parenthesis are from the original article and do not correspond with the current bibliography.

(CI: confidence interval; CV: cardiovascular; HF: heart failure; HR: hazard ratio)

Source: Raber I, McCarthy CP, Januzzi JL Jr. A Test in Context: Interpretation of High-Sensitivity Cardiac Troponin Assays in Different Clinical Settings. J Am Coll Cardiol. 2021;77(10):1357-67.

as a precipitant), interpretation of an elevated hs-cTn in the clinical setting of HF poses a huge challenge. The rise and/or fall of cTn can occur even in the absence of type 1 MI owing to mechanisms leading to demand/ supply mismatch and noncoronary myocardial injury. Troponin release can also be seen in conditions enhancing the cardiac preload without accompanying ischemia.[37] Irrespective of the cause, an increased hs-cTn concentration in the setting of acute HF predicts risk. For instance, in a study of 1,499 patients with acute HF, patients with K = hs-cTnT >43 ng/L had higher rates of all-cause death at 6, 12, and 24 months.[38] Similar cardiovascular outcomes with hs-cTn concentrations can also be seen in patients with chronic HF. A meta-analysis of 10 studies showed a strong association between hs-cTn values and risk of cardiovascular hospitalizations (HR: .42; 95% CI: 1.36–1.49), cardiovascular mortality (HR: 1.40; 95% CI: 1.33–1.48), and all-cause mortality (HR: 1.48; 95% CI: 1.41–1.55)[39] even in the absence of CAD. Patients with heart failure with reduced ejection fraction (HFrEF) and chronically elevated hs-cTn are likely to have a further decline in the left ventricular function during a year of follow-up as reported by Motiwala SR, et al.[40] Although most studies have examined the prognostic utility of hs-cTn in patients with HFrEF, a small number of studies have demonstrated its utility in predicting adverse clinical outcomes in patients with heart failure with preserved ejection fraction (HFpEF) as well.[28,41]

HIGH-SENSITIVITY CARDIAC TROPONIN IN RENAL DISEASE

Patients living with renal dysfunction have chronically elevated troponin level.[8] As a result, interpreting hs-cTn

Flowcharts 1A and B: European Society of Cardiology (ESC) 0/1-hour algorithm using high-sensitivity cardiac troponin T in patients with and without renal dysfunction.

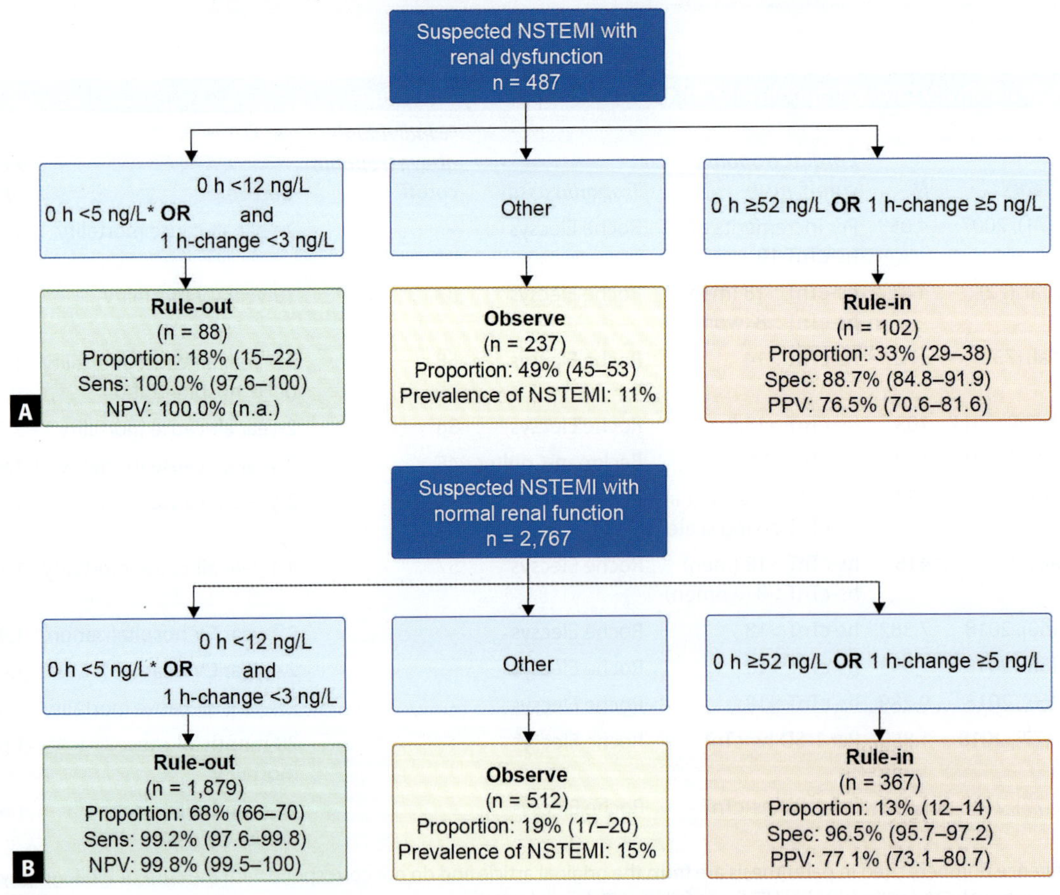

*Limit of detection

(NPV: negative predictive value; NSTEMI: non-ST-segment elevation myocardial infarction; PPV: positive predictive value)

Source: Adapted from Twerenbold R, et al.[47]

levels in this population becomes very challenging. Since these individuals exhibit a higher incidence and prevalence of MI and carry a worse prognosis in comparison to their counterparts,[42] it becomes extremely important and relevant to recognize MI in this subset of patients and ensure appropriate treatment in order to improve the outcome. The pathophysiology of chronic troponin elevation in patients with CKD, though not fully understood, is likely to be multifactorial as patients with CKD often have coexistent coronary atherosclerosis,[43] left ventricular hypertrophy,[44] HF,[39] and hypertension,[7] all of which can contribute to elevation of hs-cTn. Notably, among patients with impaired renal function, cTnT concentrations are more commonly elevated when compared with cTnI using both conventional and high-sensitivity assays.[45,46] Abnormal hs-cTn level in patients with CKD reduces the specificity of the assay for MI using both hs-cTnT and hs-cTnI assays, thereby making it difficult to diagnose MI in this subset of patients.[47] However, despite difficulties in interpreting troponins in CKD, the 0/1-hour and 0/2-hour algorithms can be applied for diagnosis of AMI with appropriate clinical symptoms and ECG changes suggestive of ischemia. Elevated troponins should not be dismissed as irrelevant in patients with CKD as incidence of ACS is quite high, requiring a thorough judgement for early treatment. The 0/1-hour and 0/2-hour protocols have been tested in CKD and found to be equally effective compared to patients without renal disease[47] **(Flowcharts 1 and 2)**.

Flowcharts 2A and B: European Society of Cardiology (ESC) 0/1-hour algorithm using high-sensitivity cardiac troponin I in patients with and without renal dysfunction.

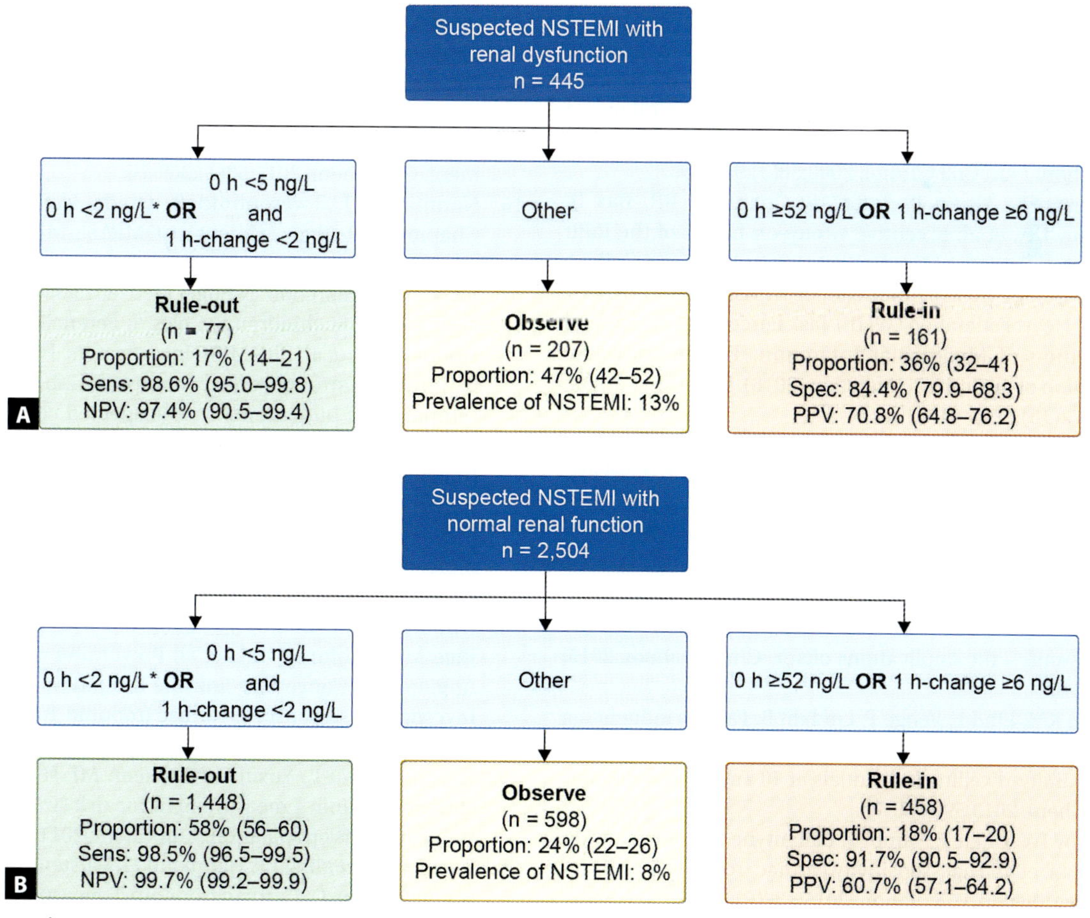

*Limit of detection

(NPV: negative predictive value; NSTEMI: non-ST-segment elevation myocardial infarction; PPV: positive predictive value)

Source: Adapted from Twerenbold R, et al.[47]

CONCLUSION

Measurement of hs-cTn has improved our understanding of cardiac as well as noncardiac conditions causing myocyte necrosis both in acute and chronic settings. It is particularly relevant to mention that the use of hs-cTn should be preferred, but diagnosis of MI should not be assumed just on the basis of a laboratory value. A good patient history, ECG findings, and an astute clinical judgement is required to differentiate a type 1 infarction from myriad conditions causing elevated troponins. The value of troponins is strongly associated with prognosis, irrespective of pathology, and calls for appropriate investigations and implementation of modern therapies.

REFERENCES

1. Katus HA, Remppis A, Scheffold T, Diederich KW, Kuebler W. Intracellular compartmentation of cardiac troponin T and its release kinetics in patients with reperfused and nonreperfused myocardial infarction. Am J Cardiol. 1991; 67:1360-7.
2. Alpert JS, Thygesen K, Antman E, Bassand JP. Myocardial infarction redefined—a consensus document of the Joint European Society of Cardiology/American College of Cardiology committee for the redefinition of myocardial infarction. J Am Coll Cardiol. 2000;36(3):959-69.
3. Thygesen K, Alpert JS, Jaffe AS, Chaitman BR, Bax JJ, Morrow DA, et al; Executive Group on behalf of the Joint European Society of Cardiology (ESC)/American College of Cardiology (ACC)/American Heart Association (AHA)/ World Heart Federation (WHF) Task Force for the Universal Definition of Myocardial Infarction. Fourth universal definition of myocardial infarction (2018). J Am Coll Cardiol. 2018;72(18):2231-64.
4. Apple FS, Sandoval Y, Jaffe AS, Ordonez-Llanos J; IFCC Task Force on Clinical Applications of Cardiac Bio-Markers. Cardiac troponin assays: guide to understanding analytical characteristics and their impact on clinical care. Clin Chem. 2017;63(1):73-81.
5. Eggers KM, Johnston N, Lind L, Venge P, Lindahl B. Cardiac troponin I levels in an elderly population from the community—the implications of sex. Clin Biochem. 2015; 48:751-6.
6. Eggers KM, Lind L, Venge P, Lindahl B. Factors influencing the 99th percentile of cardiac troponin I evaluated in community-dwelling individuals at 70 and 75 years of age. Clin Chem. 2013;59:1068-73.
7. McEvoy JW, Chen Y, Nambi V, Ballantyne CM, Sharrett AR, Appel LJ, et al. High-sensitivity cardiac troponin T and risk of hypertension. Circulation. 2015;132(9):825-33.
8. deFilippi C, Seliger SL, Kelley W, Duh SH, Hise M, Christenson RH, et al. Interpreting cardiac troponin results from high-sensitivity assays in chronic kidney disease without acute coronary syndrome. Clin Chem. 2012;58(9):1342-51.
9. Faiz KW, Thommessen B, Einvik G, Brekke PH, Omland T, Rønning OM. Determinants of high sensitivity cardiac troponin T elevation in acute ischemic stroke. BMC Neurol. 2014;14:96.
10. Røsjø H, Varpula M, Hagve TA, Karlsson S, Ruokonen E, Pettilä V, et al; FINNSEPSIS Study Group. Circulating high sensitivity troponin T in severe sepsis and septic shock: distribution, associated factors, and relation to outcome. Intensive Care Med. 2011;37(1):77-85.
11. Metkus TS, Sokoll LJ, Barth AS, Czarny MJ, Hays AG, Lowenstein CJ, et al. Myocardial injury in severe COVID-19 compared to non-COVID acute respiratory distress syndrome. Circulation. 2021;143(6):553-65.
12. Collet JP, Thiele H, Barbato E, Barthélémy O, Bauersachs J, Bhatt DL, et al.; ESC Scientific Document Group. 2020 ESC guidelines for the management of acute coronary syndromes in patients presenting without persistent ST-segment elevation. Eur Heart J. 2021;42(14):1289-367.
13. Ottani F, Galvani M, Nicolini FA, Ferrini D, Pozzati A, Di Pasquale G, et al. Elevated cardiac troponin levels predict the risk of adverse outcome in patients with acute coronary syndromes. Am Heart J. 2000;140(6):917-27.
14. Sandoval Y, Smith SW, Shah ASV, Anand A, Chapman AR, Love SA, et al. Rapid rule-out of acute myocardial injury using a single high-sensitivity cardiac troponin I measurement. Clin Chem. 2017;63(1):369-76.
15. Neumann JT, Twerenbold R, Ojeda F, Sörensen NA, Chapman AR, Shah ASV, et al; COMPASS-MI Study Group. Application of high-sensitivity troponin in suspected myocardial infarction. N Engl J Med. 2019;380(26):2529-40.
16. Januzzi JL Jr, Suchindran S, Coles A, Ferencik M, Patel MR, Hoffmann U, et al; PROMISE Investigators. High-sensitivity troponin I and coronary computed tomography in symptomatic outpatients with suspected coronary artery disease: Insights from the PROMISE Trial. JACC Cardiovasc Imaging. 2019;12(6):1047-55.
17. Januzzi JL Jr, Suchindran S, Hoffmann U, Patel MR, Ferencik M, Coles A, et al; PROMISE Investigators. Single-molecule hsTnI and short-term risk in stable patients with chest pain. J Am Coll Cardiol. 2019;73(3):251-60.
18. Omland T, de Lemos JA, Sabatine MS, hristophi CA, Rice MM, Jablonski KA, et al; Prevention of Events with Angiotensin Converting Enzyme Inhibition (PEACE) Trial Investigators. A sensitive cardiac troponin T assay in stable coronary artery disease. N Engl J Med. 2009;361(26):2538-47.
19. Kavsak PA, Xu L, Yusuf S, McQueen MJ. High-sensitivity cardiac troponin I measurement for risk stratification in a stable high-risk population. Clin Chem. 2011;57:1146-53.
20. Koenig W, Breitling LP, Hahmann H, Wüsten B, Brenner H, Rothenbacher D. Cardiac troponin T measured by a high-sensitivity assay predicts recurrent cardiovascular events in stable coronary heart disease patients with 8-year follow-up. Clin Chem. 2012;58:1215-24.

21. Beatty AL, Ku IA, Christenson RH, DeFilippi CR, Schiller NB, Whooley MA. High-sensitivity cardiac troponin T levels and secondary events in outpatients with coronary heart disease from the Heart and Soul Study. JAMA Intern Med. 2013;173:763-9.
22. Samman Tahhan A, Sandesara P, Hayek SS, Hammadah M, Alkhoder A, Kelli HM, et al. High-sensitivity troponin I levels and coronary artery disease severity, progression, and long-term outcomes. J Am Heart Assoc. 2018;7(5):e007914.
23. McCarthy CP, Vaduganathan M, Singh A, Song Z, Blankstein R, Gaggin HK, et al. Type 2 myocardial infarction and the hospital readmission reduction program. J Am Coll Cardiol. 2018;72(10):1166-70.
24. Cavender MA, White WB, Jarolim P, Bakris GL, Cushman WC, Kupfer S, et al. Serial measurement of high-sensitivity troponin I and cardiovascular outcomes in patients with type 2 diabetes mellitus in the EXAMINE Trial (Examination of Cardiovascular Outcomes With Alogliptin Versus Standard of Care). Circulation 2017;135(20):1911-21.
25. Sharma A, Vaduganathan M, Ferreira JP, Liu Y, Bakris GL, Cannon CP, et al. Clinical and biomarker predictors of expanded heart failure outcomes in patients with type 2 diabetes mellitus after a recent acute coronary syndrome: Insights from the EXAMINE Trial. J Am Heart Assoc. 2020; 9(1):e012797.
26. Nakamura Y, Yoshihisa A, Takiguchi M, Shimizu T, Yamauchi H, Iwaya S, et al. High-sensitivity cardiac troponin T predicts noncardiac mortality in heart failure. Circ J. 2014;78(4):890-5.
27. Felker GM, Mentz RJ, Teerlink JR, Voors AA, Pang PS, Ponikowski P, et al. Serial high sensitivity cardiac troponin T measurement in acute heart failure: insights from the RELAX-AHF study. Eur J Heart Fail. 2015;17(12):1262-70.
28. Fudim M, Ambrosy AP, Sun JL, Anstrom KJ, Bart BA, Butler J, et al. High-sensitivity troponin I in hospitalized and ambulatory patients with heart failure with preserved ejection fraction: insights from the Heart Failure Clinical Research Network. J Am Heart Assoc. 2018;7(24):e010364.
29. Latini R, Masson S, Anand IS, Missov E, Carlson M, Vago T, et al; Val-HeFT Investigators. Prognostic value of very low plasma concentrations of troponin t in patients with stable chronic heart failure. Circulation. 2007;116(11):1242-9.
30. Alehagen U, Dahlström U, Rehfeld JF, Goetze JP. Prognostic assessment of elderly patients with symptoms of heart failure by combining high-sensitivity troponin T and N-terminal pro-B-type natriuretic peptide measurements. Clin Chem. 2010;56:1718-24.
31. Tentzeris I, Jarai R, Farhan S, Perkmann T, Schwarz MA, Jakl G, et al. Complementary role of copeptin and high-sensitivity troponin in predicting outcome in patients with stable chronic heart failure. Eur J Heart Fail. 2011; 13(7):726-33.
32. Eggers KM, Nygren M, Venge P, Jernberg T, Wikström BG. High-sensitive troponin T and I are related to invasive hemodynamic data and mortality in patients with left-ventricular dysfunction and precapillary pulmonary hypertension. Clin Chim Acta. 2011;412:1582-8.
33. Egstrup M, Schou M, Tuxen CD, Kistorp CN, Hildebrandt PR, Gustafsson F, et al. Prediction of outcome by highly sensitive troponin t in outpatients with chronic systolic left ventricular heart failure. Am J Cardiol. 2012;110(4):552-7.
34. Diez M, Talavera ML, Conde DG, Campos R, Acosta A, Trivi MS. High-sensitivity troponin is associated with high risk clinical profile and outcome in acute heart failure. Cardiol J. 2016;23:78-83.
35. Welsh P, Kou L, Yu C, Anand I, van Veldhuisen DJ, Maggioni AP, et al. Prognostic importance of emerging cardiac, inflammatory, and renal biomarkers in chronic heart failure patients with reduced ejection fraction and anaemia: RED-HF study. Eur J Heart Fail. 2018;20(2):268-77.
36. Masson S, Anand I, Favero C, Barlera S, Vago T, Bertocchi F, et al; Valsartan Heart Failure Trial (Val-HeFT) and Gruppo Italiano per lo Studio della Sopravvivenza nell'Insufficienza Cardiaca–Heart Failure (GISSI-HF) Investigators. Serial measurement of cardiac troponin T using a highly sensitive assay in patients with chronic heart failure: data from 2 large randomized clinical trials. Circulation. 2012;125(2):280-8.
37. Feng J, Schaus BJ, Fallavollita JA, Lee TC, Canty JM Jr. Preload induces troponin I degradation independently of myocardial ischemia. Circulation. 2001;103(16):2035-7.
38. Aimo A, Januzzi JL Jr, Mueller C, Mirò O, Pascual Figal DA, Jacob J, et al. Admission high-sensitivity troponin T and NT-proBNP for outcome prediction in acute heart failure. Int J Cardiol. 2019;293:137-42.
39. Aimo A, Januzzi JL Jr, Vergaro G, Ripoli A, Latini R, Masson S, et al. Prognostic value of high-sensitivity troponin T in chronic heart failure: An individual patient data meta-analysis. Circulation. 2018;137(3):286-97.
40. Motiwala SR, Gaggin HK, Gandhi PU, Belcher A, Weiner RB, Baggish AL, et al. Concentrations of highly sensitive cardiac troponin-I predict poor cardiovascular outcomes and adverse remodeling in chronic heart failure. J Cardiovasc Transl Res. 2015;8(3):164-72.
41. Gohar A, Chong JPC, Liew OW, den Ruijter H, de Kleijn DPV, Sim D, et al. The prognostic value of highly sensitive cardiac troponin assays for adverse events in men and women with stable heart failure and a preserved vs. reduced ejection fraction. Eur J Heart Fail. 2017;19(12):1638-47.
42. Gibson CM, Pinto DS, Murphy SA, Morrow DA, Hobbach HP, Wiviott SD, et al; TIMI Study Group. Association of creatinine and creatinine clearance on presentation in acute myocardial infarction with subsequent mortality. J Am Coll Cardiol. 2003;42(9):1535-43.
43. deFilippi C, Wasserman S, Rosanio S, Tiblier E, Sperger H, Tocchi M, et al. Cardiac troponin T and C-reactive protein for predicting prognosis, coronary atherosclerosis, and cardiomyopathy in patients undergoing long-term hemodialysis. JAMA. 2003;290(3):353-9.

44. Mishra RK, Li Y, DeFilippi C, Fischer MJ, Yang W, Keane M, et al; CRIC Study Investigators. Association of cardiac troponin T with left ventricular structure and function in CKD. Am J Kidney Dis. 2013;61(5):701-9.
45. Lippi G, Cervellin G. High-sensitivity troponin T is more susceptible than high-sensitivity troponin I to impaired renal function. Am J Cardiol. 2013;112:1985.
46. Apple FS, Murakami MM, Pearce LA, Herzog CA. Predictive value of cardiac troponin I and T for subsequent death in end-stage renal disease. Circulation. 2002;106:2941-5.
47. Twerenbold R, Badertscher P, Boeddinghaus J, Nestelberger T, Wildi K, Puelacher C, et al. 0/1-hour triage algorithm for myocardial infarction in patients with renal dysfunction. Circulation. 2018;137(5):436-51.

CHAPTER 3

Newer Antiplatelet Drugs

Bhukya Anji Babu, Dayasagar Rao V

INTRODUCTION

Antiplatelet drugs are used as first line antithrombotic therapy in management of acute ischemic events in addition to prevention of secondary complications in vascular disease. Currently available antiplatelet agents have inadequate efficacy, variability in response, and are associated with risk of bleeding. Thus, there is need for more effective and safe antiplatelet drugs for therapy.

Vascular injury—either spontaneous or postintervention leads platelets to reach subendothelium in an attempt to repair, by adhesion, activation, and aggregation. This process occurs through complex interplay between platelet receptors and their ligands. Following vascular injury platelet adhesion occurs through interactions between GP (glycoproteins)—GPIb and Von Willebrand factors (VWF), GPV1 and subendothelial collagen. Platelet activation occurs through interaction of soluble agonists such as thromboxane A2 (TXA_2) and adenosine diphosphate (ADP) promoting platelet aggregation. Intracellular signaling, through various soluble agonists—leads to conformational changes and activation of GP-IIb/IIIa receptors which avidly bind to fibrinogen—thus forming link for inter platelet connectivity (aggregation).

Physiologically vascular endothelium inhibits platelet activation in circulation by:

- Release of NO (nitric oxide), prostaglandin I2 (PGI2) (prostacyclin)
- Release of adenosine—by breakdown of ADP, adenosine triphosphate (ATP) by endonucleotidases
- Expression of thrombomodulin—which binds thrombin—a powerful activator of platelets.

ANTIPLATELET DRUGS

Currently available antiplatelet drugs essentially act by one of following mechanisms:

- Preventing formation of secondary messengers—(TXA_2-by cyclooxygenase inhibitors cox-1-aspirin)
- Interfering with intracellular signaling pathways (PDE inhibitors—dipyridamol, cilostazol, and PGI2 analogues)
- *Blocking membrane receptors*
  - Purinergic 2Y type 12 (P2Y12) receptors antagonist—clopidogrel, prasugrel, and ticagrelor)
  - Protease-activated receptors (PAR) antagonist—vorapaxar
- *Inhibiting platelet aggregation*
  - GPIIb/IIIa inhibition—tirofiban, eptifibatide, and abciximab.

Incomplete protection and bleeding complication associated with currently available antiplatelet agents represent areas of further investigation for more effective and safe antiplatelet therapy.

Characteristics of ideal antiplatelet drug include following:

- Predictable pharmacodynamics profile (making monitoring unnecessary)
- Rapid onset and off set of action
- Availability of antidote (for respective antiplatelet drug)
- Potent antiplatelet effect but with low risk of bleeding
- Ideally low cost—for better long term drug compliance.

Novel antiplatelet drugs are directed against platelet glycoproteins GPVI, GPibA, GPIIb/IIIa receptors, purinergic receptors P2Y1 and P2Y12, PAR, receptors such as PAR1 and PAR-4, newer target—inhibit thrombus propagation (without effect on thrombus initiation) and include, PI3 kinase B, PDI (protein disulfide isomerase), 12-lipoxygenase inhibitors.

PURINERGIC 2Y TYPE RECEPTOR ANTAGONISTS

Purinergic 2Y type receptors are purinergic receptors belonging to P2 family and basically consists of two types of receptors—P2Y1 and P2Y12 that regulate many cellular responses to extracellular nucleotides such as ATP, ADP, uridine diphosphate (UDP), and uridine triphosphate (UTP). These receptors mediate—vasodilatation, platelet aggregation, and immune responses.

Purinergic P2Y1 (P2Y1) receptor initiates ADP-induced platelet aggregation and shape change which is amplified and stabilized by P2Y12 receptor. The potential of P2Y1 inhibition as an antiplatelet strategy has been explored which showed equal efficacy but with less bleeding compared to P2Y12 inhibition. Potential of combined P2Y12 and P2Y1 receptors inhibition—diadenosine tetraphosphate—which in preclinical studies showed to be highly potent with minimal increase in bleeding time.

The P2Y12 receptor stabilizes the platelet aggregates and amplify secretion of platelet dense granules and has selective tissue distribution that makes it attractive molecular target for therapeutic development.

Oral P2Y12[1] antagonists clopidogrel, prasugrel, ticagrelor, and intravenous cangrelor are well established in routine clinical practice with proven efficacy and will not be discussed further.

PURINERGIC 2Y TYPE 12 NOVEL INHIBITORS

Newer P2Y12 antiplatelet drug—ELINOGREL is a direct acting reversible P2Y12 inhibitor that can be administered orally and intravenously. The drug is well absorbed, with terminal half-life of 12 hours and inhibits thrombus growth, starting at 30 mg dose and in conjunction with ASPIRIN prevents formation of large platelet aggregator in two trials—ERASE—MI[2] and INNOVATE—MI.[3] In ERASE-MI trial—intravenous elinogrel (10–60 mg) before percutaneous coronary intervention (PCI) in patients with ST-elevation myocardial infarction (STEMI) was given to evaluate safety and tolerability. In INNOVATE-PCI randomized, double blind, triple dummy clopidogrel controlled study of oral and intravenous elinogrel in patients undergoing non-urgent PCI was studied, to evaluate efficacy and safety and tolerability of this novel antiplatelet agent.

SELATOGREL—novel P2Y12 inhibitor has to be administered subcutaneously reaches its peak concentration in 30 minutes after single injection and provides, prompt, potent, and consistent P2Y12 inhibition sustained for >8 hours and reversible in 24 hours. This drug is tested in both acute coronary syndrome (ACS) and chronic coronary syndrome in small clinical trials showing effective antithrombotic efficacy with lesser bleeding. This drug is well tolerated up to highest tested dose of 32 mg. Main reported adverse events were headache dizziness and dyspnea (known risk with reversible P2Y12 inhibitors). The usual dose is 16 mg SC. No major bleeding events are reported, with most bleeding events confined to injection site bruising 1.7–2.6% compared to placebo (none). Transient mild-to-moderate dyspnea is reported in 5.3% patients as is seen in all reversible P2Y12 inhibitors.[4]

NOVEL GLYCOPROTEIN IIB/IIIA RECEPTOR ANTAGONISTS

Glycoprotein IIb/IIIa (GPIIb/IIIa) receptors are highly abundant platelet receptors and are final common pathway of platelets in binding to soluble fibrinogen. The existing IIb/IIIa blockers—*abciximab, tirofiban,* and *eptifibatide* are highly potent with bleeding risk that limits its long-term utility. Once the ligand (fibrinogen) binds to GPIIb/IIIa receptor, new chain of events occurs inside platelet that promotes thrombus propagation. Thus, these parenteral GPIIb/IIIa blockers not only prevent platelet aggregation but also paradoxically potentiate platelet activation. New molecules have been identified which are specific to alpha IIb subunit of GPIIb/IIIa which maintain the receptor in low affinity state preventing the binding to ligand and does not cause platelet activation. Thus, these molecules RUC-1 and RUC-4 act powerful antiplatelet drugs without any increase in platelet activation.

RUC-4—second generation small molecule of GP2B3A inhibitors, known as *zalunfiban* specifically designed to inhibit fibrinogen binding, platelet aggregation and platelet thrombus formation that locks receptors into inactive state consequently does not cause conformational change in receptors and exposing hidden epitopes on receptors. This molecule is biologically active when given subcutaneously, with an injection volume of <1.0 mL. This molecule provides rapid (<15 minutes) and high-grade (80%) inhibition of platelet aggregation that returns to baseline values in 2 hours and does not have serious undesirable adverse events, such as thrombocytopenia bleeding and injection site reactions. It has the potential to improve infarct vessel patency and clinical outcomes if administration at first medical contact, before primary PCI by decreasing total ischemic time.[5]

This drug is being tested in STEMI and chronic coronary artery disease. We have to wait for a randomized controlled trial (RCT) before it can be recommended as routine pharmacotherapy for ACS-CAD (coronary artery disease).

PROTEASE-ACTIVATED RECEPTOR ANTAGONISTS—THROMBIN RECEPTOR ANTAGONISTS

Thrombin is the most potent platelet agonist, through its receptors on platelets PAR-1 and PAR-4, with different affinities to thrombin. The former PAR-1 being sensitive to nanomolar concentration while PAR-4 requires higher concentration to exhibit proteolytic self-activation mechanism. Thus targeting PAR-1 receptor, could inhibit platelet activation (by thrombin) without impairing other coagulant function of thrombin. Two compounds—*atopaxar* and *vorapaxar* have entered clinical trials.

Activation of PAR -1 and PAR-4 on platelet by thrombin may lead to platelet aggregation and contribute to recurrent thrombotic events in spite of dual antiplatelet therapy (DAPT) therapy. *Vorpaxar*[6] is highly selective antagonist of PAR-1, reversibly blocking thrombin-mediated platelet activation. Phase-III clinical trial TRACER[5] (thrombin receptor antagonist for clinical event reduction) in ACS on top of DAPT did not reduce primary composite endpoint but significantly reduced secondary endpoint (CV death, MI, Stroke).

TRAP – TIMI 50[7]

In TRA2P (thrombin receptor antagonist secondary prevention of atherothrombotic ischemic events)—TIMI-50 (thrombolysis in myocardial infarction 50) trial in addition to standard antiplatelet therapy significantly reduced composite endpoint of CV death, MI, stroke at 3 years in patients with history of ACS, ischemic stroke, PAD (peripheral arterial disease), but with increase in major bleeding including intracerebral hemorrhage (ICH). Based on the above studies PAR-1 inhibitors may be considered in therapy of vascular disease in patients with high residual risk but with low bleeding risk.

OTHER GLYCOPROTEINS

Glycoprotein VI (GPVI) is principal collagen receptor of platelet mediating platelet activation through binding of GPVI to collagen, that promotes crosslinking of GPVI receptors facilitating aggregation and activation through release of platelet agonist such as ADP and TXA_2. GPVI could be the most ideal for antiplatelet action as these receptors are unique to platelets and interaction with collagen leads to platelet adhesion and activation.

Genetic disorder of GPVI deficiency leads to reduced thrombosis without major bleeding complications. Thus, GPVI has been target for development of antiplatelet drugs. *Revacept*—a fusion protein comprising extracellular domain of GPVI and Fc immunoglobulin of human origin and *glenzocimab* another drug—humanized Fab fragment with GPVI with high specificity and affinity to GPVI have been studied. Initial studies reveal that both these agents decrease thrombus formation without increase in bleeding.

Revacept has been tested in patients undergoing PCI—stable CAD (ISAR-PLASTER) and in patients with symptomatic carotid stenosis, in addition to standard therapy, did not reveal any incremental benefits in reducing primary and secondary events. Both these agents—*revacept*, and *glenzocimab*—given single IV infusion decreased thrombus formation without any increase in bleeding.[8]

GLYCOPROTEIN 1B INHIBITION (GLYCOPROTEIN 1B-IX-V COMPLEX)

This receptor binds to VWF and allows early platelet adhesion to subendothelium during high shear stress. Owing to critical function of glycoprotein 1b (GP1b)-IX-V complex and VWF in thrombosis, antiplatelet drugs targeting this receptor complex have been developed *caplacizumab*[7]—humanized nano antibody against VWF has been shown to improve endothelial function in patients undergoing PCI in stable CAD. *Anafibtide* purified drug from snake venom (Agkistrodon acters) inhibits both VWF and alpha thrombin binding to GP1b. These GP1b antagonists, with high specificity to VWF and thus are effective in thrombotic thrombocytopenic purpura (TTP), as this is associated with ultra large VWF multimers.[9]

The need for newer antiplatelet drugs is influenced by weaker efficacy, with recurrent events in spite of drug therapy of presently available drugs and risk of bleeding with long term usage. Consequently, increased potency of drugs to overcome the poor efficacy is associated with increased bleeding. This observation of potency linked to bleeding has led to paradigm shift of targeting thrombosis pathway while preserving hemostasis which is expected to result in maintaining efficacy with improving safety (compared to existing antiplatelet therapy).

Developing thrombus consists of two distinct regions—core of fully activated platelets, located close to lesion (of injury) and dependent on soluble agonists such as thrombin and propagating thrombus composed primarily of platelet in lower activation states which are less susceptible to standard antiplatelet drugs. This understanding of distinction between hemostatic response which relies on thrombus core and thrombotic responses (thrombus propagation) led to focus on drugs that prevent propagation of thrombus.

NEWER TARGETS—ANTIPLATELET DRUGS

Phosphatidyl Inositol 3 Kinase B–PI3 Kinase B[10]

This lipid kinase is important for mediating platelet activation at sites of thrombus propagation. Recent evidence suggests that this enzyme has critical role in maintaining integrity of formed thrombus and inhibition of this pathway might theoretically increase risk of thrombus embolization. AZD6482 is inhibitor of PI3 kinase B enzyme and has shown in canine models, antithrombotic effects without increase in bleeding time or blood loss. In human volunteers the drug demonstrated moderate platelet inhibition (at levels between aspirin and clopidogrel) without increase in bleeding. No RCT in humans has been published.

Protein Disulfide-Isomerase–Protein Disulfide Isomerase[11]

These PDI exist on platelet surface and also in granules and are involved in thrombosis through their action on several intravascular targets. The PDI inhibitor—*isoquercetin*—is a blocker of platelet factor Va and is undergoing clinical trials for prevention of venous thrombosis in onco (oncology) patients. The role of PDI inhibitor in arterial thrombosis is not yet established.

12-Lipoxgenase Inhibitors

Lipoxygenase utilizes arachidonic acid as substrate to form bioactive metabolites that play role in platelet activation and granule secretion. Inhibitors of this enzyme mL-355 demonstrated dose dependent inhibition of human platelet aggregation, comparable to that of ASPIRIN. Further this molecule ML 355 also impaired thrombus growth with minimal bleeding.[12]

These novel antiplatelet, unlike the currently available antiplatelet agents that suppress autocrine events, they are directed against other platelet activation process such as adhesion, signaling and pro-coagulant activity.

CONCLUSION

Antiplatelet drugs remain as important pharmacological tools in therapy of established vascular disease—coronary, cerebrovascular, and PAD strategies to improve efficacy should be complemented by decreased bleeding—i.e., targeting thrombosis while preserving hemostasis should be aim of newer antiplatelet drug and we have yet to achieve it. Newer antiplatelet drugs include old targets—P2Y12, GPIIb/IIIa, with different mechanism of action, making then safer and effective. Additionally, newer targets such as inhibitors PAR, GP VI and GPIb/V/PX which are still in evolution. Newer drugs with different mechanism of action, targeting, propagation of thrombus, instead of thrombus initiation resulting in effective antiplatelet drugs, with better safety profile by reducing bleeding risk, are on the horizon, with better efficacy and safety.

REFERENCES

1. Patrono C, Baigent C, Hirsh J, Roth G. Antiplatelet drugs: American College of Chest Physicians Evidence-Based Clinical Practice Guidelines (8th Edition). Chest. 2008;133(6 Suppl):199S-233S.
2. Berger JS, Roe MT, Gibson CM, Kilaru R, Green CL, Melton L, et al. Safety and feasibility of adjunctive antiplatelet therapy with intravenous elinogrel, a direct-acting and reversible P2Y12 ADP-receptor antagonist, before primary percutaneous intervention in patients with ST-elevation myocardial infarction: the Early Rapid ReversAl of platelet thromboSis with intravenous Elinogrel before PCI to optimize reperfusion in acute Myocardial Infarction (ERASE MI) pilot trial. Am Heart J. 2009;158(6):998-1004.
3. Welsh RC, Rao SV, Zeymer U, Thompson VP, Huber K, Kochman J, et al. A randomized, double-blind, active-controlled phase 2 trial to evaluate a novel selective and reversible intravenous and oral P2Y12 inhibitor elinogrel versus clopidogrel in patients undergoing nonurgent percutaneous coronary intervention: The INNOVATE-PCI Trial. Circ Cardiovasc Interv. 2012;5(3):336-46.
4. Gehin M, Storey RF, Bernaud C, Dingemanse J. Clinical pharmacology of selatogrel for self-administration by patients with suspected acute myocardial infarction. Expert Opin Drug Metab Toxicol. 2023;19(10):697-708.
5. Valgimigli M, Landi A. Subcutaneous RUC-4 for acute myocardial infarction: a new treatment on the horizon for pre-hospital care? EuroIntervention. 2021;17(5):e362-3.
6. Tricoci P, Huang Z. Thrombin-receptor antagonist vorapaxar in acute coronary syndromes. N Engl J Med. 2012;366(1):20-33.

7. Gilchrist IC Jr, Morrow DA, Creager MA, Olin JW, Scirica BM, Goodrich EL, et al. Efficacy and safety of vorapaxar by intensity of background lipid-lowering therapy in patients with peripheral artery disease: insights from the TRA2P-TIMI 50 trial. J Am Heart Assoc. 2021;10(20):e021412.
8. Mayer K, Hein-Rothweiler R, Schüpke S, Janisch M, Bernlochner I, Ndrepepa G, et al. Efficacy and safety of revacept, a novel lesion-directed competitive antagonist to platelet glycoprotein VI, in patients undergoing elective percutaneous coronary intervention for stable ischemic heart disease: the randomized, double-blind, placebo-controlled ISAR-PLASTER phase 2 trial. JAMA Cardiol. 2021;6(7):753-61.
9. Li BX, Dai X, Xu XR, Adili R, Neves MAD, Lei X, et al. In vitro assessment and phase I randomized clinical trial of anfibatide a snake venom derived anti-thrombotic agent targeting human platelet GPIbα. Sci Rep. 2021; 11(1):11663.
10. Nylander S, Wågberg F, Andersson M, Skärby T, Gustafsson D. Exploration of efficacy and bleeding with combined phosphoinositide 3-kinase β inhibition and aspirin in man. J Thromb Haemost. 2015;13(8):1494-502.
11. Stopa JD, Zwicker JI. The intersection of protein disulfide isomerase and cancer associated thrombosis. Thromb Res. 2018;164(Suppl 1):S130-5.
12. Adili R, Tourdot BE, Mast K, Yeung J, Freedman JC, Green A, et al. First selective 12-LOX inhibitor, ML355, impairs thrombus formation and vessel occlusion in vivo with minimal effects on hemostasis. Arterioscler Thromb Vasc Biol. 2017;37(10):1828-39.

Blood Pressure Measurement Methods: Which One is the Best in Clinical Day-to-day Practice?

Abhishek Garg, Gurpreet Singh Wander

INTRODUCTION

India, with a population of >1.30 billion, is experiencing a rising burden of cardiovascular disease (CVD) along with increasing mortalities, primarily driven by uncontrolled hypertension. Hypertension directly accounts for 24% of all coronary artery disease deaths and 57% of all stroke deaths in India.[1] It is a common condition that lacks specific clinical symptoms until target organ damage develops.[2-4] Hypertension poses a significant risk for CVD, much of which is at least partially reversible with appropriate treatment. Screening adults to detect hypertension at an early stage and initiating treatment before the onset of target organ damage is crucial.[4,5] However, the teaching, training, and knowledge of blood pressure (BP) measurement and the use of related apparatus among healthcare professionals remain suboptimal.[6-8] These gaps in training are prevalent among medical students, nurses, and other paramedical staff, who need to be experts in the correct measurement technique.[1]

BLOOD PRESSURE MEASUREMENT DEVICES

Accurate BP measurement is essential for effective hypertension management and for reducing cardiovascular morbidity and mortality.[9] Overestimation of BP can result in psychological distress from misdiagnosis, unnecessary side effects of antihypertensive medications, increased treatment costs, and higher insurance premiums. On the other hand, underestimation of BP may deprive patients of necessary therapy, potentially leading to higher rates of fatal strokes and myocardial infarctions.[10] One of the primary causes of inaccurate BP measurement is the equipment used.[11,12] The three most widely accepted devices for BP measurement are the mercury sphygmomanometer, the aneroid sphygmomanometer, and the automatic digital monitor.

The mercury sphygmomanometer **(Fig. 1)** has been regarded as the gold standard for BP measurement for over 100 years. Its key advantages include high accuracy, minimal calibration requirements, and infrequent breakdowns. However, mercury devices are being phased out, not due to the advent of superior BP measurement technologies, but because of the harmful environmental and health effects of mercury. An advisory issued as early as 2010 recommended avoiding the use and procurement of mercury sphygmomanometer,[10] and India aimed to ban them by the end of 2020.[10] Despite these measures, mercury sphygmomanometer devices remain widely used in India due to the lack of a more reliable replacement. Aneroid and oscillometric devices have not yet matched the reliability of mercury sphygmomanometers,

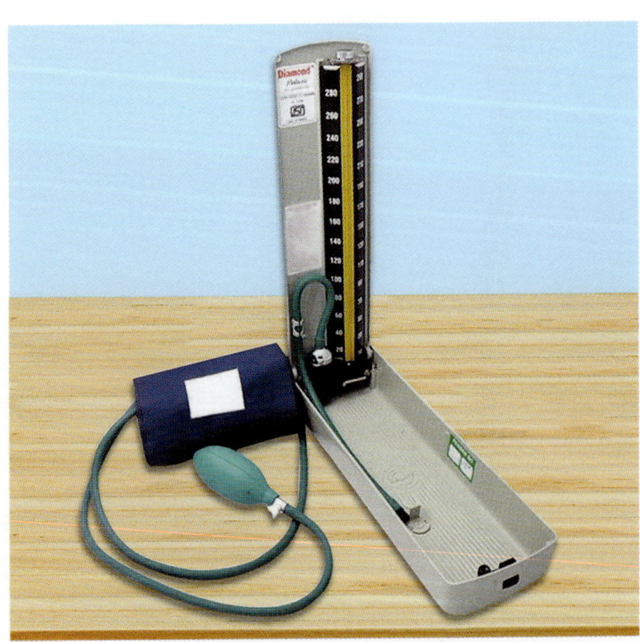

Fig. 1: Mercury sphygmomanometer.

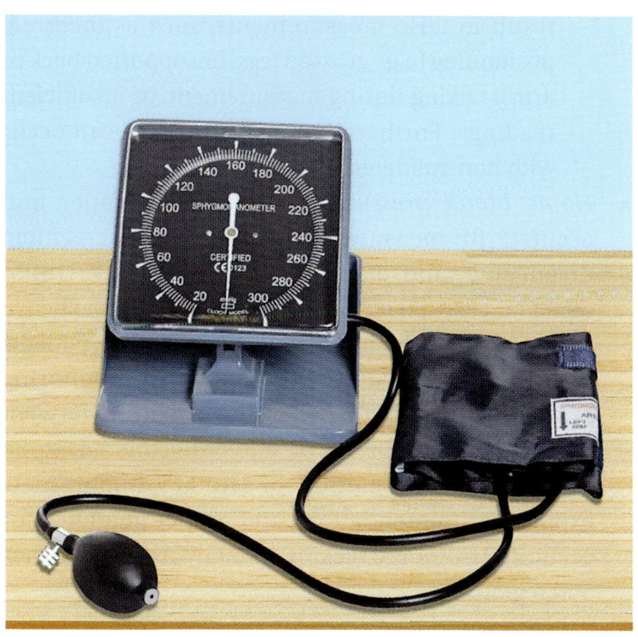

Fig. 2: Aneroid sphygmomanometer.

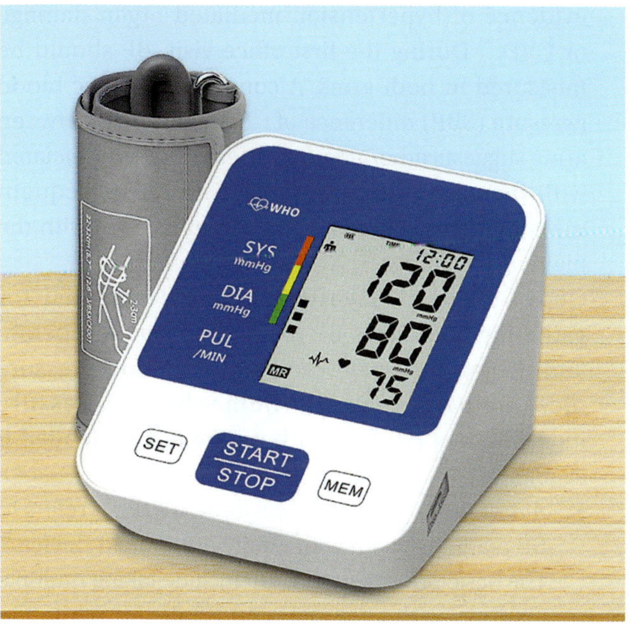

Fig. 3: Automatic digital sphygmomanometers.

contributing to clinicians' continued reliance on mercury sphygmomanometer devices.

The aneroid sphygmomanometer **(Fig. 2)** operates using mechanical springs and dashpot systems. It employs the same auscultatory method of measurement as the mercury sphygmomanometer but is prone to calibration issues, particularly in heavy-use hospital environments. These devices often lose calibration within 6 months to a year due to the loosening of springs.[13-15] Once the springs become loose, recalibration is nearly impossible. In a study conducted by McKay et al.[16] involving 114 physicians, it was found that nearly 40% of aneroid sphygmomanometer were out of calibration by at least 4 mm Hg, compared to only 8% of mercury sphygmomanometers exhibiting the same degree of error.

Automatic digital sphygmomanometers (oscillometric devices) **(Fig. 3)** are the most popular choice for home use and self-monitoring of BP. These devices use the oscillometric method, which accurately measures mean arterial pressure, while systolic and diastolic pressures are derived using various empirical and signal processing methods. These methods differ among manufacturers and are often proprietary trade secrets.[17] In a comparison between aneroid and digital BP monitors, the aneroid device demonstrated higher sensitivity and specificity than the digital device by 6.7% and 31%, respectively.[18] Despite their widespread use, both aneroid and oscillometric devices remain less accurate and reliable compared to mercury sphygmomanometers.[19]

The European Society of Hypertension (ESH) 2023 guidelines[20] recommend automatic electronic upper-arm cuff devices as Class 1 tool for both office and out-of-office BP measurement, including home and ambulatory monitoring.

BLOOD PRESSURE MEASUREMENT LOCATION

- *Office blood pressure measurement (OBPM):* It is performed using a brachial pressure cuff and auscultation of the brachial artery to detect the appearance and disappearance of Korotkoff sounds. OBPM is recommended for diagnosing hypertension, as it is the primary method used to assess hypertension-related risks, the benefits of antihypertensive treatment, and treatment-related BP thresholds and goals.[20] Triplicate measurements should be taken, and the average of the last two should be used as the representative value.[20] Hypertension should be diagnosed during at least two separate office visits (within 4 weeks), unless office BP indicates grade 3 hypertension (≥180/110 mm Hg), the patient presents with hypertension-related symptoms, or there is evidence of hypertension-mediated organ damage or CVD.[20] During the first office visit, BP should be measured in both arms. A consistent systolic blood pressure (SBP) difference of >15–20 mm Hg between arms suggests atheromatous disease and is associated with increased cardiovascular risk. All subsequent measurements should be taken from the arm with the higher BP readings.[20]

Out-of-office BP measurements are essential for gathering additional BP-related information before and during treatment. Ambulatory blood pressure measurement (ABPM), home blood pressure measurement (HBPM), or both are recommended if available.[20]

- *Automated office blood pressure (AOBP):* It refers to BP readings taken with a fully automated device.[19] The basic principles of AOBP include taking multiple readings with an automated BP device while the patient is resting alone in a quiet room. When these principles are followed, white coat hypertension is eliminated, and AOBP shows a much stronger correlation with awake ambulatory BP than routine manual BP measurements. Additionally, AOBP correlates as well with left ventricular mass as does awake ambulatory BP.[21] Over recent years, automated BP measurement devices have become widely available, but they are still expensive and not recommended for widespread use.
- *Devices:* Mercury sphygmomanometers, aneroid sphygmomanometers, and automated blood pressure measurement devices.
- *Advantages:* OBPM has been the cornerstone of hypertension diagnosis and management for over 100 years and remains the method of choice in most research, including major trials such as SPRINT and HOPE-3.[16,17] It is the recommended method for diagnosing hypertension because it serves as the basis for assessing hypertension-related risks, the benefits of antihypertensive treatments, and treatment-related BP thresholds and goals.[20]
- *Disadvantages:* A single office BP reading does not accurately represent a patient's typical BP. Errors may arise due to factors such as clinic ambiance, leading to white-coat hypertension. OBPM offers a snapshot of BP at a single visit but lacks information on BP during normal daily activities or sleep. It is also more prone to procedural errors that may result in false measurements, such as incorrect positioning (e.g., crossed legs, unsupported back or arm), talking during measurement, or insufficient readings. Furthermore, false readings can occur with non-validated devices.

- *Home blood pressure measurement:* Proper and accurate BP measurement is critical for screening, diagnosing, and managing hypertension.[22] HBPM offers an easy, reliable, convenient, and cost-effective method for measuring BP. In previous studies, patients who were more comfortable with self-monitoring at home ranked higher than those who underwent repeated measurements by staff or doctors.[22] Despite the growing recognition of HBPM's importance, explicit recommendations and proper guidance for accurate HBPM are lacking in many Asian countries and regions.[22]
    - *Device and measurement technique:* The standard monitor for home use is an oscillometric device that records BP from the brachial artery. The arm cuff is preferred over wrist or finger monitors.[23] HBPM should be measured twice daily for a 3–7-day period to diagnose hypertension; the first-day values are typically not used to allow patients to acclimatize to the process. A good regimen includes measuring BP twice in the morning (after 5 minutes of rest before breakfast, preferably between 6:00 and 10:00 AM) and twice in the evening (also preferably between 6:00 and 10:00 PM), with the patient sitting at rest for 5 minutes and with an empty bladder.[23] The Japanese Society of Hypertension guidelines recommend measuring BP after 1–2 minutes of rest, as shown in **Box 1**. Equipment must be calibrated against a mercury manometer, with the difference between measurements compared to the auscultatory method being ≤5 mm Hg. The device should also be calibrated annually. Each measurement should be documented with the pulse rate, time, and date; devices with an attached printer or integrated memory help prevent selection bias.[23]
    - *Advantages:* HBPM eliminates white coat hypertension and can help diagnose masked hypertension. It also provides BP data during activity, which OBPM cannot offer. HBPM is less influenced by observer bias, and its reproducibility is better

BOX 1: Japanese Society of Hypertension guidelines for home blood pressure monitoring.[24]

- Arm-cuffs based on the oscillometric method devices are recommended. They should be validated and confirmed for accuracy in each individual
- Blood pressure should be measured in the upper arm. Finger cuff devices and wrist-cuff devices should not be used for home blood pressure measurements
- Devices for home BP measurement should be validated by the American Association Medical Instrumentation standards and the British Hypertension Society guidelines. In addition, the difference between the blood pressure measured by the auscultatory method and that measured using the device should be 5 mm Hg or less
- The morning blood pressure measurement should be made within 1 hour after waking, after micturition, sitting after 1–2 minutes of rest, before drug ingestion, and before breakfast. The evening measurement should be made just before going to bed, sitting after 1–2 minutes of rest
- All home BP measurements should be documented without selection or omission and include the date, time, and pulse rate. Use of a device with a printer or an integrated circuit memo is useful to avoid selection bias

than that of office measurements.[23] Integrating HBPM into practice can aid in diagnosing and treating hypertension and assessing cardiovascular risk and complications related to hypertension.[23] It can be beneficial in patients with chronic kidney disease and diabetes, helping to diagnose resistant or refractory hypertension. HBPM is also valuable in research, such as studying the onset and duration of antihypertensive drugs and their side effects. Furthermore, it plays a key role in detecting or preventing hypertension-mediated organ damage. Beyond its diagnostic and prognostic value, HBPM promotes awareness of treatment and encourages active BP management.[23]

- *Disadvantages:* Despite its advantages, HBPM has some drawbacks. It requires awareness of device use and measurement techniques. Poverty and illiteracy are common barriers to HBPM, especially in countries with high poverty rates like India. A significant limitation is that HBPM cannot measure night-time BP, thus lacking prognostic value regarding dipping patterns.

- *Ambulatory blood pressure measurement:* ABPM involves automatic BP measurements at regular intervals (typically every 20 minutes during the day and every 30 minutes at night) over 24–72 hours.
  - *Device and techniques:* Patients are provided with an ABPM device, which measures BP at predefined intervals over a 24–72-hour period. If one arm shows higher readings at baseline, it should be used for subsequent measurements.[25] However, the non-dominant arm is often preferred to minimize interference with daily activities. ABPM devices include a cuff and bladder connected to electronic sensors, which detect changes in cuff pressure and allow BP to be measured oscillometrically. Systolic and diastolic pressure readings are derived from the shape of the oscillometric pressure changes using a specific algorithm. The cuff is inflated by a battery-powered compressor. Devices vary in size, weight, noise level, data manipulation, and cost, and should be validated and internationally recommended.[25] The recommended frequency of measurements is every 20 minutes during both day and night to ensure accurate readings.[20]
  - *Advantages*: ABPM overcomes the limitations of both OBPM and HBPM methods. It provides a comprehensive profile of BP behavior during daily activities, including night-time measurements. ABPM is not influenced by clinic ambiance and is superior to office BP measurements. It is recommended to identify white-coat hypertension, masked hypertension, and nocturnal BP phenotypes. Repeated ABPM may be necessary, as these phenotypes have limited reproducibility.[20] ABPM is also used to diagnose true resistant hypertension and is considered the best method for predicting cardiovascular event risk based on BP.[26] The relationship between ABPM and cardiovascular event risk is continuous, consistent, and independent of other risk factors.[26]
  - *Disadvantages*: The main disadvantage of ABPM is its cost and limited availability. Additionally, it can cause discomfort to patients, especially during sleep or sexual activity, and some patients may be reluctant to use it.

Figure 4 summarizes the uses of OBPM, HBPM, and ABPM in clinical practice according to the guidelines.

BLOOD PRESSURE MEASUREMENT TECHNIQUE

Failure to standardize the technique of measurement is one of the most common errors in BP measurement.

Previous Indian studies have shown that training, teaching, and knowledge of BP apparatus and measurement techniques for healthcare professionals are suboptimal.[1] A study conducted by Mohan B et al.[1] found that, out of 400 individuals, only 5.8% of medical staff had excellent knowledge, 74.5% had good knowledge, and 19.6% had poor knowledge of correct measurement techniques.

Office BP
Basis for hypertension diagnosis and evaluation
Home BP
For most treated individuals follow-up
Ambulatory BP
For resistant and nocturnal BP phenotypes

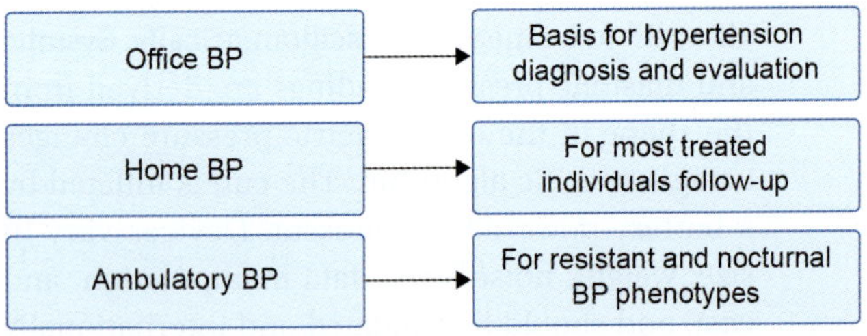

Fig. 4: Uses of office blood pressure measurement (OBPM), home blood pressure measurement (HBPM), and ambulatory blood pressure measurement (ABPM) in clinical practice according to the guidelines.

However, only 1.47% of the medical staff demonstrated accurate practices, and among paramedical staff, only 0.5% followed accurate practices. This indicates that while the knowledge of the correct BP measurement method is relatively reasonable, the actual practice is inadequate, and the necessary precautions are often not followed.

Figure 5 illustrates the various precautions that must be taken to ensure accurate BP readings. The different aspects of these precautions are discussed below:

Posture

- Blood pressure should be measured in a sitting position. If measured in a supine position, SBP may increase by 3 mm Hg, while diastolic blood pressure (DBP) may be recorded at 3 mm Hg lower.[1]
- The patient should sit comfortably with the arm at heart level. The legs should be uncrossed, feet flat on the floor, and the back supported. The arm should rest on a desk or table.[1]

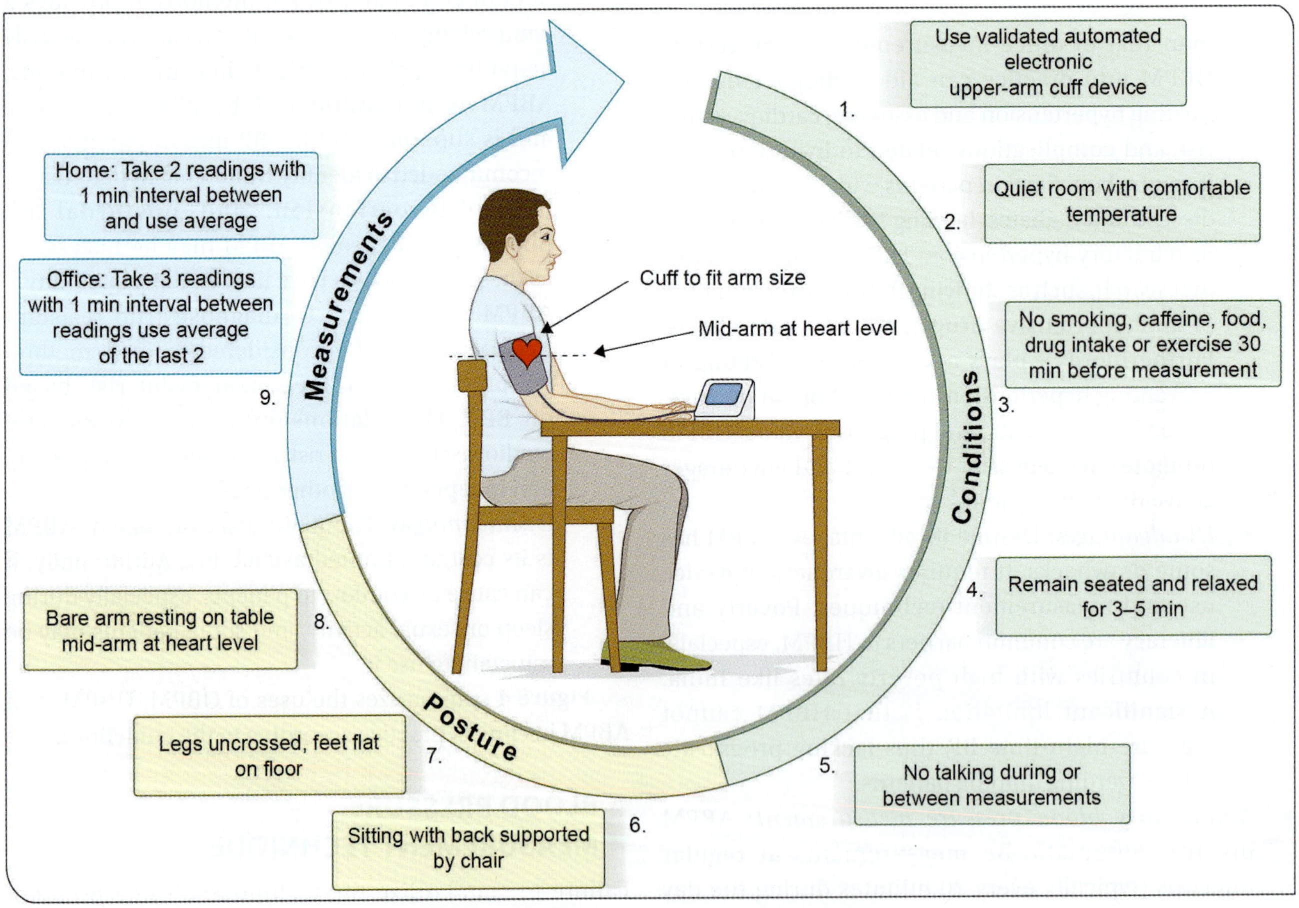

1.
Use validated automated electronic upper-arm cuff device
2.
Quiet room with comfortable temperature
3.
No smoking, caffeine, food, drug intake or exercise 30 min before measurement
Conditions
4.
Remain seated and relaxed for 3–5 min
5.
No talking during or between measurements
6.
Sitting with back supported by chair
7.
Legs uncrossed, feet flat on floor
Posture
8.
Bare arm resting on table mid-arm at heart level
9.
Office: Take 3 readings with 1 min interval between readings use average of the last 2
Home: Take 2 readings with 1 min interval between and use average
Measurements
Cuff to fit arm size
Mid-arm at heart level

Fig. 5: Technique of blood pressure measurement.

Conditions

- The patient should rest comfortably for at least 5 minutes in a quiet room before the measurement.
- Pain, strenuous exercise, cold temperatures, food consumption, smoking, caffeine ingestion, and emotional stress should be avoided for at least 30 minutes before measurements.
- The urinary bladder should be emptied before taking the measurement.

Measurements

- The BP cuff should cover 2/3 of the arm circumference. If the cuff size is too small, as in the case of obese individuals, SBP may be falsely elevated (up to 8 mm Hg).[1]
- Systolic pressure should first be estimated through palpation to ensure that the systolic gap, which may be present in some individuals, is not missed. This also helps diagnose pseudo hypertension, which is often seen in elderly individuals with significant artery calcifications.
- Blood pressure should be measured in both arms during the initial visit. The arm with the higher reading should be used for subsequent measurements.[20]
- The cuff should be inflated to 30 mm Hg above the estimated SBP.
- The deflation rate should be 2 mm Hg per second.
- The first appearance of sound (phase I) defines SBP.
- The disappearance of sound (phase V) defines DBP.

Innovative Blood Pressure Measurement Devices

Recent advancements address the limitations of traditional BP measurement methods. Cuffless BP devices utilize sensors, signal processing, and machine learning technologies integrated into wearables, pocket devices, and smartphones. These devices provide continuous BP monitoring and reduce errors from inappropriate cuff sizes. However, they require periodic calibration, and current validation protocols are inapplicable. The ESH 2023 guidelines recommend against using cuffless devices for clinical diagnosis and treatment until standardized validation protocols are established, though their future remains promising.[20]

The Auscl-D combines digital technology with manual auscultation, offering a cost-effective solution for BP measurement, particularly in resource-limited settings[27] **(Fig. 6A)**. Its digital display enables clinicians to visualize readings while simultaneously detecting Korotkoff sounds. Constructed from easily available materials, Auscl-D performs comparably to mercury sphygmomanometers in laboratory settings and to aneroid and oscillometric devices in clinical trials **(Fig. 6B)**. Preliminary trials with 30 participants showed good agreement between Auscl-D and conventional devices based on Bland-Altman analysis[27] **(Fig. 6C)**.

To replace mercury sphygmomanometers banned under the Minamata Convention, the Merkfree device employs Galinstan, a non-toxic alloy of Gallium, Indium, and Tin, as a substitute[28] **(Fig. 7A)**. Galinstan-based devices retain the design and functionality of traditional mercury sphygmomanometers while being safer and environmentally friendly **(Fig. 7B)**. In a clinical trial involving 252 participants, Merkfree demonstrated measurement accuracy comparable to mercury sphygmomanometers and validated oscillometric devices. It showed excellent correlation (0.9999) with mercury

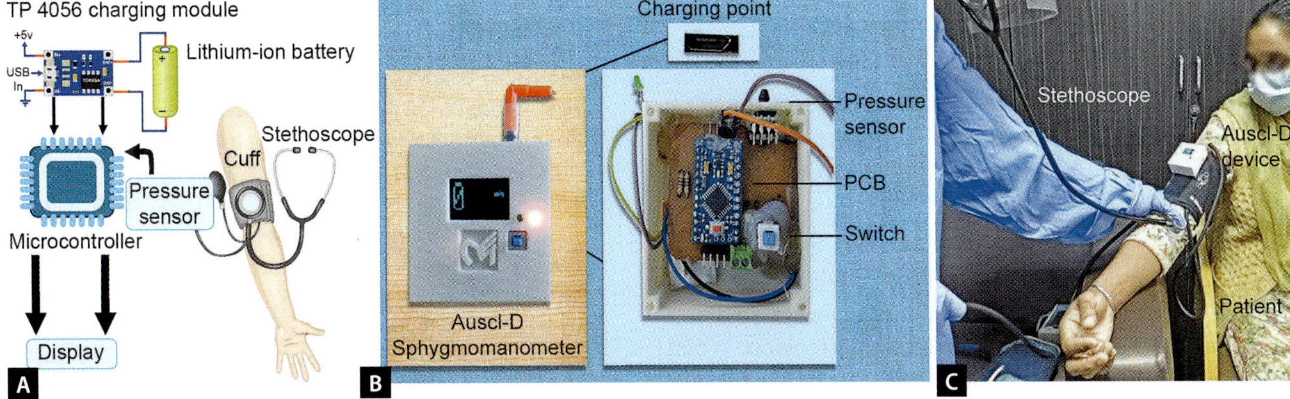

Figs. 6A to C: (A) The components of the digital BP device Auscl-D and their functioning; (B) The actual image of Auscl-D and its internal components; (C) Auscl-D being used clinically for measurement of BP; the small and convenient size of the device is visible.

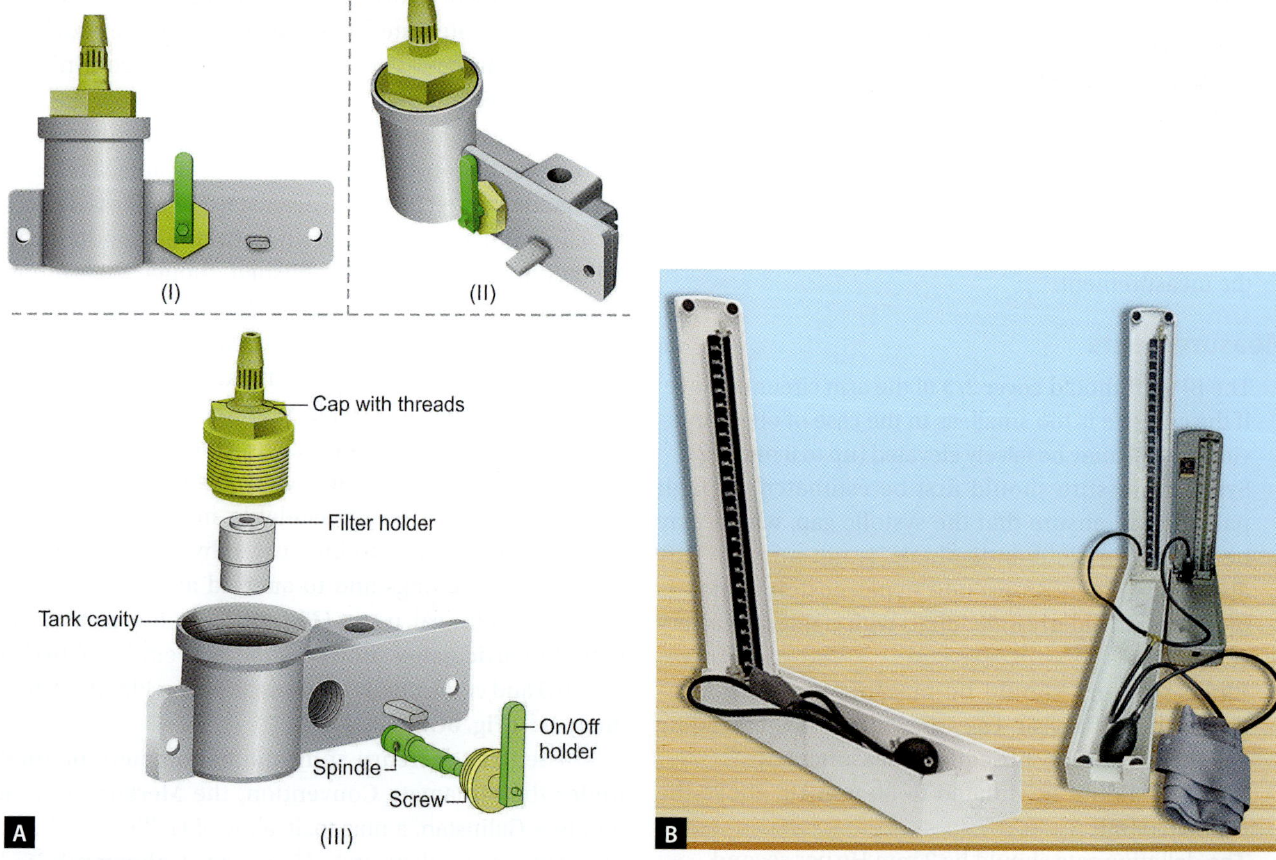

Figs. 7A and B: (A) The Merkfree device components. Container tank for Galinstan and the on-off knobs; (B) The size of the Merkfree device is double of the mercury sphygmomanometer which is seen in the picture.

devices and zero bias in the Bland-Altman analysis, confirming its reliability.[28]

These innovations highlight the transition toward safer, more accessible, and technologically advanced BP measurement tools while emphasizing the need for rigorous validation before widespread adoption.

CONCLUSION

Accurate BP measurement is essential for diagnosing and managing hypertension, the most common non-communicable disease. The recent 2023 ESH guidelines acknowledge OBPM as a reliable method for diagnosing hypertension. However, the 2024 ESC guidelines emphasize the importance of out-of-office BP measurement for more accurate diagnosis, particularly in detecting white-coat and masked hypertension. When out-of-office monitoring is not feasible due to logistical or economic constraints, repeated office BP measurements using standardized techniques are recommended to confirm the diagnosis. Clinicians should transition from mercury sphygmomanometers to validated oscillometric devices, as international guidelines recommend. Reliable devices, a quiet environment, and multiple readings are crucial for accurate results.

REFERENCES

1. Mohan B, Aslam N, Ralhan U, Sharma S, Gupta N, Singh VP, et al. Office blood pressure measurement practices among community health providers (medical and paramedical) in northern district of India. Indian Heart J. 2014;66(4):401-7.
2. Miura K, Daviglus ML, Dyer AR, Liu K, Garside DB, Stamler J, et al. Relationship of blood pressure to 25-year mortality due to coronary heart disease, cardiovascular disease, and all causes in young adult men: the Chicago Heart Association Detection Project in Industry. Arch Intern Med. 2001;161:1501-8.
3. Wang G, Grosse SD, Schooley MW. Conducting research on the economics of hypertension to improve cardiovascular health. Am J Prev Med. 2017;53(6 Suppl 2):S115-7.

4. McAlister FA, Straus SE. Measurement of blood pressure: an evidence-based review. BMJ. 2001;322:908-11.
5. Litenberg BA. Practice guidelines revisited: screening for hypertension. Ann Intern Med. 1995;122:937-9.
6. Gleichmann SI, Gleichmann UM, Mannebach HJ, Mellwig KP, Philippi HH. Educating nurses in blood pressure measurement and hypertension control. J Hypertens Suppl. 1989;7:S99-102.
7. Feher M, Harris-St John K, Lant A. Blood pressure measurement by junior hospital doctors: a gap in medical practice. Health Trends. 1992;24:59-61.
8. Wingfield D, Pierce M, Feher M. Blood pressure measurement in the community: do guidelines help? J Hum Hypertens. 1996;10:805-9.
9. Muntner P, Shimbo D, Carey RM, Charleston JB, Gaillard T, Misra S, et al. Measurement of blood pressure in humans: a scientific statement from the American Heart Association. Hypertension. 2019;73:e35-e66.
10. Kumar R, Sahani AK, Wander GS. A survey to gauge confidence of Indian clinicians on three primary devices for blood pressure measurement. Blood Press Monit. 2020;26(3):196-9.
11. Sharman JE, Marwick TH. Accuracy of blood pressure monitoring devices: a critical need for improvement that could resolve discrepancies in hypertension guidelines. J Hum Hypertens. 2019;33:89-93.
12. Campbell NR, McKay DW. Accurate blood pressure measurement: why does it matter? CMAJ. 1999;161:277-8.
13. Buchanan S, Orris P, Karliner J. Alternatives to the mercury sphygmomanometer. J Public Health Policy. 2011;32: 107-20.
14. Murray A. In praise of mercury sphygmomanometers. BMJ. 2001;322:1248-9.
15. Waugh JJ, Gupta M, Rushbrook J, Halligan A, Shennan AH. Hidden errors of aneroid sphygmomanometers. Blood Press Monit. 2002;7:309-12.
16. McKay DW, Campbell NR, Parab LS, Chockalingam A, Fodor JG. Clinical assessment of blood pressure. J Hum Hypertens. 1990;4:639-45.
17. van Montfrans GA. Oscillometric blood pressure measurement: progress and problems. Blood Press Monit. 2001;6:287-90.
18. Shahbabu B, Dasgupta A, Sarkar K, Sahoo SK. Which is more accurate in measuring blood pressure? A digital or an aneroid sphygmomanometer. J Clin Diagn Res. 2016;10:LC11-LC14.
19. Jones DW, Frohlich ED, Grim CM, Grim CE, Taubert KA. Mercury sphygmomanometers should not be abandoned: an advisory statement from the Council for High Blood Pressure Research, American Heart Association. Hypertension. 2001;37:185-6.
20. Mancia G, Kreutz R, Brunström M, Burnier M, Grassi G, Januszewicz A, et al. 2023 ESH Guidelines for the management of arterial hypertension. J Hypertens. 2023; 41(12):1874-2071.
21. National Clinical Guideline Centre (UK). Hypertension: the clinical management of primary hypertension in adults: update of clinical guidelines 18 and 34. London: Royal College of Physicians; 2011.
22. Wander GS, Salman E, Matsushita N, Verma N. Awareness and recommendation of home blood pressure measurement among physicians in India: Results from the Asia HBPM survey 2020. Indian Heart J. 2023;75(3):169-76.
23. Mallick S, Kanthety R, Rahman M. Home blood pressure monitoring in clinical practice: a review. Am J Med. 2009;122(9):803-10.
24. Japanese Society of Hypertension. Japanese Society of Hypertension guidelines for the management of hypertension (JSH 2004). Hypertens Res. 2006; 29(Suppl):S1-S105.
25. Myers MG, Godwin M. Automated office blood pressure. Can J Cardiol. 2012 May 1;28(3):341-6.
26. Roerecke M, Kaczorowski J, Myers MG. Comparing automated office blood pressure readings with other methods of blood pressure measurement for identifying patients with possible hypertension: a systematic review and meta-analysis. JAMA Intern Med. 2019;179(3):351-62.
27. Kumar V, Kumar R, Wander GS, Wander GS, Sahani A. Auscl-D: a mercury-free digital auscultatory sphygmomanometer. J Med Eng Technol. 2021;45(8):656-63.
28. Kumar R, Kumar M, Wander GS, Sahani AK. Concept, hardware development, and clinical trials of a Galinstan-based mercury-free sphygmomanometer: Merkfree. Sci Rep. 2022;12(1):15813.

Hypertension and Cognitive Impairment: Mechanisms, Evidence, and Interventions

A Muruganathan

INTRODUCTION

Hypertension (high blood pressure) is a major public health concern, affecting over 1.3 billion people worldwide.[1] While its role in cardiovascular diseases is well-documented, growing evidence suggests that chronic hypertension significantly contributes to cognitive impairment and dementia, including Alzheimer's disease (AD) and vascular dementia (VaD). The relationship between hypertension and cognitive decline is complex, involving vascular damage, reduced cerebral blood flow, and neurodegenerative processes. This article explores the pathophysiological mechanisms, clinical evidence, and potential interventions to mitigate cognitive decline in hypertensive individuals.

MECHANISMS LINKING HYPERTENSION TO COGNITIVE IMPAIRMENT

Cerebral Small Vessel Disease

Chronic hypertension damages small cerebral arteries and arterioles, leading to white matter hyperintensities (WMH), microbleeds, and lacunar infarcts.[2] These changes disrupt neural connectivity, particularly in regions responsible for memory, attention, and executive function. Studies using MRI have shown that hypertensive individuals exhibit greater white matter lesions, which correlate with slower processing speed and poorer executive function.[3]

Reduced Cerebral Blood Flow and Hypoperfusion

The brain relies on a steady blood supply, but hypertension impairs cerebrovascular autoregulation, leading to chronic hypoperfusion.[4] Reduced blood flow affects the hippocampus and prefrontal cortex, increasing the risk of memory deficits and executive dysfunction. Over time, this can accelerate neurodegeneration and synaptic loss, contributing to dementia pathology.[5]

Blood-brain Barrier Dysfunction

Hypertension increases oxidative stress and inflammation, weakening the blood-brain barrier (BBB).[6] A leaky BBB allows neurotoxic substances (e.g., fibrinogen and thrombin) to enter the brain, triggering neuroinflammation and neuronal damage.[7] This process is particularly harmful in Alzheimer's disease, where BBB dysfunction may promote amyloid-β accumulation.[8]

Amyloid Deposition and Alzheimer's Pathology

Some studies suggest that hypertension accelerates amyloid-beta (Aβ) plaque formation.[9] Animal models show that chronic high blood pressure increases Aβ deposition, possibly due to impaired clearance mechanisms.[10] This may explain why midlife hypertension is strongly linked to late-life dementia (Launer et al., 2000).

CLINICAL EVIDENCE SUPPORTING THE HYPERTENSION-COGNITIVE DECLINE LINK

Longitudinal Population Studies

- The Framingham Heart Study found that midlife hypertension (aged 45–65 years) predicts late-life cognitive decline.[11]
- The Rotterdam Study reported that uncontrolled hypertension increases dementia risk by 60%.[12]

Neuroimaging Findings

- MRI studies show that hypertensive individuals have greater brain atrophy, particularly in the hippocampus and frontal lobes (Knopman et al., 2015).
- White matter lesions are more severe in hypertensive patients, correlating with poorer cognitive performance.[3]

Hypertension and Dementia Risk

A meta-analysis by Walker et al. (2020) found:

- 50% increased risk of vascular dementia (VaD)
- 20% increased risk of Alzheimer's disease (AD)

INTERVENTIONS TO REDUCE COGNITIVE DECLINE IN HYPERTENSIVE PATIENTS

Blood Pressure Control

- The SPRINT-MIND trial (2019) demonstrated that intensive BP control (<120 mm Hg) reduces mild cognitive impairment (MCI) risk by 19%.[13]
- Angiotensin-converting enzyme (ACE) inhibitors and angiotensin receptor blockers (ARBs) may have neuroprotective effects beyond blood pressure lowering (Hajjar et al., 2020).

Lifestyle Modifications

- *Diet:* The DASH and Mediterranean diets improve vascular health and cognition (Morris et al., 2015).
- *Exercise:* Aerobic activity enhances cerebral blood flow and neurogenesis (Erickson et al., 2011).
- Smoking cessation and alcohol moderation reduce oxidative stress and inflammation.

Early Detection and Monitoring

- Cognitive screening in hypertensive patients can detect early decline.
- Ambulatory blood pressure monitoring (ABPM) helps to identify nocturnal hypertension, which is strongly linked to cognitive impairment (Yano et al., 2018).

CONCLUSION

Hypertension is a modifiable risk factor for cognitive impairment and dementia.[14] Early and aggressive blood pressure management, combined with lifestyle interventions, can significantly reduce the risk of cognitive decline. Future research should explore "personalized treatment approaches to optimize brain health in hypertensive individuals".

REFERENCES

1. World Health Organization. (2021). Hypertension. [online] Available from https://www.who.int/news-room/fact-sheets/detail/hypertension [Last accessed Sept. 2025].
2. Pantoni L. Cerebral small vessel disease: From pathogenesis and clinical characteristics to therapeutic challenges. Lancet Neurol. 2010;9(7):689-701.
3. Debette S, Markus HS. The clinical importance of white matter hyperintensities on brain magnetic resonance imaging: Systematic review and meta-analysis. BMJ. 2010;341:c3666.
4. Gorelick PB, Scuteri A, Black SE, Decarli C, Greenberg SM, Iadecola C, et al. Vascular contributions to cognitive impairment and dementia: A statement for healthcare professionals. Stroke. 2011;42(9):2672-713.
5. Iadecola C. The pathobiology of vascular dementia. Neuron. 2013;80(4):844-66.
6. Farrall AJ, Wardlaw JM. Blood-brain barrier: Ageing and microvascular disease—Systematic review and meta-analysis. Neurobiol Aging. 2009;30(3):337-52.
7. Nation DA, Sweeney MD, Montagne A, Sagare AP, D'Orazio LM, Pachicano M, et al. Blood-brain barrier breakdown is an early biomarker of human cognitive dysfunction. Nat Med. 2015;21(9):1094-9.
8. Montagne A, Nation DA, Sagare AP, Barisano G, Sweeney MD, Chakhoyan A, et al. APOE4 leads to blood-brain barrier dysfunction predicting cognitive decline. Nature. 2017;581:71-6.
9. Kelleher RJ, Soiza RL. Evidence of endothelial dysfunction in the development of Alzheimer's disease: Is Alzheimer's a vascular disorder? Am J Cardiovasc Dis. 2013;3(4):197-226.
10. Carnevale D, Mascio G, D'Andrea I, Fardella V, Bell RD, Branchi I, et al. Hypertension induces brain β-amyloid accumulation, cognitive impairment and memory deterioration through activation of receptor for advanced glycation end products in brain vasculature. Hypertension. 2012;60(1):188-97.
11. Seshadri S, Beiser A, Selhub J, Jacques PF, Rosenberg IH, D'Agostino RB, et al. Plasma homocysteine as a risk factor for dementia and Alzheimer's disease. N Engl J Med. 2004;346:476-83.
12. Ruitenberg A, Skoog I, Ott A, Aevarsson O, Witteman JC, Lernfelt B, et al. Blood pressure and risk of dementia: Results from the Rotterdam Study and the Gothenburg H-70 Study. Dement Geriatr Cogn Disord. 2005;22(1):24-33.
13. SPRINT MIND Investigators for the SPRINT Research Group; Williamson JD, Pajewski NM, Auchus AP, Bryan RN, Chelune G, et al. Effect of intensive vs standard blood pressure control on probable dementia: A randomized clinical trial. JAMA. 2019;321(6):553-61.
14. Peters R, Booth A, Rockwood K, Peters J, D'Este C, Anstey KJ. Combining modifiable risk factors and risk of dementia: A systematic review and meta-analysis. BMJ Open. 2019;9(1):e022846.

Clinical Evaluation and Management of Resistant Hypertension

Girish G, Geetha Priya V, Iyengar SS

INTRODUCTION

Hypertension (HTN), aptly called the "silent killer," is a leading preventable cause of cardiovascular disease (CVD) and associated morbidity and mortality. Resistant hypertension (RH) is a significant challenge in cardiovascular medicine, affecting approximately 3–30% of hypertensive patients globally.[1] Indian data shows that RH is found in 11–16.13% of hypertensive patient.[2,3] With 234 million hypertensive patients, around 23 million are likely to have RH due to nonadherence to treatment and therapeutic inertia.[4]

The pathophysiological mechanism implicated in true RH is an interplay between factors like raised levels of aldosterone, endothelin 1, vasopressin, and increased sympathetic activity.[5-7]

Patients with RH have a worse prognosis and a higher risk of myocardial infarction, stroke, end-stage renal disease, and death that may be two- to sixfold higher.[8] Secondary causes of hypertension are also more likely in the presence of resistant hypertension.

Patients with RH necessarily need frequent assessment and may require hospitalization leading to enhanced healthcare costs.

DEFINITION

True RH is defined as BP above goal [systolic BP (SBP) or diastolic BP (DBP) that remains ≥140 or ≥90 mm Hg, respectively as per ESH guidelines[9] and ≥130 or ≥80 mm Hg, respectively as per ACC/AHA guidelines[1]] despite appropriate use of lifestyle intervention and optimal doses of three drugs comprising a renin-angiotensin-aldosterone (RAAS) blocker (either an angiotensin-converting enzyme inhibitor or an angiotensin receptor blocker), a calcium-channel blocker, and a thiazide/thiazide-like diuretic.

Incidentally, none of the definitions mention about the duration of the drug therapy to be received by the patient before considering RH.

The prerequisites for true RH are:
- All RH definitions require a diuretic in the treatment.
- One has to exclude pseudoresistance including poor adherence, white coat hypertension, and evaluation of adherence.

Other terms:
- *Controlled RH:* It includes high BP that is controlled on ≥4 antihypertensive medications.
- *Refractory hypertension:* It is referred to as uncontrolled BP despite five or more drugs of different classes, including a diuretic.

DIAGNOSTIC EVALUATION OF RESISTANT HYPERTENSION

It comprises the following steps:
- *Step 1:* Confirm that the patient has to be evaluated for "resistant hypertension". He should have three drugs, i.e., he should have received calcium-channel blocker, RAS blocker, and a diuretic in maximal or maximally tolerated dose for an adequate period.
- *Step 2:* Exclude apparent resistant (or pseudoresistant) hypertension, by measuring BP by proper technique, by excluding white coat effect with the help of home BP monitoring or preferably by 24-hour ambulatory BP monitoring, and by ensuring that the patient is adherent to the therapy **(Table 1)**.
- *Step 3:* Carefully evaluate if the patient is consuming certain drugs which contribute to elevation of BP, the common ones being nonsteroidal anti-inflammatory drugs, steroids, oral contraceptives, cyclosporin, etc. **(Table 1)**.
- *Step 4:* Secondary hypertension should be excluded in all patients with RH **(Table 1)**. After confirming RH, assessment for secondary hypertension, which can partly be guided by medical history and physical examination, is required. Screening tests for common secondary causes should be carried out depending on the clinical suspicion **(Table 2)**.

TABLE 1: Causes of resistant hypertension.

Causes of pseudoresistant hypertension	*Use of drugs or substances that may increase BP*
• Poor adherence to treatment • White-coat phenomenon • Improper technique of BP measurement • Pseudohypertension (Osler phenomenon) • Clinician inertia (inadequate doses and inappropriate combinations of BP-lowering drugs)	• Non-steroidal anti-inflammatory drugs • Selective cyclooxygenase-2 (COX-2) inhibitors • Oral contraceptives • Glucocorticoids and mineralocorticoids • *Sympathomimetic amines*: Amphetamine, ephedrine, pseudoephedrine, phenylpropanolamine • Antidepressants • Erythropoietin-stimulating agents • Cocaine • Cyclosporine, tacrolimus • Vascular endothelial growth factor (VEGF) inhibitors
Causes of resistant hypertension	
Behavioral factors: • Overweight/obesity • Physical inactivity • Excess daily dietary sodium • Excess habitual alcohol consumption	
Often underdiagnosed conditions	
Endocrine causes	*Metabolic disease*
• Primary aldosteronism • Pheochromocytoma • Cushing syndrome	• Obstructive sleep apnea • *Renal causes:* – Renal parenchymal disease, e.g., glomerulonephritis, polycystic kidney disease, and chronic kidney disease – Renal artery stenosis • *Cardiovascular causes:* Coarctation of aorta

TABLE 2: Screening for some common causes of secondary hypertension.

Cause	*Screening test*
1. Primary aldosteronism	Aldosterone-to-renin ratio (Hypokalemia is a clue.)
2. Renovascular hypertension	Renal Doppler ultrasound abdominal CT angiography or MRI
3. Pheochromocytoma	24-hour urinary and/or plasma metanephrine and normetanephrine
4. Obstructive sleep apnea	Overnight ambulatory polysomnography
5. Renal parenchymal disease	• Serum creatinine, Na/K, eGFR, urine RE • Urinary albumin/creatinine ratio, renal ultrasound
6. Coarctation of the aorta	Echocardiogram aortic CT angiogram

(eGFR: estimated glomerular filtration rate; RE: routine examination)

Among the secondary causes of RH, primary aldosteronism is one of the most common causes, which is often underdiagnosed. Spontaneous or diuretic-induced hypokalemia are often suggestive of primary aldosteronism. Every patient with RH should be screened for primary aldosteronism with the measurement of plasma renin and aldosterone levels.[10]

Obstructive sleep apnea syndrome (OSAS) is prevalent in RH, with studies indicating that up to 60% of patients with RH have features of OSAS.[11] OSAS should be suspected in patients with hypertension and suggestive history like snoring, day-time somnolence, and in nondippers on 24-hour BP monitoring, especially if obese.

MANAGEMENT OF RESISTANT HYPERTENSION

Nonpharmacological Interventions

The lifestyle measures should be an integral and essential component of the management of RH patients. Regular exercise, reduction in salt intake, quitting smoking and alcohol abstinence contribute favorably. Weight reduction in obese patients has to be ensured. The Treating Resistant Hypertension Using Lifestyle Modification to Promote Health (TRIUMPH) study showed significant clinic and ambulatory BP reductions in patients with RH participating in a lifestyle intervention program.[12]

Pharmacological Interventions

It is reasonable to adopt a stepwise approach to institute drugs for true RH.

1. Optimization of the existing treatment. Use maximally tolerated recommended doses of the drugs. Single-pill combination is recommended to reduce the pill burden, thereby increasing drug adherence and persistence.[13]
2. Use an appropriate diuretic. If eGFR is <30 mL/min/ 1.73 m^2 chlorthalidone is the preferred diuretic. In the CLICK trial, in patients with eGFR 15–29 mL/min/ 1.73 m^2 and true RH, chlorthalidone exhibited a better response (SBP reduction of 10 mm Hg in 24 hours) as compared to placebo.[14] In end-stage renal disease (ESRD), loop diuretics need to be used.
3. Add one or more of the following drugs to intensify the antihypertensive therapy so that BP should be reduced below 140/90 mm Hg and below 130/80 mm Hg, if well tolerated.

Mineralocorticoid Receptor Antagonists

Spironolactone: Most patients with RH require the addition of non-first-line BP-lowering drugs of these, low-dose spironolactone (25–50 mg daily) should be considered first.[15-17]

In PATHWAY-2 trial, 8,335 patients of RH were randomly assigned to spironolactone, doxazosin, bisoprolol, and placebo. Spironolactone was clearly superior to placebo, doxazosin, and bisoprolol in reducing home SBP, and the treatment was well tolerated.[18] In patients with RH and type 2 diabetes mellitus, spironolactone (25–50 mg daily) reduced BP and albuminuria.[19] Spironolactone may have side effects such as breast tenderness, gynecomastia (in about 6%), and sexual impotence in men, and menstrual irregularities in women. eGFR and serum potassium should be closely monitored. Steroidal MRAs are contraindicated in patients with an eGFR < 30/min/1.73 m^2.

Eplerenone: If spironolactone is not tolerated due to antiandrogen side effects, eplerenone may be used. If eplerenone is used, higher doses (i.e., 50–200 mg daily) and twice-daily dosing may be necessary to achieve a BP-lowering effect.[20]

Finerenone: Finerenone is a potent, selective, and nonsteroidal MRA. In a post-hoc analysis, the authors concluded that in comparison to patients with true RH and chronic kidney disease treated with spironolactone with or without patiromer, finerenone was associated with a lower SBP reduction, lower risk of hyperkalemia, and lower treatment discontinuation, during 4 months of treatment.[21]

Sacubitril–Valsartan

The post-hoc analysis of PARAGON-HF trial showed that 731 heart failure with preserved ejection fraction (HFpEF) patients (15.2%) had apparent RH and 135 (2.8%) had apparent mineralocorticoid receptor antagonist (MRA)-resistant' hypertension. These patients had a poor outcome as compared to those with well-controlled hypertension. It was also noted that patients of RH on angiotensin receptor-neprilysin inhibitor (ARNI) had greater reduction in SBP at 1 and 4 months than with valsartan. With ARNI, 47.9% of RH patients had controlled BP versus 34.3% who received valsartan.[22].

Other Commonly Used Drugs

Hydralazine and minoxidil are direct vasodilators that are not favored much in RH, as they are known to cause reflex sympathetic activation, tachycardia, and fluid retention.

Adrenergic blockers: A small observational study involving 8,639 patients with RH received MRAs, β-blockers (BBs), and α-1-blockers. The results showed that there was a nonsignificant benefit in favor of BBs and α-blockers.[23] These drugs, vasodilating BBs and α-blockers, are useful additions to achieve the goal BP in patients with true RH.

Newer Drugs

Aldosterone synthase inhibitors: Baxdrostat blocks aldosterone synthase, and thus reduces synthesis of aldosterone. It is highly selective and reduces plasma aldosterone levels but not cortisol levels. In a multicenter, placebo-controlled trial, 248 patients with RH received baxdrostat or placebo for 12 weeks. In these patients with RH, baxdrostat showed dose-related significant reductions in systolic and diastolic BP, without serious adverse events and instances of adrenocortical insufficiency. Hyperkalemia seen in two patients did not recur after withdrawal and reinitiation of the drug.[7]

Endothelin receptor antagonists

Aprocitentan: Endothelin-1 is a powerful vasoconstrictor that regulates vascular tone, remodeling, and BP. Aprocitentan is a dual endothelin-1 antagonist of ET-A and ET-B receptors. The "PRECISION" a multicenter, blinded, randomized, parallel-group, phase 3 study involved 730 patients of RH. At baseline, mean office BP was 153/88 mm Hg and mean 24-hour ambulatory BP was 138/83 mm Hg. Patients were randomized to receive daily oral aprocitentan or placebo, plus three drugs comprising amlodipine, valsartan, and hydrochlorothiazide. The study concluded that in patients with RH, aprocitentan was well tolerated and superior to placebo in lowering BP at week 4 with a sustained effect at week 40. Edema, a common side effect, was seen in about 10% of patients. In March 2024, the US Food and Drug Administration (FDA) approved aprocitentan as a new drug for treating patients with RH.[6]

RNA Interference Therapeutics

Angiotensinogen, the precursor of angiotensin peptides, plays a key role in the pathogenesis of hypertension. Zilebesiran is an RNA interference therapeutic agent, has a prolonged duration of action, and interferes with angiotensinogen synthesis in liver. It is expected that zilebesiran will exert a sustained reduction of BP over a 24-hour period for months, with twice-yearly or quarterly subcutaneous administration. In a phase 1 study, 107 patients with hypertension were enrolled. Single dose of zilebesiran (≥200 mg) showed a decrease in SBP (>10 mm Hg) and diastolic blood pressure (>5 mm Hg) by 8 weeks, the reduction being consistent throughout diurnal cycle and was sustained up to 24 weeks. It showed an augmented effect when irbesartan was coadministered. There were no adverse events such as hypotension, hyperkalemia, or worsening of renal function, requiring intervention. Mild injection site reactions were reported.[15] Applicability of these results in a broader population with hypertension needs to be studied.[24]

Device-based Intervention

Catheter-based Renal Denervation (Table 3)

Sympathetic nervous system overactivity contributes to the development and progression of hypertension. Renal denervation aims to interrupt afferent and efferent sympathetic nerves in the adventitia and perivascular tissue of the renal arteries.[25]

Recent data from sham-controlled trials showed second-generation radiofrequency and ultrasound catheters demonstrated a BP-lowering efficacy in a broad range of patients, with and without concomitant BP-lowering medications, including those with RH. Long-term, nonrandomized, follow-up data from the Global Symplicity Registry,[26] Spyral HTN-ON MED pilot trial,[27] Symplicity HTN-3 trial,[27] and A Study of the Recor Medical Paradise System in Clinical Hypertension (RADIANCE-HTN) SOLO[28] trial indicate a sustained BP-lowering effect for up to 3 years.

There are no reported procedure-related serious safety signals beyond the usual risk of femoral arterial access procedures. After renal denervation, there is a 0.25–0.5% rate of renal artery stenosis/dissection requiring stenting.[29]

TABLE 3: Selection of patients for renal denervation.

Patient selection	
Likely to be useful	***Contraindications***
• Patient with uncontrolled hypertension • Patient at elevated cardiovascular risk • Patients with a preference for the procedure over adding more drugs, or who have experienced side effects from medications • Patients for whom drug adherence is challenge	• Pregnancy • Fibromuscular dysplasia • Stented renal artery • Renal artery aneurysm • Significant renal artery stenosis • Known kidney or secreting adrenal tumors
Conditions with limited data	
• Stage 1 hypertension • Isolated systolic hypertension • Stages 4 and 5 chronic kidney disease • Single kidney • Kidney transplant recipients	

WHAT DO THE GUIDELINES SAY?

The recent guidelines of European Society of Hypertension 2024 recommend the following drugs for true RH.

- In patients with RH and uncontrolled BP despite use of first-line BP lowering therapies, the addition of spironolactone to existing treatment should be considered (Class IIa).
- In patients with RH in whom spironolactone is not effective or tolerated, treatment with eplerenone instead of spironolactone, or the addition of a β-blocker if not already indicated and, next, a centrally acting an α-blocker, hydralazine, or a potassium-sparing diuretic should be considered (Class IIa).
- To reduce BP, and if performed at a medium-to-high volume center, catheter-based renal denervation may be considered for RH patients who have RH and who express a preference to undergo renal denervation (Class IIb).

Flowchart 1: An approach to the management of resistant hypertension (RH).

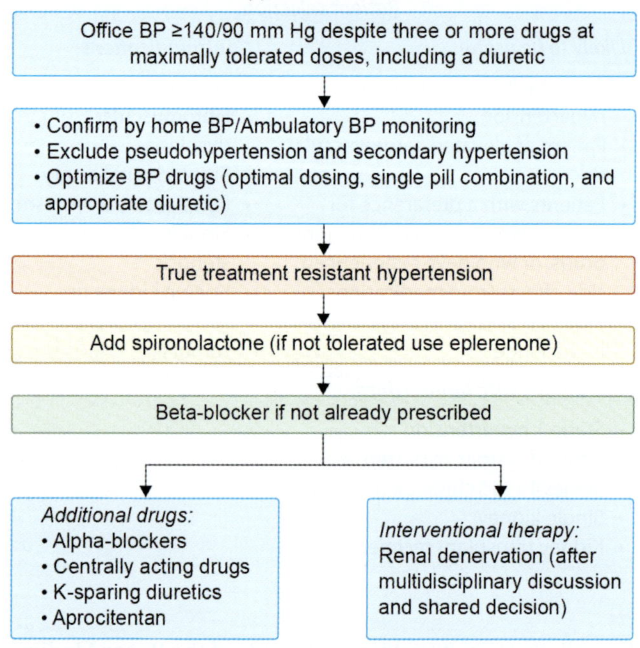

The approach to management of patients with RH is given in **Flowchart 1**.

CONCLUSION

Resistant hypertension remains a significant clinical challenge. Diagnosis of true RH should be established after a careful evaluation. Various pharmacologic and nonpharmacologic measures should be instituted judiciously. Newer drugs and devices appear promising. Artificial intelligence is likely to play a role in assisting clinicians in diagnosis and management of true RH in near future, leading to improved outcomes and better health for patients with RH.

REFERENCES

1. Whelton PK, Carey RM, Aronow WS, Casey DE Jr, Collins KJ, Dennison Himmelfarb C, et al. 2017 ACC/AHA/AAPA/ABC/ACPM/AGS/APHA/ASH/ASPC/NMA/PCNA guideline for the prevention, detection, evaluation, and management of high blood pressure in adults: executive summary: a report of the American College of Cardiology/American Heart Association Task Force on clinical practice guidelines. Hypertension. 2018;71(6):e13-115.
2. Mahapatra R, Kaliyappan A, Chinnakali P, Hanumanthappa N, Govindarajalou R, Bammigatti C. Prevalence and risk factors for resistant hypertension: cross-sectional study from a tertiary care referral hospital in South India. Cureus. 2021;13:e18779.
3. Basavanagowdappa H, Basavanagowdappa N, Ravikumar YS, Kulkarni P, Devegowda D. Magnitude of resistant hypertension and impact of aldosterone to renin ratio in resistant hypertension. J Cardiovasc Dis Res. 2016;7:133-8.
4. Ramakrishnan S, Zachariah G, Gupta K, Shivkumar Rao J, Mohanan PP, Venugopal K, et al. Prevalence of hypertension among Indian adults: results from the great India blood pressure survey. Indian Heart J. 2019;71:309-13.
5. Mancia G, Kreutz R, Brunström M, Burnier M, Grassi G, Januszewicz A, et al. 2023 ESH Guidelines for the management of arterial hypertension. The Task Force for the management of arterial hypertension of the European Society of Hypertension: Endorsed by the International Society of Hypertension (ISH) and the European Renal Association (ERA). J Hypertens. 2023;41(12):1874-2071.
6. Schlaich MP, Bellet M, Weber MA, Danaietash P, Bakris GL, Flack JM, et al. Dual endothelin antagonist aprocitentan for resistant hypertension (PRECISION): A multicentre, blinded, randomised, parallel-group, phase 3 trial. Lancet. 2022;400:1927-37.
7. Freeman MW, Halvorsen YD, Marshall W, Pater M, Isaacsohn J, Pearce C, et al. Phase 2 trial of baxdrostat for treatment-resistant hypertension. N Engl J Med. 2023;388(5):395-405.
8. Carey RM, Calhoun DA, Bakris GL, Brook RD, Daugherty SL, Dennison-Himmelfarb CR, et al. Resistant hypertension: detection, evaluation, and management: a scientific statement from the American Heart Association. Hypertension. 2018;72:e53-90.
9. McEvoy JW, McCarthy CP, Bruno RM, Brouwers S, Canavan MD, Ceconi C, et al. 2024 ESC Guidelines for the management of elevated blood pressure and hypertension. Eur Heart J. 2024;45(38):3912-4018..
10. Jaffe G, Gray Z, Krishnan G, Stedman M, Zheng Y, Han J, et al. Screening rates for primary aldosteronism in resistant hypertension: a cohort study. Hypertension. 2020;75:650-9.
11. Pedrosa RP, Drager LF, Gonzaga CC, Sousa MG, de Paula LK, Amaro AC, et al. Obstructive sleep apnea: the most common secondary cause of hypertension associated with resistant hypertension. Hypertension. 2011;58:811-7.
12. Blumenthal JA, Hinderliter AL, Smith PJ, Mabe S, Watkins LL, Craighead L, et al. Effects of lifestyle modification on patients with resistant hypertension: results of the TRIUMPH randomized clinical trial. Circulation. 2021;144:1212-26.
13. Parati G, Kjeldsen S, Coca A, Cushman WC, Wang J. Adherence to single-pill versus free-equivalent combination therapy in hypertension: a systematic review and meta-analysis. Hypertension. 2021;77:692-705.
14. Agarwal R, Sinha AD, Cramer AE, Balmes-Fenwick M, Dickinson JH, Ouyang F, et al. Chlorthalidone for

hypertension in advanced chronic kidney disease. N Engl J Med. 2021;385(27):2507-19.

15. Chen C, Zhu XY, Li D, Lin Q, Zhou K. Clinical efficacy and safety of spironolactone in patients with resistant hypertension: a systematic review and meta-analysis. Medicine (Baltimore). 2020;99:e21694.
16. Zhao D, Liu H, Dong P, Zhao J. A meta-analysis of add-on use of spironolactone in patients with resistant hypertension. Int J Cardiol. 2017;233:113-7.
17. Bazoukis G, Thomopoulos C, Tsioufis C. Effect of mineralocorticoid antagonists on blood pressure lowering: overview and meta-analysis of randomized controlled trials in hypertension. J Hypertens. 2018;36:987-94.
18. Williams B, MacDonald TM, Morant S, Webb DJ, Sever P, McInnes G, et al. Spironolactone versus placebo, bisoprolol, and doxazosin to determine the optimal treatment for drug-resistant hypertension (PATHWAY-2): A randomised, double-blind, crossover trial. Lancet. 2015;386:2059-68.
19. Oxlund CS, Henriksen JE, Tarnow L, Schousboe K, Gram J, Jacobsen IA. Low dose spironolactone reduces blood pressure in patients with resistant hypertension and type 2 diabetes mellitus: a double blind randomized clinical trial. J Hypertens. 2013;31:2094-102.
20. Tam TS, Wu MH, Masson SC, Tsang MP, Stabler SN, Kinkade A, et al. Eplerenone for hypertension. Cochrane Database Syst Rev. 2017;2:CD008996.
21. Agarwal R, Pitt B, Palmer BF, Kovesdy CP, Burgess E, Filippatos G, et al. A comparative post hoc analysis of finerenone and spironolactone in resistant hypertension in moderate-to-advanced chronic kidney disease. Clin Kidney J. 2023;16(2):293-302.
22. Jackson AM, Jhund PS, Anand IS, Düngen HD, Lam CSP, Lefkowitz MP, et al. Sacubitril-valsartan as a treatment for apparent resistant hypertension in patients with heart failure and preserved ejection fraction. Eur Heart J. 2021;42(36):3741-52.
23. Sinnott SJ, Smeeth L, Williamson E, Perel P, Nitsch D, Tomlinson LA, et al. The comparative effectiveness of fourth-line drugs in resistant hypertension: An application in electronic health record data. Pharmacoepidemiol Drug Saf. 2019;28(9):1267-77.
24. Desai AS, Webb DJ, Taubel J, Casey S, Cheng Y, Robbie GJ, et al. Zilebesiran, an RNA interference therapeutic agent for hypertension. N Engl J Med. 2023;389(3):228-38.
25. DiBona GF, Esler M. Translational medicine: the antihypertensive effect of renal denervation. Am J Physiol Regul Integr Comp Physiol. 2010;298:R245-53.
26. Mahfoud F, Böhm M, Schmieder R, Narkiewicz K, Ewen S, Ruilope L, et al. Effects of renal denervation on kidney function and long-term outcomes: 3-year follow-up from the global SYMPLICITY registry. Eur Heart J. 2019; 40:3474-82.
27. Mahfoud F, Kandzari DE, Kario K, Townsend RR, Weber MA, Schmieder RE, et al. Long-term efficacy and safety of renal denervation in the presence of antihypertensive drugs (SPYRAL HTN-ON MED): a randomised, sham-controlled trial. Lancet. 2022;399(10333):1401-10.
28. Rader F, Kirtane AJ, Wang Y, Daemen J, Lurz P, Sayer J, et al. Durability of blood pressure reduction after ultrasound renal denervation: three-year follow-up of the treatment arm of the randomised RADIANCE-HTN SOLO trial. EuroIntervention. 2022;18:e677-85.
29. Townsend RR, Walton A, Hettrick DA, Hickey GL, Weil J, Sharp ASP, et al. Review and meta-analysis of renal artery damage following percutaneous renal denervation with radiofrequency renal artery ablation. EuroIntervention. 2020;16:09-96.

Etiology and Management of Heart Failure in Pediatric Population

Anita Saxena

INTRODUCTION

Heart failure is defined as an abnormality of cardiac structure or function leading to failure of the heart to deliver oxygen at a rate commensurate with the requirements of the metabolizing tissues, despite normal filling pressures (or only at the expense of increased filling pressures). Since underlying congenital heart disease (CHD) is the cause in majority, surgical, or transcatheter treatment can resolve symptoms with normalization of structure and function of the heart. Myocardial causes such as myocarditis, genetic cardiomyopathies, and metabolic diseases have different clinical course and require long-term therapies.

ETIOLOGY

The various causes of heart failure in children are shown in **Box 1**. The underlying etiology tends to vary at different ages. The various causes which are more likely at different ages are shown in **Table 1**. Acquired heart disease is more common in toddlers or in older children. Arrhythmias are also important cause of heart failure and may be missed as neonates and infants tend to have high heart rates even normally.

BOX 1: Etiology of pediatric heart failure.

Volume overload with preserved systolic ventricular function (over circulation HF)
- *Large left to right shunt:* VSD, AVSD, and PDA
- *Admixture lesions with high PBF:* TGA, TAPVC, and truncus
- *Regurgitant lesions:* MR, AR (Rheumatic/Congenital/IE)
- Anemia, AV fistula, beriberi, etc.

Myocyte dysfunction with abnormal ventricular contractile function (pump failure)
- *Pressure overload:* Severe LVOT, RVOT obstruction, CoA
- *DCM:* Idiopathic, neuromuscular, familial, and metabolic
- *Inflammatory:* Myocarditis, Chaga's, HIV-related
- *Rhythm disturbances:* Tachycardiomyopathy and CHB
- *Ischemic:* ALCAPA
- *Postoperated:* Fontan, ToF with severe PR
- *Others:* LV noncompaction, hypocalcemia, anthracycline toxicity, and sepsis

(ALCAPA: anomalous origin of left coronary artery from pulmonary artery; AR: aortic regurgitation; AV: arteriovenous; AVSD: atrioventricular septal defect; CHB: complete heart block; HIV: human immunodeficiency viruses; IE: infective endocarditis; LV: left ventricle; LVOT: left ventricular outflow tract; MR: mitral regurgitation; PDA: patent ductus arteriosus; PR: pulmonary regurgitation; RVOT: right ventricular outflow tract; TGA: transposition of great arteries; ToF: tetralogy of Fallot; TAPVC: total anomalous pulmonary venous connection; VSD: ventricular septal defect)

TABLE 1: Causes of heart failure at different ages.

Day 1 of life/fetal	
• Asphyxia • Systemic AV fistula • Myocarditis	• Metabolic arrhythmias • Ebstein anomaly
1st week of life (after day 1)	
• Critical AS/PS HLHS • Adrenal insufficiency	• Obstructed TAPVC • Coarctation • Hypertension • TGA IVS
2nd week of life	
• Large VSD • AV septal defect • Unobstructed TAPVC	• Large PDA • Persistent truncus arteriosus
1–2 months	
• VSD, AVSD • Transposition, and malposition complexes ALCAPA	• PDA • Aortopulmonary window • Unobstructed TAPVC
2–6 months	
• Causes at 1–2 months, coarctation, critical AS/PS • *Metabolic:* Hypocalcemia/beriberi	
Older children	
• Rheumatic heart disease • Cardiomyopathies • Palliated CHD/postoperative • Corrected transposition great arteries • Severe PS/AS with ventricular dysfunction • Severe hypertension and aortoarteritis	

Note: Tachycardiomyopathy can present at any age.
Abbreviations as in Box 1. (AS: aortic stenosis; IVS: intact ventricular septum; HLHS: hypoplastic left heart syndrome; PS: pulmonary stenosis)

CLINICAL FEATURES

Common signs and symptoms of heart failure in children are given in **Table 2**. These symptoms may be mistaken for pneumonia, sepsis, bronchiolitis, acute gastroenteritis, etc. The conventional New York Heart Association (NYHA) functional classification is not applicable to children under 6 years of age. For this reason, modified Ross classification is used for assessment of younger children.[1] A comparison of two classifications is given in **Table 3**.

DIAGNOSTIC WORKUP

Chest X-ray: Cardiac silhouette, severity of cardiac enlargement, pulmonary vasculature, pulmonary artery dilatation and associated skeletal abnormalities **(Figs. 1A and B)**.

TABLE 2: Common signs and symptoms of heart failure in children.

Age	*Common signs and symptoms*	*Less common signs and symptoms*
Infant	Growth failure, persistent tachypnea, tachycardia, feeding difficulties, diaphoresis, subcostal recession, hepatomegaly	Cyanosis, palpitation, syncope, seizures, and wheeze
Toddlers	Respiratory distress, tachypnea, tachycardia, fatigue, and hepatomegaly	Poor appetite, palpitations, and edema
School age	Fatigues, effort intolerance, poor appetite, orthopnea, abdominal pain, nausea, vomiting, hepatomegaly, and raised JVP	Palpitations, chest pain, leg edema, ascites, and basal crepts
Adolescents	Effort intolerance, poor appetite, abdominal pain, orthopnea, and hepatomegaly	Nausea, vomiting, leg edema, and ascites

TABLE 3: New York Heart Association (NYHA) and modified Ross heart failure classification for children.

Class	*NYHA*	*Modified Ross*
Class I	No limitations of physical activity	No limitations or symptoms
Class II	May experience fatigue, palpitations, dyspnea, or angina during moderate exercise but not during rest	*Infants:* Mild tachypnea or diaphoresis with feeding *Older children:* Mild-to-moderate dyspnea on exertion
Class III	Symptoms with minimal exertion that interfere with normal daily activity	*Infants:* Growth failure and marked tachypnea or diaphoresis with feeding *Older children:* Marked dyspnea on exertion
Class IV	Unable to carry out any physical activity because they typically have symptoms at rest that worsen with any exertion	Symptoms at rest such as tachypnea, retractions, grunting, or diaphoresis

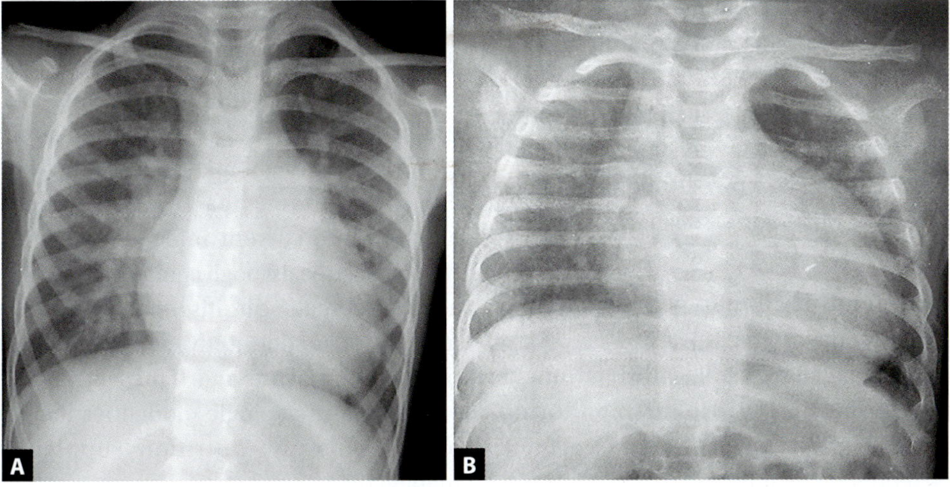

Figs. 1A and B: X-ray chest from two infants with heart failure. (A) Secondary to a large ventricular septal defect; (B) Secondary to dilated cardiomyopathy.

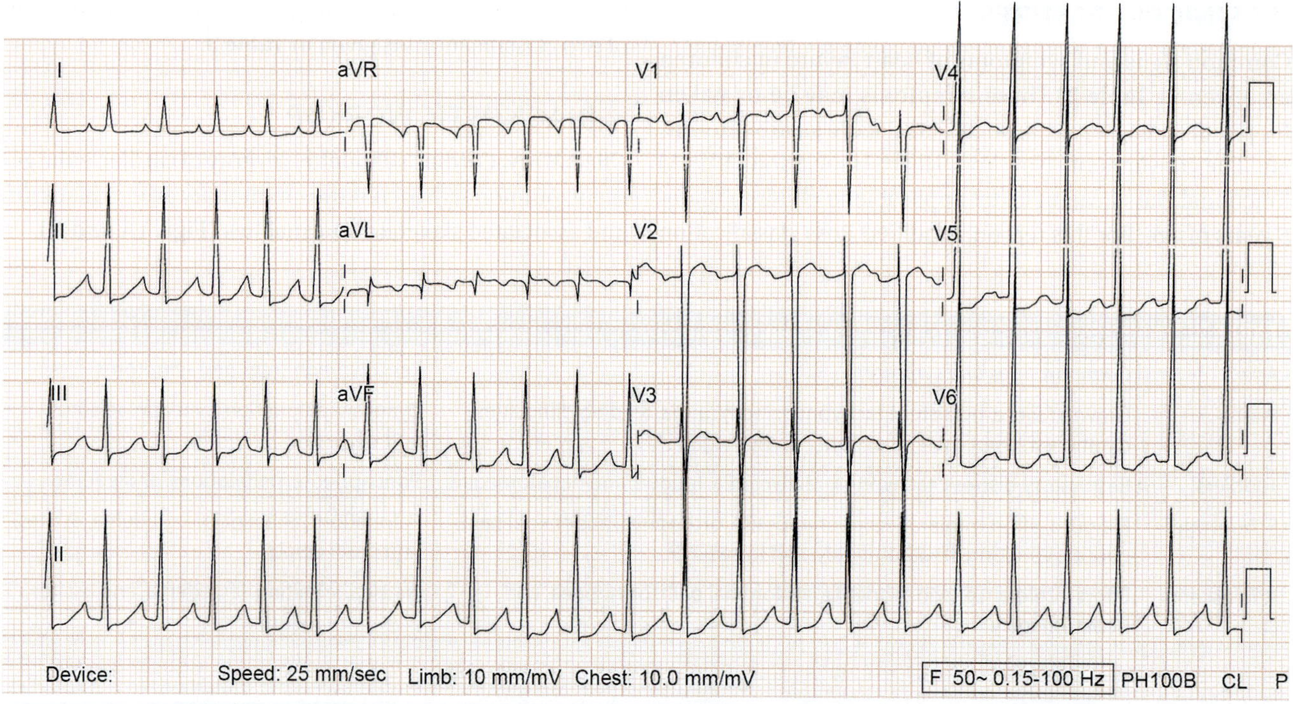

Fig. 2: ECG from a 10-year-old boy showing supraventricular tachycardia at a rate of 150 beats/min.

ECG: It can diagnose some of the treatable causes of heart failure, e.g., sustained tachyarrhythmia **(Fig. 2)**, coronary anomalies (anomalous origin of left coronary artery from pulmonary artery, ALCAPA), Pompe's disease, hypocalcemia, etc.

Echocardiography: Very important for precise diagnosis and to guide appropriate management.

Blood tests: Complete blood count, electrolytes, blood urea nitrogen (BUN), creatinine, calcium, C-reactive protein (CRP) (sepsis), liver function test, antistreptolysin titer, erythrocyte sedimentation rate (ESR) and CRP may be required in rheumatic heart disease (RHD) cases. Other blood tests which may be required in specific cases include thyroid function test, cardiac enzymes [troponin I, T, and creatine kinase-MB (CK-MB)] and in suspected cases of viral myocarditis.

Serum biomarkers: Brain-natriuretic peptide (BNP) is useful in monitoring response to therapy.

More advanced tests include cardiac MRI, CT angiography, endomyocardial biopsy, Holter monitoring, metabolic and genetic testing, viral pathogenic screening, etc. These may be required in a minority of patients.

MANAGEMENT OF HEART FAILURE

The main goals of therapy are to improve hemodynamics, functional status, and quality of life, correct the underlying cause, and reduce morbidity and mortality. In infant and children with heart failure, therapy should allow for somatic growth and development. Therapy should reduce congestion and improve cardiac output and end-organ perfusion. The preload should be optimized without causing volume depletion. In patients with dilated cardiomyopathy, treatment should halt the progression of disease through improved ventricular modeling.

Main principles of management include treatment of underlying cause, e.g., shunts, valvar stenosis/regurgitation, coronary anomaly, etc. A number of comorbidities can precipitate heart failure and these include anemia, intercurrent infections, electrolyte imbalance (hypocalcemia, hypoglycemia, and acidosis), arrhythmias, active rheumatic carditis, infective endocarditis, and drug toxicity/interaction. Active search should be made for these precipitating factors and, if present, appropriately treated.

Nonpharmacologic modalities include supplemental oxygen therapy, nutrition supplements, and fluid management.

Nutrition: In infants calorie intake of 120–150 kcal/kg/day is recommended with a fluid intake of 100 mL/kg/day. Many patients are unable to tolerate this amount of fluid. Calorie dense food, adding fat to feeds (coconut oil or medium chain triglyceride), frequent small feeding, and at times feeding through the nasogastric tube may achieve adequate calories. Nutrition supplementation is easier in older children where protein content of the diet is increased along with optimal fats and carbohydrates. Calcium and vitamin D_3 supplements should be prescribed. Unlike in adults, dietary restriction of sodium is generally not recommended in children unless there is severe edema which is not responding to diuretic therapy. Frequent weight measurement is encouraged, especially in infants, to assess their nutritional status.

Fluid management: Fluid intake is generally not restricted unless child has acute heart failure with significant lung congestion, edema despite diuretics. Fluid restriction may also be required in cases with hyponatremia.

Bed rest: This is generally not required. In fact, some amount of physical activity should be encouraged in children with controlled heart failure.

Correction of anemia: A large proportion of these children are anemic due to various reasons and these should receive iron and vitamin supplements. If Hb is <7 or 8 g/dL, blood transfusion is recommended.

PHARMACOLOGICAL THERAPY

Most of the recommendations for chronic pediatric heart failure therapy are extrapolated from adult heart failure trials. Medical therapy for heart failure has been based on the neurohormonal paradigm. Impairment of heart function activates the compensatory mechanisms. The adrenergic nervous system, the renin-angiotensin system, and the cytokine system are activated leading to secondary end-organ damages which worsen symptoms and a vicious cycle is set up leading to decompensation and heart failure. Drugs which can block this pathway can break this cycle and prevent the further deterioration and may improve symptoms of heart failure, hospitalization, and even death. **Figure 3** depicts the pharmacologic targets for treatment of heart failure.

Despite the lack of such robust data in pediatrics, drugs commonly used in adults, i.e., diuretics, ACE inhibitors, ARBs, and aldosterone antagonists (spironolactone and eplerenone) are the current standard of care therapy for chronic heart failure. The addition of a β-adrenergic receptor antagonist (β-blocker) for both asymptomatic and symptomatic patients with chronic heart failure is less well-supported in the pediatric literature, but is being increasingly used in practice. Digoxin is not routinely recommended, but it can be reserved for patients who remain symptomatic despite maximum doses of above-stated drugs and in those with tachyarrhythmia such as atrial fibrillation.

Table 4 provides the most common pediatric heart failure drugs and doses. **Table 5** provides information on

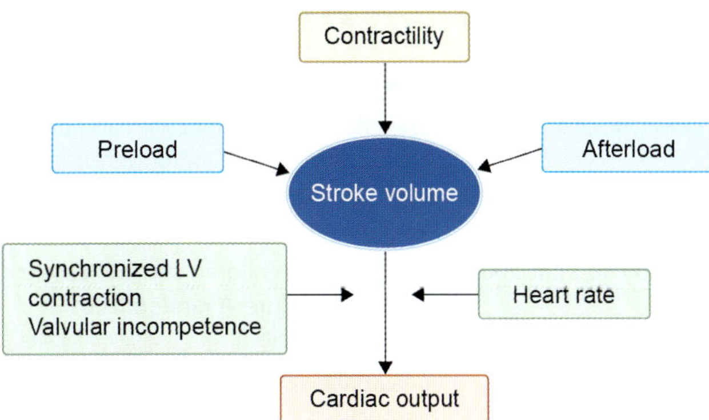

Fig. 3: Pharmacologic targets for treatment of heart failure. (LV: left ventricular)

TABLE 4: Conventional pharmacotherapy of chronic heart failure in children.

Drug	*Standard dose*
Captopril	0.5–2 mg/kg/dose, 2–5 times/day (maximum 25 mg/dose)
Enalapril	0.1–0.5 mg/kg/day (maximum 20 mg/dose)
Lisinopril	0.05–2 mg/kg/day once or twice/day
Losartan	0.5–2 mg/kg/day
Metoprolol	0.1 mg/kg two times/day (maximum 1 mg/kg dose)
Bisoprolol	0.05–0.2 mg/kg/day 1–2 times/day
Propranolol	0.2–0.5 mg/kg/dose three times/day
Carvedilol	0.025 mg/kg/dose twice a day, maximum 0.5 mg/kg/dose BD
Furosemide	0.5–2 mg/kg/day
Spironolactone	0.5–2 mg/kg/day twice a day, maximum 200 mg/day
Hydrochlorothiazide	0.5–1 mg/kg/day
Digoxin	3 to 5 μg/kg dose twice a day

TABLE 5: Randomized controlled trials for pediatric heart failure.

Author/year	*Title*	*Key findings*
Lewis AB, et al. 1993[2]	The effect of treatment with angiotensin-converting enzyme inhibitors on survival of pediatric patients with dilated cardiomyopathy	*n* = 80; (26 = ACEi, 54 = digoxin plus diuretics). 1-year and 2-year survival with ACEi was better than digoxin group
Shaddy RE, et al. 2007[3]	Carvedilol for children and adolescent with heart failure: A randomized controlled trial	*n* = 161; No significant difference between treatment versus placebo group in primary endpoint (clinical improvement) or secondary endpoint (ventricular function or serum BNP)
Hsu DT, et al. 2010[4]	Enalapril in infants with single ventricle	*n* = 230; No improvement in somatic growth, ventricular function, heart failure severity. Routine use of enalapril in SV CHD patients with RV is not recommended as systemic ventricle
Bonnet D, et al. 2017[5]	Ivabradine in children with dilated cardiomyopathy and symptomatic chronic heart failure	*n* = 116; Primary endpoint reached by 51 out of 73 children taking ivabradine (70%); ivabradine safely reduced the resting heart rate of children with chronic HF and dilated cardiomyopathy; improvement in ejection fraction, functional class, and NT-pro-BNP was noted
Shaddy R, et al. 2024[6]	Sacubitril/Valsartan in pediatric heart failure (PANORAMA-HF): A randomized, multicenter, double-blind trial	*n* = 375, randomized to sacubitril/valsartan (*n* = 187) or enalapril (*n* = 188). At week 52, clinically meaningful reductions observed in both treatment arms in NYHA/Ross, PGIS, Patient Global Impression of Change, and NT-pro-BNP, without significant differences between groups. Adverse events were similar. Safety profile was acceptable

(ACEi: angiotensin-converting enzyme inhibitor; BNP: brain natriuretic peptide; CHD: congenital heart disease; HF: heart failure; SV: single ventricle)

five randomized clinical trials on drugs, with key findings, which have been performed in children with heart failure till date.[2-6]

NEW DRUGS FOR HEART FAILURE

Several children, especially those with reduced left ventricular function, continue to deteriorate despite therapy. A number of new drugs have been added to the armamentarium of heart failure therapy for adults, but evidence for pediatric age group is lacking. These may be useful in cases with progressive disease. Some of the newer drugs are discussed below.

Ivabradine

Ivabradine is an inhibitor of the funny channels located in the sinoatrial node that slows the rate of phase-4 depolarization, thereby reducing the heart rate. Ivabradine has been well-studied in adult population with heart failure, in the SHIFT and BEAUTIFUL trials.[7] A randomized, double-blind, placebo-controlled, phase II/III clinical trial of children with stable HF reported safety of ivabradine in children.[5] The trial showed reduction of the resting heart rate and an increase in the left ventricular ejection fraction. Following this trial, ivabradine has been approved by the Food and Drug Administration (FDA) in the year 2019 for treatment in children with symptomatic heart failure >6 months of age. The recommended dose is 0.02–0.05 mg/kg twice a day for children under 40 kg and 2.5 mg twice a day for children >40 kg.

Sacubitril-Valsartan

This drug is a combination of a neprilysin inhibitor with an angiotensin II receptor antagonist. A large trail conducted in adults, PARDIGM-HF (2009–2014), showed a reduction of 3.7% in the primary endpoint of death from cardiovascular causes or hospitalization for heart failure and a 3.2% reduction in overall mortality.[8] Recently, the results of PANORAMA-HF study conducted in pediatric patients have been published. 375 children were randomized to sacubitril/valsartan or enalapril. At week 52, clinically meaningful reductions were observed in both treatment arms in NYHA/Ross, Patient

Global Impression of Change, and NT-pro-BNP, without significant differences between groups. Adverse events were also similar. The safety profile of sacubitril/valsartan was acceptable.[6] Based on a preliminary 12-week findings from PANORAMA-HF, US-FDA approved sacubitril/valsartan in ≥1-year-old pediatric patients with HF secondary to systemic left ventricular systolic dysfunction. The starting dose for children <40 kg is 1.6 mg/kg of the combined amount of both valsartan and sacubitril. The dose is titrated upward every 2 weeks from 2.3 mg/kg up to a maximum dose of 3.1 mg/kg based on tolerance.

Sodium-Glucose Co-transporter-2 Inhibitors

Drugs included under this group are canagliflozin, dapagliflozin, and empagliflozin. These were initially developed for patients with diabetes mellitus. The mechanism of action is to inhibit the sodium/glucose cotransporter situated in the kidney, and to promote glucose excretion and improve sugar control in a diabetic patient. However, the trial also showed a reduction in heart failure-related events in these patients and this led to further trials, specifically addressing the issue of improvement in heart failure and reducing other cardiovascular events. In a large trial, named EMPEROR-Reduced confirmed the finding of improved outcome in heart failure patients, seen as early as within 12 weeks of therapy.[9] Similar results have been seen with canagliflozin in the CHIEF-HF trial where 476 adults with heart failure were randomized.[10] The first description of use of sodium-glucose co-transporter-2 (SGL-T2) inhibitor use in pediatric age group was reported in the year 2021.[11] Around 38 patents were included and dapagliflozin was added to the heart failure therapy regimen. The drug was well-tolerated and there were no reports of experiencing hypovolemia or hypoglycemia. However, six patients reported a symptomatic urinary tract infection requiring antibiotic treatment. The left ventricular function improved in 26 patients who had dysfunction initially. The ejection fraction of left ventricle significantly improved from 32 to 37.2%. More data in pediatric heart failure is required before recommending this drug for heart failure. The dose in pediatric age group is 0.1–0.2 mg/kg once daily with a maximum of 10 mg.

Vericiguat

Vericiguat is a novel oral soluble guanylate cyclase stimulator, an enzyme responsible for the production of nitrogen monoxide (NO). This enzyme plays a role in arteriolar vasodilation and inhibits fibrosis. It is also known to reduce mechanical and oxidative vascular stress. In a recent trial in adult patients (VICTORIA) with chronic symptomatic heart failure, this drug reduced the risk of cardiovascular death, all-cause death, and hospitalization due to heart failure.[12] No data are currently available for children. A clinical trial about the safety, efficacy, and pharmacokinetics of vericiguat in pediatric heart failure is being initiated. No information on pediatric dosing is available.

Omecamtiv Mecarbil

This drug is the first small molecule which is an activator of cardiac myosin. It improves myocardial function by directly augmenting cardiac sarcomere function and increases the systolic function of ventricle in patients with reduced ejection fraction. A trial in adult patients (GALACTIC-HF trial) demonstrated that "omecamtiv mecarbil" significantly decreased the primary endpoint (time-to-first heart failure event or death due to cardiovascular causes), more so in the group of patients with ejection fraction of <22%. Overall, there was a 16% reduction in the time-to-first heart failure event or cardiovascular death (HR: 0.84; 95% CI: 0.77–0.92; $p = 0.0003$).[13] However, no data is currently available for children and there is no ongoing trial. No information on pediatric dosing is available.

ADVANCED NONPHARMACOLOGIC THERAPY

Device therapy: Device therapy in heart failure includes pacemaker therapy, cardiac resynchronization therapy (CRT), and mechanical circulatory support.

Cardiac resynchronization therapy: CRT may be useful in adolescents and young adults as per 2013 EHRA and AEPC guidelines. The QRS duration should be >98th percentile for age and patient should have a systemic left ventricle, complete left bundle branch block pattern. A specific evaluation for mechanical dyssynchrony should be made before CRT is offered.[14]

Implantable cardioverter defibrillator (ICD): This device is implanted for patients with a history of cardiac arrest or symptomatic sustained ventricular tachycardia in association with CHD. Some pediatric patients with a history of severe left ventricular dysfunction (LVEF < 30%) with or without documented ventricular arrhythmias may benefit from a combination of CRT and ICD, so called defibrillator-associated cardiac resynchronization therapy (CRT-D).

Extracorporeal membrane oxygenation (ECMO) and ventricular assist device (VAD): This approach has been widely used in acute settings of cardiopulmonary arrest, especially when the cause of heart failure is likely to be reversible, such as fulminant myocarditis. ECMO or a VAD are used as a temporizing measure allowing ventricular function to recover. ECMO is also often used in emergency during perioperative period if there is ventricular pump failure. Patients who require a long-term support as a bridge to cardiac transplantation, VAD is increasingly being used. VAD devices can offer isolated left or right ventricular support or biventricular circuit support. However, VADs have high complication rates including thrombosis, bleeding, infections, and more so in infants with a body weight of <10 kg.

CARDIAC TRANSPLANTATION

The most common indication is cardiomyopathy, other indication is uncorrectable CHD, such as hypoplastic left heart syndrome or failed Fontan due to ventricular dysfunction. Approximately 600–700 pediatric heart transplantation procedures are performed worldwide each year. Complications include systemic viral infections (cytomegalovirus, Epstein–Barr virus, and adenovirus), acute rejection, vasculopathy with graft failure, and hypertension. Malignancy-like lymphoproliferative disorders are other major complications of cardiac transplantation in children. Survival is >70% at 5 years, a large number of children survive for over 20 years. Major limitation is the inadequate donor supply.

PULMONARY ARTERY BANDING

Recently, it has been used in selected infants or toddlers with dilated cardiomyopathy, as a bridge-to-recovery or to more definitive therapy such as cardiac transplantation. The mechanism of action of pulmonary artery band in improving left ventricular function has been described by Schranz et al.[15] Band results in right ventricular pressure overload, which straightens the interventricular septum, thereby improving the filling of left ventricle, its end-diastolic volume, and pressure. This improves left ventricular ejection fraction. A multicenter survey reported 70 patients from 15 centers in 11 countries.[16] Approximately 60% of the patients showed a clinical improvement after pulmonary artery banding, and 48% showed a functional recovery in 1 year. Right ventricular function must be normal for this modality of pulmonary artery banding to be of use. The best response is obtained in children <1 year, normal pulmonary artery pressure, and normal or mild left atrial dilatation.

CONCLUSION

Heart failure in children is a complex syndrome resulting from diverse etiologies and varied clinical presentation. Correction of underlying heart disease can reverse heart failure in a large number of cases. Treatment has evolved, however, most of pharmacotherapy for heart failure in children is extrapolated from data in adults. In future, pediatric specific data should be developed with the goal of identifying individualized management regimen.

REFERENCES

1. Ross RD. The Ross classification for heart failure in children after 25 years: a review and an age-stratified revision. Pediatr Cardiol. 2012;33:1295-300.
2. Lewis, AB, Chabot M. The effect of treatment with angiotensin-converting enzyme inhibitors on survival of pediatric patients with dilated cardiomyopathy. Pediatr Cardiol. 1993;14:9-12.
3. Shaddy RE, Boucek MM, Hsu DT, Boucek RJ, Canter CE, Mahony L, et al. Carvedilol for children and adolescent with heart failure: A randomized controlled trial. J Am Med Assoc. 2007;298:1171-9.
4. Hsu DT, Mahony L, Sleeper LA. Enalapril in infants with single ventricle. Circulation. 2010;122:333-40.
5. Bonnet D, Berger F, Jokinen E, Kantor PF, Daubeney PEF. Ivabradine in Children with Dilated Cardiomyopathy and Symptomatic Chronic Heart Failure. J Am Coll Cardiol. 2017;70:1262-72.
6. Shaddy R, Burch M, Kantor PF, Solar-Yohay S, Garito T, Zhang S, et al. Sacubitril/Valsartan in Pediatric Heart Failure (PANORAMA-HF): A Randomized, Multicenter, Double-Blind Trial. Circulation. 2024;150:1756-66.
7. Fox K, Komajda M, Ford I, Robertson M, Böhm M, Borer JS, et al. Effect of ivabradine in patients with left-ventricular systolic dysfunction: A pooled analysis of individual patient data from the BEAUTIFUL and SHIFT trials. Eur Heart J. 2013;34:2263-70.
8. McMurray JJ, Packer M, Desai AS, Gong J, Lefkowitz MP, Rizkala AR, et al. Angiotensin–Neprilysin Inhibition versus Enalapril in Heart Failure. N Engl J Med. 2014;11:993-1004.
9. Packer M, Butler J, Zannad F, Filippatos G, Ferreira JP, Pocock SJ, et al. Effect of Empagliflozin on Worsening Heart Failure Events in Patients with Heart Failure and Preserved Ejection Fraction: EMPEROR-Preserved Trial. Circulation. 2021;144:1284-94.

10. Spertus JA, Birmingham MC, Nassif M, Damaraju CV, Abbate A, Butler J, et al. The SGLT2 inhibitor canagliflozin in heart failure: The CHIEF-HF remote, patient-centered randomized trial. Nat Med. 2022;28:809-13.
11. Newland DM, Hong BJ, Albers EL, Friedland-Little JM, Kemna MS, Law YM. Safety of Dapagliflozin in Children with Heart Failure. J Heart Lung Transplant. 2021;40:S280.
12. Armstrong PW, Pieske B, Anstrom KJ, Ezekowitz J, Hernandez AF, Butler J, et al. Vericiguat in Patients with Heart Failure and Reduced Ejection Fraction. N Engl J Med. 2020;382:1883-93.
13. Teerlink JR, Diaz R, Felker GM, McMurray JJV, Metra M, Solomon SD, et al. Effect of Ejection Fraction on Clinical Outcomes in Patients Treated with Omecamtiv Mecarbil in GALACTIC-HF. J Am Coll Cardiol. 2021;78:97-108.
14. Brugada J, Blom N, Sarquella-Brugada G, Blomstrom-Lundqvist C, Deanfield J, Janousek J, et al. EHRA/AEPC CONSENSUS STATEMENT Pharmacological and non-pharmacological therapy for arrhythmias in the pediatric population: EHRA and AEPC-Arrhythmia Working Group joint consensus statement. Europace. 2013;15:1337-82.
15. Schranz D, Rupp S, Müller M, Schmidt D, Bauer A, Valeske K, et al. Pulmonary artery banding in infants and young children with left ventricular dilated cardiomyopathy: A novel therapeutic strategy before heart transplantation. J Heart Lung Transplant. 2013;32:475-81.
16. Schranz D, Akintuerk H, Bailey L. Pulmonary Artery Banding for Functional Regeneration of End-Stage Dilated Cardiomyopathy in Young Children: World Network Report. Circulation. 2018;137:1410-2.

Implication of Rapid Initiation of Quadruple Therapy in Heart Failure

Abraham Oomman, Narra Lavanya

INTRODUCTION

Heart failure (HF) is a complex clinical syndrome presenting with signs and symptoms of underlying cardiac abnormality with evidence of systemic and/or pulmonary congestion and evidence of elevated filling pressures on laboratory testing or objective findings. HF is one of the leading causes of morbidity and mortality worldwide, with fatality rates equal to or even worse than some of the malignancies. HF with reduced ejection fraction (HFrEF) with EF <40% comprises >50% of the HF patients.

The management of HFrEF has come a long way from only diuretics and digoxin to the current guideline-directed medical therapy (GDMT) comprising the four pillars of HF therapy. These include the renin-angiotensin-aldosterone inhibitors (RAASi); the angiotensin converting enzyme inhibitors (ACEi), angiotensin receptor blockers (ARB) or angiotensin receptor neprolysin inhibitor (ARNI), β-blockers (BB), mineralocorticoid receptor antagonists (MRA), and the sodium-glucose cotransportor-2 (SGLT-2) inhibitors. Despite evidence that use of GDMT instead of conventional therapy with ACEi/ARB, and BB could further reduced the cardiovascular (CV) mortality by 50% in HFrEF,[1] the initiation and uptitration of these drugs has not been satisfactory. The discussion on how and when to initiate and uptitrate these drugs has been a topic of much debate. In this review we would like to describe the rapid initiation of quadruple therapy and the challenges associated with it.

DESCRIPTION

Once the diagnosis of HF is made, the mortality is roughly 50% in the next 5 years. Even though HF carries a dismal prognosis similar to some cancers, the aggressive treatment protocols followed in cancer treatment are not yet implemented in HF care. Despite guideline recommendations and availability of GDMT which has been proven to reduce HF morbidity and mortality, there is significant inertia in initiating and titrating HF medications.[2]

BENEFITS OF GUIDELINE-DIRECTED MEDICAL THERAPY

The goal of GDMT is to reduce the mortality, re-hospitalization rates, and improve the functional status and quality of life.[3] Triple therapy with ACEi/ARB, BB, and the MRA is recommended by guidelines as cornerstone therapies for HFrEF patients, unless they are contraindicated or not tolerated. These drugs should be titrated to the doses used in trials or to maximum tolerated doses. In patients symptomatic on this triad, ACEi/ARB may be replaced by an ARNI; however, ARNI may still be considered as first-line instead of ACEi. The SGLT2i in addition to the triple therapy further reduces CV death and hospitalization in HFrEF patients irrespective of their diabetic status.[4]

The use of quadruple therapy has been shown to reduce the CV morality by 73% over 2 years.[5] The 2022 ACC guidelines have described a 16–17% relative risk reduction in mortality with the use of ACEi/ARB/ARNI, 34% with BBs, 30% with MRA and 17% with SGLT2i.[6] Despite these benefits, a significant number of HFrEF patients are either not on quadruple therapy or do not receive the target doses of GDMT.

ELIGIBILITY FOR GUIDELINE-DIRECTED MEDICAL THERAPY

Utilizing the Get With The Guidelines–Heart Failure registry, a retrospective cohort study was done among 33,000 patients hospitalized for newly diagnosed HFrEF to characterize the degree to which these patients are eligible for quadruple medical therapy and their associated benefits. Although four out of five patients were eligible for in-hospital initiation of GDMT, only 15.3% were prescribed quadruple therapy and 41.5% were prescribed triple therapy. If the full potential of the trial data is realized with rapid in-hospital initiation of quadruple medical therapy for newly diagnosed HFrEF, one death can be prevented by treating four patients over a period of 1 year compared to those with no treatment.[7]

The change the management of patients with heart failure (CHAMP-HF) registry studied 3,518 chronic HFrEF patients on at least one medication for HF. Although eligible for HF therapy, ACEI/ARB/ARNI was not prescribed to 27% of the patients, 33% were not prescribed BB and 67% were not prescribed the MRA therapy. Even in those prescribed GDMT it was at a much lower doses and <25% received all three medications simultaneously, showing the glaring disparity in implementation of HF therapy even in eligible patients.[8]

GAPS IN IMPLEMENTING GUIDELINE-DIRECTED MEDICAL THERAPY

The probable reasons for the inertia in implementing GDMT is probably due to two opposing misconceptions that is: the patient is "too sick" for the treatment of that the patient is "too stable" for therapy. The most common reasons for not initiating or uptitrating GDMT are the fear of side effects including hypotension, hyperkalemia and worsening renal failure; whereas frailty and recent hospitalization for HF especially in those patients who were on inotropes or in those with prolonged hospital stay are the reasons to not initiate GDMT in the hospital setting.[9]

Meanwhile, some patients often get misclassified as stable HF as they are doing well on one or two pillars of GDMT. In such cases, physician inertia gets in the way of implementing all four pillars under the false notion that the patient is stable and may not need the entire treatment. It has to be emphasized that HF is a chronic condition which has certain stable periods but ultimately the prognosis is poor and delay in initiating and uptitrating the therapy in early stages will have worse outcomes in the future in which case we would have already missed the bus.[9]

In an observational study by Saverese et al., among 68,172 new users of HF drugs across Sweden, UK, and US, it was found that the GDMT doses at the initiation of therapy followed the guideline recommendations. The achievement of target dose was limited (10–30%) and drug discontinuation was common (24–55%) over 12 months from the initiation of therapy. Suboptimal dosing was more common in elderly and in those with CKD. Importantly, even while optimization of HF medical therapy was ongoing, patients were at high risk of heart failure hospitalization (HHF) and death, emphasizing the need for rapid uptitration and reaching target/tolerable doses of GDMT.[10]

SEQUENTIAL INITIATION OF GUIDELINE-DIRECTED MEDICAL THERAPY

Traditionally, once the diagnosis of HFrEF has been made, the initiation of GDMT is often a serial and selective process wherein one medication is often initiated or titrated at a time. Patients were initially started on a combination of ACEi/ARB and a BB and slowly titrated to maximum tolerated doses over weeks. Those patients who were still symptomatic then became eligible for the addition of an MRA which was again slowly titrated to maximum tolerated doses. Only in those patients where symptoms persisted despite the maximum doses triple therapy, ACEi/ARB was replaced with ARNI.[11]

Considering the safety profile, the then guidelines suggested slow initiation and uptitration of GDMT and it would approximately take 4–6 weeks for each step of this algorithm to be implemented and assessed thereafter taking months to reach maximum tolerated doses in the background of progressing pathophysiology of HF. In cases where the patient was stable/asymptomatic the guidelines would indicate limiting treatment to the drugs initiated and the patient might never receive the full treatment. This approach considerably slows down the process of GDMT uptitration and by the time quadruple therapy is implemented at target or maximally tolerated doses, 6–12 months may be lost. Even eligible patients might not receive optimal GDMT in long-term follow-up period.[12]

RAPID INITIATION OF GUIDELINE-DIRECTED MEDICAL THERAPY

In a meta-analysis by Tromp et al., triple therapy with ACEi/ARB, MRA, and BB reduced all-cause mortality by 48%, CV mortality and HF hospitalization by 42% and CV mortality by 53%. When SGLT2i was added to this combination, the risk reduction of the same outcomes was 61, 64, and 67% each showing the dramatic difference between outcomes of triple and quadruple therapy. Thus current guidelines recommend the rapid initiation of quadruple therapy for all eligible patients with HFrEF.[13]

The safety, tolerability, and efficacy of uptitration of guideline-directed medical therapies for acute heart failure (STRONG-HF) was a multinational, open-labeled randomized control trial (RCT) which compared usual care versus high-intensity care with rapid uptitration of GDMT over 180 days in de novo acute HF patients. The high-intensity care group was monitored closely at 1, 2, 3, and 6 weeks and assessed clinically and biochemically. The high-intensity care group patients achieved higher doses of the GDMT with greater reduction in New York Heart Association (NYHA) class, weight, blood pressure, and NT-proBNP levels and lower HF readmissions and all-cause death. The study was prematurely terminated due to a greater than expected difference in the primary endpoint favoring the high-intensity care group.[14]

Based on the STRONG-HF data, the 2023 focused update of the 2021 European Society of Cardiology guidelines for the diagnosis and treatment of acute and chronic HF gave a class I level B recommendation for an intensive strategy of initiation and rapid uptitration of evidence-based treatment before discharge. This was to be followed up with frequent and careful follow-up visits in the first 6 weeks following an HF hospitalization to reduce the risk of rehospitalization or death. Even though SGLT2i were not approved and not widely used (<10%) in the STRONG-HF trial, latest guidelines recommend their use as a class I recommendation.[15]

CONCLUSION

There has tremendous progress in the treatment of HF in the recent years improving quality of life (QOL) and reducing morbidity and mortality. Sadly, implementation of these therapies had been far from optimal either due to unfounded fears regarding adverse effects or physician inertia. Latest clinical trials have given profound evidence that rapid implementation of quadruple therapy is not only effective and safe but very much required to get the maximum benefits of GDMT keeping in mind the patients' tolerance.

For successful implementation of GDMT, the patients should have close follow-up of after initiation of treatment to evaluate tolerance, identify adverse effects and to uptitrate GDMT to maximal doses. For most patients, starting quadruple therapy at half-doses with uptitration to full doses in 2 weeks seems reasonable. For patients in whom tolerance or adverse events are a concern initiating two medications first, with early follow-up for reassessment of tolerance and initiation of the rest of the treatment within a month might be a reasonable option. Close follow-up and careful uptitration of GDMT might help us to offer a faster and much needed therapy to our HF patients.

REFERENCES

1. Vaduganathan M, Claggett BL, Jhund PS, Cunningham JW, Pedro Ferreira J, Zannad F, et al. Estimating lifetime benefits of comprehensive disease-modifying pharmacological therapies in patients with heart failure with reduced ejection fraction: a comparative analysis of three randomised controlled trials. Lancet. 2020;396(10244):121-8.
2. Taylor CJ, Ordóñez-Mena JM, Roalfe AK, Lay-Flurrie S, Jones NR, Marshall T, et al. Trends in survival after a diagnosis of heart failure in the United Kingdom 2000-2017: population-based cohort study. BMJ. 2019;364:l223.
3. Ambrosy AP, Fonarow GC, Butler J, Chioncel O, Greene SJ, Vaduganathan M, et al. The global health and economic burden of hospitalizations for heart failure: lessons learned from hospitalized heart failure registries. J Am Coll Cardiol. 2014;63(12):1123-33.
4. McDonagh TA, Metra M, Adamo M, Gardner RS, Baumbach A, Böhm M, et al. 2021 ESC Guidelines for the diagnosis and treatment of acute and chronic heart failure: Developed by the Task Force for the diagnosis and treatment of acute and chronic heart failure of the European Society of Cardiology (ESC) With the special contribution of the Heart Failure Association (HFA) of the ESC. Eur Heart J. 2021;42(36):3599-726.
5. Bassi NS, Ziaeian B, Yancy CW, Fonarow GC. Association of optimal implementation of sodium-glucose cotransporter 2 inhibitor therapy with outcome for patients with heart failure. JAMA Cardiol. 2020;5(8):948-51.
6. Heidenreich PA, Bozkurt B, Aguilar D, Allen LA, Byun JJ, Colvin MM, et al. 2022 AHA/ACC/HFSA Guideline for the Management of Heart Failure: A Report of the American College of Cardiology/American Heart Association Joint Committee on Clinical Practice Guidelines. Circulation. 2022;145(18):e895-e1032.
7. Greene SJ, Ayodele I, Pierce JB, Khan MS, Lewsey SC, Yancy CW, et al. Eligibility and projected benefits of rapid initiation of quadruple therapy for newly diagnosed heart failure. JACC Heart Fail. 2024;12(8):1365-77.
8. Greene SJ, Butler J, Albert NM, DeVore AD, Sharma PP, Duffy CI, et al. Medical therapy for heart failure with reduced ejection fraction: The CHAMP-HF registry. J Am Coll Cardiol. 2018;72(4):351-66.
9. Carrizales-Sepúlveda EF, Ordaz-Farías A, Vargas-Mendoza JA, Vera-Pineda R, Flores-Ramírez R. Initiation and up-titration of guideline-directed medical therapy for patients with heart failure: Better, Faster, Stronger! Card Fail Rev. 2024;10:e03.

10. Savarese G, Bodegard J, Norhammar A, Sartipy P, Thuresson M, Cowie MR, et al. Heart failure drug titration, discontinuation, mortality and heart failure hospitalization risk: a multinational observational study (US, UK and Sweden). Eur J Heart Fail. 2021;23(9):1499-511.
11. Ponikowski P, Voors AA, Anker SD, Bueno H, Cleland JG, Coats AJ, et al. 2016 ESC Guidelines for the diagnosis and treatment of acute and chronic heart failure: The Task Force for the diagnosis and treatment of acute and chronic heart failure of the European Society of Cardiology (ESC). Developed with the special contribution of the Heart Failure Association (HFA) of the ESC. Eur J Heart Fail. 2016;18(8):891-975.
12. Khan MS, Butler J, Greene SJ. Simultaneous or rapid sequence initiation of medical therapies for heart failure: seeking to avoid the case of 'too little, too late.' Eur J Heart Fail. 2021;23(9):1514-7.
13. Tromp J, Ouwerkerk W, van Veldhuisen DJ, Hillege HL, Richards AM, van der Meer P, et al. A systematic review and network meta-analysis of pharmacological treatment of heart failure with reduced ejection fraction. JACC Heart Fail. 2022;10(2):73-84.
14. Mebazaa A, Davison B, Chioncel O, Cohen-Solal A, Diaz R, Filippatos G, et al. Safety, tolerability and efficacy of up-titration of guideline-directed medical therapies for acute heart failure (STRONG-HF): a multinational, open-label, randomised, trial. Lancet. 2022;400(10367):1938-52.
15. McDonagh TA, Metra M, Adamo M, Gardner RS, Baumbach A, Böhm M, et al. 2023 Focused Update of the 2021 ESC Guidelines for the diagnosis and treatment of acute and chronic heart failure: Developed by the task force for the diagnosis and treatment of acute and chronic heart failure of the European Society of Cardiology (ESC) with the special contribution of the Heart Failure Association (HFA) of the ESC. Eur Heart J. 2023;44(37):3627-39.

Sodium-glucose Cotransporter 2 Inhibitors in Acute Decompensated Heart Failure

AK Pancholia

INTRODUCTION

Heart failure (HF) is a global pandemic that is estimated to affect >64 million people, representing 1–3% of adult human population. HF is a progressive disease, characterized by variable durations of symptomatic stability, often punctuated by episodes of worsening despite continued therapy. Patients with heart failure experience frequent hospitalizations. The 5-year mortality rate in heart failure remains >50%, which is significantly affected by outpatient worsening episodes as well as recurrent hospitalizations.

In the clinical trajectory of heart failure, worsening heart failure (WHF) is defined as worsening signs and symptoms in a patient with chronic HF after a period of clinical stability that requires escalation of therapy. This definition includes the need for a hospitalization for HF, or treatment of HF in the emergency department (ED), or receipt of intravenous diuretic therapy in the outpatient setting.[1-5]

INDIAN SCENARIO

The critical impact of WHF is well recognized. The large HF registries of India suggest that 1 out of every 3 patients are rehospitalized + within 1 year of initial hospitalization for HF.[6] Further, 1 event of re-hospitalization occurs for every 8 patients, within 90 days of initial hospital discharge.[7] A particular vulnerable phase is recognized within 30–90 days of hospital discharge, after the initial hospitalization for HF.[8] This period is associated with increased risk of rehospitalization and death. This high risk during the vulnerable period stems from worsening of hemodynamics due to subclinical congestion, with progressive increase in left ventricular filling pressures. Even modest increases in filling pressures can potentially result in clinical deterioration, due to the poor hemodynamic reserve during this period. This leads to persistent hemodynamic congestion, and multiorgan

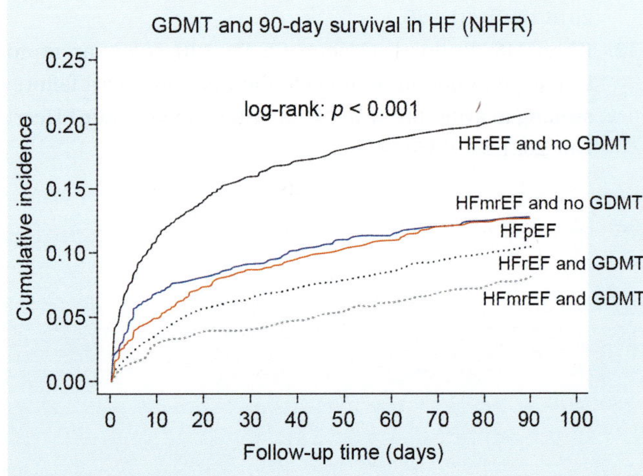

Fig. 1: National Heart Failure Registry (NHFR) of India suggests high mortality risk in 90-days post initial hospitalization, by the use of guideline-directed medical therapy (GDMT).[9]

injury. The worsening of signs and symptoms due to congestion predisposes to subsequent rehospitalizations and also death during this vulnerable phase. **Figure 1** represents evidence from National Heart Failure Registry (NHFR), on 90-day outcomes in patients with acute HF, from 53 tertiary care hospitals of India.[9]

In the NHFR, 14.2% of patients died and 8.4% of patients required a rehospitalization, during the 90-day vulnerable period after initial hospitalization. The 90-day survival rate was significantly improved in patients of heart failure with reduced (HFrEF) or mildly reduced (HFmrEF) ejection fraction, who had received GDMT of a β-blocker, renin-angiotensin system inhibitor, and aldosterone antagonist. There was no defined GDMT for patients with heart failure and preserved ejection fraction (HFpEF) in the NHFR. The use of sodium-glucose cotransporter-2 inhibitor (SGLT2-i) was not proven and indicated for treatment of HF, at the time of this initial NHFR analysis.[9]

OPTIMIZING MANAGEMENT OF ADHF OR WHF: EVIDENCE AND PLACE OF SGLT2 INHIBITION

Despite therapeutic advances in chronic heart failure (CHF), WHF has a dismal prognosis owing to multiple factors that may prohibit optimization of care. Loop diuretics are the mainstay of therapy for controlling signs and symptoms in WHF, but have a negative impact on renal function as well as potential neurohormonal imbalance.[10-12]

Over the past few years, the sodium-glucose cotransporter 2 inhibitors (SGLT2-i) have demonstrated compelling evidence of improving clinical outcomes in patients with chronic HF, across the categories of left-ventricular ejection fraction.[13] These SGLT2-i agents have also been shown to consistently reduce the risk of cardiovascular death or hospitalization for HF, in patients with type-2 diabetes mellitus and high cardiovascular risk, as well as in patients with chronic kidney disease.[14,15] The recent guidelines from the European Society of Cardiology (ESC) represent a class I recommendation supported by level A evidence, for the SGLT2-i agents with proven evidence of reducing the risk of heart-failure hospitalizations or cardiovascular death, as foundational therapies in patients of HFrEF, HFmrEF, as well as HFpEF.[16,17] **Figure 2** summarizes these evidence-based recommendations for SGLT2-i agents in heart-failure.

The major trials of SGLT2-i largely represent patients with chronic stable HF.[13,10-21] However, the overall evidence also consistently demonstrates clinical benefits with SGLT2-i agents, across the clinical trajectory of HF, including WHF.[18-27]

The *SOLOIST-WHF*[22] trial evaluated the effect of sotagliflozin, a dual SGLT2 and SGLT1 inhibitor, initiated either during or soon after hospitalization for worsening heart-failure. The study represented only patients with type-2 diabetes. The use of sotagliflozin resulted in significant 33% lesser risk for cardiovascular deaths or HF-related hospitalizations or urgent visits. The use of sotagliflozin resulted in significant 33% lesser risk for cardiovascular deaths or HF-related hospitalizations or urgent visits.[22]

The *EMPUSE*[23] study was a dedicated randomized controlled trial, aimed to study the effect of early initiation of empagliflozin in acute stable HF, prior to hospital discharge. The study involved 530 patients hospitalized for acute HF, who had been stabilized hemodynamically. At randomization, the hemodynamic stability criteria included systolic blood-pressure ≥100 mm Hg, with no increase in intravenous diuretic dose in past 6-hours, no intravenous vasodilator use in past 6-hours, and no intravenous inotrope use in past 24-hours. These patients were randomized to receive empagliflozin 10 mg OD ($n = 265$) or placebo ($n = 265$), on top of standard treatment prior to hospital discharge. Over 90 days of follow-up, empagliflozin use was associated with significant 36% greater likelihood of clinical benefit (p value 0.0054). The clinical benefit was consistent across patients with *de-novo* acute HF or decompensated acute on chronic HF, those with left ventricular ejection fraction ≤40% and >40%, and those with or without diabetes. Over 90 days, death occurred in 22 (8.3%) patients receiving placebo vis-a-vis 11 (4.2%) patients receiving empagliflozin. The events of worsening of HF (including hospitalization, urgent HF visit, or unplanned outpatient visit) occurred in

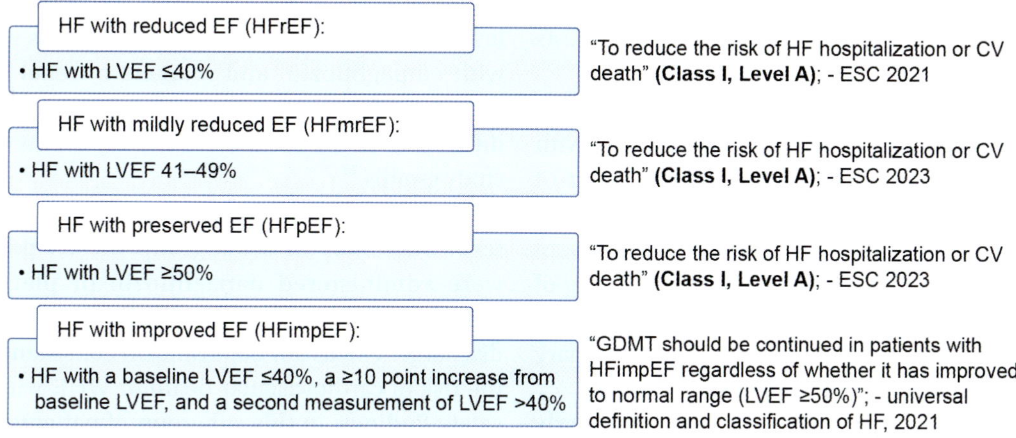

Fig. 2: Evidence-based recommendations for SGLT2-i therapy in heart failure.[2,16,17]

TABLE 1: Safety of empagliflozin use in acute stable heart failure, from EMPULSE study.[23]

Summary of adverse events	*Empagliflozin*		*Placebo*	
MedDRA preferred term	*n (%)*	*Rate/100 patients-years*	*n (%)*	*Rate/100 patients-years*
Number of patients	260 (100.0)		264 (100.0)	
Acute renal failure (narrow SMQ)	20 (7.7)	34.69	32 (12.1)	55.69
Acute kidney injury	10 (3.8)	16.9	19 (7.2)	32.28
Renal impairment	9 (3.5)	15.38	11 (4.2)	18.58
Renal failure	2 (0.8)	3.34	2 (0.8)	3.33
Serious	12 (4.6)	20.37	23 (8.7)	39.35
Leading to discontinuation of study medication	6 (2.3)	10.02	4 (1.5)	6.64
Urinary tract infection	11 (4.2)	18.8	17 (6.4)	29.23
Cystitis	8 (3.1)	13.62	5(1.9)	8.36
Urinary tract infection	3 (1.2)	5.01	6 (2.3)	10.1
Urinary tract infection bacterial	1 (0.4)	1.67	6 (2.3)	10.07
Escherichia urinary tract infection	1 (0.4)	1.67	0	–
Bacteriuria	0	–	1 (0.4)	1.66
Complicated (renal infections or urosepsis or serious UTI)	1 (0.4)	1.67	2 (0.8)	3.33

(MedDRA: Medical Dictionary for Regulatory Activities; SMQ: Standardized MedDRA query; UTI: urinary tract infection)

39 (14.7%) patients receiving placebo vis-a-vis 28 (10.6%) patients receiving empagliflozin. The total number of such worsening HF events was 52 in the placebo group, and 36 in the empagliflozin group, over these 90 days. The use of empagliflozin also showed greater reduction in NT-proBNP concentration, and grater diuretic response. The benefit was unaffected by the eGFR status in acute setting. Further, the use of empagliflozin prior to hospital discharge was relatively safe, and not associated with unexpected increase in the risk of adverse events, as summarized in **Table 1.**[23]

The *EMPA-RESPONSE AHF*[24] was a small randomized controlled trial, involving 80 patients hospitalized with acute heart-failure. The study evaluated the effect of empagliflozin versus placebo on top of standard treatment for acute HF. Over 60 days of follow-up, empagliflozin use was associated with a reduced risk of worsening of HF, including the combination of in-hospital worsening, rehospitalizations, and mortality events. A visual summary of the study results is described in **Figure 3.**[24]

The *EMPAG-HF*[25] study further revealed that early addition of empagliflozin to standard diuretic therapy, in patients with acute decompensated HF, increases urine output without affecting markers of renal function. The study included 60 patients with acute decompensated HF, who were randomized to receive either empagliflozin 25 mg daily or placebo, in addition to standard decongestive treatment within 12 hours of hospitalization. The addition of empagliflozin resulted in significant 25% increase in cumulative urine output over 5 days, along with significant improvements in loop-diuretic efficiency, NT-proBNP levels, and NYHA class. The uric acid levels were lowered with empagliflozin, and markers of renal dysfunction were not different between the two groups. There were no differences in the incidence of safety events between the study groups.[25]

The *DELIVER*[21,26] study demonstrated similar long-term outcomes in a subgroup of 654 patients, who were administered dapagliflozin or placebo during hospitalization for HF or within 30 days of hospital discharge. The use of dapagliflozin consistently improved the risk of cardiovascular death or WHF, with consistent safety findings, in this subgroup of patients with recent hospitalization for HF.[21,26]

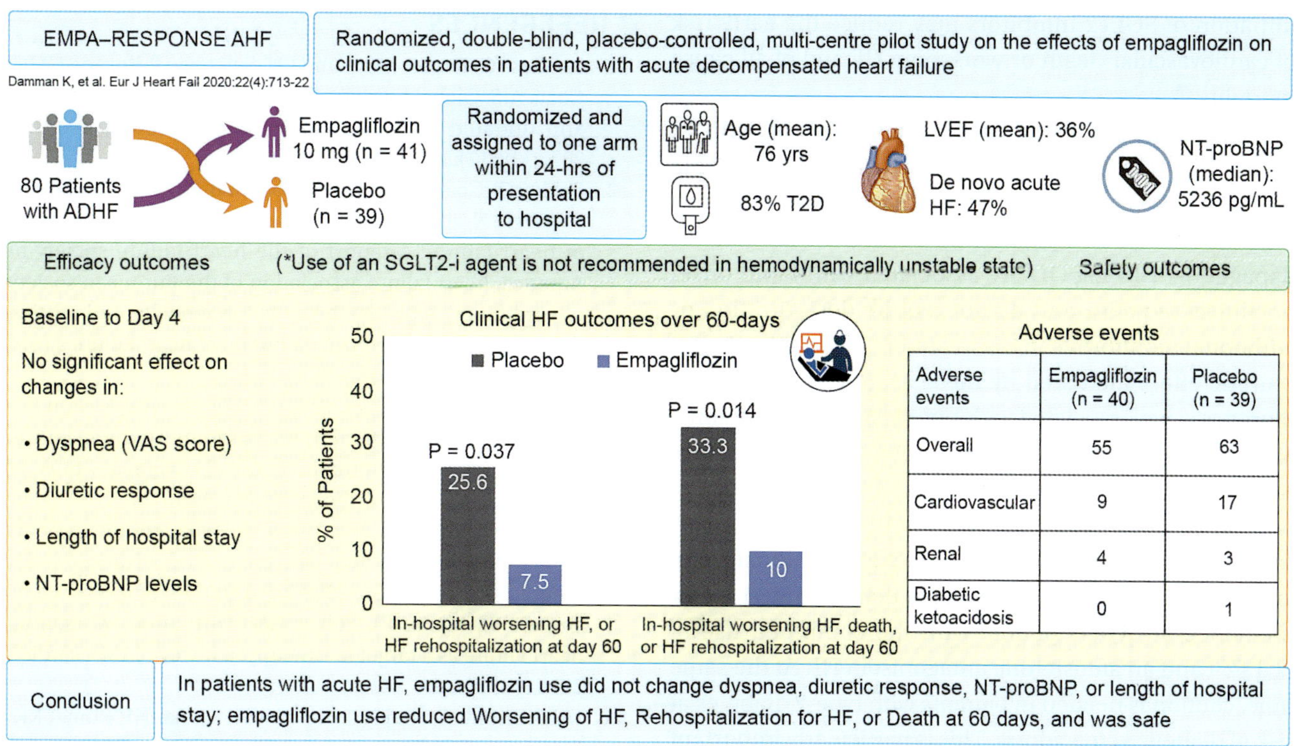

Adverse events	Empagliflozin (n = 40)	Placebo (n = 39)
Overall	55	63
Cardiovascular	9	17
Renal	4	3
Diabetic ketoacidosis	0	1

Fig. 3: Visual abstract of EMPA-RESPONSE AHF study findings.[24]

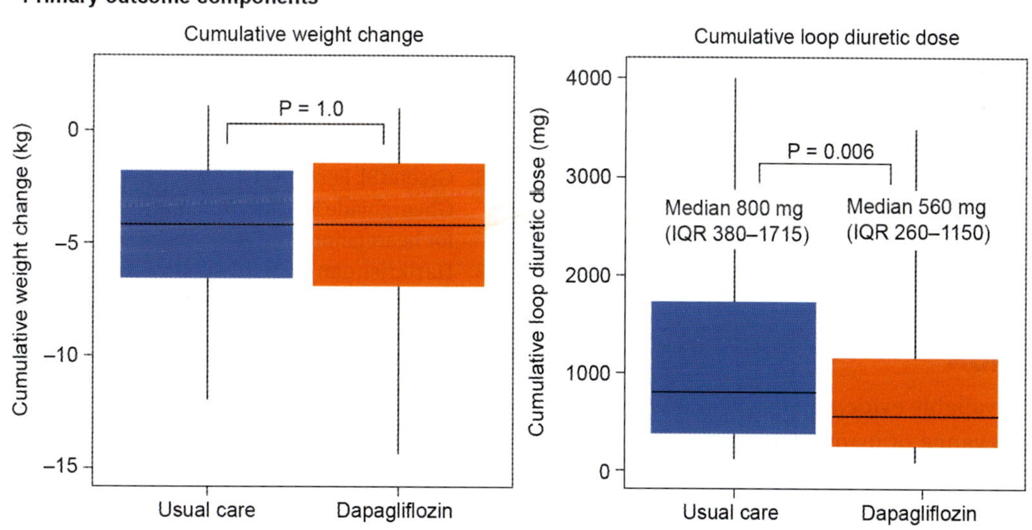

Fig. 4: DICTATE-AHF trial.

Source: Presented by Dr. Zachary Cox at the European Society of Cardiology Congress, Amsterdam, Netherlands, August 28, 2023.

The recently presented *DICTATE AHF*[27] study in the ESC congress 2023 showed a trend toward increased diuretic efficiency with dapagliflozin in patients hospitalized with acute decompensated HF requiring intravenous loop-diuretic therapy[27] **(Fig. 4)**. Recently published DAPA ACT HF TIMI 68 trial concluded that in-hospital initiation of dapagliflozin did not significantly reduce the risk of cardiovascular death or worsening HF through 2 months in hospitalized HF patients. However, the totality of randomized clinical trial data suggests that in-hospital initiation of SGLT2 inhibitors may reduce the early risk of cardiovascular death or worsening HF and of all cause mortality.[28]

Apart from these studies, the major trials of SGLT2-i agents in patients that largely represent chronic stable HF have consistently demonstrated risk reduction in WHF events.[18-21] Empagliflozin 10 mg OD as well as dapagliflozin 10 mg OD are associated with rapid onset of clinical benefits, and do not require dose-titration or additional monitoring, in the treatment of HF. The modest diuretic effect mediated by these agents on top of loop diuretics is not associated with significant neurohormonal activation. Further, the benefits provided by these drugs are consistently observed either as first-line agents in new-onset HF, or on top of other foundational treatments including sacubitril valsartan, as well as aldosterone antagonists. The studies have also demonstrated lesser incidence of hyperkalemia, with the combined use of SGLT2-i and an aldosterone antagonist in HF. At the same time, caution is needed in patients with type-2 diabetes at risk of diabetic ketoacidosis. This is particularly important in patients treated with insulin when carbohydrate intake is reduced or when insulin is not adequately replenished. These agents also need to be discontinued during acute severe medical illness, 3-days before any major surgery, and should be avoided with starvation or excessive alcohol drinking. These agents are not indicated in patients with type 1 diabetes. Further, the known general risks associated with these agents, including volume depletion, urogenital infection, as well as the need for appropriate dose-titration of concomitantly used insulin, sulfonylurea, or loop diuretic, need to be considered.[13,16-22]

CONCLUSION

The presently available evidence suggests consistent and compelling relevance of using SGLT2-i agents early, in patients with acute stable HF, to reduce the risk of clinical worsening and death. Based on the critical importance of this vulnerable phase of worsening in the trajectory of heart-failure, the recent ESC guidelines recommend that "An intensive strategy of initiation and rapid up-titration of evidence-based treatment before discharge and during frequent and careful follow-up visits in the first 6 weeks following a HF hospitalization is recommended to reduce the risk of HF rehospitalization or death (*Class I, Level B*)".[16]

REFERENCES

1. Savarese G, Becher PM, Lund LH, Seferovic P, Rosano GMC, Coats AJS. Global burden of heart failure: a comprehensive and updated review of epidemiology. Cardiovasc Res. 2023;118(17):3272-87.
2. Bozkurt B, Coats AJ, Tsutsui H, Abdelhamid M, Adamopoulos S, Albert N, et al. Universal definition and classification of heart failure: a report of the heart failure society of America, heart failure association of the European society of cardiology, Japanese heart failure society and writing committee of the universal definition of heart failure. J card fail. 2021;27(4):387-413.
3. Greene SJ, Bauersachs J, Brugts JJ, Ezekowitz JA, Lam CS, Lund LH, et al. Worsening heart failure: nomenclature, epidemiology, and future directions: JACC review topic of the week. J Am Coll Cardiol. 2023;81(4):413-24.
4. Greene SJ, Fonarow GC, Butler J. Risk profiles in heart failure: baseline, residual, worsening, and advanced heart failure risk. Circulation. 2020;13(6):e007132.
5. Greene SJ, Mentz RJ, Felker GM. Outpatient worsening heart failure as a target for therapy: a review. JAMA cardiol. 2018;3(3):252-9.
6. Harikrishnan S, Sanjay G, Agarwal A, Kumar NP, Kumar KK, Bahuleyan CG. One-year mortality outcomes and hospital readmissions of patients admitted with acute heart failure: Data from the Trivandrum Heart Failure Registry in Kerala, India. Am Heart J. 2017:189:193-9.
7. Joseph S, Panniyammakal J, Abdullakutty J, Sujithkumar S, Vaikathuseril JL, Joseph J, et al. The Cardiology Society of India-Kerala Acute Heart Failure Registry: poor adherence to guideline-directed medical therapy. Eur Heart J. 2021;ehab793. Online ahead of print.
8. Greene SJ, Fonarow GC, Vaduganathan M, Khan SS, Butler J, Gheorghiade M. The vulnerable phase after hospitalization for heart failure. Nat Rev Cardiol. 2015;12(4):220-9.
9. Harikrishnan S, Bahl A, Roy A, Mishra A, Prajapati J, Manjunath CN, et al. NHFR investigators. Clinical profile and 90 day outcomes of 10 851 heart failure patients across India: National Heart Failure Registry. ESC Heart Fail. 2022;9(6):3898-908.
10. Mullens W, Damman K, Harjola V, Mebazaa A, Brunner-La Rocca H, Martens P, et al. The Use of Diuretics in Heart Failure with Congestion - A Position Statement from the Heart Failure Association of the European Society of Cardiology. Eur J Heart Fail. 2019;21(2):137-55.
11. Felker GM, O'Connor CM, Braunwald E. Loop Diuretics in Acute Decompensated Heart Failure: Necessary? Evil? A Necessary Evil? Circ Heart Fail. 2009;2(1):56-62.
12. Chiong JR, Cheung RJ. Loop Diuretic Therapy in Heart Failure: The Need for Solid Evidence on a Fluid Issue. Clin Cardiol. 2010;33(6):345-52.
13. Vaduganathan M, Docherty KF, Claggett BL, Jhund PS, de Boer RA, Hernandez AF, et al. SGLT-2 inhibitors in

patients with heart failure: a comprehensive meta-analysis of five randomised controlled trials. Lancet. 2022; 400(10354):757-67.

14. McGuire DK, Shih WJ, Cosentino F, Charbonnel B, Cherney DZ, Dagogo-Jack S, et al. Association of SGLT2 inhibitors with cardiovascular and kidney outcomes in patients with type 2 diabetes: a meta-analysis. JAMA Cardiol. 2021;6(2):148-58.
15. The Nuffield Department of Population Health Renal Studies Group and the SGLT2 inhibitor Meta-Analysis Cardio-Renal Trialists' Consortium. Impact of diabetes on the effects of sodium glucose co-transporter-2 inhibitors on kidney outcomes: collaborative meta-analysis of large placebo-controlled trials. Lancet. 2022;400(10365): 1788-801.
16. ESC Scientific Document Group. 2023 Focused Update of the 2021 ESC Guidelines for the diagnosis and treatment of acute and chronic heart failure. Eur Heart J. 2023;44(37):3627-39.
17. ESC Scientific Document Group. 2021 ESC Guidelines for the diagnosis and treatment of acute and chronic heart failure. Eur Heart J. 2021;42(36):3599-726.
18. Packer M, Anker SD, Butler J, Filippatos G, Ferreira JP, Pocock SJ, et al. Effect of Empagliflozin on the Clinical Stability of Patients With Heart Failure and a Reduced Ejection Fraction: The EMPEROR-Reduced Trial. Circulation. 2021;143(4):326-36.
19. Packer M, Butler J, Zannad F, Filippatos G, Ferreira JP, Pocock SJ, et al. Effect of empagliflozin on worsening heart failure events in patients with heart failure and preserved ejection fraction: EMPEROR-Preserved trial. Circulation. 2021;144(16):1284-94.
20. McMurray JJV, Solomon SD, Inzucchi SE, Køber L, Kosiborod MN, Martinez FA, et al. DAPA-HF Trial Committees and Investigators. Dapagliflozin in patients with heart failure and reduced ejection fraction. N Engl J Med. 2019;381:1995-2008.
21. Cunningham JW, Vaduganathan M, Claggett BL, Kulac IJ, Desai AS, Jhund PS, et al. Dapagliflozin in Patients Recently Hospitalized With Heart Failure and Mildly Reduced or Preserved Ejection Fraction. J Am Coll Cardiol. 2022;80(14):1302-10.
22. Bhatt DL, Szarek M, Steg PG, Cannon CP, Leiter LA, McGuire DK, et al. SOLOIST-WHF Trial Investigators. Sotagliflozin in Patients with Diabetes and Recent Worsening Heart Failure. N Engl J Med. 2021 Jan 14;384(2):117-28.
23. Voors AA, Angermann CE, Teerlink JR, Collins SP, Kosiborod M, Biegus J, et al. The SGLT2 inhibitor empagliflozin in patients hospitalized for acute heart failure: a multinational randomized trial. Nature med. 2022;28(3):568-74.
24. Damman K, Beusekamp JC, Boorsma EM, Swart HP, Smilde TD, Elvan A, et al. Randomized, double-blind, placebo-controlled, multicentre pilot study on the effects of empagliflozin on clinical outcomes in patients with acute decompensated heart failure (EMPA-RESPONSE-AHF). Eur J Heart Fail. 2020;22(4):713-22.
25. Schulze PC, Bogoviku J, Westphal J, Aftanski P, Haertel F, Grund S, et al. Effects of early empagliflozin initiation on diuresis and kidney function in patients with acute decompensated heart failure (EMPAG-HF). Circulation. 2022;146(4):289-98.
26. Chatur S, Vaduganathan M, Claggett BL, Cunningham JW, Docherty KF, Desai AS, et al. Outpatient Worsening Among Patients With Mildly Reduced and Preserved Ejection Fraction Heart Failure in the DELIVER Trial. Circulation. 2023;148(22):1735-45.
27. Cox Z. Efficacy and Safety of Dapagliflozin in Acute Heart Failure (DICTATE-AHF). Presented at the ESC Congress, Amsterdam, Netherlands, August 28, 2023.
28. David D Berg, et al. DAPA ACT HF TIMI 68 Circulation. 2025;152:1411-22.

Management of Worsening Heart Failure

Satyanarayan Routray, Sradhananda Rout, Ravi Ranjan Kindo

INTRODUCTION

Worsening heart failure (WHF) is an actively debated fate on the journey of chronic heart failure (CHF) in recent times. Its definition is still at dawn, which may be stated as per the recent clinical consensus statement by the Heart Failure Association of the European Society of Cardiology[1] as given in **Table 1**.

Worsening heart failure definition is derived from treatment point of view rather than molecular mechanism or biologic process. It also highlights challenge of drug compliance and secondary insults that are excluded from the skeleton of definition.

Once the diagnosis of WHF is ascertained, there are three primary point of care as where escalation/intensification of heart failure (HF) therapy normally undertaken as given in **Table 2**.

MANAGEMENT

The standard four pillars of heart failure management as enumerated in **Figure 1**[2] are the cornerstone of pharmacological management of WHF.

TABLE 1: WHF definition as per clinical consensus statement by the Heart Failure Association of the European Society of Cardiology June, 2023.[1]

	Includes	*Excludes*
Definition	• Worsening symptoms and signs of HF – Requiring intensification of treatment, generally including diuretic therapy • Occurring in patients with pre-existing HF	• New-onset HF • Episodes with concomitant factors, including comorbidities and/or poor compliance, as primary cause
Pathophysiology	• Disease progression • Congestion	Precipitating factors as main cause
Site of care	• *Hospital:* – Emergency department – *Ambulatory:* - With IV therapy - With escalation of oral therapy	Episodes requiring no changes in HF treatment

(HF: heart failure; IV: intravenous therapy; WHF: worsening heart failure)

TABLE 2: Point-of-care for escalation/intensification of heart failure (HF) therapy in WHF.

Serial number	*Point-of-care*	*Patient phenotype*
1	In hospital	Patients with WHF needing intravenous (IV) medications
2	Emergency department (ED) visit	Patients of WHF who are discharged without hospitalization
3	Outdoor patients department (OPD) visits	WHF outpatients treated with an escalation of their oral diuretic therapy

(WHF: worsening heart failure)

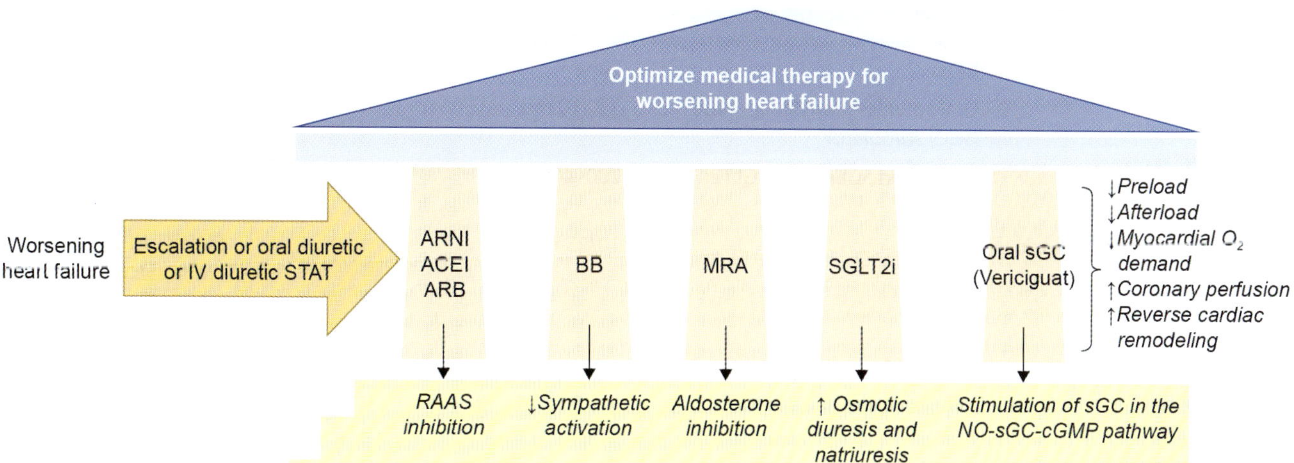

Fig. 1: Optimization of Medical Therapy for WHF.
Source: Seth S, Chopra VK, Mantri RR, Modi SK, Mittal S, Balagopalan JP, et al. Strategies to Optimize Management of Outpatient Worsening Heart Failure: A National Consensus from India. J Pract Cardiovasc Sci. 2025;11(1):14-26.

TABLE 3: Drugs dose escalation strategy in worsening heart failure.

Drug	*First visit (3–7 days)*	*Second visit (day 14)*	*Third visit (day 21)*	*Fourth visit (day 45, i.e., at 1.5 months)*	*Fifth visit (day 60, i.e., at 2 months)*	*Sixth visit (day 90, i.e., at 3 months)*
ACEi/ARB/ARNi	Ramipril 2.5 mg (1.25 mg OD/BID if BP <90 mm Hg) or nitrate hydralazine if renal failure	Higher dose ACEi or switch to ARNI	Uptitrate ACEi/ARNi or TID if BP falls	Clinical improvement? • Can walk 2–3 minutes • Reduction in BNP • Less edema		
Loop diuretics + MRA	Torsemide + spironolactone 10 + 50 mg OD/BID depending on patient's clinical condition (can go up to 2–4 tabs)	Adjust dose (up/down based on edema or SOB)	Continue	Yes ↓	No ↓	
SGLT2i	Dapagliflozin or Empagliflozin 10 mg (if RFT reasonable)	Continue	Continue	Continue current treatment	Consider the following: • Digoxin • Massive dosage of diuretics • Bed rest	
BB (β-blockers)	Small dose of BB carvedilol 3.125 mg (half or full tab OD/BID depending on patient's clinical condition)	Increase dose	BID to max possible dose			
sGC stimulators	Vericiguat 2.5 mg in this visit or start next visit if decompensation occurred	Double the dose	Increase dose to 5/10 mg			

(ACEi: angiotensin-converting enzyme inhibitor; ARB: angiotensin receptor blocker; ARNi: angiotensin receptor-neprilysin inhibitor; SGLT2i: sodium-glucose cotransporter-2 inhibitor; sGC: soluble guanylate cyclase)
Source: Seth S, Chopra VK, Mantri RR, Modi SK, Mittal S, Balagopalan JP, et al. Strategies to Optimize Management of Outpatient Worsening Heart Failure: A National Consensus from India. J Pract Cardiovasc Sci. 2025;11(1):14-26.

The starting dose and time period of escalation is always individualized as per patient tolerance and cardiologists interpretation and advise. A good guidance is provided by consensus statement by Seth et al.[2] as the following **Table 3**.

RECENT ADVANCES OF PHARMACOLOGICAL MANAGEMENT OF WORSENING HEART FAILURE

In **Table 4**, we have tried to give comprehensive drugs and its doses with referenced trials.

TABLE 4: Recent advances on pharmacological management of WHF.

Drugs	Class	Dose	Trials
Vericiguat	Oral soluble guanylate cyclase (sGC) stimulator	2.5–10 mg	VICTORIA trial
Sotagliflozin	Combined SGLT1 and SGLT2i inhibitor	200–400 mg	• SCORED trial • SOLOIST-WHF trial
Dapagliflozin/empagliflozin	SGLT1i	10/25 mg	• EMPAG-HF trial • EMPULSE trial • DAPA HF trial • DELIVER trial
Finerenone	Nonsteroidal antagonist of mineralcorticoid receptors	20–40 mg OD	• FIDELIO-DKD trial • FIGARO-DKD trial • FINEARTS-HF trial
Levosimendan	Inodilator, calcium sensitizer	Weight-based IV infusion—weekly	• LevoRep trial • LION-HEART trial • LeoDOR trial • LAICA study
Omecamtiv mecarbil	Cardiac myosin activator	25–50 mg	• GALACTIC-HF trial • METEORIC-HF trial • COSMIC-HF trial
Acetazolamide	Carbonic anhydrase inhibitor	IV 500 mg OD	ADVOR trial

(SGLT: sodium-glucose cotransporter; WHF: worsening heart failure)

Vericiguat is a cyclic guanosine monophosphate (cGMP) pathway enhancer, which acts by directly stimulating soluble guanylate cyclase (sGC) and increases endothelial NO. The VICTORIA trial[3] of Vericiguat in 2020, which included 5050 patients with chronic HF, a left ventricular ejection fraction (LVEF) <45%, and an episode of recent worsening HF, showed that, among patients with high-risk HF, the incidence of the primary endpoint, a composite of death from cardiovascular causes or first hospitalization for HF, was significantly less in those who received Vericiguat compared to those who received placebo. Vericiguat was also proven to be safe and well tolerated, with no significant effects on kidney function and electrolytes, showing minimal effects on blood pressure upon treatment initiation, and, overall, few side effects compared to placebo. Based on the VICTORIA trial results, Vericiguat has been approved for the treatment of symptomatic chronic HF with an LVEF <45%, following a worsening HF event, with the objective of reducing cardiovascular death and HF hospitalization risk. Considering the high mortality and hospitalization rate of patients with WHF, and, considering the persistently high risk of adverse events despite optimal GDMT, Greene et al.[4] recommended that the adjunct use of Vericiguat, added to standard quadruple GDMT, is to be considered. In clinical practice, patients currently often do not achieve uptitration to the target dosage of GDMT. However, the benefits of Vericiguat on mortality or HF hospitalization seem to be consistent independent of GDMT use and dose.[4] Moreover, as it has been largely demonstrated that the benefits of the current four pillars of GDMT are additive, this applies to Vericiguat as well. So, the initiation of Vericiguat can be considered either while reaching GDMT target doses or simultaneously with GDMT uptitration.

Sotagliflozin is a combined sodium-glucose cotransporter-1 inhibitor (SGLT1i) and sodium-glucose cotransporter-2 inhibitor (SGLT2i), with predominantly SGLT2 inhibitory capacity.[5] SGLT1 mediates the reabsorption of glucose in the gastrointestinal tract, resulting in a reduction in glycemia and increase in plasma glucagon-like peptide 1 (GLP-1). SGLT2 is expressed in the first proximal convoluted tubule segment, reabsorbing about 90% of the glucose in the peritubular capillaries. The dual inhibition of SGLT1 and SGLT2 may provide a combined effect, causing the decrease in serum glucose levels through reduced intestinal absorption and increased urinary output. SGLTi also have a myocardial antiremodeling effect, reduces inflammation and oxidative stress, and induces a cardiomyocytes metabolic shift. Given the great impact of SGLT2i on HF treatment, the effects of Sotagliflozin were studied in the SOLOIST-WHF trial.[5] The patients enrolled in the trial were affected by T2DM and had experienced a recent worsening in HF, including both patients with HFrEF and with HF with preserved ejection fraction (HFpEF). In patients treated with Sotagliflozin, the primary endpoint, a combination of the total number of cardiovascular deaths, hospitalizations, and urgent visits for HF, resulted in being significantly lower, and the benefits of an early initiation, before or immediately after hospital discharge, was highlighted. In the SCORED trial[6] aimed to evaluate the role of Sotagliflozin in preventing cardiovascular adverse events in patients with diabetes mellitus and chronic kidney disease, Bhatt et al.[6] demonstrated that Sotagliflozin reduced the composite endpoint of HF hospitalization, urgent ambulatory visit, and cardiovascular death, along with the major incidence of adverse events such as ketoacidosis, infections, and volume depletion, compared to placebo.

Dapagliflozin and empagliflozin act by inhibiting selectively the function of SGLT2. These drugs being one of the four pillars in the treatment of HFrEF and being indicated in the treatment of HFmrEF and HFpEF. As evidenced by the EMPAG-HF,[7] the EMPA-RESPONSE-AHF,[8] and the EMPULSE trials,[9] SGLT2i should be considered as an add-on therapy to loop diuretics in order to improve diuretic efficacy and, therefore, further facilitate decongestion in patients affected by WHF. Empagliflozin was shown to lead to a 25% increase in cumulative urine output, greater reduction in NT-proBNP and lower body weight when combined with diuretic therapy, without increased renal derangement.[7-9] Also, the use of Dapagliflozin in the DAPA-RESPONSE-AHF trial was associated with improvement in urinary output and symptoms in patients with acute HF.[10]

Finerenone is a nonsteroidal antagonist of mineral-corticoid receptors which inhibits renin-angiotensin-aldosterone system (RAAS) activation, reducing the risk of myocardial and kidney fibrosis as well as inflammation. Its more selectivity and better safety profile with lesser hyperkalemic properties, renal function depression, and less gynecomastia makes it a good candidate drug for WHF. FIDELIO-DKD trial,[11] which demonstrated that finerenone reduced the risk of kidney disease progression and cardiovascular events, including HF hospitalization, in patients with diabetes mellitus and chronic kidney disease. The FIGARO-DKD trial[12] showed that finerenone reduced the incidence of new HF and improved HF outcomes in patients with diabetes mellitus and chronic kidney disease, regardless of HF presence in ARTS-HF trial that demonstrated that finerenone was well tolerated and determined a significant reduction in NT-proBNP levels in patients with WHF and diabetes mellitus and/or chronic kidney disease.[13]

Levosimendan is an inodilator having a calcium sensitizer properties with pleiotropic effects. It is acetylated in the liver into an active metabolite with a long half-life named OR-1896 having a half-life of 75–80 hours. Its cardiovascular effects persist for 7–9 days following discontinuation of drug. The inotropic action of Levosimendan is performed by sensitizing cardiac troponin C (cTnC) to calcium (Ca^{2+}) binding. The calcium sensitizer enhances the contractility of cTnC exclusively in the Ca^{2+} activated conformation, thereby improving systolic function without affecting diastolic relaxation or augmenting the risk of adverse effects related to the increased Ca^{2+} concentration. It also causes vasodilation of pulmonary, coronary, and peripheral arteries and its metabolite are also found to be selective inhibitors of phosphodiesterase isoenzyme 3 (PDE 3), potentially resulting in an increase in intracellular Ca^{2+} concentration. The LevoRep trial[14] was a multicentre, randomized, prospective, double-blind trial whose primary endpoint was a composite of at least a 20% improvement in the 6-minute walk test (6MWT) and at least a 15% improvement in the Kansas City Cardiomyopathy Questionnaire (KCCQ-12) following repetitive infusions of levosimendan in an acute HF outpatient setting. Altenberger et al.[14] reported that the intermittent outpatient treatment did not significantly improve patients' functional capacity and quality of life when compared to placebo administration. The LION-HEART trial[15] was a multicenter, randomized, double-blind trial which included 69 patients who underwent randomization at a 2:1 ratio to be treated either with Levosimendan or with placebo. Comín-Colet et al.[15] demonstrated that the intermittent administration of levosimendan was effective in decreasing the serum concentration of NT-proBNP and was associated with improvement in clinical symptoms in comparison to the placebo group. The LAICA study[16] was a multicentre trial aimed at evaluating the efficacy and safety of intermittent administration of levosimendan as a continuous, 24-hour, intravenous infusion in patients with advanced HF.

García-González et al.[16] demonstrated the beneficial impact of repetitive levosimendan infusion in reducing the HF hospitalization rate and HF worsening in patients with advanced HF, compared with placebo. The LeoDOR trial[17] was a multicenter trial with the aim of evaluating the efficacy and safety of intermittent intravenous levosimendan therapy, administered in addition to standard therapy, for 12 weeks, either as a 6-hour continuous infusion or as a 24-hour continuous infusion. The trial found that the repetitive administration of levosimendan in patients with a recent HF hospitalization did not result in post-hospitalization clinical stability. In summary, the repetitive administration of levosimendan and its role to achieve the hemodynamic stabilization in patients with worsening HF remain controversial, and further studies are needed with adequate sample size.

Omecamtiv mecarbil (OM) is a cardiac myosin activator, a small molecule that enhances cardiac contractility by binding to myosin. OM is an oral inotropic agent which stimulates myosin heads that are ready to bind actin filaments. It improves systolic function, cardiac contractility, and systolic ejection time, without increasing myocardial oxygen consumption. The dose and the effects of OM administration were studied in various trials, such as the COSMIC-HF trial,[18] the GALACTIC-HF trial,[19] and the METEORIC-HF trial.[20] The GALACTIC-HF trial[21] aimed to examine the effects of OM administration in terms of improving symptoms, preventing clinical HF events, and delaying cardiovascular death. The primary composite endpoint of hospitalization or urgent visit for HF and death from cardiovascular causes appeared to be reduced in the intervention group when compared to placebo.[18-21]

Loop diuretics are the fundamental therapy in the management of cardiac congestion. They reduce NaCl reabsorption at the level of the ascending limb of the loop of Henle by inhibiting the Na^+-K^+-$2Cl^-$ channel in its basal membrane. The DOSE trial,[22] despite not meeting its primary end points, did reveal benefits in secondary endpoints, with improvements in terms of dyspnea, congestion, and NT-proBNP.

Acetazolamide can also be considered as an add-on therapy to diuretics. Acetazolamide is a carbonic anhydrase inhibitor, which acts by reducing proximal tubular sodium reabsorption. The ADVOR trial[23] demonstrated the beneficial effects of decongesting patients with acute HF that resulted from the combination of intravenous acetazolamide and loop diuretics.

Figure 2 provides a timeline of dose titration of various drugs in management of WHF.

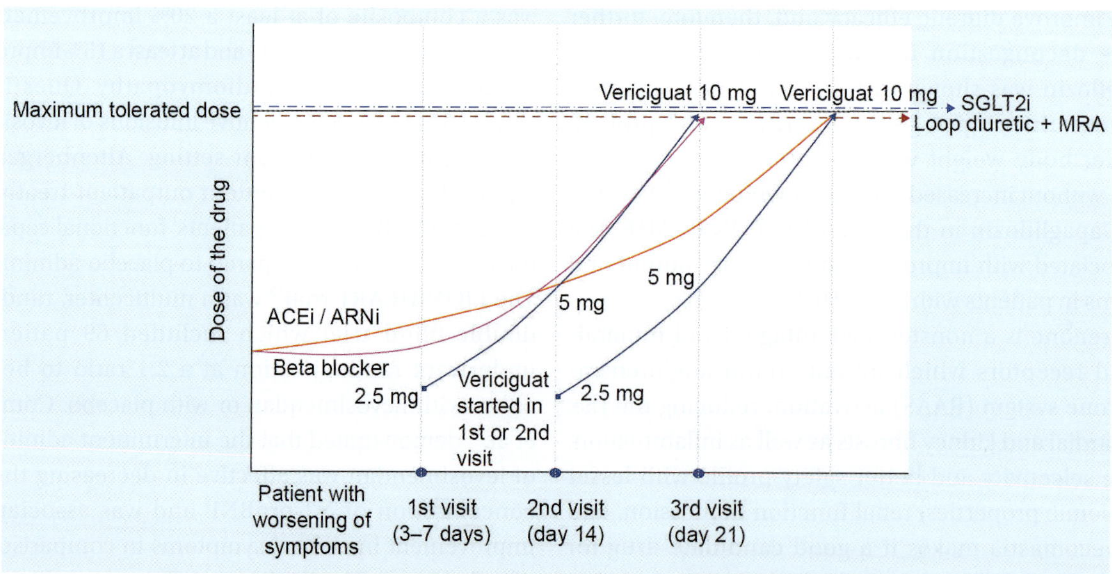

Fig. 2: Dose titration in WHF. (ACEi: angiotensin-converting enzyme inhibitor; ARNI: angiotensin receptor-neprilysin inhibitor; WHF: worsening heart failure)

Source: Seth S, Chopra VK, Mantri RR, Modi SK, Mittal S, Balagopalan JP, et al. Strategies to Optimize Management of Outpatient Worsening Heart Failure: A National Consensus from India. J Pract Cardiovasc Sci. 2025;11(1):14-26.

DEVICES IN MANAGEMENT OF WORSENING HEART FAILURE

CardioMEMS system measures pulmonary artery pressure (PAP) and wirelessly transmits these data to a healthcare provider. The CHAMPION Trial[24] was a large trial which included 550 patients with chronic HF in NYHA class III with a hospital admission for HF in the previous 12 months. The trial demonstrated a significant reduction in HF hospital admissions in patients with daily PAP monitoring; during the 18-months follow-up, patients treated with the usual care had a significantly higher rate of hospitalization compared to the CardioMEMS group. CardioMEMS was found to be successful from a safety point of view as well, showing freedom from device- or system-related complications equal to 98.6% and freedom from sensor failures of 100%. patients treated with both GDMT and CardioMEMS, the hospitalization was significantly lower. Additionally, in the MONITOR HF trial,[25] 348 patients were randomized in a 1:1 fashion, with 179 being assigned to the CardioMEMS group and 178 being assigned to the control group (being treated with GDMT and diuretics). The trial has shown that CardioMEMS improved the QoL of HF patients, with a significant increase in KCCQ-12 scores when compared to controls.

The SIRONA,[26] a multicentre, open-label, first-in-human, feasibility study to evaluate the usability of the comprehensive Cordella™ Heart Failure System (CHFS) showed that implantation of the Cordella Sensor **(Figs. 3A and B)** was feasible and safe with excellent accuracy of the Cordella Sensor PAP measurements for predicting HF Worsening. Select population with Cardiac resynchronization therapy and the implantable cardioverter-defibrillator offer diagnostic features for early detection of WHF.

The high filling pressures in the left atrium (LA) contribute to congestion and the worsening of HF symptoms, mainly in patients with HFpEF, making it reasonable to monitor its changes through LA pressure sensors (Heart POD and V-LAP devices). The V-LAP system incorporates a sensory implant that wirelessly measures and transmits left atrial pressure (LAP) to an external unit. The VECTOR-HF study[27] showed that V-LAP safely provided reliable measurements in patients with NYHA Class III may allow the remote tailoring of the therapy, and preliminary data showed promising results in increasing NYHA functional status and QoL.

Cardiac contractility modulation (CCM) represents a device-based therapy suitable for a wide range of HF patients that do not meet the criteria for CRT. This device is reserved for those with LVEF between 25 and 45% who remain symptomatic (NYHA II–IV) despite OMT and who do not have a left bundle branch block (LBBB) morphology. The CCM device physically resembles a pacemaker, as it is constituted by a generator and two leads; the generator, containing the battery and electronic circuits, similar to any other cardiac implantable electronic device (CIED) generator, can be positioned in the left or right pectoral region, in a pocket located under the skin. However, the CCM function differs from pacemakers as it generates an electrical signal specifically and exclusively during the absolute refractory period of the myocardium for 5–7 hours a day. It does not capture the myocardium in order to obtain heart contractions. CCM manages to enhance Ca_2^+ handling through the upregulation of RYR2 and SERCA2a, restoring the function of the $Na^+/Ca2^+$ exchanger and normalizing the levels of phospholamban phosphorylation. The trials with the most encouraging

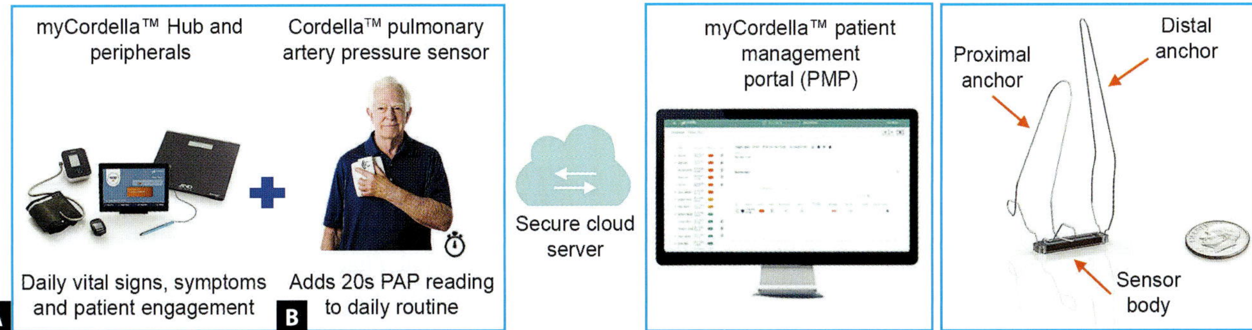

Figs. 3A and B: The Cordella™ Heart Failure System. (A) The Cordella™ system securely transmits daily health information (weight, blood pressure, saturations, heart rate) as well as pulmonary artery pressure (PAP) data to clinicians from the patient's home; (B) The Cordella™ pulmonary artery pressure sensor.

TABLE 5: Invasive monitoring systems and device therapy used in WHF.

Device	*Class*	*Trials*
CardioMEMS	Measures pulmonary artery pressure (PAP)	CHAMPION trial MONITOR-HF trial EMBRACE-HF trial
Cordella device	Measures pulmonary artery pressure (PAP)	SIRONA study
CCM	*Cardiac contractility modulation*	FIX-HF-4 study FIX-HF-5 study
V-LAP	Left atrial pressure (LAP) measurements	VECTOR-HF study
BAT	Baroreflex activation therapy	BeAT-HF study, HOPE4HF study

(BAT: baroreflex activation therapy; CCM: cardiac contractility modulation; WHF: worsening heart failure)

results are the FIX-HF-4 study[28] and the FIX-HF-5 trial,[29] which examined CCM as an addition to OMT compared to OMT alone, demonstrating that CCM is safe and effective in improving exercise tolerance and QoL, while reducing HF hospitalizations.

Baroreflex activation therapy (BAT) consists of a device implanted to electrically stimulate the baroreceptors responsible for autonomic nervous system modulation. The Barostim Neo™ device has shown promising results in safely improving clinical symptoms and NYHA functional class in patients with worsening HF.[30] The BeAT-HF study[31] and the HOPE4HF study[32] have revealed that BAT therapy significantly improved QoL and exercise capacity, and reduced NT-proBNP levels.

A summary of the main trials regarding invasive monitoring systems and device therapy used in WHF is represented in **Table 5**.

CONCLUSION

In the era of heart failure pandemic, the treatment and prevention of WHF is at its dawn as is its definition, waiting to see a bright morning. Besides the guideline-directed four pharmacological pillars, acetazolamide, vericiguat, and finerenone all have shown candidacy for future WHF management. The new concept of "door to furosemide time" must be shortened and well emphasized for WHF management. Some patients category that frequently need hospitalization (termed as frequent flyers by some authors) may get benefited by combining left ventricular assist device (LVAD) and monitoring device implantations.

REFERENCES

1. Metra M, Tomasoni D, Adamo M, Bayes-Genis A, Filippatos G, Abdelhamid M, et al. Worsening of chronic heart failure: definition, epidemiology, management and prevention. A clinical consensus statement by the Heart Failure Association of the European Society of Cardiology. Eur J Heart Fail. 2023;25(6):776-791.
2. Seth S, Chopra VK, Mantri RR, Modi SK, Mittal S, Balagopalan JP, et al. Strategies to Optimize Management of Outpatient Worsening Heart Failure: A National Consensus from India. J Pract Cardiovasc Sci. 2025;11(1):14-26.
3. Armstrong PW, Pieske B, Anstrom KJ, Ezekowitz J, Hernandez AF, Butler J, et al. Vericiguat in Patients with Heart Failure and Reduced Ejection Fraction. N Engl J Med. 2020;382:1883-93.
4. Greene SJ, Bauersachs J, Brugts JJ, Ezekowitz JA, Filippatos G, Gustafsson F, et al. Management of Worsening Heart Failure with Reduced Ejection Fraction: JACC Focus Seminar 3/3. J Am Coll Cardiol. 2023;82:559-71.
5. Bhatt DL, Szarek M, Steg PG, Cannon CP, Leiter LA, McGuire DK, et al. Sotagliflozin in Patients with Diabetes and Recent Worsening Heart Failure. N Engl J Med. 2021;384:117-28.
6. Bhatt DL, Szarek M, Pitt B, Cannon CP, Leiter LA, McGuire DK, et al. Sotagliflozin in Patients with Diabetes and Chronic Kidney Disease. N Engl J Med. 2021;384: 129-39.
7. Schulze PC, Bogoviku J, Westphal J, Aftanski P, Haertel F, Grund S, et al. Effects of Early Empagliflozin Initiation on Diuresis and Kidney Function in Patients with Acute Decompensated Heart Failure (EMPAG-HF). Circulation. 2022;146:289-98.
8. Damman K, Beusekamp JC, Boorsma EM, Swart HP, Smilde TDJ, Elvan A, et al. Randomized, double-blind, placebo-controlled, multicentre pilot study on the effects of empagliflozin on clinical outcomes in patients with acute decompensated heart failure (EMPA-RESPONSE-AHF). Eur J Heart Fail. 2020;22:713-22.
9. Biegus J, Voors AA, Collins SP, Kosiborod MN, Teerlink JR, Angermann CE, et al. Impact of empagliflozin on decongestion in acute heart failure: The EMPULSE trial. Eur Heart J. 20231;44:41-50.
10. Emara AN, Wadie M, Mansour NO, Shams MEE. The clinical outcomes of dapagliflozin in patients with acute heart failure: A randomized controlled trial (DAPA-RESPONSE-AHF). Eur J Pharmacol. 2023;961:176-9.
11. Bakris GL, Agarwal R, Anker SD, Pitt B, Ruilope LM, Rossing P, et al. Effect of Finerenone on Chronic Kidney Disease Outcomes in Type 2 Diabetes. N Engl J Med. 2020; 383:2219-9.
12. Filippatos G, Anker SD, Agarwal R, Ruilope LM, Rossing P, Bakris GL, et al. Finerenone Reduces Risk of Incident Heart Failure in Patients with Chronic Kidney Disease and

Type 2 Diabetes: Analyses From the FIGARO-DKD Trial. Circulation. 2022;145:437-47.
13. Filippatos G, Anker SD, Bohm M, Gheorghiade M, Kober L, Krum H, et al. A randomized controlled study of finerenone vs. eplerenone in patients with worsening chronic heart failure and diabetes mellitus and/or chronic kidney disease. Eur Heart J. 2016;37:2105-14.
14. Altenberger J, Parissis JT, Costard-Jaeckle A, Winter A, Ebner C, Karavidas A, et al. Efficacy and safety of the pulsed infusions of levosimendan in outpatients with advanced heart failure (LevoRep) study: A multicentre randomized trial. Eur J Heart Fail. 2014;16:898-906.
15. Comín-Colet J, Manito N, Segovia-Cubero J, Delgado J, García Pinilla JM, Almenar L, et al. Efficacy and safety of intermittent intravenous outpatient administration of levosimendan in patients with advanced heart failure: The LION-HEART multicentre randomised trial. Eur J Heart Fail. 2018;20:1128-36.
16. García-González MJ, de Mora-Martín M, López-Fernández S, López-Díaz J, Martínez-Sellés M, Romero-García J, et al. Rationale and design of a randomized, double-blind, placebo controlled multicenter trial to study efficacy, security, and long term effects of intermittent repeated levosimendan administration in patients with advanced heart failure: LAICA study. Cardiovasc Drugs Ther. 2013; 27:573-9.
17. Polzl G, Altenberger J, Comín-Colet J, Delgado JF, Fedele F, García-González MJ, et al. Repetitive levosimendan infusions for patients with advanced chronic heart failure in the vulnerable post-discharge period: The multinational randomized LeoDOR trial. Eur J Heart Fail. 2023;25:2007-17.
18. Teerlink JR, Felker GM, McMurray JJ, Solomon SD, Adams KF Jr, Cleland JG, et al. Chronic Oral Study of Myosin Activation to Increase Contractility in Heart Failure (COSMIC-HF): A phase 2, pharmacokinetic, randomised, placebo-controlled trial. Lancet. 2016;388:2895-903.
19. Teerlink JR, Diaz R, Felker GM, McMurray JJV, Metra M, Solomon SD, et al. Omecamtiv Mecarbil in Chronic Heart Failure with Reduced Ejection Fraction: Rationale and Design of GALACTIC-HF. JACC Heart Fail. 2020;8:329-40.
20. Lewis GD, Voors AA, Cohen-Solal A, Metra M, Whellan DJ, Ezekowitz JA, et al. Effect of Omecamtiv Mecarbil on Exercise Capacity in Chronic Heart Failure with Reduced Ejection Fraction: The METEORIC-HF Randomized Clinical Trial. JAMA. 2022;328:259-69.
21. Felker GM, Solomon SD, Claggett B, Diaz R, McMurray JJV, Metra M, et al. Assessment of Omecamtiv Mecarbil for the Treatment of Patients with Severe Heart Failure: A Post Hoc Analysis of Data From the GALACTIC-HF Randomized Clinical Trial. JAMA Cardiol. 2022;7:26-34.
22. Felker GM, Lee KL, Bull DA, Redfield MM, Stevenson LW, Goldsmith SR, et al. Diuretic strategies in patients with acute decompensated heart failure. N Engl J Med. 2011; 364:797-805.
23. Mullens W, Dauw J, Martens P, Verbrugge FH, Nijst P, Meekers E, et al. Acetazolamide in Acute Decompensated Heart Failure with Volume Overload. N Engl J Med. 2022;387:1185-95.
24. Abraham WT, Stevenson LW, Bourge RC, Lindenfeld JA, Bauman JG, Adamson PB. Sustained efficacy of pulmonary artery pressure to guide adjustment of chronic heart failure therapy: Complete follow-up results from the CHAMPION randomised trial. Lancet. 2016;387:453-61.
25. Brugts JJ, Radhoe SP, Clephas PRD, Aydin D, van Gent MWF, Szymanski MK, et al. Remote haemodynamic monitoring of pulmonary artery pressures in patients with chronic heart failure (MONITOR-HF): A randomised clinical trial. Lancet. 2023;401:2113-23.
26. Mullens W, Sharif F, Dupont M, Rothman AMK, Wijns W. Digital health care solution for proactive heart failure management with the Cordella Heart Failure System: results of the SIRONA first-in-human study. Eur J Heart Fail. 2020;22(10):1912-9.
27. D'Amario D, Meerkin D, Restivo A, Ince H, Sievert H, Wiese A, et al. Safety, usability, and performance of a wireless left atrial pressure monitoring system in patients with heart failure: The VECTOR-HF trial. Eur J Heart Fail. 2023;25:902-11.
28. Borggrefe MM, Lawo T, Butter C, Schmidinger H, Lunati M, Pieske B, et al. Randomized, double blind study of non-excitatory, cardiac contractility modulation electrical impulses for symptomatic heart failure. Eur Heart J. 2008;29:1019-28.
29. Abraham WT, Kuck KH, Goldsmith RL, Lindenfeld J, Reddy VY, Carson PE, et al. A Randomized Controlled Trial to Evaluate the Safety and Efficacy of Cardiac Contractility Modulation. JACC Heart Fail. 2018;6:874-83.
30. Blanco C, Madej T, Mangner N, Hommel J, Grimm S, Knaut M, et al. Baroreflex activation therapy in patients with heart failure with reduced ejection fraction: A single-centre experience. ESC Heart Fail. 2023;10:3373-84.
31. Zile MR, Lindenfeld JA, Weaver FA, Zannad F, Galle E, Rogers T, et al. Baroreflex Activation Therapy in Patients with Heart Failure with Reduced Ejection Fraction. J Am Coll Cardiol. 2020;76:1-13.
32. Abraham WT, Zile MR, Weaver FA, Butter C, Ducharme A, Halbach M, et al. Baroreflex Activation Therapy for the Treatment of Heart Failure with a Reduced Ejection Fraction. JACC Heart Fail. 2015;3:487-96.

CHAPTER 11

Revascularization for Heart Failure

Vivekanand S Gajapati

INTRODUCTION

Coronary artery disease (CAD) remains the most common cause of heart failure with reduced ejection fraction (HFrEF). Ischemic etiology is estimated to account for over two thirds of all heart failure (HF) cases and is associated with impaired quality of life and poor prognosis.[1,2] Pharmacological and device therapy are the main modalities of treatment of HFrEF.

Revascularization should be offered to patients with impaired left ventricular (LV) function who present with angina or acute coronary syndrome.

There is limited evidence to support revascularization in patients with stable ischemic HF and minimal symptoms. Separating true ischemic HF from bystander CAD in nonischemic HF is frequently challenging. The preferred choice of revascularization [percutaneous coronary intervention (PCI) or coronary artery bypass grafting (CABG)] depends on age, sex, comorbidities, and coronary anatomy. Severe LV dysfunction is associated with increased procedural mortality and morbidity following surgical or percutaneous revascularization. CABG surgery has been an important mode of revascularization in patients with multivessel CAD and HFrEF. However, recent advances in interventional cardiology led to overall increase in PCI in treatment of ischemic HFrEF.

It is essential to understand the better modality for coronary revascularization in this unique and growing patient population to improve outcomes.

ROLE OF REVASCULARIZATION

Ischemic cardiomyopathy (ICM) is a LV dysfunction due to atherosclerotic CAD. It incorporates many clinical, imaging, and angiographic features. While the evidence of guideline-directed medical treatment (GDMT) in HFrEF is strong, there is more controversy surrounding the ideal approach and timing of coronary revascularization in ICM.

Revascularization, particularly CABG, is recommended for patients with ischemic HFrEF based on the assumption that blood flow restoration of viable but ischemic myocardium might reverse the LV dysfunction.[3] The potential mechanism of improving pumping function is the reversal of myocardial hibernation, an adaptive process triggered by repeated episodes of ischemia. Myocardial viability testing is the prospective identification of myocardium, which is likely to be hibernating, and it is one of the important considerations when adopting revascularization strategy. A large meta-analysis demonstrated a strong association between myocardial viability and improved survival after revascularization in patients with chronic CAD and LV dysfunction.[4]

TYPES OF REVASCULARIZATION

Surgical Revascularization (Coronary Artery Bypass Grafting)

Patients with ICM frequently present with complex and extensive CAD, which often makes surgical revascularization the preferred mode of invasive treatment.

The contemporary evidence on the role of CABG comes from the results of the STICH (Surgical Treatment of Ischemic Heart Failure) trial which randomized 1,212 patients with ICM <35% left ventricular ejection fraction (LVEF) to either CABG or medical therapy.[5,6] At the first prespecified analysis at 5 years, there was no significant difference in primary outcomes of all-cause mortality between groups. There was only borderline significance in the secondary end point of cardiovascular mortality. When followed up for 10 years, there was significant reduction of all-cause mortality in CABG arm (7% absolute reduction), which translated into to 17 months median increase in survival.

The STICH trial remains a landmark trial, but there were several limitations which limits us to generalize its conclusions in routine clinical practice. Increasing age is known to be an important predictor of worse outcomes in patients with HF. Patients in STICH trial were younger than most contemporary registries of HF (the mean age was 60 years). Younger cohorts derived more beneficial outcomes than those over the age of 65 years. The use of medical and device therapy did not reflect contemporary practice with very low rates of implantable cardioverter-defibrillator (ICD) implantations and poor adherence to medical therapy. Presence of three vessel disease, LVEF < 27%, and LV end-systolic volume >79 mL/m^2 were associated with greater benefit from CABG. Surprisingly the presence of angina, ischemia, viability, and diabetes did not appear to benefit more from CABG. Myocardial viability testing was not mandatory in STICH trial. Moreover, the evidence of viability was not associated with improved outcomes in HF patients undergoing CABG.[7,8] In conclusion, CABG is an effective mode of revascularization in selected cases and its modest benefit can be distinguished from the increased mortality due to the surgical procedure beyond 5 years.

Percutaneous Coronary Intervention

Percutaneous coronary intervention is now emerging as an important mode of revascularization in patients with ICM due to technological development and advancing experience. The role of PCI has expanded to more complex cases such as left main disease, multivessel disease, and chronic total occlusions. The number of patients with ischemic HF undergoing PCI has increased compared to those referred for CABG,[9,10] even though most randomized clinical trials comparing CABG and PCI in stable patients have excluded patients with reduced LVEF.[11,12] The long-term outcomes are unknown in patients undergoing PCI for ischemic HF.[13] The theoretical advantage of PCI compared to CABG cannot be extrapolated as the mechanism of revascularization is substantially different. PCI may not achieve complete revascularization compared to CABG. Although PCI is considered to be associated with lesser mortality and morbidity than CABG, no robust comparisons have been made in patients with HF.

The United States and European Society of Cardiology (ESC) guidelines recommend CABG as the preferred revascularization option in patients with ischemic HF.[14,15] CABG is superior to PCI according to ESC guidelines, while the US guidelines do not comment on PCI but recommend CABG. Still PCI is extensively performed in daily practice due to preference of patients, refusal by surgeons, and feasibility of PCI.

More recently published large, randomized Revascularization for Ischemic Ventricular Dysfunction (REVIVED) trial provided critical evidence on the possible role of PCI in patients with ICM. It showed no significant prognostic impact of PCI over optimal medical therapy (OMT).[16] A total of 700 patients with LVEF ≤ 35% with extensive CAD, suitable for PCI and confirmed myocardial viability, were enrolled in the study. The primary outcome (composite of all-cause mortality and HF hospitalization) over a median of 41 months was comparable between the groups (PCI: 37.2% vs. OMT: 38.0%). Furthermore, there was no difference in LVEF between the groups at 6 and 12 months. Longer-term follow-up is planned, but late benefit is unlikely to emerge as 3.4-year follow-up did not show any discernible effect. However, the results need to be interpreted carefully as there are some major concerns. The trial included only patients with confirmed myocardial viability but previous studies did not demonstrate the benefit of revascularization guided by viability testing. Scar burden, but not viability, predicts the likelihood of LV function recovery. Therefore, based on myocardial viability alone, it is difficult to identify patients with HFrEF who might benefit from PCI.[17,18] Patients enrolled in REVIVED-British Cardiovascular Intervention Society (BCIS)-2 were 10 years older than those enrolled in the STICH trial. Further analyses of REVIVED data are awaited, which will answer some of the questions, for example, the extent of ischemia versus myocardial jeopardy (67% of patients had no angina). BCIS Jeopardy score which was used by investigators to define angiographic eligibility was not validated in HFrEF patients. It was hypothesized that PCI on top of optimal medical treatment would offer the benefits of revascularization without the early mortality associated with CABG.

In the REVIVED trial, despite inclusion of patients with left main disease, PCI was not associated with increased early mortality. Periprocedural myocardial infarction (MI) constituted approximately 40% of all MIs in PCI arm. Twofold increase of spontaneous MI was observed in the optimal medical treatment group when compared to PCI (5.2% vs. 9.3%). Therefore, the overall MI rates at the end were similar in both the groups (OMT 10.8% vs. PCI 10.7%). Moreover, there was no significant difference between the groups in the incidence of automatic implantable cardioverter-defibrillator (AICD) therapy

TABLE 1: CABG versus PCI in ischemic heart failure.

	STICH trial	*REVIVED-BCIS-2 trial*
Number of patients	1,212	700
Mean age	60 years	70 years
Mean LVEF	30%	27%
Revascularization modality	CABG	PCI
Viability imaging	Not mandatory	Mandatory
Patients with viability imaging	50%	100%
Modality used	• CMR: 21% • Remaining SPECT/DSE	• CMR: 70% • Remaining DSE/SPECT/PET
Guideline-directed medical therapy	ACEi/ARB, beta-blockers	• ACEi/ARB/ARNI • Beta-blockers, MRA/SGLT2i
Median follow-up	9.8 years	3.4 years
Primary end point	All-cause mortality	• All-cause mortality • HF hospitalization
Outcome	Favors CABG	No difference

(ACEi: angiotensin-converting enzyme inhibitors; ARB: angiotensin receptor blockers; ARNI: angiotensin receptor neprilysin inhibitors; CABG: coronary artery bypass grafting; CMR: cardiac magnetic resonance; DSE: dobutamine stress echocardiography; HF: heart failure; LVEF: left ventricular ejection fraction; MRA: mineralocorticoid receptor antagonists; PCI: percutaneous coronary intervention; PET: positron emission tomography; REVIVED-BCIS-2: Revascularization for Ischemic Ventricular Dysfunction-British Cardiovascular Intervention Society 2; SLGT2i: sodium–glucose cotransporter 2 inhibitors; SPECT: single-photon emission computed tomography; STICH: Surgical Treatment of Ischemic Heart Failure)

and risk of all-cause mortality or aborted sudden cardiac death, indicating that PCI did not reduce the incidence of potentially fatal ventricular arrhythmias.[19]

The concept of recovery of myocardial hibernation with revascularization has been challenged by this trial. The medical management of HF is evolving rapidly with the introduction of new therapies such as sodium–glucose cotransporter 2 (SGLT2) inhibitors. The important role of OMT in HFrEF patients has emerged as one of the significant findings of the REVIVED trial, but the role of SGLT2 inhibitors has not been addressed by this trial. The key findings in REVIVED-BCIS2 and STICH trial are summarized in **Table 1**.

CONCLUSION

Ischemic cardiomyopathy is associated with high morbidity and mortality and the identification of an ischemic substrate can help in the decision-making process and improve patient's outcomes. To date, the evidence basis for coronary revascularization in ischemic LV dysfunction is largely informed by observational data. There is an absence of direct randomized controlled trial evidence comparing revascularization strategies in these patient populations. This may illustrate why, despite the guidelines and the large body of observational evidence supporting CABG in favor of PCI, high PCI rates have been observed in this patient population in the real world. Better understanding of this discrepancy between theory and practice will require direct randomized evidence of PCI versus CABG in this specific patient population.

Revascularization decisions in patients with reduced LVEF have so far been largely based on STICH trial that showed a benefit of CABG over OMT alone. The beneficial effect of CABG is observed after extended observation (10 years) and therefore it should be performed in carefully selected patients with acceptable perioperative risk. The REVIVED trial confirmed the importance of contemporary pharmacological treatment in the HFrEF setting. But it demonstrated that in stable asymptomatic patients with confirmed myocardial viability, PCI added no benefit in reduction of all-cause mortality or HF hospitalization rates.

Therefore, extended follow-up and more detailed analyses of this study are crucial to confirm these results in the long-term observation and identify potential subgroups of patients in whom PCI might be beneficial.

Flowchart 1: Tailored management algorithm for patients with ischemic heart failure with reduced ejection fraction (HFrEF).

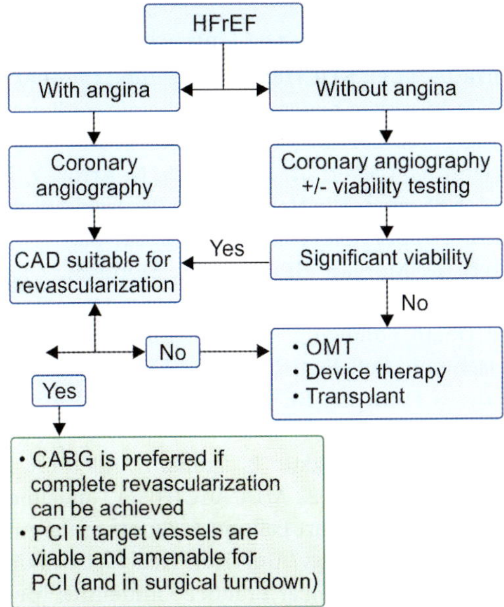

(CABG: coronary artery bypass grafting; CAD: coronary artery disease; OMT optimal medical therapy; PCI: percutaneous coronary intervention)

Both REVIVED-BCIS-2 and STICH trials challenge the hypothesis of hibernating myocardium, amenable to functional improvement following successful revascularization that would ultimately improve prognosis. Assessment of myocardial viability does not aid the selection of patients who will benefit or not from PCI for ICM. So REVIVED-BCIS-2 also challenged long-held beliefs on myocardial viability prior to PCI. The United States and ESC guidelines provide a class 2b recommendation for noninvasive stress imaging to assess myocardial ischemia and viability.[14,20]

The decision on revascularization in ICM often cannot be made based on the guidelines. Therefore, tailored treatment approach is essential with multidisciplinary approach **(Flowchart 1)**. These decisions should be based on the ability to achieve complete revascularization, which may not be accomplished in certain patients.

REFERENCES

1. Mosterd A, Hoes AW. Clinical epidemiology of heart failure. Heart. 2007;93(9):1137-46.
2. Johansson I, Dahlström U, Edner M, Näsman P, Rydén L, Norhammar A. Prognostic implications of type 2 diabetes mellitus in ischemic and nonischemic heart failure. J Am Coll Cardiol. 2016;68(13):1404-16.
3. Wolff G, Dimitroulis D, Andreotti F, Kołodziejczak M, Jung C, Scicchitano P, et al. Survival benefits of invasive versus conservative strategies in heart failure in patients with reduced ejection fraction and coronary artery disease: a meta-analysis. Circ Heart Fail. 2017;10(1):e003255.
4. Allman KC, Shaw LJ, Hachamovitch R, Udelson JE. Myocardial viability testing and impact of revascularization on prognosis in patients with coronary artery disease and left ventricular dysfunction: a meta-analysis. J Am Coll Cardiol. 2002;39(7):1151-8.
5. Neumann FJ, Sousa-Uva M, Ahlsson A, Alfonso F, Banning AP, Benedetto U, et al; ESC Scientific Document Group. 2018 ESC/EACTS Guidelines on myocardial revascularization. Eur Heart J. 2019;40(2):87-165.
6. Velazquez EJ, Lee KL, Deja MA, Jain A, Sopko G, Marchenko A, et al; STICH Investigators. Coronary-artery bypass surgery in patients with left ventricular dysfunction. N Engl J Med. 2011;364(17):1607-16.
7. Panza JA, Ellis AM, Al-Khalidi HR, Holly TA, Berman DS, Oh JK, et al. Myocardial viability and long-term outcomes in ischemic cardiomyopathy. N Engl J Med. 2019; 381(8):739-48.
8. Bonow RO, Maurer G, Lee KL, Holly TA, Binkley PF, Desvigne-Nickens P, et al; STICH Trial Investigators. Myocardial viability and survival in ischemic left ventricular dysfunction. N Engl J Med. 2011;364(17):1617-25.
9. Nieminen MS, Brutsaert D, Dickstein K, Drexler H, Follath F, Harjola VP, et al. EuroHeart Survey Investigators; Heart Failure Association, European Society of Cardiology. EuroHeart Failure Survey II (EHFS II): a survey on hospitalized acute heart failure patients: description of population. Eur Heart J. 2006;27(22):2725-36.
10. Marui A, Kimura T, Nishiwaki N, Komiya T, Hanyu M, Shiomi H, et al; CREDO-Kyoto PCI/CABG Registry Cohort-2 Investigators. Three-year outcomes after percutaneous coronary intervention and coronary artery bypass grafting in patients with heart failure: from the CREDO-Kyoto percutaneous coronary intervention/coronary artery bypass graft registry cohort-2. Eur J Cardiothorac Surg. 2015;47(2):316-21; discussion 321.
11. Serruys PW, Morice MC, Kappetein AP, Colombo A, Holmes DR, Mack MJ, et al; SYNTAX Investigators. Percutaneous coronary intervention versus coronary-artery bypass grafting for severe coronary artery disease. N Engl J Med. 2009;360(10):961-72.
12. Stone GW, Sabik JF, Serruys PW, Simonton CA, Généreux P, Puskas J, et al; EXCEL Trial Investigators. Everolimus-Eluting Stents or Bypass Surgery for Left Main Coronary Artery Disease. N Engl J Med. 2016;375(23):2223-35.
13. Sun LY, Gaudino M, Chen RJ, Bader Eddeen A, Ruel M. Long-term outcomes in patients with severely reduced left ventricular ejection fraction undergoing percutaneous coronary intervention vs coronary artery bypass grafting. JAMA Cardiol. 2020;5(6):631-41.

14. McDonagh TA, Metra M, Adamo M, Gardner RS, Baumbach A, Böhm M, et al; ESC Scientific Document Group. 2021 ESC Guidelines for the diagnosis and treatment of acute and chronic heart failure. Eur Heart J. 2021;42(36):3599-3726.
15. Fihn SD, Gardin JM, Abrams J, Berra K, Blankenship JC, Dallas AP, et al; American College of Cardiology Foundation; American Heart Association Task Force on Practice Guidelines; American College of Physicians; American Association for Thoracic Surgery; Preventive Cardiovascular Nurses Association; Society for Cardiovascular Angiography and Interventions; Society of Thoracic Surgeons. 2012 ACCF/AHA/ACP/AATS/PCNA/SCAI/STS Guideline for the diagnosis and management of patients with stable ischemic heart disease: a report of the American College of Cardiology Foundation/American Heart Association Task Force on Practice Guidelines, and the American College of Physicians, American Association for Thoracic Surgery, Preventive Cardiovascular Nurses Association, Society for Cardiovascular Angiography and Interventions, and Society of Thoracic Surgeons. J Am Coll Cardiol. 2012;60(24):e44-e164.
16. Perera D, Clayton T, O'Kane PD, Greenwood JP, Weerackody R, Ryan M, et al; REVIVED-BCIS2 Investigators. Percutaneous Revascularization for Ischemic Left Ventricular Dysfunction. N Engl J Med. 2022; 387(15):1351-60.
17. Velazquez EJ, Lee KL, Jones RH, Al-Khalidi HR, Hill JA, Panza JA, et al; STICHES Investigators. Coronary-artery bypass surgery in patients with ischemic cardiomyopathy. N Engl J Med. 2016;374(16):1511-20.
18. Cleland JG, Calvert M, Freemantle N, Arrow Y, Ball SG, Bonser RS, et al. The Heart Failure Revascularisation Trial (HEART). Eur J Heart Fail. 2011;13(2):227-33.
19. Perera D, Morgan HP, Ryan M, Dodd M, Clayton T, O'Kane PD, et al; REVIVED-BCIS2 Investigators. Arrhythmia and Death Following Percutaneous Revascularization in Ischemic Left Ventricular Dysfunction: Prespecified Analyses From the REVIVED-BCIS2 Trial. Circulation. 2023;148(11):862-71.
20. Heidenreich PA, Bozkurt B, Aguilar D, Allen LA, Byun JJ, Colvin MM, et al. 2022 AHA/ACC/HFSA Guideline for the Management of Heart Failure: A Report of the American College of Cardiology/American Heart Association Joint Committee on Clinical Practice Guidelines [published correction appears in J Am Coll Cardiol. 2023;81(15):1551]. J Am Coll Cardiol 2022;79(17):e263-e421.

Recent Advances in Guidelines-directed Management of Acute Coronary Syndrome

Viveka Kumar, Sangeeta Dhir, Mitendra Singh Yadav

INTRODUCTION

Acute coronary syndromes (ACS) comprise a spectrum of conditions with patients presenting recent changes in clinical symptoms or signs, possible electrocardiogram (ECG) changes and elevation in cardiac troponin (cTn) concentrations. Pathologically ACS are typically caused by the disruption (rupture or erosion) of an unstable coronary artery atherosclerotic plaque with associated partial or complete coronary artery thrombosis and/or microemboli, that results in reduced. Based on severity ACS presents three clinical conditions—unstable angina, non-ST-segment elevation myocardial infarction (NSTEMI) and ST-segment elevation myocardial infarction (STEMI). Classical definition of unstable angina is transient myocardial ischemia leading to diminished flow in the absence of significant myocardial necrosis detected by circulating troponin. Patients with severe myocardial ischemia are diagnosed with myocardial infarction (MI) and have elevated inflammatory biomarker troponin. NSTEMI may present with a partially occluded vessel causing subendocardial ischemia. In contrast STEMI presents a completely occluded vessel leading to transmural myocardial ischemia and infarction. Underlying pathogenesis of the inflammation leads to increased accumulation of lipids within an atherosclerotic plaque which causes plaque instability, its rupture and exposure of the plaque contents to circulation. This causes activation of the coagulation cascade and subsequent thrombosis. The presence of thrombus may compromise flow to the myocardium, leading to myocardial ischemia and necrosis. borne by low- and middle-income countries. ACS is often the first clinical manifestation of cardiovascular disease (CVD). In 2019, there were an estimated 5.8 million new cases of ischemic heart disease worldwide. Ischemic heart disease is the most common cause of cardiovascular death with 38% of all CVD deaths in females and 44% in males. This chapter reviews the management of patients suffering from ACS based on the recently published guideline.[1]

DIAGNOSIS OF ACUTE CORONARY SYNDROME

Acute chest discomfort (presented by patient—pain, pressure, tightness, heaviness, or burning) is the chief symptom. Chest pain can be classified as cardiac, possibly cardiac, and likely non-cardiac. It can be described as—dyspnea, epigastric pain, and pain in the left or right arm or neck/jaw. The initial ECG, history, examination, biomarkers, and other aids are essential for evaluation.

RECOMMENDATIONS FOR PATIENT ASSESSMENT IN HOSPITAL (FOR POSSIBLE ACS/CONFIRMED ACS)[2]

- *Suspected ACS:* ECG to be done ECG within 10 minutes is recommended to help guide patient management.
- *Suspected ACS with deteriorating symptoms:* Initial ECG may be nondiagnostic, serial 12-lead ECGs should be performed (detects ischemic changes).
- *Suspected ACS:* High-sensitivity cTn assay should be measured at earliest.

MANAGEMENT OF PATIENT PRESENTING WITH CARDIAC ARREST

Emergency medical services transfer approximately 10% patients with out-of-hospital cardiac arrest. Literature states that timely recognition of STEMI in resuscitated patients and direct transfer to a percutaneous transluminal coronary angioplasty (PTCA) center improves the survival rate of the patients.[3] Postcardiac arrest resuscitation of patients with STEMI are comparable to patients with STEMI with no cardiac arrest. Former section of patients (resuscitated postcardiac arrest) are candidates for

BOX 1: Recommendations for management of patients presenting with cardiac arrest.

- Resuscitated arrest patients with ST-segment elevation myocardial infarction (STEMI) should be transferred by EMS to angioplasty facility hospital[4]
- Resuscitated noncomatose/comatose cardiac arrest patients with favorable prognostic features and with evidence of STEMI, should be treated with angioplasty for improve survival rate[5]
- Comatose cardiac arrest patients, with unfavorable prognosis and evidence of STEMI, angioplasty may be done after assessment[6]
- Angiography is not recommended in resuscitated comatose cardiac arrest patients without STEMI (stable on electrical and hemodynamic parameters otherwise) due to lack of benefit

primary percutaneous coronary intervention (PPCI), i.e., coronary angioplasty. Stable ST-segment elevation patients with out-of-hospital cardiac arrest, do not require immediate coronary angiography. It can be deferred until risk assessment is done **(Box 1)**.

MEDICAL TREATMENT RECOMMENDATIONS FOR PATIENTS WITH STEMI AND NSTE-ACS (BOXES 2 AND 3)

- *Oxygen therapy:* In patients with ACS and confirmed hypoxia (oxygen saturation <90%), supplemental oxygen to increase oxygen saturations to ≥90% is recommended to improve myocardial oxygen supply and decrease angina symptoms.[7,8]
- *Analgesics:* Patients presenting with known or suspected ACS often experience chest pain or other uncomfortable symptoms. Rapid and effective pain relief remains an important treatment goal to prevent sympathetic activation and adverse clinical sequelae. Analgesic therapies may provide symptomatic relief, but they have not been shown to improve clinical outcomes in patients with ACS.
- *Antiplatelet:* Aspirin has long been considered an integral part of antiplatelet therapy to prevent recurrent atherothrombotic events among patients with ACS. In patients with ACS, an initial oral loading dose of aspirin, followed by aspirin should be initiated with a loading dose (162–325 mg) in patients with ACS irrespective of final management strategy (invasive or noninvasive), followed by a daily low maintenance dose daily low-dose aspirin, is recommended to reduce death and major adverse cardiovascular events (MACE).[9] Current evidence supports the use of uncoated low-dose aspirin (75–100 mg) for daily maintenance therapy. The 75–100 mg daily dose of aspirin exceeds the minimal effective dose required for platelet thromboxane A2 suppression.[9] Oral inhibitors of the platelet purinergic receptor P2Y, G-protein coupled, 12 protein ($P2Y_{12}$) receptor antagonize adenosine diphosphate-mediated activation of platelets. Across the spectrum of ACS, the addition of a $P2Y_{12}$ inhibitor to aspirin significantly reduces platelet aggregation and has been shown to reduce the incidence of recurrent MACE but with an increased risk of bleeding.[10,11] Popular oral $P2Y_{12}$ inhibitors include clopidogrel, prasugrel, and ticagrelor **(Table 1)**.
- *Intravenous glycoprotein 2b/3a inhibitors:* Glycoprotein IIb/IIIa receptor inhibitors are parenterally administered drugs that block platelet aggregation by preventing platelet crosslinking via fibrinogen or von Willebrand factor binding to the glycoprotein

BOX 2: Recommendations for standard of care—reperfusion strategies—ST-segment elevation myocardial infarction (STEMI) PCI-enabled hospitals.

- In patients with STEMI presenting <12 hours after symptom onset, primary percutaneous coronary intervention (PPCI) should be performed with a goal of first medical contact (FMC) to device activation of ≤90 minutes, or ≤120 minutes in patients requiring hospital transfer, to improve survival[21]
- In patients with acute coronary syndrome (ACS) and cardiogenic shock or hemodynamic instability, emergency revascularization of the culprit vessel by PCI or coronary artery bypass graft (CABG) is indicated to improve survival, irrespective of time from symptom onset
- In patients who are stable with STEMI who have a totally occluded infarct-related artery >24 hours after symptom onset and are without evidence of ongoing ischemia, acute severe HF, or life-threatening arrhythmia, PPCI should not be performed due to lack of benefit

BOX 3: Recommendations for standard of care—reperfusion strategies—ST-segment elevation myocardial infarction (STEMI) non-PCI-enabled Hospitals.

- In patients with STEMI and an estimated time from first medical contact (FMC) to device activation of ≤120 minutes or those with a contraindication to fibrinolytic therapy, transfer to a PCI-capable hospital for PPCI is recommended to reduce MACE[22]
- In patients with STEMI and symptom onset of <12 hours and anticipated delay to PPC >120 minutes from FMC, fibrinolytic therapy should be administered in patients without contraindication to reduce MACE[23]

TABLE 1: Recommendations for antiplatelet therapy (aspirin and $P2Y_{12}$ inhibitors).[1,2]

All patients with acute coronary syndrome (ACS) [ST-segment elevation myocardial infarction (STEMI) and NSTE-ACS]	• Patients with ACS, an oral $P2Y_{12}$ inhibitor, should be administered in addition to aspirin to reduce MACE • In patients with a history of stroke or transient ischemic attack, prasugrel should not be administered because of worse net clinical outcomes
Management in patients with STEMI and NSTE-ACS	• In patients with NSTE-ACS undergoing percutaneous coronary intervention (PCI), prasugrel or ticagrelor is recommended to reduce • Major adverse cardiovascular events (MACE) and stent thrombosis • Clopidogrel is recommended to reduce MACE when prasugrel or ticagrelor are (unavailable, cannot be tolerated, or are contraindicated) • In patients with NSTE-ACS planned for an invasive strategy with timing of angiography anticipated to be >24 hours, upstream treatment with clopidogrel or ticagrelor may be considered to reduce MACE • In patients with STEMI managed with fibrinolytic therapy, clopidogrel should be administered concurrently to reduce death and MACE
Intravenous $P2Y_{12}$ inhibition	Among patients with ACS undergoing PCI who have not received a $P2Y_{12}$ inhibitor, intravenous cangrelor may be reasonable to reduce periprocedural ischemic events

IIb/IIIa receptor. However, limited data is available on its use. In patients with ACS, glycoprotein IIb/IIIa inhibitors should not be administered routinely due to lack of ischemic benefit and increased risk of bleeding.[12,13]

- *Parenteral anticoagulation:* Parenteral anticoagulation is recommended for all patients with ACS, irrespective of the initial treatment strategy, to treat the underlying pathophysiologic process (coronary atherothrombosis) and reduce the risk of recurrent MACE **(Table 2)**.
- *Lipid management:* Atherosclerotic cardiovascular disease (ASCVD) event rates are substantially higher (10–15%) in patients with recent ACS hospitalization. These events include rates of cardiovascular death, MI, and ischemic stroke.[17] Higher risk among patients with ACS supports more aggressive management of LDL-cholesterol (LDL-c). Multiple therapeutic drugs are available which include statins and non-statins **(Table 3)**.

TABLE 2: Recommendations for parenteral anticoagulation.[1]

NSTE-acute coronary syndrome (ACS) anticoagulant therapy	• In patients with NSTE-ACS, intravenous unfractionated heparin (UFH) is useful to reduce ischemic events[14] • When early invasive approach is not anticipated, either enoxaparin or fondaparinux are recommended alternatives to UFH to reduce ischemic event[15]
Anticoagulant therapy in patients undergoing coronary revascularization	Patients with ACS undergoing coronary revascularization [coronary artery bypass graft (CABG) or percutaneous coronary intervention (PCI)] in the same admission, parenteral anticoagulation should be continued until revascularization to reduce ischemic event[16]
Anticoagulant therapy to support PCI in ACS [ST-segment elevation myocardial infarction (STEMI) and NSTE-ACS]	• In patients with STEMI undergoing PCI, bivalirudin is useful as an alternative to UFH to reduce mortality and bleeding • In patients with ACS, fondaparinux should not be used to support PCI because of the risk of catheter thrombosis
STEMI: Anticoagulant therapy treated with fibrinolytic therapy	• Enoxaparin and fondaparinux are the recommended anticoagulants to reduce ischemic events in patients with STEMI who are not intended to undergo an invasive approach • STEMI treated with fibrinolytic therapy, parenteral anticoagulation should be continued for the duration of the hospital stay (maximum of 8 days) or until revascularization is performed to reduce ischemic events

- *Beta blockers:* The clinical benefits of beta blockers in patients with left ventricular ejection fraction (LVEF) <40% and stabilized HF are well established, including patients post-MI. Beta blockers decrease myocardial oxygen demand by reducing the heart rate, blood pressure, and myocardial contractility.[18] In patients with ACS without contraindications, early (<24 hours) initiation of oral beta-blocker therapy is recommended to reduce risk of reinfarction and ventricular arrhythmias.[19]

TABLE 3: Statin classification.

High intensity	*Moderate intensity*	*Low intensity*
• Atorvastatin 40–80 mg • Rosuvastatin 20–40 mg	• Atorvastatin 10–20 mg • Rosuvastatin 5–10 mg • Simvastatin 20–40 mg • Pravastatin 40–80 mg • Lovastatin 40 mg • Fluvastatin XL 80 mg • Fluvastatin 40 mg BID • Pitavastatin 1–4 mg	• Simvastatin 10 mg • Pravastatin 10–20 mg • Lovastatin 20 mg • Fluvastatin 20–40 mg

- *Renin-angiotensin aldosterone system inhibitors:* In high-risk patients with ACS (LVEF ≤40%, hypertension, diabetes mellitus, or STEMI with anterior location), an oral angiotensin-converting enzyme inhibitor (ACEi) or an angiotensin receptor blocker (ARB) is indicated to reduce all-cause death and MACE.[20] In patients with ACS who are not considered high risk, an oral ACEi or an ARB is reasonable to reduce MACE.[20]

TIMING AND CHOICE OF FIBRINOLYTIC THERAPY

The benefit of fibrinolytic therapy in patients who present >12 hours after symptom onset has not been established.[24] Patients should be transferred to a PCI-capable hospital after initiation of fibrinolytic therapy for routine coronary angiography.

RECOMMENDATION FOR CORONARY ANGIOGRAPHY AND PERCUTANEOUS CORONARY INTERVENTION AFTER FIBRINOLYTIC THERAPY

Failure of reperfusion and risk of reocclusion after successful fibrinolytic therapy are important limitations of fibrinolytic therapy. Hence, patients are transferred to PCI-capable hospital to facilitate immediate or early catheterization depending on the clinical circumstances **(Box 4)**.

BOX 4: Recommendations for coronary angiography (CAG) and percutaneous coronary intervention (PCI) after fibrinolytic therapy.

- In patients with ST-segment elevation myocardial infarction (STEMI), transfer to a PCI-capable center immediately after fibrinolytic therapy is recommended[25]
- Patients with STEMI with suspected failed reperfusion after fibrinolytic therapy, immediate angiography with rescue PCI is recommended to reduce the risk of death or recurrent MI
- In patients with STEMI treated with fibrinolytic therapy, early angiography between 2 and 24 hours with the intent to perform PCI is recommended to reduce the rates of death or MI

CONSIDERATIONS FOR CATHETERIZATION IN ACUTE CORONARY SYNDROME

- *Vascular approach:* In patients with ACS undergoing PCI, a radial approach is preferred to a femoral approach to reduce bleeding, vascular complications, and death.[26]
- *Intracoronary imaging:* In patients with ACS undergoing coronary stent implantation in left main artery or in complex lesions, intracoronary imaging with intravascular ultrasound (IVUS) or optical coherence tomography (OCT) is recommended for procedural guidance to reduce ischemic events.[27]
- *Multivessel coronary artery disease (CAD) in STEMI ACS:* In selected hemodynamically stable patients with STEMI and multivessel disease (MVD), after successful PCI of the infarct-related artery, PCI of significantly stenosed noninfarct-related arteries is recommended to reduce the risk of death or MI and improve angina-related quality of life.[28]
- *Multivessel CAD in NSTEMI ACS:* In stable patients with NSTE-ACS with MVD but without left main stenosis who are not intended for coronary artery bypass graft (CABG) surgery and undergoing culprit-lesion PCI, PCI of significant non-culprit lesions (at the time of the index procedure or as a staged procedure) is recommended to reduce the risk of MACE.[29]

IN-HOSPITAL CONCERNS: ACUTE CORONARY SYNDROME MANAGEMENT (TABLE 4)

Patients with ACS and with ongoing angina, hemodynamic instability, uncontrolled arrhythmias, suboptimal reperfusion, or cardiogenic shock should be admitted to a cardiac intensive care unit (CICU) to reduce cardiovascular events.

HOSPITAL DISCHARGE PLANNING: RECOMMENDATIONS

General Recommendations

Patients with ACS should be referred to an outpatient Cardiac Rehabilitation program prior to hospital discharge

TABLE 4: Recommendations for acute coronary syndrome (ACS) complications.

Mechanical complications	Patients with a mechanical complication of ACS should be managed in a facility with cardiac surgical expertise
Electrical complications	• *Ventricular arrhythmia:* In patients post MI, implantable cardioverter defibrillator (ICD) implantation is recommended. In selected patients with a left ventricular ejection fraction (LVEF) ≤40% at least 40 days post MI and at least 90 days post-revascularization to reduce death[30] • *Bradyarrhythmia:* In patients presenting with an acute myocardial infarction (AMI) with sustained evidence of second-degree Mobitz type II atrioventricular block, high-grade atrioventricular block, alternating bundle-branch block, or third-degree atrioventricular block (persistent or infranodal), permanent pacing is indicated[31]

to reduce death, MI, hospital readmissions, and improve functional status and quality of life.

Post-discharge Strategy—dual Antiplatelet Therapy and Anticoagulant Therapy First 12 months

- In patients with ACS who are not at high bleeding risk, dual antiplatelet therapy (DAPT) with aspirin and an oral $P2Y_{12}$ inhibitor should be administered for at least 1 year to reduce MACE.[32]
- In patients with ACS who have tolerated DAPT with ticagrelor, transition to ticagrelor monotherapy ≥1 month post PCI is useful to reduce bleeding risk.[33]
- In patients at high risk of gastrointestinal bleeding, a proton pump inhibitor (PPI) is recommended in combination with DAPT, oral anticoagulants, or both to reduce risk of bleeding.[34]
- In patients with ACS who require oral anticoagulant therapy, aspirin should be discontinued after 1–4 weeks of triple antithrombotic therapy, with continued use of a $P2Y_{12}$ inhibitor (preferably clopidogrel) and an oral anticoagulant to reduce bleeding risk.[35]

CONCLUSION

ACS is a potentially life-threatening condition. It affects millions of patients. Timely identification and prevention of ACS continues to be important public health concern. Preliminary ACS management should include risk stratification, appropriate medical management including DAPT, anticoagulation and appropriate adjuvant therapies, and a decision to pursue early invasive or conventional treatment strategy. Effective long-term management of ACS involves following evidence-based recommendation.

REFERENCES

1. Rao SV, O'Donoghue ML, Ruel M, Rab T, Tamis-Holland JE, Alexander JH, et al. 2025 ACC/AHA/ACEP/NAEMSP/SCAI guideline for the management of patients with acute coronary syndromes: a report of the American College of Cardiology/American Heart Association Joint Committee on Clinical Practice Guidelines. Circulation. 2025;151:e771-e862.
2. Gulati M, Levy PD, Mukherjee D, Amsterdam E, Bhatt DL, Birtcher KK, et al. 2021 AHA/ACC/ASE/CHEST/SAEM/SCCT/SCMR Guideline for the Evaluation and Diagnosis of Chest Pain: A Report of the American College of Cardiology/American Heart Association Joint Committee on Clinical Practice Guidelines. Circulation. 2021;144:e368-e454.
3. Kragholm K, Lu D, Chiswell K, Al-Khalidi HR, Roettig ML, Roe M, et al. Improvement in care and outcomes for emergency medical service-transported patients with ST-elevation myocardial infarction (STEMI) with and without prehospital cardiac arrest: a Mission: Lifeline STEMI Accelerator study. J Am Heart Assoc. 2017;6:e005717.
4. Wnent J, Seewald S, Heringlake M, Lemke H, Brauer K, Lefering R, et al. Choice of hospital after out-of hospital cardiac arrest-a decision with far-reaching consequences: a studying large German city. Crit Care. 2012;16:R164.
5. Gorjup V, Radsel P, Kocjancic ST, Erzen D, Noc M. Acute ST-elevation myocardial infarction after successful cardiopulmonary resuscitation. Resuscitation. 2007;72:379-85.
6. Desch S, Freund A, Akin I, Behnes M, Preusch MR, Zelniker TA, et al. Angiography after out-of-hospital cardiac arrest without ST-segment elevation. N Engl J Med. 2021;385:2544-53.
7. Sukumalchantra Y, Levy S, Danzig R, Rubins S, Alpern H, Swan HJ. Correcting arterial hypoxemia by oxygen therapy in patients with acute myocardial infarction. Effect on ventilation and hemodynamics. Am J Cardiol. 1969;24:838-52.
8. CURRENT-OASIS 7 Investigators; Mehta SR, Bassand JP, Chrolavicius S, Diaz R, Eikelboom JW, et al. Dose comparisons of clopidogrel and aspirin in acute coronary syndromes. N Engl J Med. 2010;363:930-42.
9. Patrono C, Garcia Rodriguez LA, Landolfi R, Baigent C. Low-dose aspirin for the prevention of atherothrombosis. N Engl J Med. 2005;353:2373-83.

10. Yusuf S, Zhao F, Mehta SR, Chrolavicius S, Tognoni G, Fox KK, et al. Effects of clopidogrel in addition to aspirin in patients with acute coronary syndromes without ST-segment elevation. N Engl J Med. 2001;345:494-502.
11. Steg PG, James S, Harrington RA, Ardissino D, Becker RC, Cannon CP, et al. Ticagrelor versus clopidogrel in patients with ST-elevation acute coronary syndromes intended for reperfusion with primary percutaneous coronary intervention: Platelet Inhibition and Patient Outcomes (PLATO) trial subgroup analysis. Circulation. 2010; 122:2131-41.
12. Harrington RA, Stone GW, McNulty S, White HD, Lincoff AM, Gibson CM, et al. Platelet inhibition with cangrelor in patients undergoing PCI. N Engl J Med. 2009; 361:2318-29.
13. Steg PG, Bhatt DL, Hamm CW, Stone GW, Gibson CM, Mahaffey KW, et al. Effect of cangrelor on periprocedural outcomes in percutaneous coronary interventions: a pooled analysis of patient-level data. Lancet. 2013;382:1981-92.
14. Risk of myocardial infarction and death during treatment with low dose aspirin and intravenous heparin in men with unstable coronary artery disease. The RISC Group. Lancet. 1990;336:827-30.
15. Murphy SA, Gibson CM, Morrow DA, Van de Werf F, Menown IB, Goodman SG, et al. Efficacy and safety of the low molecular weight heparin enoxaparin compared with unfractionated Heparin across the acute coronary syndrome spectrum: a meta-analysis. Eur Heart J. 2007;28:2077-86.
16. Bahit MC, Topol EJ, Califf RM, Armstrong PW, Criger DA, Hasselblad V, et al. Reactivation of ischemic events in acute coronary syndromes: results from GUSTO-IIb. Global Use of Strategies To Open occluded arteries in acute coronary syndromes. J Am Coll Cardiol. 2001;37:1001-7.
17. Ulvenstam A, Graipe A, Irewall AL, Söderström L, Mooe T. Incidence and predictors of cardiovascular outcomes after acute coronary syndrome in a population-based Cohort study. Sci Rep. 2023;13:3447.
18. Freemantle N, Cleland J, Young P, Mason J, Harrison J. Beta blockade after myocardial infarction: systematic review and meta regression analysis. BMJ. 1999;318:1730-7.
19. Dahl Aarvik M, Sandven I, Dondo TB, Gale CP, Ruddox V, Munkhaugen J, et al. Effect of oral beta-blocker treatment on mortality in contemporary post-myocardial infarction patients: a Systematic review and meta-analysis. Eur Heart J Cardiovasc Pharmacother. 2019;5:12-20.
20. ACE Inhibitor Myocardial Infarction Collaborative Group. Indications for AC inhibitors in the early treatment of acute myocardial infarction: systematic overview of individual data from 100 000 patients in randomized trials. Circulation. 1998;97:2202-12.
21. Keeley EC, Boura JA, Grines CL. Primary angioplasty versus intravenous thrombolytic therapy for acute myocardial infarction: a quantitative review of 23 randomised trials. Lancet. 2003;361:13-20.
22. French WJ, Gunderson M, Travis D, Bieniarz M, Zegre-Hemsey J, Goyal A, et al. Emergency interhospital transfer of patients with ST-segment-elevation myocardial infarction: call 9-1-1-the American Heart Association Mission: Lifeline Program. J Am Heart Assoc. 2022;11:e026700.
23. GUSTO investigators. An international randomized trial comparing four thrombolytic strategies for acute myocardial infarction. N Engl J Med. 1993;329:673-82.
24. Indications for fibrinolytic therapy in suspected acute myocardial infarction: collaborative overview of early mortality and major morbidity results from all randomised trials of more than 1000 patients. Fibrinolytic Therapy Trialists' (FTT) Collaborative Group. Lancet. 1994; 343:311-22.
25. Bohmer E, Hoffmann P, Abdelnoor M, Arnesen H, Halvorsen S. Efficacy and safety of immediate angioplasty versus ischemia-guided management after thrombolysis in acute myocardial infarction in areas with very long transfer distances results of the NORDISTEMI (NORwegian study on District treatment of ST-elevation myocardial infarction). J Am Coll Cardiol. 2010;55:102-10.
26. Valgimigli M, Frigoli E, Leonardi S, Vranckx P, Rothenbühler M, Tebaldi M, et al. Radial versus femoral access and bivalirudin versus unfractionated heparin in invasively managed patients with Acute coronary syndrome (MATRIX): final 1-year results of a multicentre, randomised controlled trial. Lancet. 2018;392:835-48.
27. Lee JM, Choi KH, Song YB, Lee JY, Lee SJ, Lee SY, et al. Intravascular imaging-guided or angiography-guided complex PCI. N Engl J Med.2023;388:1668-79.
28. Gershlick AH, Khan JN, Kelly DJ, Greenwood JP, Sasikaran T, Curzen N, et al. Randomized trial of complete versus lesion-only revascularization in patients undergoing primary percutaneous coronary intervention for STEMI and multivessel disease: the CvLPRIT trial. J Am Coll Cardiol. 2015;65:963-72.
29. Sardella G, Lucisano L, Garbo R, Pennacchi M, Cavallo E, Stio RE, et al. Single-staged compared with multistaged PCI in multivessel NSTEMI patients: the SMILE trial. J Am Coll Cardiol. 2016;67:264-72.
30. Moss AJ, Hall WJ, Cannom DS, Daubert JP, Higgins SL, Klein H, et al. Improved survival with an implanted defibrillator in patients with coronary disease at high risk for ventricular arrhythmia. N Engl J Med. 1996;335:1933-40.
31. Kim HL, Kim SH, Seo JB, Chung WY, Zo JH, Kim MA, et al. Influence of second-and third-degree heart block on 30-day outcome following acute myocardial infarction in the drug-eluting stent era. Am J Cardiol. 2014;114:1658-62.
32. Fox KA, Mehta SR, Peters R, Zhao F, Lakkis N, Gersh BJ, et al. Benefits and risks of the combination of clopidogrel and

aspirin in patients undergoing surgical revascularization for non-ST-elevation acute coronary syndrome: the Clopidogrel in Unstable angina to prevent Recurrent ischemic Events (CURE) Trial. Circulation. 2004;110:1202-8.

33. Kim BK, Hong SJ, Cho YH, Yun KH, Kim YH, Suh Y, et al. Effect of ticagrelor monotherapy vs ticagrelor with aspirin on major bleeding and cardiovascular events in patients with acute coronary syndrome: the TICO randomized clinical trial. JAMA. 2020;323:2407-16.
34. Ahn HJ, Lee SR, Choi EK, Rhee TM, Kwon S, Oh S, et al. Protective effect of proton-pump inhibitor against gastrointestinal bleeding in patients receiving oral anticoagulants: a systematic review and meta-analysis. Br J Clin Pharmacol. 2022;88:4676-87.
35. Cannon CP, Bhatt DL, Oldgren J, Lip GYH, Ellis SG, Kimura T, et al. Dual antithrombotic therapy with dabigatran after PCI in atrial fibrillation. N Engl J Med. 2017;377:1513-24.

Chronic Coronary Syndrome: Diagnosis and Management

Monotosh Panja, Arindam Pande, Madhumanti Panja

INTRODUCTION

The term "stable coronary artery disease" has been updated to "chronic coronary syndrome" (CCS), reflecting a more accurate classification of CAD, which now encompasses two primary clinical presentations: Acute coronary syndrome (ACS) and CCS. CAD is a dynamic disease process characterized by atherosclerotic plaque formation, rupture, and erosion, which can be influenced by lifestyle modifications, pharmacological therapies, and revascularization. These interventions promote plaque stabilization or regression, thereby slowing or preventing disease progression.

Chronic coronary syndrome represents an updated conceptual framework encompassing various clinical manifestations stemming from chronic structural and/or functional abnormalities in the coronary arteries and microvasculature. These pathological changes create a predisposition for transient myocardial hypoperfusion (ischemia) due to demand-supply imbalance, typically—though not exclusively—triggered by physical exertion, emotional stress, or other physiological stressors. Clinical presentations may include angina pectoris, atypical chest discomfort, dyspnea, or remain entirely asymptomatic. While often clinically stable for extended periods, CCS reflects an inherently progressive disease process that carries the constant risk of acute destabilization manifesting as ACS. Importantly, this nomenclature distinguishes between the underlying coronary pathology and its clinical manifestations.

DIAGNOSIS OF CHRONIC CORONARY SYNDROME

Coronary artery disease primarily results from athero-sclerotic plaque accumulation in the major epicardial coronary arteries, leading to progressive luminal obstruction. The hallmark symptom of angina pectoris occurs when this obstruction creates an imbalance between myocardial oxygen demand and supply, resulting in transient myocardial ischemia. This pathophysiological mechanism underlies both CCSs and acute coronary events.

Patients typically report substernal chest discomfort characterized by pressure or heaviness, often radiating to the jaw, shoulder, back, or arm, with episodes lasting several minutes. This symptomatology demonstrates classic provocation by physical exertion, emotional stress, cold exposure, or heavy meals, and typically resolves with rest or sublingual nitroglycerin within 2–5 minutes. Some patients may present with anginal equivalents, including epigastric discomfort, exertional dyspnea, unexplained fatigue, or presyncope. Based on symptom characteristics, presentations are clinically categorized as:

1. Typical angina (meeting all classic features)
2. Atypical angina (partial symptom correspondence), or
3. Noncardiac chest pain (lacking ischemic features)

The different clinical scenarios in patients with suspected or established CCS are:

- Patients with suspected CAD and "stable" anginal symptoms, and/or dyspnea
- Patients with new onset of heart failure (HF) or left ventricular (LV) dysfunction and suspected CAD
- Asymptomatic and symptomatic patients with stabilized symptoms <1 year after an ACS, or patients with recent revascularization
- Asymptomatic and symptomatic patients >1 year after initial diagnosis or revascularization[1]
- Patients with angina and suspected vasospastic or microvascular disease, and
- Asymptomatic subjects in whom CAD is detected at screening.

The pretest probability of CAD is based on age, gender, and nature of symptoms which have undergone major revisions in the European Society of Cardiology (ESC)

Guidelines 2024. A new phrase *"Clinical likelihood of CAD"* that utilizes various risk factors of CAD which have also been updated. The application of various diagnostic tests in different patient groups to rule-in or rule-out CAD has been updated.

RECENT GUIDELINES OF CHRONIC CORONARY SYNDROME[2]

Recent guidelines of chronic coronary syndrome are shown in **Table 1**.

TABLE 1: New major recommendations in 2024.

Recommendations	*Class[a]*	*Level[b]*
History taking and risk factor assessment and resting electrocardiogram in individuals with suspected chronic coronary syndrome—Section 3		
In individuals reporting symptoms of suspected myocardial ischemic origin, a detailed assessment of cardiovascular risk factors, medical history, and symptom characteristics (including onset, duration, type, location, triggers, relieving factors, and time of day) is recommended	I	C
Symptoms such as chest pain triggered by emotional stress; dyspnea or dizziness on exertion; pain in the arms, jaw, neck, or upper back; or fatigue should be considered as potential angina equivalents	IIa	B
Basic biochemistry in the initial diagnostic management of individuals with suspected chronic coronary syndrome—Section 3		
Additionally, high-sensitivity C-reactive protein and/or fibrinogen plasma levels should be considered	IIa	B
Likelihood of obstructive atherosclerotic coronary artery disease in the initial diagnostic management of individuals with suspected chronic coronary syndrome—Section 3		
It is recommended to estimate the pretest likelihood of obstructive epicardial CAD using the risk factor-weighted clinical likelihood model	I	B
It is recommended to use additional clinical data (e.g., examination of peripheral arteries, resting ECG, resting echocardiography, presence of vascular calcifications on previously performed imaging tests) to adjust the estimate yielded by the "Risk Factor-weighted Clinical Likelihood" model	I	C
In individuals with a *very low* (≤5%) pretest likelihood of obstructive CAD, deferral of further diagnostic tests should be considered	IIa	B
In individuals with a *low* (>5–15%) pretest likelihood of obstructive CAD, CACS should be considered to reclassify subjects and to identify more individuals with very low (≤5%) CACS-weighted clinical likelihood	IIa	B
In individuals with an initially low (>5–15%) likelihood of obstructive CAD, exercise ECG and detection of atherosclerotic disease in noncoronary arteries may be considered to adjust the pretest likelihood estimate	IIb	C
Ambulatory electrocardiogram in the initial diagnostic management of individuals with suspected chronic coronary syndrome—Section 3		
Ambulatory ECG monitoring should be considered in subjects with suspected vasospastic angina	IIa	B
Noninvasive anatomical imaging tests in the initial diagnostic management of individuals with suspected obstructive coronary artery disease—coronary computed tomography angiography, if available and supported by local expertise—Section 3		
In individuals with suspected CCS and low or moderate (>5–50%) pretest likelihood of obstructive CAD, CCTA is recommended to diagnose obstructive CAD and to estimate the risk of MACE	I	A
Noninvasive tests in the initial diagnostic management of individuals with suspected chronic coronary syndrome—stress echocardiography, if available and supported by local expertise—Section 3		
In individuals with suspected CCS and moderate or high (>15–85%) pretest likelihood of obstructive CAD, stress echocardiography is recommended to diagnose myocardial ischemia and to estimate the risk of MACE	I	B
During stress echocardiography, when two or more contiguous myocardial segments are not visualized, it is recommended to use commercially available intravenous ultrasound contrast agents (microbubbles) to improve diagnostic accuracy	I	B
During stress echocardiography, myocardial perfusion using commercially available intravenous ultrasound contrast agents (microbubbles) is recommended to improve diagnostic accuracy and to refine risk stratification beyond wall motion	I	B

Contd...

Contd...

Recommendations	*Class*[a]	*Level*[b]
During stress echocardiography, Doppler left anterior descending coronary artery flow reserve may be considered to improve risk stratification beyond wall motion and to assess microvascular function	IIb	B
Noninvasive functional myocardial imaging tests in the initial diagnostic management of individuals with suspected chronic coronary syndrome—resting and stress single-photon emission computed tomography/positron emission tomography—cardiac magnetic resonance imaging, if available and supported by local expertise—Section 3		
In individuals with suspected CCS and moderate or high (>15–85%) pretest likelihood of obstructive CAD, SPECT or, preferably, PET myocardial perfusion imaging is recommended to: • Diagnose and quantify myocardial ischemia and/or scar • Estimate the risk of MACE • Quantify myocardial blood flow (PET)	I	B
In patients selected for PET or SPECT myocardial perfusion imaging, it is recommended to measure CACS from unenhanced chest CT imaging (used for attenuation correction) to improve detection of both nonobstructive and obstructive CAD	I	B
In individuals with suspected CCS and moderate or high (>15–85%) pretest likelihood of obstructive CAD, CMR perfusion imaging is recommended to diagnose and quantify myocardial ischemia and/or scar and estimate the risk of MACE	I	B
Definition of high risk of adverse events		
An initial stratification of risk of adverse events is recommended based on basic clinical assessment (e.g., age, ECG, anginal threshold, diabetes, CKD, and LVEF)	I	B
The use of one or more of the following test results is recommended to identify individuals at high risk of adverse events: • *Exercise ECG:* Duke Treadmill Score < –10 • *Stress SPECT or PET perfusion imaging:* Area of ischemia ≥10% of the LV myocardium • *Stress echocardiography:* ≥3 of 16 segments with stress-induced hypokinesia or akinesia • *Stress CMR:* – ≥2 of 16 segments with stress perfusion defects, or – ≥3 dobutamine-induced dysfunctional segments • *CCTA:* – Left main disease with ≥50% stenosis – Three-vessel disease with ≥70 stenosis, or – Two-vessel disease with 70% stenosis, including the proximal LAD, or – One-vessel disease of the proximal LAD with ≥70% stenosis and FFR-CT ≤0.8	I	B
Cardiovascular risk, lifestyle changes, and exercise interventions in patients with established chronic coronary syndrome—Section 4		
An informed discussion on CVD risk and treatment benefits tailored to individual patient needs is recommended	I	C
Multidisciplinary behavioral approaches to help patients to achieve healthy lifestyles, in addition to appropriate pharmacological management, are recommended	I	A
Aerobic physical activity of at least 150–300 mins/week of moderate intensity or 75–150 mins/week of vigorous intensity and reduction in sedentary time are recommended	I	B
Home-based cardiac rehabilitation and mobile health interventions should be considered to increase patients' long-term adherence to healthy behaviors, and to reduce hospitalizations or cardiac events	IIa	B
Antianginal drugs in patients with chronic coronary syndrome—Section 4		
It is recommended to tailor the selection of antianginal drugs to the patient's characteristics, comorbidities, concomitant medications, treatment tolerability, and underlying pathophysiology of angina, also considering local drug availability and cost	I	C
Ivabradine should be considered as add-on antianginal therapy in patients with left ventricular systolic dysfunction (LVEF <40%) and inadequate control of symptoms, or as part of initial treatment in properly selected patients	IIa	B
Ivabradine is not recommended as add-on therapy in patients with CCS, LVEF > 40%, and no clinical heart failure	III	B
Combination of ivabradine with non-DHP-CCB or other strong *CYP3A4* inhibitors is not recommended	III	B

Contd...

Contd...

Recommendations	***Class***[a]	***Level***[b]
Antithrombotic therapy in patients with chronic coronary syndrome—Section 4		
Long-term antithrombotic therapy in patients with chronic coronary syndrome and no clear indication for oral anticoagulation		
In CCS patients with a prior MI or PCI, clopidogrel 75 mg daily is recommended as a safe and effective alternative to aspirin monotherapy	I	A
After CABG, aspirin 75–100 mg daily is recommended lifelong	I	A
In CCS patients *without* prior MI or revascularization but with evidence of significant obstructive CAD, aspirin 75–100 mg daily is recommended lifelong	I	B
Lipid-lowering drugs in patients with chronic coronary syndrome—Section 4		
Lipid-lowering treatment with an LDL-C goal of <1.4 mmol/L (55 mg/dL) and a ≥50% reduction in LDL-C vs. baseline is recommended	I	A
For patients who are statin intolerant and do not achieve their goal on ezetimibe, combination with bempedoic acid is recommended	I	B
For patients who do not achieve their goal on a maximum tolerated dose of statin and ezetimibe, combination with bempedoic acid should be considered	IIa	C
Sodium-glucose cotransporter-2 inhibitors and/or glucagon-like peptide-1 receptor agonists in patients with chronic coronary syndrome—Section 4		
SGLT-2 inhibitors with proven CV benefit are recommended in patients with T2DM and CCS to reduce CV events, independent of baseline or target HbA1c and independent of concomitant glucose-lowering medication	I	A
The GLP-1 receptor agonist semaglutide should be considered in CCS patients without diabetes, but with overweight or obesity (BMI >27 kg/m^2), to reduce CV mortality, MI, or stroke	IIa	B
Anti-inflammatory drugs in patients with chronic coronary syndrome—Section 4		
In CCS patients with atherosclerotic CAD, low-dose colchicine (0.5 mg daily) should be considered to reduce myocardial infarction, stroke, and need for revascularization	IIa	A
Revascularization in patients with chronic coronary syndrome—Section 4		
Informed and shared decisions		
For complex clinical cases, to define the optimal treatment strategy, in particular when CABG and PCI hold the same level of recommendation, a Heart Team discussion is recommended, including representatives from interventional cardiology, cardiac surgery, noninterventional cardiology, and other specialties if indicated, aimed at selecting the most appropriate treatment to improve patient's outcomes and quality of life	I	C
It is recommended that the decision for revascularization and its modality be patient-centered, considering when possible patient's preferences, health literacy, cultural circumstances, and social support	I	C
Revascularization to improve outcomes		
In CCS patients with LVEF ≤35%, it is recommended to choose between revascularization or medical therapy alone, after careful evaluation, preferably by the Heart Team, of coronary anatomy, correlation between coronary artery disease and LV dysfunction, comorbidities, life expectancy, individual risk-to-benefit ratio, and patient perspectives	I	C
Assessment of procedural risks and postprocedural outcomes		
Intracoronary imaging guidance by IVUS or OCT is recommended for performing PCI on anatomically complex lesions, in particular left main stem, true bifurcations and long lesions	I	A
Intracoronary pressure measurement (FFR or iFR) or computation (QFR):		
• Is recommended to guide lesion selection for intervention in patients with multivessel disease	I	A

Contd...

Contd…

Recommendations	*Class*[a]	*Level*[b]
• Should be considered at the end of the procedure to identify patients at high risk of persistent angina and subsequent clinical events • May be considered at the end of the procedure to identify lesions potentially amenable to treatment with additional PCI	IIa IIb	B B
Choice of revascularization modality		
It is recommended that physicians select the most appropriate revascularization modality based on patient's profile, coronary anatomy, procedural factors, LVEF, patient's preferences and outcome expectations	I	C
Mode of revascularization in patients with chronic coronary syndrome *Left main disease*		
In CCS patients at low surgical risk with significant left main coronary stenosis, CABG: • Is recommended over medical therapy alone to improve survival • Is recommended as the overall preferred revascularization mode over PCI, given the lower risk of spontaneous myocardial infarction and repeat revascularization	 I I	 A A
In CCS patients with significant left main coronary stenosis of low complexity (SYNTAX score ≤22), in whom PCI can provide equivalent completeness of revascularization to that of CABG, PCI is recommended as an alternative to CABG, given its lower invasiveness and noninferior survival	I	A
Management of chronic coronary syndrome patients with chronic heart failure—Section 5		
In HF patients with LVEF ≤35% in whom obstructive CAD is suspected, ICA is recommended with a view toward improving prognosis by CABG, taking into account the risk-to-benefit ratio of the procedures	I	B
In HF patients with LVEF >35% and suspected CCS with low or moderate (>5–50%) pretest likelihood of obstructive CAD, CCTA, or functional imaging is recommended	I	C
In patients with HFpEF with angina or equivalent symptoms and normal or nonobstructive epicardial coronary arteries. PET or CMR perfusion or invasive functional coronary testing should be considered to detect or rule out coronary microvascular dysfunction	IIa	B
In selected patients with HFrEF undergoing high-risk PCI for complex CAD, the use of a microaxial flow pump may be considered in experienced centers	IIb	C
It is recommended that CCS patients with heart failure be enrolled in a multidisciplinary heart failure management program to reduce the risk of heart failure hospitalization and to improve survival	I	A
Sacubitril/valsartan is recommended as a replacement for an ACE-I or ARB in CCS patients with HFrEF to reduce the risk of heart failure hospitalization and death	I	B
Diagnosis and management of patients with angina/ischemia with nonobstructive coronary arteries—Section 5 *Management of ANOCA/INOCA*		
In symptomatic patients with ANOCA/INOCA, medical therapy based on coronary functional test results should be considered to improve symptoms and quality of life	IIa	A
For the management of endothelial dysfunction. ACE-I should be considered for symptom control	IIa	B
For the management of microvascular angina associated with reduced coronary/myocardial blood flow reserve, β-blockers should be considered for symptom control	IIa	B
For the treatment of isolated vasospastic angina: • Calcium-channel blockers are recommended to control symptoms and to prevent ischemia and potentially fatal complications • Nitrates should be considered to prevent recurrent episodes	 I IIa	 A B
In patients with evidence of overlapping endotypes, combination therapy with nitrates, calcium-channel blockers, and other vasodilators may be considered	IIb	B

Contd…

Contd...

Recommendations	*Class*[a]	*Level*[b]
Older, female, high-bleeding risk, comorbid, and socially/geographically diverse patients—Section 5		
Similar guideline-directed cardiovascular preventive therapy is recommended in women and men	I	C
Bleeding risk assessment is recommended using the PRECISE-DAPT score, the qualitative ARC-HBR tool or other, validated methods	I	B
Attention to interaction between antiretroviral treatment and statins is recommended in patients with HIV	I	B

[a]Class of recommendation.
[b]Level of evidence.
(ACE-I: angiotensin-converting enzyme inhibitor; ANOCA, angina with nonobstructive coronary arteries; ARB: angiotensin receptor blocker; ARC-HBR: Academic Research Consortium for High Bleeding Risk; BMI: body mass index; CABG: coronary artery bypass grafting; CACS: coronary artery calcium score; CAD: coronary artery disease; CCB: calcium-channel blocker; CCS: chronic coronary syndrome; CCTA: coronary computed tomography angiography; CFC: coronary flow capacity; CFR: coronary flow reserve; CKD: chronic kidney disease; CMR: cardiac magnetic resonance; CT: computed tomography; CV: cardiovascular; CVD: cardiovascular disease; CYP3A4: cytochrome P450 3A4; DHP: dihydropyridine; dPR: diastolic pressure ratio; ECG: electrocardiogram; FFR: fractional flow reserve; FFR-CT: coronary computed tomography angiography-derived fractional flow reserve; GLP-1: glucagon-like peptide-1; HbA1c: glycated hemoglobin; HF: heart failure; HFpEF: heart failure with preserved ejection fraction; HFrEF: heart failure with reduced ejection fraction; HIV: human immunodeficiency virus; HSR: hyperemic stenosis resistance; ICA: invasive coronary angiography; iFR: instantaneous wave-free ratio; INOCA: ischemia with nonobstructive coronary arteries; IVUS: intravascular ultrasound; LAD: left anterior descending; LDL-C, low-density lipoprotein cholesterol; LV: left ventricular; LVEF: left ventricular ejection fraction; MACE: major adverse cardiovascular events; MCS: mechanical circulatory support; MI: myocardial infarction; OCT: optical coherence tomography; PCI: percutaneous coronary intervention; Pd/Pa: distal coronary pressure to aortic pressure ratio; PET: positron emission tomography; PRECISE-DAPT: PREdicting bleeding Complications In patients undergoing Stent implantation and subsEquent Dual AntiPlatelet Therapy; QFR: quantitative flow ratio; RFR: relative flow reserve; SGLT2: sodium-glucose cotransporter 2; SPECT: single-photon emission computed tomography; T2DM: type 2 diabetes mellitus)

DIAGNOSTIC MANAGEMENT OF PATIENTS WITH ANGINA AND SUSPECTED CORONARY ARTERY DISEASE

A Detailed History Including Signs and Symptoms

A detailed history is required including various symptoms and risk factors such as family history of CVD, dyslipidemia, diabetes, hypertension, smoking, and other lifestyle factors. The characteristics of chest pain may be divided into four categories: Location, character, duration, its relationship to exertion, and other exacerbating or relieving factors. Exacerbations of symptoms after a heavy meal or after waking up in the morning are classic features of angina **(Table 2)**. Angina may paradoxically be reduced with further exercise (walk-through angina) or on second exertion (warm-up angina). Sublingual nitrates rapidly relieve angina.

Classification of Different Angina Symptoms (Table 2)

The Canadian Cardiovascular Society classification is still used as a grading system for angina to quantify the threshold at which symptoms occur in relation to physical activities.[3]

TABLE 2: Classification of different angina symptoms.

Type of chest pain	*Characteristics*
Typical angina	*Meets the following three characteristics:* 1. Constricting discomfort in the front of the chest or in the neck, jaw, shoulder, or arm 2. Precipitated by physical exertion 3. Relieved by rest or nitrates within 5 minutes
Atypical angina	Meets two of these characteristics
Nonanginal chest pain	Meets only one or none of these characteristics

Physical examination of a patient with suspected CAD is important to assess the presence of anemia, hypertension, valvular heart disease, hypertrophic cardiomyopathy, or arrhythmias. Microvascular disease should also be evaluated.

Various Comorbidities

It is necessary to assess the patient's general health, comorbidities, and quality of life. Noninvasive functional imaging for ischemia is an option to verify the diagnosis. If the pain is clearly nonanginal, other diagnostic test should be indicated to diagnose gastrointestinal,

TABLE 3: Testing for suspected patients with coronary artery disease (CAD).

Recommendations	*Class*[a]	*Level*[b]
History taking and risk factor assessment		
In individuals reporting symptoms of suspected myocardial ischemic origin, a detailed assessment of cardiovascular risk factors, medical history, and symptom characteristics (including onset, duration, type, location, triggers, relieving factors, time of day) is recommended	I	C
Symptoms like chest pain triggered by emotional stress; dyspnea or dizziness on exertion; pain in the arms, jaw, neck, or upper back; or fatigue should be considered as potential angina equivalents	IIa	B
Resting ECG		
If clinical or ECG assessment suggests ACS rather than CCS, immediate referral to the emergency department and/or repeated measurement of blood troponin, preferably using high-sensitivity or ultrasensitive assays, to rule out acute myocardial injury, is recommended	I	B
A resting 12-lead ECG is recommended in all individuals reporting chest pain (unless an obvious noncardiac cause is identified), particularly during or immediately after, an episode suggestive of myocardial ischemia	I	C
Using ST-segment deviations during supraventricular tachyarrhythmias, particularly during re-entrant atrioventricular tachycardias, per se, as reliable evidence of obstructive CAD, is not recommended	III	B

[a]Class of recommendation.
[b]Level of evidence.
(ACS: acute coronary syndrome; CCS: chronic coronary syndrome; ECG, electrocardiogram)
Source: © ESC 2024

TABLE 4: Recommendations for basic biochemistry in the initial diagnostic management of individuals with suspected chronic coronary syndrome.

Recommendations	*Class*[a]	*Level*[b]
The following blood tests are recommended in all individuals to refine risk stratification, diagnose comorbidities, and guide treatment:		
• Lipid profile including LDL-C	I	A
• Full blood count (including hemoglobin)	I	B
• Creatinine with estimation of renal function	I	B
• Glycemic status with HbA1c and/or fasting plasma glucose	I	B
In patients with suspected CCS, it is recommended to assess thyroid function at least once	I	B
Additionally, hs-CRP and/or fibrinogen plasma levels should be considered	IIa	B

[a]Class of recommendation.
[b]Level of evidence.
(CCS: chronic coronary syndrome; hs-CRP: high-sensitivity C-reactive protein; ECG: electrocardiogram; HbA1c: glycated hemoglobin; LDL-C: low-density lipoprotein cholesterol)
Source: ESC 2024.

pulmonary, or musculoskeletal causes of chest pain. Risk charts such as SCORE (Systematic Coronary Risk Evaluation) can be used as a guideline for risk factor modification.[4]

Testing for Suspected Patients with Coronary Artery Disease (Table 3)

Basic testing in patients with suspected CAD **(Tables 3 to 8)** includes standard laboratory biochemical testing **(Table 4)**, a resting ECG, possible ambulatory ECG monitoring **(Table 5)**, resting echocardiography, and chest X-ray.

Table 4 *shows recommendations for basic biochemistry in the initial diagnostic management of individuals with suspected chronic coronary syndrome.*

Table 5 shows ambulatory ECG for diagnosing patients with suspected CAD.

Table 6 shows recommendations for exercise ECG in the initial diagnostic management of individuals with suspected CAD.

Table 7 shows recommendations for resting transthoracic ultrasound and cardiac magnetic resonance imaging in the initial diagnostic management of individuals with suspected chronic coronary syndrome.

TABLE 5: Ambulatory ECG for diagnosing patients with suspected coronary artery disease (CAD).

Recommendations	*Class*[a]	*Level*[b]
Ambulatory ECG monitoring is recommended in subjects with chest pain and suspected arrhythmias	I	C
Ambulatory ECG monitoring should be considered in subjects with suspected vasospastic angina	IIa	B

[a]Class of recommendation.
[b]Level of evidence.
(ECG: electrocardiogram)
Source: ESC 2024.

TABLE 6: Recommendations for exercise ECG in the initial diagnostic management of individuals with suspected coronary artery disease (CAD).

Recommendations	*Class*[a]	*Level*[b]
Exercise ECG is recommended in selected patients[c] for the assessment of exercise tolerance, symptoms, arrhythmias, BP response, and event risk	I	C
Exercise ECG may be considered as an alternative test to rule-in and rule-out CAD when noninvasive imaging tests are unavailable	IIb	B
An exercise ECG may be considered to refine risk stratification and treatment	IIb	B
In individuals with a low (>5–15%) pretest likelihood of obstructive CAD. An exercise ECG may be considered to identify patients in whom further testing can be deferred	IIb	C
Exercise ECG is not recommended for diagnostic purposes in patients with ≥0.1 mV ST-segment depression on resting ECG. Left bundle branch block or who are being treated with digitalis	III	C
In individuals with a low or moderate (>5–50%) pretest likelihood of obstructive CAD, an exercise ECG is not recommended to rule out CAD if CCTA or functional imaging tests are available	III	C

[a]Class of recommendation.
[b]Level of evidence.
[c]When this information will have an impact on diagnostic strategy or management.
(BP: blood pressure; CCTA: coronary computed tomography angiography; ECG: electrocardiogram)
Source: ESC 2024.

TABLE 7: Recommendations for resting transthoracic ultrasound and cardiac magnetic resonance imaging in the initial diagnostic management of individuals with suspected chronic coronary syndrome.

Recommendations	*Class*[a]	*Level*[b]
A resting transthoracic echocardiogram is recommended to measure LVEF, volumes, and diastolic function: • Identify regional wall motion abnormalities • Identify noncoronary cardiac disease (e.g., hypertrophy, cardiomyopathy, valve disease, and pericardial effusion) • Assess right ventricular function and estimate systolic pulmonary artery pressure; to refine risk stratification and guide treatment	I	B
CMR, if available, may be considered as an alternative imaging test in individuals with inconclusive echocardiographic evaluation	IIb	C

[a]Class of recommendation.
[b]Level of evidence.
(CMR: cardiac magnetic resonance; LVEF: left ventricular ejection fraction)
Source: ESC 2024.

Assessment of Pretest Probability and Clinical Likelihood of Coronary Artery Disease (Table 8)

If the likelihood of CAD is intermediate diagnostic testing is most useful. If the likelihood is high, a large number of patients need to be studied to identify the few patients that do not have disease, and a negative test result can seldom rule out the presence of obstructive CAD. A simple predictive model can be used to estimate the pretest probability (PTP) of obstructive CAD based on age, sex, and the nature of symptoms.[5]

Table 8 shows determinants of clinical likelihood of CAD.

Lifestyle Modification in Patients with Chronic Coronary Syndrome (Table 9)

Management of CCS aims to reduce symptoms and improve prognosis of patients through appropriate medications and interventions, and to control risk factors through lifestyle behaviors. Optimal medical therapy in the COURAGE (Clinical Outcomes Utilizing Revascularization and Aggressive Drug Evaluation) trial included the promotion of medication adherence, behavioral counseling, and support for the managing

TABLE 8: Determinants of clinical likelihood of coronary artery disease (CAD).

Decreases likelihood	*Increases likelihood*
• Normal exercise ECG[a] • No coronary calcium by CT (Agatston score = 0)[a]	• Risk factors for CVD (dyslipidemia, diabetes, hypertension, smoking, and family history of CVD) • Resting ECG changes (Q-wave or ST-segment/T-wave changes) • LV dysfunction suggestive of CAD • Abnormal exercise ECG[a] • Coronary calcium by CT[a]

[a]When available.
(CVD: cardiovascular disease; LV: left ventricular)

lifestyle risk factors delivered by nurse case managers.[6] Smoking cessation improves the prognosis in patients by 36% risk reduction in mortality for those who quit.[7]

Box 1 shows recommended diet.

Lifestyle factors and implementation of healthy behaviors (including smoking cessation, physical activity, a healthy diet **(Box 1)**, and maintaining a healthy weight, significantly decreases the risk of future cardiovascular events and death. Clinical trials have shown that psychological (e.g., counseling and/or cognitive behavioral therapy) and pharmacological interventions have a beneficial effect on depression, anxiety, and stress, with some evidence of a reduction in cardiovascular mortality.

TABLE 9: Lifestyle interventions in patients with chronic coronary syndrome (CCS).

Topic	*Recommendation and treatment goals in patients with established CCS*
Lifestyle counseling	
Immunization	Vaccination against influenza, pneumococcal disease, and other widespread infections, e.g., COVID-19
Sleep quality	Treat sleep-related breathing disorders
Sexual activity	• *Males and females:* Low risk for stable patients who are not symptomatic at low-to-moderate activity levels • *Males:* PDE-5 inhibitors are generally safe, not to be taken in combination with nitrate medications because of risk of severe hypotension
Psychosocial aspects	• Avoid psychosocial stress • Treat depression and anxiety by psychological or pharmacological interventions
Environment/pollution	• Avoid passive smoking • Reduce environmental noise • Avoid exposure to air pollution
Lifestyle interventions for risk-factor control	
Smoking and substance abuse	• Use pharmacological and behavioral strategies to assist in smoking cessation • Avoid e-cigarettes • Abstain from substance abuse
Obesity and being overweight	• Obtain and maintain a healthy weight (BMI = 18.5–25 kg/m^2) • Reduce weight through recommended energy intake and increased physical activity and through pharmacological/surgical interventions in selected patients
Hyperlipidemia	• Ultimate LDL-C goal of <1.4 mmol/L (55 mg/dL) and a ≥50% reduction in LDL-C vs. baseline is recommended
Diabetes	• HbA1c < 70% (53 mmol/mol)
Arterial hypertension	• SBP 120–129 mm Hg, provided the antihypertensive treatment is well tolerated
Diet and alcohol consumption	• Limit alcohol consumption to <100 g/week • Diet high in vegetables, fruit, and wholegrains (Mediterranean diet) • Limit saturated fat to <10% of total calorie intake
Physical activity and exercise	• 30–60 minutes moderate activity, >5 days/week • Reduce sedentary time and engage in at least light activity throughout the day

(BMI: body mass index; CCS: chronic coronary syndrome; COVID-19: coronavirus disease 2019; HbA1c: glycated hemoglobin; LDL-C: low-density lipoprotein cholesterol; PDE-5: phosphodiesterase-5; SBP: systolic blood pressure)

Pharmacological Management (Table 10)

Short-acting Nitrates

Nitroglycerin spray acts more rapidly than sublingual nitroglycerine. At the onset of angina, the patient should be in a sitting position because standing promotes syncope, and lying down enhances venous return and preload and take nitroglycerin (0.3–0.6 mg tablet sublingually, or 0.4 mg spray to the tongue) every 5 minutes until the pain disappears, or a maximum of 1.2 mg has been taken within 15 minutes. Isosorbide dinitrate (5 mg sublingually) has a slightly slower onset of action than nitroglycerin due to hepatic conversion to mononitrate.

BOX 1: Recommended diet.

Characteristics:
- Increase consumption of fruits and vegetables (≥200 g each per day)
- 35–45 g of fiber per day, preferably from wholegrains
- Moderate consumption of nuts (30 g per day, unsalted)
- 1–2 servings of fish per week (one to be oily fish)
- Limited lean meat low-fat dairy products, and liquid vegetable oils
- Saturated fats to account for <10% of total energy intake; replace with polyunsaturated fats
- As little intake of trans unsaturated fats as posable, preferably no intake from processed food, and <1% of total energy intake
- ≤5–6 g of salt per day
- If alcohol is consumed, limiting intake to ≤100 g/week or <15 g/day is recommended
- Avoid energy-dense foods such as sugar-sweetened soft drinks

Long-acting Nitrates

Long-acting nitrate formulations (e.g., nitroglycerin, isosorbide dinitrate, and isosorbide mononitrate) should be considered as second-line therapy for angina relief when initial therapy with a β-blocker or nondihydropyridine (non-DHP) is contraindicated. Nitroglycerin can be administered orally or transdermally through slow-release patch systems. It should be gradually tapered to avoid a rebound increase in angina. The most common side effects are hypotension, headache, and flushing. Contraindications include hypertrophic obstructive cardiomyopathy, severe aortic valvular stenosis, and co-administration of phosphodiesterase inhibitors such as sildenafil, tadalafil, or vardenafil or riociguat.

TABLE 10: Pharmacological management of chronic coronary syndrome (CCS).

	Standard therapy	*High heart rate (e.g., >80 bpm)*	*Low heart rate (e.g., <50 bpm)*	*LV dysfunction of heart failure*	*Low blood pressure*
1st step	BB or CCB[a]	BB or non-DHP-CCB	DHP-CCB	BB	Low-dose BB or low-dose non-DHP-CCB[c]
	↓	↓	↓	↓	↓
2nd step	BB + DHP-CCB	BB + CCB[b]	Switch to LAN	BB + LAN or BB + ivabradine	Switch to ivabradine,[d] ranolazine or trimetazidine[e]
	↓	↓	↓	↓	↓
3rd step	Add 2nd line drug	BB + ivabradine[d]	DHP-CCB + LAN	Add another 2nd line drug	Combine two 2nd line drugs
			↓		
4th step			Add nicorandil, ranolazine or trimetazidine		

[a]Combination of a BB with a DHP-CCB should be considered as first step; combination of a BB or a CCB with a second-line drug may be considered as a first step.
[b]The combination of a BB and non-DHP-CCB should initially use low doses of each drug under close monitoring of tolerance, particularly heart rate and blood pressure.
[c]Low-dose BB or low-dose non-DHP-CCB should be used under close monitoring of tolerance, particularly heart rate and blood pressure.
[d]Ivabradine should not be combined with non-DHP-CCB.
[e]Consider adding the drug chosen at step 2 to the drug tested at step 1 if blood pressure remains unchanged.
[BB: beta-blocker; bpm: beats per minute; CCB: (any class of) calcium-channel blocker; DHP-CCB: dihydropyridine calcium-channel blocker; HF: heart failure; LAN: long-acting nitrate; LV: left ventricular; non-DHP-CCB: nondihydropyridine calcium-channel blocker]

Beta-blockers

Beta-blockers can be combined with DHP CCBs to reduce DHP-induced tachycardia. A combination of β-blocker is with verapamil or diltiazem should be cautiously used due to the potential for developing worsening of HF, excessive bradycardia, and/or atrioventricular block. Combination of a β-blocker with a nitrate attenuates the reflex tachycardia. The principal side effects of β-blockers are fatigue, depression, bradycardia, heart block, bronchospasm, peripheral vasoconstriction, postural hypotension, impotence, and masking of hypoglycemia symptoms. In patients with recent MI and those with chronic HF with reduced ejection fraction, β-blockers have been associated with a significant reduction in mortality and/or cardiovascular events.

Nondihydropyridine Agents

Verapamil: It has a large range of approved indications, including all varieties of angina (effort, vasospastic, and unstable), supraventricular tachycardias, and hypertension. Risks of heart block, bradycardia, and HF. Compared with metoprolol, the antianginal activity was similar. Compared with atenonol in hypertension with CAD, verapamil is associated with fewer cases of diabetes, fewer anginal attacks, and less psychological depression. Beta-blockade combined with verapamil is not advised due to the risk of heart block.

Diltiazem: Like verapamil, it acts by peripheral vasodilation, relief of exercise-induced coronary constriction, a modest negative inotropic effect, and sinus node inhibition. Use of non-DHP CCBs in patients with LV dysfunction is not advised.

Dihydropyridine Agents

Nifedipine: ACTION (A Coronary disease Trial Investigating Outcome with Nifedipine gastrointestinal therapeutic system) trial, addition of long-acting nifedipine (60 mg o.d.) to conventional treatment of angina had no effect on major cardiovascular event-free survival.[8] Long-acting nifedipine proved to be safe, and reduced the need for coronary angiography and cardiovascular interventions. Relative contraindications to nifedipine are severe aortic stenosis, hypertrophic obstructive cardiomyopathy, or HF, and careful combination with β-blockade is usually feasible and desirable. Vasodilatory side effects include headache and ankle edema.

Amlodipine: Side effects are mainly ankle edema. In patients with CCS and normal BP, amlodipine 10 mg/day reduces coronary revascularizations and hospitalizations for angina. Exercise-induced ischemia is also reduced.

Ivabradine

Adding ivabradine 7.5 mg bd twice a day to atenolol therapy gives better control of heart rate and anginal symptoms.

Nicorandil

Nicorandil is a nitrate derivative of nicotinamide, with antianginal effects similar to those of nitrates or β-blockers. Side effects include nausea, vomiting, and severe oral, intestinal, and mucosal ulcerations. In IONA (Impact Of Nicorandil in Angina) trial, nicorandil significantly reduced the composite of coronary heart disease (CHD) death, nonfatal MI, or unplanned hospital admission for suspected anginal symptoms in patients with CCS, but there was no effect on death from ischemic heart disease or nonfatal MI.[9]

Ranolazine

Ranolazine is a selective inhibitor of the late inward sodium current. Side effects include dizziness, nausea, and constipation. In addition, ranolazine increases QTc, and should therefore be used carefully in patients with QT prolongation or on QT prolonging drugs.

Trimetazidine

Trimetazidine (35 mg b.i.d.) added to β-blockade (atenolol) improves effort-induced myocardial ischemia. It is contraindicated in Parkinson's disease, motion disorders, such as tremor, muscle rigidity, walking disorders, and restless leg syndrome.

Allopurinol

The role of allopurinol in reducing clinical events in CVD remains unclear. An observational study of 29, 298 episodes of incident allopurinol use found an association of allopurinol use with a reduction in the risk of incident MI in the elderly, particularly when used for >2 years.

Recommendation for Prevention of Event

See **Table 11**.

TABLE 11: Recommendations for antianginal drugs in patients with chronic coronary syndrome.

Recommendations	*Class*[a]	*Level*[b]
General strategy		
It is recommended to tailor the selection of antianginal drugs to the patient's characteristics, comorbidities, concomitant medications, treatment tolerability, and underlying pathophysiology of angina, also considering local drug availability and cost	I	C
Selection of antianginal medication		
Short-acting nitrates are recommended for immediate relief of angina	I	B
Initial treatment with β-blockers and/or CCBs to control heart rate and symptoms is recommended for most patients with CCS[c]	I	B
If anginal symptoms are not successfully controlled by initial treatment with a beta-blocker or a CCB alone, the combination of a β-blocker and a DHP-CCB should be considered, unless contraindicated	IIa	B
Long-acting nitrates or ranolazine should be considered as add-on therapy in patients with inadequate control of symptoms while on treatment with β-blockers and/or CCBs, or as part of initial treatment in properly selected patients[d]	IIa	B
When long-acting nitrates are prescribed, a nitrate-free or low-nitrate interval should be considered to reduce tolerance	IIa	B
Ivabradine should be considered as add-on antianginal therapy in patients with left ventricular systolic dysfunction (LVEF <40%) and inadequate control of symptoms, or as part of initial treatment in properly selected patients	IIa	B
Nicorandil or trimetazidine may be considered as add-on therapy in patients with inadequate control of symptoms while on treatment with β-blockers and/or CCBs, or as part of initial treatment in property selected patients	IIb	B
Ivabradine is not recommended as add-on therapy in patients with CCS, LVEF >40%, and no clinical heart failure	III	B
Combination of ivabradine with non-DHP-CCB or other strong *CYP3A4* inhibitors is not recommended	III	B
Nitrates are not recommended in patients with hypertrophic cardiomyopathy or in coadministration with phosphodiesterase inhibitors	III	B

[a]Class of recommendation.
[b]Level of evidence.
[c]These drugs may require caution or may be contraindicated in certain patients with low BP (β-blockers and DHP-CCB), DM (β-blockers), atrioventricular conduction disorders (β-blockers and non-DHP-CCB), chronic obstructive pulmonary disease (noncardioselective β-blockers).
[d]Consideration for initial therapy: Ivabradine, nicorandil, long-acting nitrates, ranolazine, or trimetazidine for patients with intolerance or contraindications to β-blockers and/or CCBs; ranolazine and trimetazidine for patients with microvascular angina; nicorandil or nitrates for patients with coronary artery spasm. The drugs are listed in alphabetical order.
(CCB: calcium-channel blocker; CCS: chronic coronary syndrome; *CYP3A4:* cytochrome P450 3A4; DHP: dihydropyridine; DM: diabetes mellitus; LVEF: left ventricular ejection fraction)
Source: © ESC 2024
Vrints C, Andreotti F, Koskinas KC, Rossello X, Adamo M, Ainslie J, et al.; ESC Scientific Document Group. 2024 ESC Guidelines for the management of chronic coronary syndromes. Eur Heart J. 2024;45(36):3415-537.

Recommendations for Antithrombotic Therapy in Patients with Chronic Coronary Syndrome

See **Table 12**.

Treatment for Dual Antithrombotic Therapy with Aspirin in High or Moderate Risk Patients Who do not have High Bleeding Risk

See **Table 13**.

Recommendations for Lipid-lowering Drugs in Patients with Chronic Coronary Syndrome

See **Table 14**.

Dyslipidemia

The goal of treatment is to lower LDL-C by at least 50% from baseline and to <1.4 mmol/L (<55 mg/dL) although a lower target LDL-C of <1.0 mmol/L (<40 mg/dL) may be considered in patients who have experience a second vascular event within 2 years. When this level cannot be achieved, the addition of ezetimibe has been demonstrated to decrease cholesterol and cardiovascular events in post-ACS patients, and in those with diabetes. Proprotein convertase subtilisin-kexin type 9 (PCSK9) inhibitors (evolocumab and alirocumab) are very effective at reducing cholesterol, lowering LDL-C in a stable fashion to <1.3 mmol/L (50 mg/dL).

TABLE 12: Recommendations for antithrombotic therapy in patients with chronic coronary syndrome.

Recommendations	*Class*[a]	*Level*[b]
Long-term antithrombotic therapy in patients with chronic coronary syndrome and no clear indication for oral anticoagulation		
In CCS patients with a prior MI or remote PCL aspirin 75–100 mg daily recommended lifelong after an initial period of DAPT	I	A
In CCS patients with a prior MI or remote PCL, clopidogrel 75 mg daily is recommended as a safe and effective alternative to aspirin monotherapy	I	A
Alter CABG, approximate 75–100 mg daily a recommended lifelong	I	A
In patients without prior MI or revascularization but with evidence of significant obstructive CAD, aspirin 75–100 ng daily is recommended lifelong	I	B
Adding a second antithrombotic agent to aspirin for extended long-term secondary prevention should be considered in patients at enhanced ischemic risk[c] without high bleeding risk[d]	IIa	A
In CCS or stabilized post-ACS patients who underwent PC and were initially treated with ticagrelor-based DAPT, who remain at high ischemic risk and are not at high bleeding risk, ticagrelor monotherapy 90 mg BID may be considered as an alternative to dual or other single antiplatelet therapy	IIb	C
Antithrombotic therapy postpercutaneous coronary intervention in patients with chronic coronary syndrome and no indication for oral anticoagulation		
In CCS patients with no indication for oral anticoagulation DAPT consisting of aspirin 75–100 mg and clopidogrel 75 mg daily for up to 6 months is recommended as the default antithrombotic strategy after PCI-stenting	I	A
In patients at high bleeding risk[d] but not at high ischemic risk,c it is recommended to discontinue DAPT 1–3 months after PCI and to continue with single antiplatelet therapy	I	A
Stopping DAPT alter 1–3 months from PCI stenting may be considered in patients who are not at high bleeding risk nor at high risk of ischemic events[c,d]	IIb	B
In CCS patients undergoing high-thrombotic risk stenting (e.g., complex left main stent, two-stent bifurcation, suboptimal stenting result, prior stent thrombosis, previously known CYP2C19*/*23 polymorphism), prasugrel or ticagrelor (in addition to aspirin) may be considered instead of clopidogrel, for the first month, and up to 3–6 months	IIb	C
Long-term antithrombotic therapy in patients with chronic coronary syndrome and an indication for oral anticoagulation		
In CCS patients with a long-term indicator for OAC, an AF therapeutic dose of VKA alone or, preferably of DOAC alone (unless contraindicated) is recommended lifelong	I	B
Antithrombotic therapy postpercutaneous coronary intervention in chronic coronary syndrome patients with an indication for oral anticoagulation		
In patients with an indication for OAC who undergo PCI, initial low-dose aspirin once daily recommended (loading dose when not on maintenance dose) in addition to OAC and clopidogrel	I	C
In patients who are eligible for OAC DOACs contradicted, recommended in preference to VIKA	I	A
Alter uncomplicated PCI in CCS patients with concomitant indication for OAC: • Early cessation of aspirin (≤1 week) • *Followed by the continuation of OAC and clopidogrel:* – Up to 6 months in patients not at high ischemic risk,[c] or – Up to 12 months in patients at high ischemic risk[c] – Followed by OAC alone is recommended	I	A
Continuation of aspirin up to 1 month after PCI. In addition to OAC and clopidogrel, it should be considered in patients at high ischemic risk[c] or with anatomical characteristics judged to outweigh the blending risk[e]	IIa	B
When concerns about high bleeding risk prevail over concerns about stent thrombosis or ischemic stroke: • Rivaroxaban 15 mg daily should be considered in preference to rivaroxaban 20 mg daily for the duration of concomitant antiplatelet therapy	IIa	B
• Dabigatran 110 mg twice daily should be considered in preference to dabigatran 150 mg daily for the duration of concomitant antiplatelet therapy	IIa	B

Contd...

Contd...

Recommendations	*Class*[a]	*Level*[b]
In patients with an indication for VKA in combination with single or dual antiplatelet therapy targeting VKA to an INR in the lower part of the recommended range and to a time in therapeutic range >70% should be considered	IIa	B
The use of prasugrel and ticagrelor is generally not recommended as part of antithrombotic therapy with aspirin and an OAC	III	C
Antithrombotic therapy postcoronary artery bypass grafting		
It is recommended to initiate aspirin postoperatively as soon as there is no concern over bleeding	I	B
DAFT may be considered after CABG in selected patients at greater risk of graft occlusion[f] and at low risk of bleeding	IIb	B
Use of proton-pump inhibitors		
A proton-pump inhibitor is recommended in patients at increased risk of gastrointestinal bleeding for the duration of combined antithrombotic therapy (antiplatelet therapy and for OAC)	I	A
A proton-pump inhibitor should be considered when a single antithrombotic (antiplatelet or anticoagulant drug) is used, considering the gastrointestinal bleeding risk of the individual patient	IIa	A

[a]Class of recommendation.
[b]Level of evidence.
[c]Enhanced thrombotic/ischemic risk criteria for extended treatment with a second antithrombotic agent.
[d]Bleeding-risk criteria according to PRECISE-DAPT or ARC-HBR.
[e]Anatomical/procedural thrombotic risk characteristics: stenting of left main, proximal LAD, or last remaining patent artery; suboptimal stent deployment; stent length of >60 mm; bifurcation with two stents implanted; treatment of chronic total occlusions.
[f]For example, stentectomy, endarterectomy, poor venous graft quality.

(ACS: acute coronary syndrome; AF; atrial fibrillation; ARC-HBR: Academic Research Consortium for High Bleeding Risk; b.i.d., bis in die (twice daily); CABG: coronary artery bypass grafting; CAD: coronary artery disease; CCS: chronic coronary syndrome; CKD: chronic kidney disease; CYP2C19: cytochrome P450 2C19; DAPT: dual antiplatelet therapy; DOAC: direct oral anticoagulant; INR: international normalized ratio; LAD: left anterior descending; MI: myocardial infarction; OAC: oral anticoagulant; PCI: percutaneous coronary intervention; PRECISE-DAPT: PREdicting bleeding Complications In patients undergoing Stent implantation and subsEquent Dual AntiPlatelet Therapy; VKA: vitamin K antagonist)

Source: © ESC 2024

Vrints C, Andreotti F, Koskinas KC, Rossello X, Adamo M, Ainslie J, et al.; ESC Scientific Document Group. 2024 ESC Guidelines for the management of chronic coronary syndromes. Eur Heart J. 2024;45(36):3415-537.

TABLE 13: Treatment for dual antithrombotic therapy with aspirin in high- or moderate-risk patients who do not have high bleeding risk.

Drug option	*Dose*	*Indication*	*Additional cautions*
Clopidogrel	75 mg OD	Post-MI in patients who have tolerated DAPT for 1 year	
Prasugrel	*10 mg OD or 5 mg OD*: If body weight <60 kg or age >75 years	Post-PCI for MI in patients who have tolerated DAPT for 1 year	Age >75 years
Rivaroxaban	2.5 mg BID	Post-MI >1 year or multivessel CAD	Creatinine clearance 15–29 mL/min
Ticagrelor	60 mg BID	Post-MI in patients who have tolerated DAPT for 1 year	

(CAD: chronic artery disease; DAPT: dual antiplatelet therapy; MI: myocardial infarction; PCI: percutaneous coronary intervention)

Renin Angiotensin System Blockers

ACE inhibitors can reduce mortality, MI, stroke, and HF among patients with LV dysfunction, previous vascular disease, and high-risk diabetes. It is recommended that ACE inhibitors or ARBs in cases of intolerance can be considered for the treatment of patients with CCS with coexisting hypertension, LVEF <40%, diabetes, or CKD, unless contraindicated (e.g., severe renal impairment, hyperkalemia, etc.). The first in class is *LCZ696* can be used in patients with HF (LVEF <35%) who remain symptomatic despite optimal treatment with an ACE inhibitor, a β-blocker, and a mineralocorticoid receptor antagonist (MRA), sacubitril/valsartan is recommended as a replacement for an ACE inhibitor to further reduce the risk of HF hospitalization and death in ambulatory patients.

Revascularization

Revascularization by PCI **(Fig. 1)** or CABG may effectively relieve angina, reduce the use of antianginal drugs, and improve exercise capacity and quality of life compared with a strategy of medical therapy alone. In the 5-year follow-up of the FAME 2 (Fractional Flow Reserve

TABLE 14: Recommendations for lipid-lowering drugs in patients with chronic coronary syndrome.

Recommendations	*Class*[a]	*Level*[b]
Lipid-lowering treatment with an LDL-C goal of <1.4 mmol/L (55 mg/dL) and a ≥50% reduction in LDL-C vs. baseline is recommended	I	A
A high-intensity statin up to the highest tolerated dose to reach the LDL-C goals is recommended for all patients with CCS	I	A
If a patient's goal is not achieved with the maximum tolerated dose of statin, combination with ezetimibe is recommended	I	B
For patients who are statin intolerant and do not achieve their goal on ezetimibe, combination with bempedoic acid is recommended	I	B
For patients who do not achieve their goal on a maximum tolerated dose of statin and ezetimibe, combination with a PCSK9 inhibitor is recommended	I	A
For patients who do not achieve their goal on a maximum tolerated dose of statin and ezetimibe, combination with bempedoic acid should be considered	IIa	C
For patients with a recurrent atherothrombotic event (not necessarily of the same type as the first event) while taking maximally tolerated statin therapy, an LDL-C goal of <1.0 mmol/L (<40 mg/dL) may be considered	IIb	B

[a]*Class* of recommendation.
[b]Level of evidence.
(CCS: chronic coronary syndrome; LDL-C: low-density lipoprotein cholesterol; PCSK9: proprotein convertase subtilisin/kexin type 9)
Source: ESC 2024.

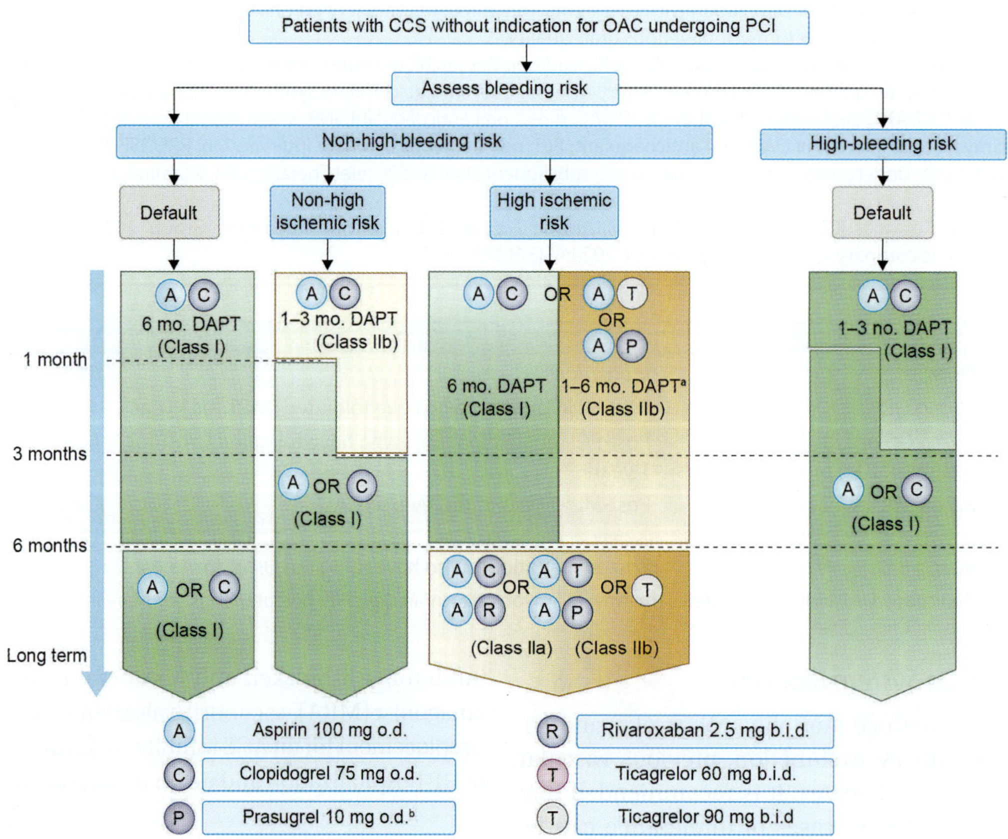

Fig. 1: Recommendation for event prevention.

[a]In CCS patients undergoing high-thrombotic risk stenting (e.g., complex left main stem, two-stent bifurcation, suboptimal stenting result, prior stent thrombosis, previously known CYP2C19*2/*3 polymorphisms), prasugrel or ticagrelor (in addition to aspirin) may be considered instead of clopidogrel for the first month, and up to 3–6 months.
[b]Prasugrel 5 mg o.d. for patients aged ≥75 years or with a body weight <60 kg.
(b.i.d.: bis in die (twice daily); CCS: chronic coronary syndrome; DAPT: dual antiplatelet therapy; mo.: months; OAC: oral anticoagulant; o.d.: once daily; PCI: percutaneous coronary intervention)
Source: European Society of Cardiology (ESC)

versus Angiography for Multivessel Evaluation 2) trial, revascularization improved quality of life, and reduced the use of antianginal drugs and associated side effects.[10] The ORBITA (Objective Randomized Blinded Investigation with optimal medical Therapy or Angioplasty in stable angina) study, entailing a sham procedure in the control group, found no significant improvement in exercise capacity with PCI[11] **(Flowchart 1)**.

Decision for Revascularization in Patients with Chronic Coronary Syndrome

See **Flowchart 1**.

Management of Patients with Ischemic Cardiomyopathy and Left Ventricular Dysfunction

See **Table 15**.

Recommendation for Patients with Longstanding Chronic Coronary Syndrome

See **Table 16**.

Microvascular Angina

Patients with microvascular angina typically have exercise-related angina, evidence of ischemia in noninvasive tests,

Flowchart 1: Decision tree for patients undergoing invasive coronary angiography. Decisions for revascularization by percutaneous coronary intervention or coronary artery bypass grafting are based on clinical presentation (symptoms present or absent), and prior documentation of ischemia (present or absent). In the absence of prior documentation of ischemia, indications for revascularization depend on invasive evaluation of stenosis severity or prognostic indications. Patients with no symptoms and ischemia include candidates for transcatheter aortic valve implantation, valve, and other surgery.

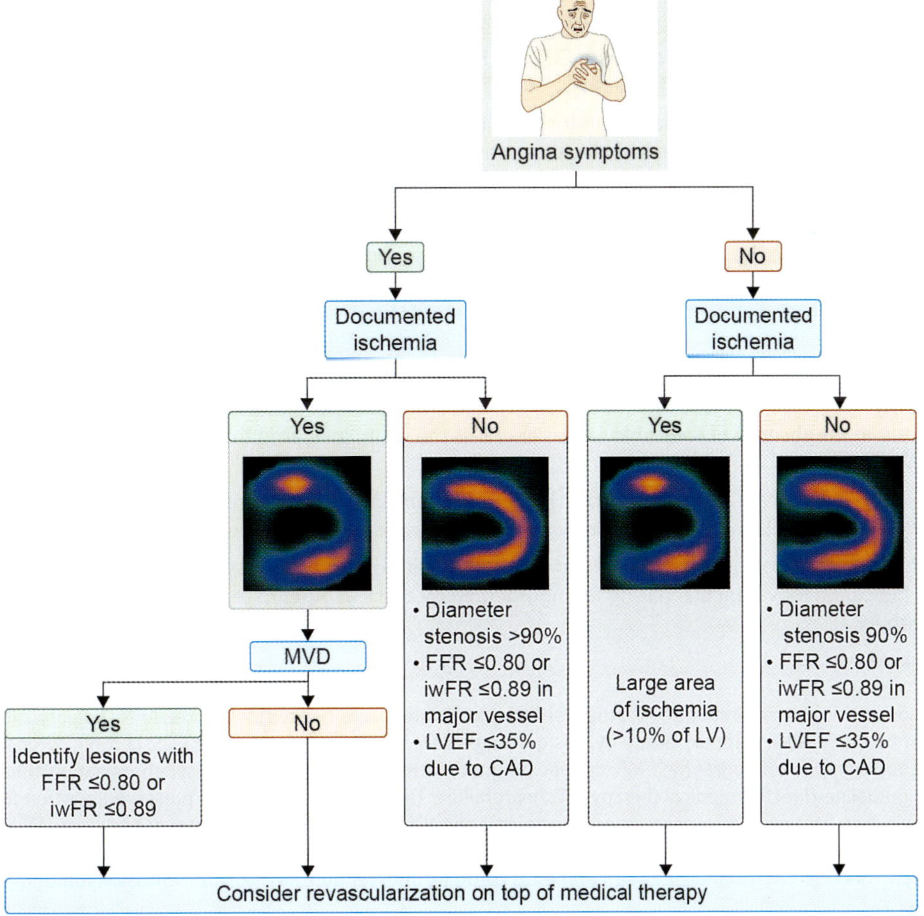

(CAD: coronary artery disease; FFR: fractional flow reserve; iwFR: instantaneous wave-free ratio; LV: left ventricle; LVEF: left ventricular ejection fraction; MVD: multivessel disease)

Source: ESC 2019.

TABLE 15: Management of patients with ischemic cardiomyopathy and LV dysfunction.

Recommendations	*Class*[a]	*Level*[b]
Managing CCS in heart failure patients		
In HF patients with LVEF < 35% in whom obstructive CAD is suspected, ICA is recommended with a view toward improving prognosis by CABG, taking into account the risk-to-benefit ratio of the procedures	I	B
In HF patients with LVEF > 35% and suspected CCS with low or moderate (>5–50%) pretest likelihood of obstructive CAD, CCTA, or functional imaging is recommended	I	C
In HF patients with LVEF > 35% and suspected CCS with very high (>85%) pretest likelihood of obstructive CAD, ICA (with FFR, iFR, or QFR when needed) is recommended	I	C
In patents with HFpEF with persistent angina or equivalent symptoms and normal or nonobstructive epicardial coronary arteries. PET or CMR perfusion or invasive coronary functional testing should be considered to detect or rule out coronary microvascular dysfunction	IIa	B
In selected patients with HFrEF undergoing high-risk PCI for complex CAD, the use of a microaxial flow pump may be considered in experienced centers	IIb	C
Managing heart failure in CCS patients		
It is recommended that CCS patients with HF be enrolled in a multidisciplinary HF management program to reduce the risk of HF hospitalization and to improve survival	I	A
An ACE-I, an MRA, an SGLT-2 inhibitor (dapagliflozin or empagliflozin) and, in stable conditions, a β-blocker is recommended for CCS patents with HFrEF to reduce the risk of HF hospitalization and death	I	A
An SGLT-2 inhibitor (dapagliflozin or empagliflozin) is recommended in patients with heart failure with mildly reduced ejection fraction (HFmrEF) or HFpEF to reduce the risk of HF hospitalization or cardiovascular death	I	A
An ARB is recommended in symptomatic patients with CCS and HFrEF unable to tolerate an ACE-I or ARNI to reduce the risk of HF hospitalization and cardiovascular death	I	B
Sacubitril/valsartan is recommended as a replacement for an ACE-I or ARB in CCS patients with HFrEF to reduce the risk of HF hospitalization and of cardiovascular and all-cause death	I	B
Diuretics are recommended in CCS patients with HF and signs and/or symptoms of congestion to alleviate symptoms, improve exercise capacity, and reduce HF hospitalizations	I	B
An ICD is recommended to reduce the risk of sudden death and all-cause mortality in patients with symptomatic HF (NYHA class II–III) of ischemic etiology (unless they have had an MI in the prior 40 days), and an LVEF <35% despite >3 months of optimized medical treatment, provided they are expected to survive substantially longer than 1 year with good functional status	I	A
An ICD is recommended to reduce the risk of sudden death and all-cause mortality in patients who have recovered from a ventricular arrhythmia causing hemodynamic instability, and who are expected to survive for >1 year with good functional status, in the absence of reversible causes or unless the ventricular arrhythmia has occurred <48 hours after an MI	I	A
CRT is recommended for CCS patients with symptomatic HF, sinus rhythm, LVEF < 35% despite GDMT, and a QRS duration >150 ms with an LBBB QRS morphology to improve symptoms and survival and to reduce morbidity	I	A
CRT rather than right ventricular pacing is recommended for patients with HFrEF regardless of NYHA class or QRS width who have an indication for ventricular pacing for high-degree AV block in order to reduce morbidity. This includes patients with AF	I	A

[a]Class of recommendation.
[b]Level of evidence.

(ACE-I: angiotensin-converting enzyme inhibitor; AF: atrial fibrillation; ARB: angiotensin-receptor blocker; ARNI: angiotensin receptor neprilysin inhibitor; AV: atrioventricular; CABG: coronary artery bypass grafting; CAD: coronary artery disease; CCS: chronic coronary syndrome; CCTA: coronary computed tomography angiography; CMR: cardiac magnetic resonance; CRT: cardiac resynchronization therapy; FFR: fractional flow reserve; GDMT: guideline-directed medical therapy; HF: heart failure; HFpEF: heart failure with preserved ejection fraction; HFrEF: heart failure with reduced ejection fraction; ICA: invasive coronary angiography; ICD: implantable cardioverter defibrillator; iFR: instantaneous wave-free ratio; LBBB: left bundle branch block; LVEF: left ventricular ejection fraction; MI: myocardial infarction; MRA: mineralocorticoid receptor antagonist; NYHA: New York Heart Association; PCI: percutaneous coronary intervention; PET: positron emission tomography; SGLT2: sodium–glucose cotransporter 2)

Source: Vrints C, Andreotti F, Koskinas KC, Rossello X, Adamo M, Ainslie J, et al.; ESC Scientific Document Group. 2024 ESC Guidelines for the management of chronic coronary syndromes. Eur Heart J. 2024;45(36):3415-537.

TABLE 16: Recommendation for patients with longstanding chronic coronary syndrome (CCS).		
Recommendations for asymptomatic patients	*Class*[a]	***Level***[b]
A periodic visit to a cardiovascular healthcare professorial is recommended to reassess any potential change in the risk status of patients, entailing clinical evaluation of lifestyle-modification measures, adherence to targets of cardiovascular risk factors, and the development of comorbidities that may affect treatments and outcomes	I	C
In patients with mild or no symptoms receiving medical treatment in whom noninvasive risk stratification indicates a high risk, and for whom revascularization is considered for improvement of prognosis, invasive coronary angiography (with FFR when necessary) is recommended	I	C
Coronary CTA is not recommended as a routine follow-up test for patients with established CAD	III	C
Invasive coronary areography is not recommended solely for risk stratification	III	C
Symptomatic patients		
Reassessment of CAD status is recommended in patents with deteriorating LV systolic function that cannot be attributed to a reversible cause (e.g., long-standing tachycardia or myocarditis)	I	C
Risk stratification is recommended in patients with new or worsening symptom levels, preferably using stress imaging or, alternatively, exercise stress ECG	I	B
It is recommended to expeditiously refer patients with significant worsening of symptoms for evaluation	I	C
Invasive coronary angiography (with FFR/iFR when necessary) is recommended for risk stratification in patients with severe CAD, particularly if the symptoms are refractory to medical treatment or if they have a high-risk clinical profile	I	C

[a]Class of recommendation.
[b]Level of evidence.

TABLE 17: Investigations to diagnose microvascular angina.		
Recommendations	***Class***[a]	***Level***[b]
Guidewire-based CFR and/or microcirculatory resistance measurements should be considered in patients with persistent symptoms, but coronary arteries that are either angiographically normal or have moderate stenoses with preserved iwFR/FFR	IIa	B
Intracoronary acetylcholine with ECG monitoring may be considered during angiography. If coronary arteries are either angiographically normal or have moderate stenoses with preserved iwFR/FFR to assess microvascular vasospasm	IIb	B
Transthoracic Doppler of the LAD, CMR, and PET may be considered for noninvasive assessment of CFR	IIb	B

[a]Class of recommendation.
[b]Level of evidence.
(CFR: coronary flow reserve; CMR: cardiac magnetic resonance; FFR: fractional flow reserve; iwFR: instantaneous wave-free ratio; LAD: left anterior descending; PET: positron emission tomography)

with no stenoses or mild-to-moderate stenoses (40–60%). Secondary microvascular angina, in the absence of epicardial obstruction, may result from cardiac or systemic conditions like hypertrophic cardiomyopathy, aortic stenosis, and hypertensive heart disease or inflammation such as myocarditis or vasculitis. Values of IMR >25 units or CFR <2.0 are indicative of abnormal microcirculatory function. Both CFR and IMR are typically measured while using intravenous vasodilators, such as adenosine or regadenoson. In patients with abnormal CFR <2.0 or IMR >25 units, and a negative acetylcholine provocation test, β-blockers, ACE inhibitors, and statins, along with lifestyle changes and weight loss, are indicated. Patients developing ECG changes and angina in response to acetylcholine testing but without severe epicardial vasoconstriction may be treated like vasospastic angina patients.

Investigations to Diagnose Microvascular Angina

See **Table 17**.

TABLE 18: Recommendations for diagnosis of patients with angina/ischemia with nonobstructive coronary arteries.

Recommendations	*Class*[a]	*Level*[b]
Diagnosis of ANOCA/INOCA endotypes		
In persistently symptomatic patients despite medical treatment with suspected ANOCA/INOCA (i.e., anginal symptoms with normal coronary arteries or nonobstructive lesions at noninvasive imaging, or intermediate stenoses with normal FFR/iFR at coronary arteriography) and poor quality of life, invasive coronary functional testing is recommended to identify potentially treatable endotypes and to improve symptoms and quality of life, considering patient's choices and preferences	I	B
In persistently symptomatic patients with documented or suspected ANOCA/INOCA, transthoracic Doppler of the LAD, stress echocardiography, CMR, and PET may be considered for the noninvasive assessment of coronary/ myocardial flow reserve	IIb	B

[a]Class of recommendation.
[b]Level of evidence.
(ANOCA: angina with nonobstructive coronary arteries; CMR: cardiac magnetic resonance; FFR: fractional flow reserve; iFR: instantaneous wave-free ratio; INOCA: ischemia with nonobstructive coronary arteries; LAD: left anterior descending; PET: positron emission tomography)
Source: Vrints C, Andreotti F, Koskinas KC, Rossello X, Adamo M, Ainslie J, et al.; ESC Scientific Document Group. 2024 ESC Guidelines for the management of chronic coronary syndromes. Eur Heart J. 2024;45(36):3415-537.

TABLE 19: Investigations for suspected vasospastic angina.

Diagnostic tests for vasospastic angina	*Class*	*Level*
In individuals with suspected vasospastic angina, a resting 12-lead ECG recording during angina is recommended	I	C
In patients with suspected vasospastic angina and repetitive episodes of rest angina associated with ST-segment changes that resolve with nitrates and/or calcium antagonists, invasive coronary functional testing is recommended to confirm the diagnosis and to determine the severity of underlying atherosclerotic disease	I	C
In individuals with suspected vasospastic angina and frequent symptoms, ambulatory ST-segment monitoring should be considered to identify ST-segment deviation during angina	IIa	B

Recommendations for Diagnosis of Patients with Angina/Ischemia with Nonobstructive Coronary Arteries

See **Table 18.**

Vasospastic Angina

Vasospastic angina should be suspected in patients with angina symptoms occurring predominantly at rest, with maintained effort tolerance. Attacks follow a circadian pattern with more episodes at night and in the early morning hours. It is suspected in patients with patent coronary stents and persistent angina. The diagnosis is based on detecting transient ischemic ST-segment changes during an angina attack usually at rest. A provocation test for coronary spasm is considered positive when it triggers: (i) anginal symptoms, (ii) ischemic ECG changes, and (iii) severe vasoconstriction of the epicardial vessel. CCBs and long-acting nitrates is the treatment of choice, control of cardiovascular risk factors, and lifestyle changes. Nifedipine has been shown to be effective in reducing coronary spasm associated with stent implantation.

Investigations for Suspected Vasospastic Angina

See **Table 19.**

Recommendation for Screening of Coronary Artery Disease in Asymptomatic Individuals

See **Table 20.**

Management of Diabetes Mellitus

See **Table 21.**

Management of Refractory Angina

See **Table 22.**

TABLE 20: Recommendation for screening of coronary artery disease (CAD) in asymptomatic individuals.

Recommendations	*Class*[a]	*Level*[b]
Opportunistic screening of healthy individuals for cardiovascular risk factors and to estimate the risk of future cardiovascular events using scoring systems, e.g., SCORE-2 and SCORE-OP, is recommended to detect individuals at high risk and guide treatment decisions	I	C
When coronary artery calcification findings are available from previous chest CT scans, using these findings to enhance risk stratification and guide treatment of modifiable risk factors should be considered	IIa	C
CACS may be considered to improve risk classification around treatment decision thresholds	IIb	C
An ultrasound of the carotid arteries may be considered as an alternative when CACS is unavailable or not feasible to detect atherosclerotic disease and to improve risk classification around treatment decision thresholds	IIb	B

[a]Class of recommendation.
[b]Level of evidence.
(CACS: coronary artery calcium scoring; CT: computed tomography, SCORE2: systematic coronary risk estimation 2; SCORE-OP: systematic coronary risk estimation 2-older persons)
Source: Vrints C, Andreotti F, Koskinas KC, Rossello X, Adamo M, Ainslie J, et al.; ESC Scientific Document Group. 2024 ESC Guidelines for the management of chronic coronary syndromes. Eur Heart J. 2024;45(36):3415-537.

TABLE 21: Management of diabetes mellitus.

Recommendations	*Class*[a]	*Level*[b]
CCS patients with type 2 diabetes mellitus (T2DM)		
SGLT-2 inhibitors with proven CV benefit[c] are recommended in patients with T2DM and CCS to reduce CV events, independent of baseline or target HbA1c and independent of concomitant glucose-lowering medication	I	A
GLP-1 receptor agonists with proven CV benefit[d] are recommended in patients with T2DM and CCS to reduce CV events, independent of baseline or target HbA1c and independent of concomitant glucose-towering medication	I	A
CCS patients without type 2 diabetes mellitus		
The GLP-1 receptor agonist semaglutide should be considered in overweight (BMI >27 kg/m^2) or obese CCS patients without diabetes to reduce CV mortality, MI, or stroke	IIa	B

[a]Class of recommendation.
[b]Level of evidence.
[c]Canagliflozin, dapagliflozin, empagliflozin, sotagliflozin (listed in alphabetical order).
[d]Dulaglutide, efpeglenatide, liraglutide, and semaglutide (listed in alphabetical order).
(BMI: body mass index; CCS: chronic coronary syndrome; CV: cardiovascular; GLP-1: glucagon-like peptide-1; HbA1c: glycated hemoglobin; MI: myocardial infarction; SGLT2: sodium–glucose co-transporter 2)
Source: Vrints C, Andreotti F, Koskinas KC, Rossello X, Adamo M, Ainslie J, et al.; ESC Scientific Document Group. 2024 ESC Guidelines for the management of chronic coronary syndromes. Eur Heart J. 2024;45(36):3415-537.

TABLE 22: Management of refractory angina.

Therapy	*Type of therapy*	*RCT*
External counter pulsation	Enhanced extremal counter pulsation	Must
Extracorporeal shockwave	Low-energy extracorporeal shockwave therapy	Not available
Coronary sinus constriction	Reducer device	COSIRA
Neuromodulation	Spinal cord stimulation	STARTSTIMS
	Transcutaneous electrical neural stimulation	Not available
	Subcutaneous electrical neural stimulation	Not available
	Sympathectomy	Denby et al.

Contd…

Contd...

Recommendations	*Class*[a]	*Level*[b]
Gene therapy	Adenovirus fibroblast growth factor 5	Not available
Autologous cell therapy	Mononuclear bone marrow-derived hematopoietic progenitor cells	RENEW
In patients with refractory angina leading to poor quality of life and with documented or suspected ANOCA/INOCA invasive coronary functional testing is recommended to define ANOCA/INOCA endotypes and appropriate treatment considering patient choices and preferences	I	B
In patients with debilitating angina and obstructive CAD refractory to optimal medical and revascularization strategies, a reducer device for coronary sinus constriction may be considered to improve symptoms, in experienced centers	IIb	B

[a]Class of recommendation.
[b]Level of evidence.
(ANOCA: angina with nonobstructive coronary arteries; CAD: coronary artery disease; NOCA: ischemia with nonobstructive coronary arteries)
Source: Vrints C, Andreotti F, Koskinas KC, Rossello X, Adamo M, Ainslie J, et al.; ESC Scientific Document Group. 2024 ESC Guidelines for the management of chronic coronary syndromes. Eur Heart J. 2024;45(36):3415-537.

CONCLUSION

An initial trial of medical therapy alone is the cornerstone of treatment for CCS. Revascularization is required in patients with persistent symptoms. Ischemia should be established with a noninvasive stress test before angiography. In patients undergoing angiography without a previous noninvasive stress test, FFR may be used to make appropriate decisions regarding revascularization. Revascularization with PCI or CABG is a very effective treatment for CAD.

The method of choice for revascularization depends on the angiographic characteristics of the lesions causing ischemia, LV dysfunction, comorbid conditions, suitability of the patient for surgery. The physician's ultimate decisions regarding patient care must include current evidence-based medicine as well as the patient's preferences and quality-of-life expectations.

In summary, the management of CAD, particularly in patients with CCS and conditions like ANOCA/INOCA, requires a multifaceted approach that encompasses precise diagnostic strategies, guideline-directed medical therapy, and individualized treatment pathways. The emphasis on shared decision-making and patient's education is critical to optimize risk-factor control and long-term outcomes. While advanced imaging techniques and functional testing play pivotal roles in guiding interventions, ongoing research is essential to enhance the understanding of disease endotypes and to develop effective lifestyle modification strategies. Ultimately, a holistic approach that integrates lifestyle changes, evidence-based therapies, and tailored revascularization strategies will be vital in improving patient's outcomes and reducing the burden of cardiovascular disease.

REFERENCES

1. SCOT-HEART Investigators. CT coronary angiography in patients with suspected angina due to coronary heart disease (SCOT-HEART): an open-label, parallel-group, multicentre trial. Lancet. 2015;385(9985):2383-91.
2. Vrints C, Andreotti F, Koskinas KC, Rossello X, Adamo M, Ainslie J, et al. 2024 ESC Guidelines for the management of chronic coronary syndromes: developed by the Task Force for the management of chronic coronary syndromes of the European Society of Cardiology (ESC). Eur Heart J. 2024;45(36):3415-537.
3. Campeau L. Letter: grading of angina pectoris. Circulation. 1976;54(3):522-3.
4. Mark DB, Shaw L, Harrell FE Jr, Hlatky MA, Lee KL, Bengtson JR, et al. Prognostic value of a treadmill exercise score in outpatients with suspected coronary artery disease. N Engl J Med. 1991;325(12):849-53.
5. Diamond GA, Forrester JS. Analysis of probability as an aid in the clinical diagnosis of coronary-artery disease. N Engl J Med. 1979;300(24):1350-8.
6. Maron DJ, Boden WE, O'Rourke RA, Hartigan PM, Calfas KJ, Mancini GB, et al. Intensive multifactorial intervention for stable coronary artery disease: optimal medical therapy in the COURAGE (Clinical Outcomes Utilizing

Revascularization and Aggressive Drug Evaluation) trial. J Am Coll Cardiol. 2010;55(13):1348-58.
7. Critchley JA, Capewell S. Mortality risk reduction associated with smoking cessation in patients with coronary heart disease: a systematic review. JAMA. 2003;290(1):86-97.
8. Poole-Wilson PA, Lubsen J, Kirwan BA, van Dalen FJ, Wagener G, Danchin N, et al.; ACTION investigators. Effect of long-acting nifedipine on mortality and cardiovascular morbidity in patients with stable angina requiring treatment (ACTION trial): randomised controlled trial. Lancet. 2004;364(9437):849-57.
9. IONA Study Group. Effect of nicorandil on coronary events in patients with stable angina: the Impact Of Nicorandil in Angina (IONA) randomised trial. Lancet. 2002;359(9314):1269-75.
10. Xaplanteris P, Fournier S, Pijls NHJ, Fearon WF, Barbato E, Tonino PAL, et al. Five-year outcomes with PCI guided by fractional flow reserve. N Engl J Med. 2018;379(3):250-9.
11. Al-Lamee R, Thompson D, Dehbi HM, Sen S, Tang K, Davies J, et al. Percutaneous coronary intervention in stable angina (ORBITA): a double-blind, randomised controlled trial. Lancet. 2018;391(10115):31-40.

Cardiac Toxicity of Oncology Drugs

Asha Moorthy, Supraja Moorthy, Prashant Moorthy

INTRODUCTION

Cardiovascular complications in patients with cancer represent a major challenge for cardiologists and oncologists with considerable advances in cancer treatment. As a result, there is a dramatic increase in the number of patients presenting with a combination of cancer and cancer treatment-related cardiovascular diseases.[1] Several international guidelines and position articles have been published on the cardiovascular monitoring and management of patients treated with cancer drugs.[2] A panel, from the French Working Group of Cardio-Oncology, analyzed and compared the key components of the pathways recommended by the most recent guidelines from the American and European societies of both oncology and cardiology. They then proposed pragmatic approaches based on harmonization of these guidelines and the most recent published studies.

The guidelines from the American Society of Clinical Oncology (ASCO-2017 and ASCO-2018), the European Society for Medical Oncology (ESMO-2017 and ESMO-2020), and the European Society of Cardiology (ESC-2016) give a clear-cut approach to these subsets of patients. The ESMO-2017 and ASCO-2018 guidelines were specific to immune checkpoint inhibitor (ICI)-related toxicity. For cardiovascular monitoring strategies, only the cancer drugs associated with a high risk of cardiovascular toxicity were analyzed, including anthracyclines, human epidermal growth factor-2 inhibitors (HER2Is), vascular endothelial growth factor inhibitors (VEGFIs), Bcr-Abl kinase inhibitors, proteasome inhibitors (proteasomes), ICIs, and ibrutinib. Cardiovascular complications related to anticancer hormonotherapy and radiotherapy are not addressed. This work does not provide detailed information regarding the cardiovascular toxicities associated with each cancer treatment because these data are available in the existing guidelines; rather, it provides a more practical harmonization that can be useful in daily clinical practice for physicians who care for patients with cancer.

CARDIOVASCULAR MONITORING DURING CANCER TREATMENT

It is mandatory to identify patients with increased risk of developing cardiovascular toxicity. However, differences exist in the definition of high-risk patients and the recommended strategies for investigation. All of the definitions include patients with previous cardiovascular diseases or risk factors, high-dose anthracycline, and combination therapy based on several studies.[3] The pragmatic harmonized definition proposed by the working group is shown in **Box 1**.

BOX 1: Patients with increased risk of developing cardiovascular toxicity.

- High-dose anthracycline (e.g., doxorubicin ≥250 mg/m^2, epirubicin ≥600 mg/m^2)
- High-dose radiotherapy (≥30 Gy) where the heart is in the treatment field
- Lower-dose anthracycline (e.g., doxorubicin <250 mg/m^2, epirubicin <600 mg/m^2) or HERIs or VEGFIs or proteasomes (proteasome inhibitors) or Bcr-Abl inhibitors and presence of any of the following factors:
  - Age ≥60 years
  - Lower-dose radiotherapy (<30 Gy) where the heart is in the treatment field
  - ≥2 risk factors, including smoking, hypertension, diabetes mellitus, dyslipidemia, chronic renal insufficiency, and obesity
- Previous heart disease
  - Elevated cardiac biomarkers before initiation of anticancer therapy
- This parameter should be measured during the first evaluation but will be rechecked during follow-up only with cancer treatments that may modify them (e.g., Bcr-Abl inhibitors or mammalian target of rapamycin inhibitors)

(Bcr-Abl: Bcr-Abl kinase; HERIs: human epidermal growth factor-2 inhibitors; VEGFIs: vascular endothelial growth factor inhibitors)

N-terminal Pro-B-type Natriuretic Peptide (or B-type Natriuretic Peptide) and/or Troponin

For a long time, cardiological assessment of patients receiving cancer therapy has been limited to the measurement of left ventricular ejection fraction (LVEF). It is now clearly established that this evaluation is insufficient and should include a more comprehensive cardiovascular risk evaluation allowing earlier detection of myocardial toxicities as well as other cardiovascular toxicities (e.g., hypertension, QTc interval prolongation, arrhythmias, and vascular diseases) **(Box 2)**.

Anthracyclines

Box 3 shows pragmatic approach for monitoring patients treated with anthracyclines and HER2Is.

Anthracyclines should not be used in patients with LVEF <40% unless there is no effective alternative cancer treatment. In patients with LVEF <50% but ≥40% and those exposed to multiple cardiotoxic cancer treatments who have a normal LVEF and associated cardiovascular risk factors, anthracyclines can be used with a cardio protective strategy using angiotensin-converting enzyme inhibitors (ACEIs) [or angiotensin receptor blockers (ARBs)] and/or beta blockers (BBs). Regarding monitoring during therapy, the use of troponin to predict left ventricular systolic dysfunction (LVSD) is highly variable because of conflicting results.[4,5] Hence, troponin assay is indicated in situations which it has most clearly demonstrated its value, namely, high-cumulative-dose anthracycline (doxorubicin ≥250 mg/m^2 or epirubicin ≥600 mg/m^2), lower-cumulative-dose anthracycline in association with other cardiotoxic therapy, or cardiovascular risk factors.

Human Epidermal Growth Factor-2 Inhibitors

A cardiological assessment before HER2I initiation is recommended, including physical examination, electrocardiogram (ECG), and cardiac imaging, preferably

BOX 2: Cardiovascular assessment included in the "cardio-oncological evaluation".

- Clinical consultation (including BP measurement)
- ECG
- Blood glucose, lipid profile, glomerular filtration rate calculation
- Cardiovascular global risk assessment using guidelines
- TTE including measurements of LVEF measurements (ideally three-dimensional but at least two-dimensional Simpson biplane method) and GLS; in the absence of GLS quantification of LV longitudinal function, use mitral annular displacement by M-mode echocardiography and/or peak systolic velocity of the mitral annulus by pulsed-wave DTI
- LV contrast agents could be potentially useful in two-dimensional echocardiography
- CMR is recommended if the quality of TTE is suboptimal.
- Use the same imaging modality for monitoring
- Actively manage modifiable cardiovascular risk factors and diseases
- Encourage exercise on a regular basis and healthy dietary habits

(BP: blood pressure; CMR: cardiac magnetic resonance; DTI: Doppler tissue imaging; ECG: electrocardiogram; GLS: global longitudinal strain; LV: left ventricular; LVEF: left ventricular ejection fraction; TTE: transthoracic echocardiogram)

BOX 3: Pragmatic approach for monitoring patients treated with anthracyclines and human epidermal growth factor-2 inhibitors (HER2Is).

The cardio-oncological evaluation will systematically include at least one visit with:

- Clinical consultation (including BP measurement)
- ECG
- Blood glucose, lipid profile, and glomerular filtration rate calculation should be evaluated before initiation of anthracyclines and HER2Is. Recheck at least at 1 year, 2 years, and periodically thereafter for patients who received anthracyclines
- TTE including measurements of LVEF measurements (ideally three-dimensional but at least two-dimensional Simpson biplane method) and GLS; In the absence of GLS quantification of LV longitudinal function, use mitral annular displacement by M-mode echocardiography and/or peak systolic velocity of the mitral annulus by pulsed-wave DTI
- LV contrast agents could be potentially useful in two-dimensional echocardiography
- CMR is recommended if the quality of TTE is suboptimal
- Use the same imaging modality for monitoring
- Actively manage modifiable cardiovascular risk factors and diseases
- Encourage exercise on a regular basis and healthy dietary habits
- For monitoring, assays should be performed by the same laboratory (same type of troponin, same method of measurement) and at the same time (before or within 24 hours after each cycle). Troponin+ if >99th percentile of the upper reference limit or significantly increased compared with baseline

(BP: blood pressure; CMR: cardiac magnetic resonance; DTI: Doppler tissue imaging; ECG: electrocardiogram; GLS: global longitudinal strain; LV: left ventricular; LVEF: left ventricular ejection fraction; TTE: transthoracic echocardiogram)

transthoracic echocardiogram. However, there are important differences regarding initial and subsequent evaluation of cardiac biomarkers and pretherapeutic introduction of ACEIs (or ARBs) and/or BBs in high-risk patients. While most guidelines recommend cardiac imaging monitoring every 3 months during treatment, the ASCO-2016 guidelines leave the choice of timing to the physician's discretion. No specific recommendations for HER2Is are proposed by the guidelines regarding the long-term follow-up in survivors.

These inhibitors should not be used in patients with LVEF <40% unless there is no effective alternative cancer treatment. In patients with LVEF <50% but ≥40% and those exposed to multiple cardiotoxic cancer treatments with a normal LVEF and associated cardiovascular risk factors, HER2Is can be used with a cardioprotective strategy using ACEIs (or ARBs) and/or BBs. A complete cardio-oncological evaluation is recommended every 3 months during HER2I treatment in all patients. The benefit of troponins to predict intravenous or subcutaneous HER2 is that cardiotoxicity is somewhat equivocal and appears to be more helpful, especially in patients with prior exposure to anthracyclines. Troponin evaluation may be used after each infusion in patients at higher risk of cardiotoxicity.

Vascular Endothelial Growth Factor Inhibitors

Initial cardiovascular evaluation includes screening and management of cardiovascular risk factors, baseline blood pressure (BP) value, and LVEF measurement. During VEGFI therapy, the guidelines recommend the same general rules as for other cancer treatments with potential cardiotoxicity but highlight the importance of performing appropriate and close BP monitoring and screening of early signs and symptoms of heart failure (HF). However, there is no consensus on the use of cardiac biomarkers or the timing of evaluations.

Bcr-Abl Kinase Inhibitors

The Bcr-Abl kinase inhibitors (imatinib, dasatinib, nilotinib, bosutinib, and ponatinib) are associated with accelerated atherosclerosis, peripheral artery disease development, acute coronary syndrome, stroke, hypertension, hyperglycemia, hypercholesterolemia, pericardial effusion, pulmonary arterial hypertension, QTc prolongation, and occasionally LVSD.

A monitoring strategy based on the specific risk of toxicity for each Bcr-Abl inhibitor drug and the individual global cardiovascular risk should be performed. Special attention should be paid to patients at very high or high individual cardiovascular risk and those treated with nilotinib and ponatinib. Indeed, previously unrecognized and severe peripheral atherosclerosis has emerged as a critical concern with nilotinib, along with serious arterial thrombotic events with ponatinib. The results of several studies support the utilization of the ankle-brachial index in this setting. An abnormal ankle-brachial index (<0.9) is sensitive and specific for peripheral artery disease and could indicate systemic atherosclerotic disease.

Proteasome Inhibitors

Proteasomes (carfilzomib, bortezomib, and ixazomib) are associated mainly with LVSD, HF, arterial hypertension, and myocardial ischemia.

All patients eligible for proteasomes and particularly for carfilzomib should have a baseline cardio-oncological evaluation before treatment begins. This initial evaluation should also contain a baseline measurement of natriuretic peptides and baseline home BP monitoring. This proposal is based on the fact that median time to first cardiovascular adverse event (AE) from proteasomes start was 31 days, with 86% of cardiovascular events occurring within the first 3 months, and that baseline natriuretic peptides were also predictive of cardiovascular events. After the baseline evaluation, it is suggested to repeat cardio-oncological evaluation, including natriuretic peptides, and home BP monitoring every 3 months in the first year, and every 6 months thereafter, throughout the course of proteasome therapy.[6]

Ibrutinib

Ibrutinib has been associated with atrial fibrillation (AF) since the early drug development phases. More recently, other cardiovascular toxicities were described, including hypertension, HF, ventricular arrhythmias, and conduction disorders.

All patients eligible for ibrutinib therapy should have a baseline cardio-oncological evaluation. After the baseline evaluation, asymptomatic patients should receive repeat cardio-oncological evaluation every 3 months in the first year (and every 6 months afterward) associated with home BP monitoring during all ibrutinib therapy. The decision to perform cardio-oncological evaluations every 3 months during the first year is based on the fact that conduction disorders mainly develop during the first 30 days, and AF, ventricular arrhythmias, and HF have a peak incidence at 2–3 months, whereas hypertension occurs mainly after 4–5 months. Overall, cardiac AEs steadily occur during the first year after ibrutinib initiation. In symptomatic patients, repeated Holter-ECG monitoring for AF screening is suggested.

Immune Checkpoint Inhibitors

Immune checkpoint inhibitors are associated with the occurrence of immune-related myocarditis, which has a high mortality of ≈50%. Pericarditis, supraventricular arrhythmias, acute coronary syndrome, and Takotsubo syndrome are other potential cardiovascular immune-related AEs.

Clinical suspicion of ICI-associated myocarditis is usually made by oncologists during patient monitoring. Hence, the proposed algorithm should be available in the oncology department, easy to perform, and easy for a non-cardiologist to analyze. It is the proposal of the working group to consider two strategies that best reflect the entire possible clinical scenario. Strategy 1 considers baseline cardiovascular signs/symptoms, ECG, and troponin I or T for each patient deemed to receive ICI therapy. Strategy 2 considers that only cardiovascular signs/symptoms be checked before each ICI administration, and only patients with new cardiovascular signs/symptoms or non-cardiovascular immune-related AEs be evaluated with ECG and troponin. Strategies 1 and 2 consider that asymptomatic patients with a rise in troponin or new ECG abnormalities or patients with new cardiovascular signs/symptoms who are rapidly referred to a cardio-oncology unit should be able to confirm or deny the diagnosis of ICI-related myocarditis.

CONCLUSION

Cancer therapy-related cardiac dysfunction (CTRCD) affects an increasing population of oncology patients. It can be classified as direct (dose-dependent vs. dose-independent) or indirect, either case being potentially permanent or reversible. Risk assessment, recognition, and prevention of CTRCD are crucial.

Traditional cardiac risk factors, as well as therapy-related risk factors, may be predictive of CTRCD. Anthracyclines, alkylating agents, HER2Is, taxanes, and fluoropyrimidines are traditional cancer therapies with the risk of cardiotoxicity, with more targeted therapies including tyrosine kinase inhibitors (TKIs) and immunotherapy more recently being described as culprits.

Troponin assessment has been shown to be of high negative and positive predictive values for CTRCD. Although cardiac magnetic resonance imaging (MRI) is the gold standard to evaluate cardiac function, echocardiography is the first-line screening tool and may be of greater value when global longitudinal strain (GLS) and three-dimensional echocardiography for ejection fraction (EF) are used.

We recommend screening all patients before starting cancer therapeutics with the potential for cardiac dysfunction with an ECG, troponin level, and left ventricular (LV) function assessment with an echocardiogram including GLS, echo contrast, and, if possible, three-dimensional EF.

Beta blockers, renin-angiotensin inhibitors, aldosterone antagonist therapy, and statins can preserve LV systolic function in patients at risk. Dexrazoxane in patients who are planned to exceed the recommended cumulative dose of anthracyclines and steroids in the event of immunotherapy-related cardiac dysfunction are important cancer therapy-specific considerations.

Results indicate that relative reduction of GLS >15% from the baseline is a sensitive marker for predicting early planned to exceed the recommended cumulative dose of anthracyclines and steroids in the event of immunotherapy-related cardiac dysfunction are important cancer therapy-specific considerations.

Results indicate that relative reduction of GLS >15% from the baseline is a sensitive marker for predicting early planned to exceed the recommended cumulative dose of anthracyclines and steroids in the event of immunotherapy-related cardiac dysfunction are important cancer therapy-specific considerations.

REFERENCES

1. Cautela J, Lalevée N, Ammar C, Ederhy S, Peyrol M, Debourdeau P, et al. Management and research in cancer treatment-related cardiovascular toxicity: Challenges and perspectives. Int J Cardiol. 2016;224:366-75.
2. Plana JC, Galderisi M, Barac A, Ewer MS, Ky B, Scherrer-Crosbie M, et al. Expert consensus for multimodality imaging evaluation of adult patients during and after cancer therapy: a report from the American Society of Echocardiography and the European Association of Cardiovascular Imaging. Eur Heart J Cardiovascular Imaging. J Am Soc Echocardiogr. 2014;27(9):911-39.
3. Brahmer JR, Lacchetti C, Schneider BJ, Atkins MB, Brassil KJ, Caterino JM, et al. National Comprehensive

Cancer Network. Management of immune-related adverse events in patients treated with immune checkpoint inhibitor therapy: American Society of Clinical Oncology Clinical Practice Guideline. J Clin Oncol. 2018;36:1714-68.

4. Cardinale D, Ciceri F, Latini R, Franzosi MG, Sandri MT, Civelli M, et al. ICOS-ONE Study Investigators. Anthracycline-induced cardiotoxicity: A multicenter randomised trial comparing two strategies for guiding prevention with enalapril: The International Cardio Oncology Society-one trial. Eur J Cancer. 2018;94:126-37.
5. Cardinale D, Colombo A, Sandri MT, Lamantia G, Colombo N, Civelli M, et al. Prevention of high-dose chemotherapy-induced cardiotoxicity in high-risk patients by angiotensin-converting enzyme inhibition. Circulation. 2006;114:2474-81.
6. Bringhen S, Milan A, D'Agostino M, Ferri C, Wäsch R, Gay F, et al. Prevention, monitoring and treatment of cardiovascular adverse events in myeloma patients receiving carfilzomib A consensus paper by the European Myeloma Network and the Italian Society of Arterial Hypertension. J Intern Med. 2019;286:63-74.

Two-Stent Strategy for Bifurcation: Current Best Practices

Ajit G Desai, Nikesh D Jain

INTRODUCTION

Coronary bifurcation lesions (CBLs) are encountered in ~15–20% of percutaneous coronary interventions (PCIs).[1] Their unique geometry increases the complexity and risk of target lesion failure (TLF), side-branch (SB) closure, restenosis, and stent thrombosis compared to nonbifurcation lesions.

Though the provisional stent (PS) approach remains the preferred strategy with comparable outcomes compared to two-stent strategy,[2,3] anatomy characterized by large SB vessels (>2.5 mm), ostial and SB lesions (>10 mm), and difficult SB access often necessitate upfront two-stent strategies.[4,5] Also, in PS strategy, a second stent may still be required in 4–31% of cases.[6-8] Emerging evidence supports the superiority of specific two-stent techniques—particularly double kissing (DK) crush and culotte—in select lesions, challenging the one-size-fits-all provisional paradigm.

CURRENT INDICATIONS OF TWO-STENT TECHNIQUE

Two-stent strategy is recommended as an upfront strategy with the following anatomical characteristics:[6-9]

- Side branch with diameter >2.5 mm
- SB lesion extending 10–20 mm beyond the ostium (>10–20 mm)
- An unfavorable angle for recrossing after main branch (MB) stenting
- A narrow angle between MB and SB causing increased risk of carina shift

In Definition II study,[10] a systematic two-stent strategy was clearly associated with better outcomes than PS strategy in complex bifurcation lesions. Similar outcomes were seen in Nordic-Baltic IV[11] and DK crush II trials.[12]

CURRENT TWO-STENT TECHNIQUES

Currently used two-stent techniques are:

- Culotte technique
- Mini-crush technique
- DK crush technique
- T and small protrusion (TAP) technique
- T technique—less commonly used
- V or simultaneous kissing stent (SKS) technique—less commonly used

There is a lack of comparative data amongst different two-stent techniques. A particular two-stent technique should be decided based on clinical manifestation, anatomical characteristics, and operator experience. In any two-stent technique (except V and SKS technique), final kissing inflation (FKI)[13,14] and proximal optimization technique (POT) should be mandatory **(Table 1)**.

TABLE 1: Advantages and disadvantages of various two-stent techniques.

Stent strategy	*Advantages*	*Disadvantages*
T and TAP techniques **(Fig. 1)**[15]	• Suitable for angle close to 90° • Easy FKI	• Not suitable for wide angle • Invariable protrusion of SB stent
Mini-crush technique **(Figs. 2A to C)**[16]	Ensures complete coverage of SB ostium	• Difficulty in SB reaccess due to multiple layers of stent • Rewiring for FKI is a challenge sometimes • Not suitable for wide angle

Contd...

Contd...

Stent strategy	*Advantages*	*Disadvantages*
DK crush technique **(Fig. 3)**[15]	• 6Fr compatible • Facilitated SB access • More complete coverage of anatomy with less stent deformation	Multiple steps involved
Culotte technique **(Fig. 4)**[15]	• Complete coverage of SB ostium • Homogeneous metal and drug distribution at ostium, carina, and proximal MB • Suitable for wide angle • Avoids triple-layered stent segment in proximal MV	• Rewiring to MB is sometimes difficult • Excessive metal at MB • Requires SB and distal MB of equal diameters
V stenting	• Suitable for normal proximal MB • Short procedure time • No need for SB recrossing • Both branch patency maintained throughout the procedure	• 7 or 8Fr guide required • Proximal MB needs to be disease-free • Geographical miss or protrusion of struts in MB
SKS	• Suitable for large proximal MB • Short procedure time • No need for SB recrossing • Both branch patency maintained throughout the procedure	• Non-left main bifurcation usually not suitable • 7 or 8Fr guide required • Proximal MB has excessive metal with 2 barrels

(DK: double kissing; FKI: final kissing inflation; MB: main branch; MV: main vessel; SB: side branch; SKS: simultaneous kissing stent; TAP: T and small protrusion)

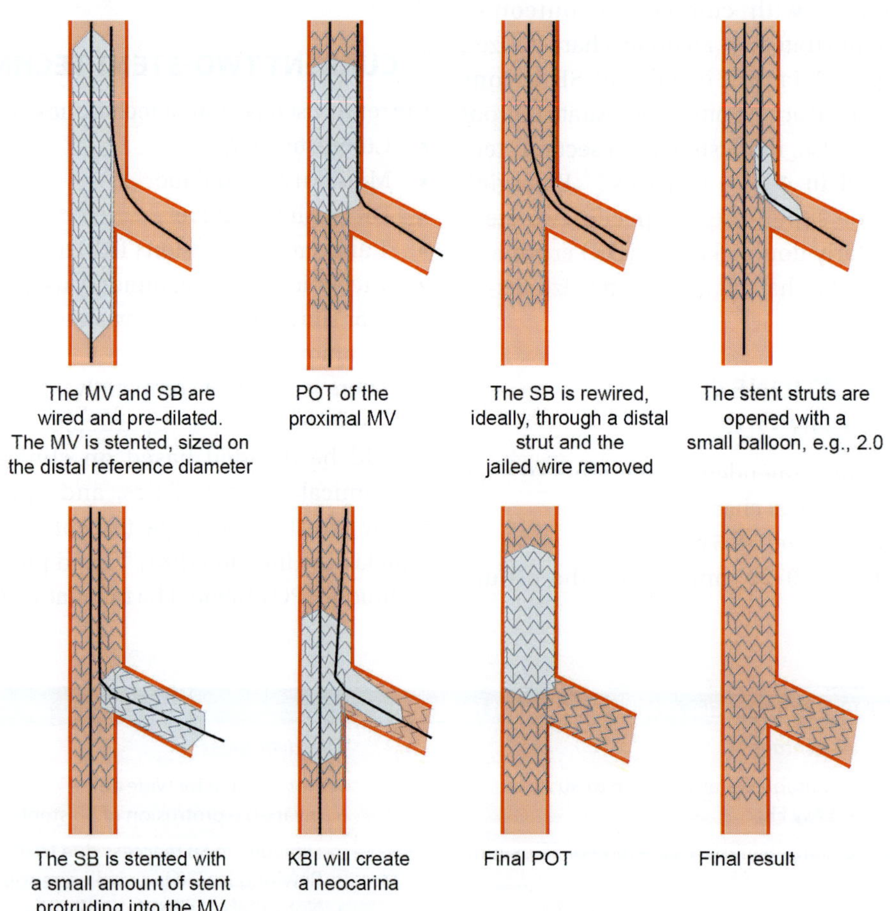

Fig. 1: T stent/TAP, treating MV first.[15] (KBI: kissing balloon inflation; MV: main vessel; POT: proximal optimization technique; TAP: T and small protrusion; SB: side branch)

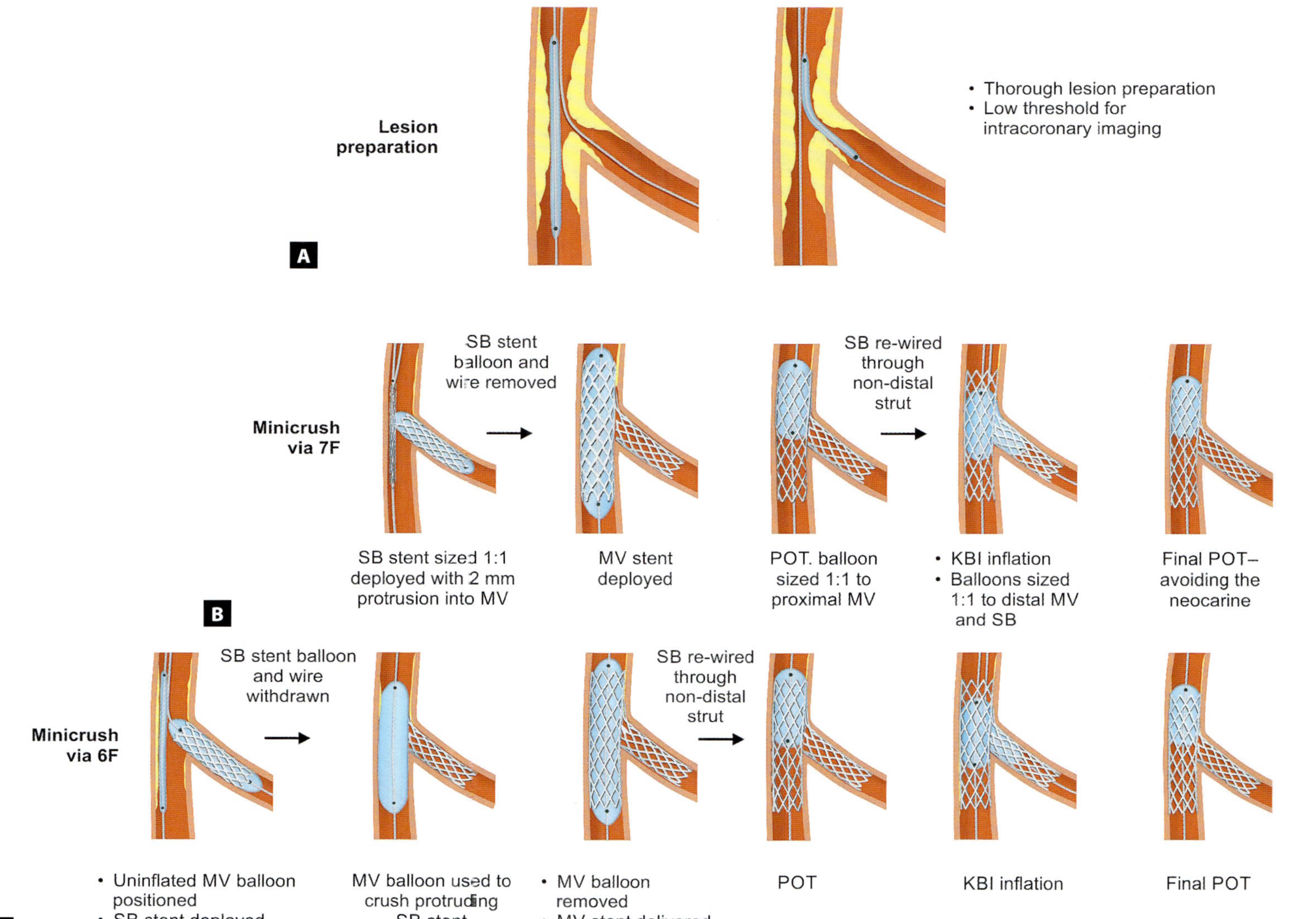

Figs. 2A to C: Mini-crush stepwise technique.[16] (KBI: kissing balloon inflation; MV: main vessel; POT: proximal optimization technique; SB: side branch)

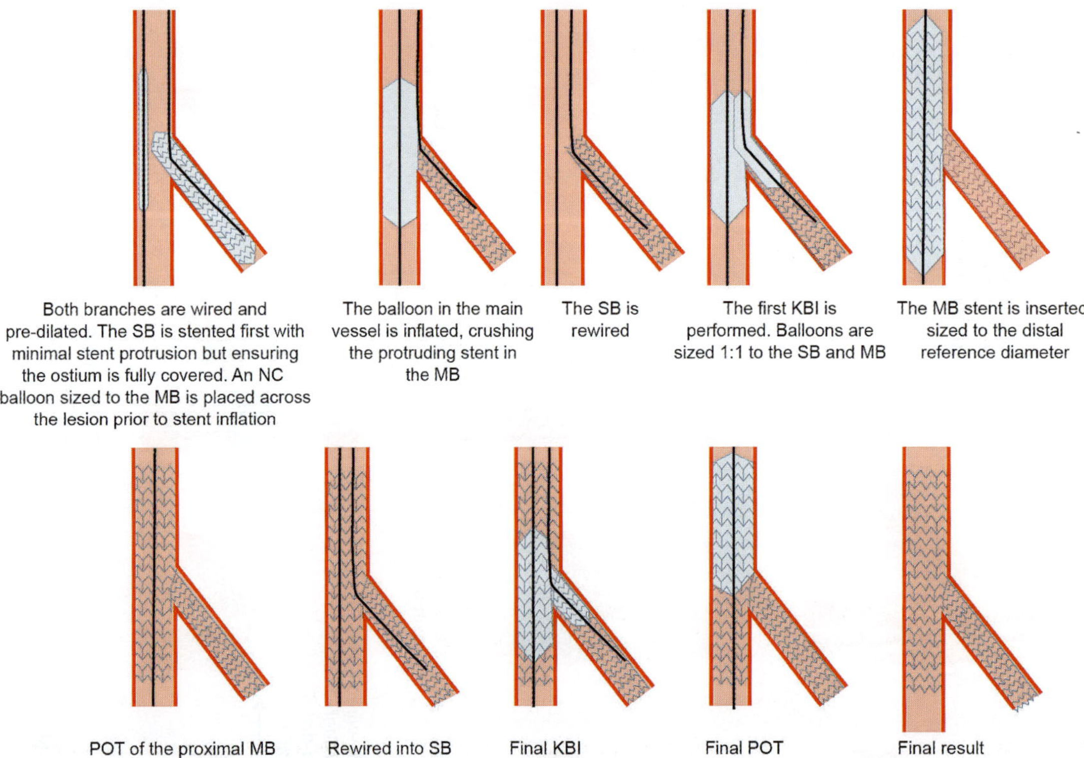

Fig. 3: DK crush technique. Two KBI (unlike classic or mini-crush) are performed, which increases the success of recross after main vessel stenting.[15] (DK: double kissing; KBI: kissing balloon inflation; MB: main branch; NC: non-compliant; POT: proximal optimization technique; SB: side branch)

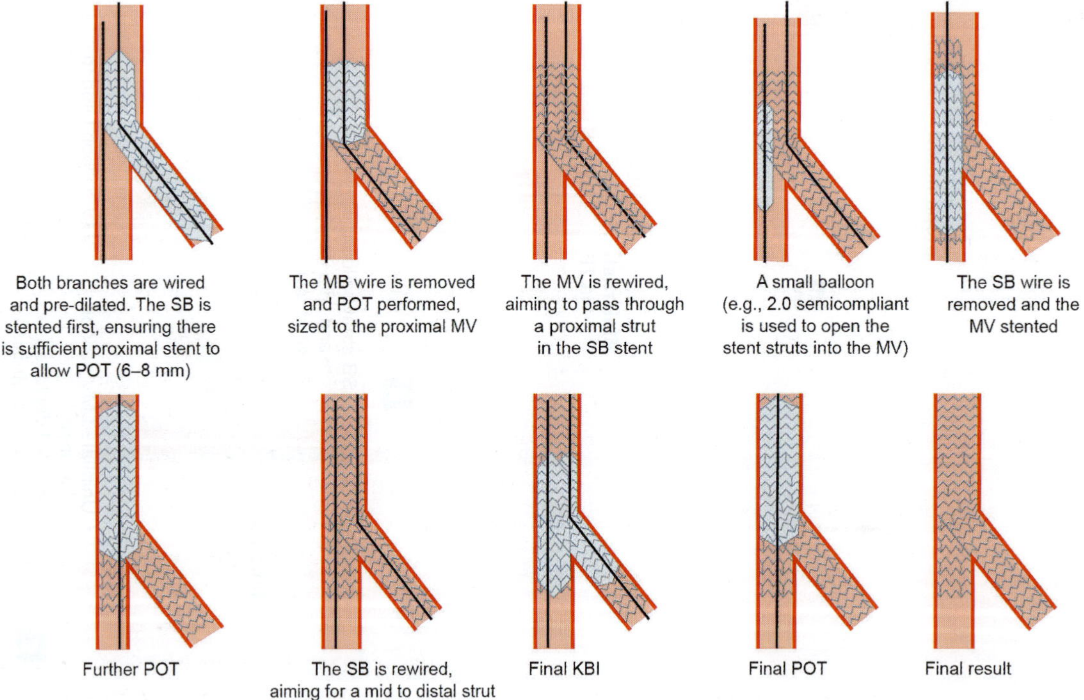

Fig. 4: The culotte technique.[15] (KBI: kissing balloon inflation; MV: main vessel; POT: proximal optimization technique; SB: side branch)

Flowcharts. 1A and B: Decision-making algorithm for optimal bifurcation stenting strategy.[17,18]

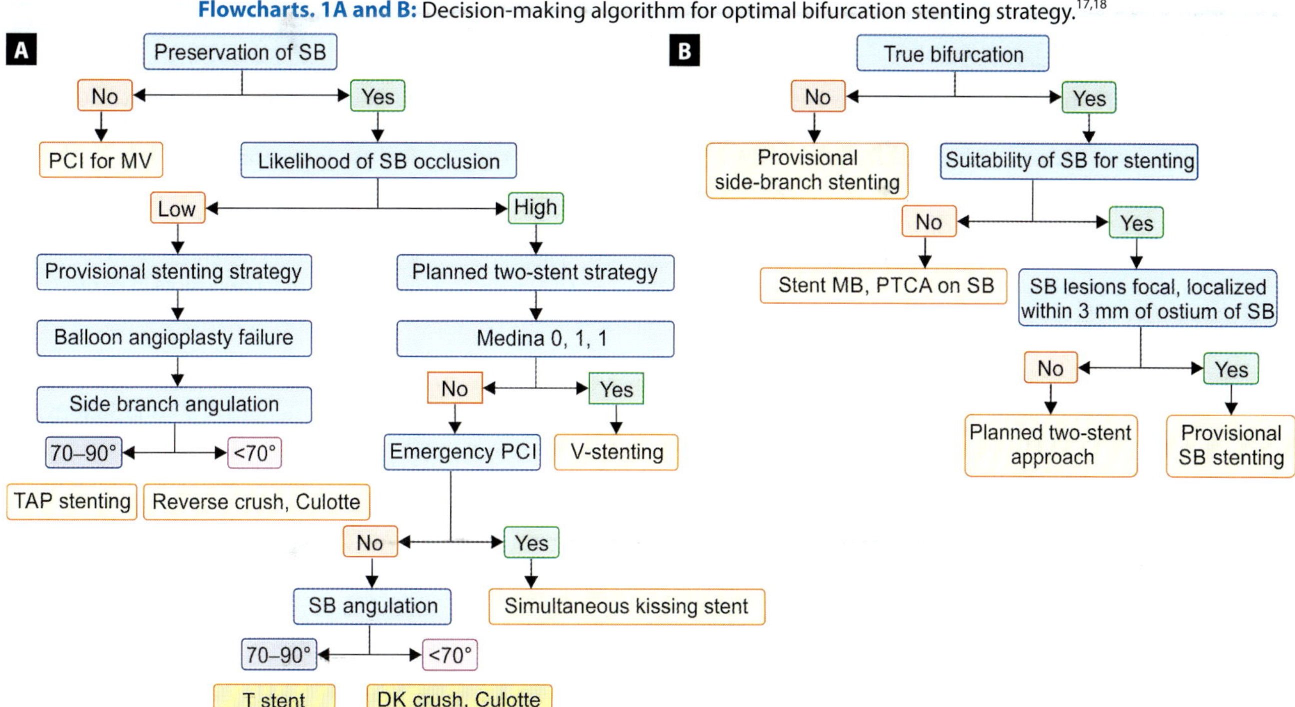

(DK: double kissing; MB: main branch; MV: main vessel; PCI: percutaneous coronary intervention; PTCA: percutaneous transluminal coronary angioplasty; SB: side branch; TAP: T and small protrusion)

Of the above two-stent techniques, DK crush, mini-crush, and culotte are commonly used techniques. Bifurcation angle is an important determinant of choice of technique. A 90° angle facilitates use of T stenting, whereas an acute angle will favor TAP technique. A wide angle will be unfavorable to perform culotte stenting. In angle >80°, there may be incomplete stent apposition in SB with crush techniques.

In DK crush, care should be taken to rewire SB through a proximal strut, unlike in provisional or culotte which require distal strut crossing, to avoid incomplete SB coverage. Some modifications suggested in culotte stenting are mini-culotte, referring to minimal protrusion of stent strut into proximal main vessel (MV) and DK culotte, in which KBI is performed after the first rewiring.

A decision algorithm for selecting optimal bifurcation stenting strategy can be summarized in **Flowcharts 1A and B**.

SELECTING TWO-STENT STRATEGY BASED ON EVIDENCE

Performing trials on bifurcation stenting is difficult due to anatomical variations, definitions used for significant SB, operator experience, and regional preference of practice. Improved techniques of bifurcation stenting, newer stent designs, and improved pharmacotherapy have improved outcomes of two-stent techniques. Previous bifurcation trials used first-generation stents, different inclusion and significant SB definition used, and outcomes measured varied like clinical/angiographic follow-up.

STUDIES ON NON-LEFT MAIN BIFURCATION

Studies mostly involved left anterior descending (LAD)/ diagonal bifurcation lesions. Majority of SB in non-left main bifurcation do not supply >10% of myocardium, limiting the benefits of stenting SB. Studies have clearly shown that with nonsignificant SB disease (<2.5 mm diameter, disease length <10 mm), there was no benefit with two-stent techniques, instead it did more harm **(Table 2)**.

In conclusion, DK crush provides an edge over other two-stent techniques, including PS in true bifurcation lesions with significant diseased SB. This was further substantiated by Definition II study,[10] which categorized bifurcation lesions into simple and complex based on specific anatomical criteria. In simple bifurcation lesion,

TABLE 2: Trials performed with true bifurcation lesions and outcomes.

Study name	*Study details*	*Procedural details*	*Outcome*
EBC TWO[19]	• 200 patients with SB ≥2.5 mm and lesion length >5 mm • *Technique:* Culotte vs. provisional	• KBI - 95% in provisional group, 98% in Culotte group • 16% required second stent in PS group	• MACE rates similar; 7.7% in PS vs. 10.3% in culotte • Trial was underpowered
Nordic-Baltic bifurcation study IV[11]	• 450 patients with SB ≥2.75 mm and lesion length up to 15 mm • Second-generation stent used	• Culotte 66%, mini-crush 21% • 3.7% in PS group required second stent	• 8-month angiography follow-up showed increased binary restenosis of SB • MACE was numerically more in PS group, though not significant 12.9% vs. 8.4%, $p = 0.12$
DK crush II[12]	• 370 patients with Medina 1, 1, 1 or 0, 1, 1 with SB lesion length up to 15 mm • PS compared to DK crush • Second-generation stent used	29% of PS group received second stent	• 8-month angiography follow-up showed increased restenosis in MV and SB with PS group • MACE at 12 months and 5 years were similar, but TVR and TLR were significantly less with DK crush

(DK: double kissing; EBC: European Bifurcation Club; MACE: major adverse cardiovascular event; MV: main vessel; PS: provisional stent; TLR: target lesion revascularization; TVR: target vessel revascularization; SB: side branch)

PS group showed lower in-hospital stent thrombosis and 12-month target lesion revascularization (TLR). In complex bifurcation lesions, DK crush was performed in 77.8%, and culotte in 17.9% of patients. SB stenting was required in 23% of PS group. TLF was lower in two-stent group—6.1% versus 11.4%, $p = 0.019$.

Definition II study further stressed upon tailoring strategy based on anatomy of each patient. For non-left main bifurcation, DK crush technique performed better in complex bifurcation lesion. Other techniques to consider are culotte technique and its modifications, and mini-crush technique **(Fig. 5)**.

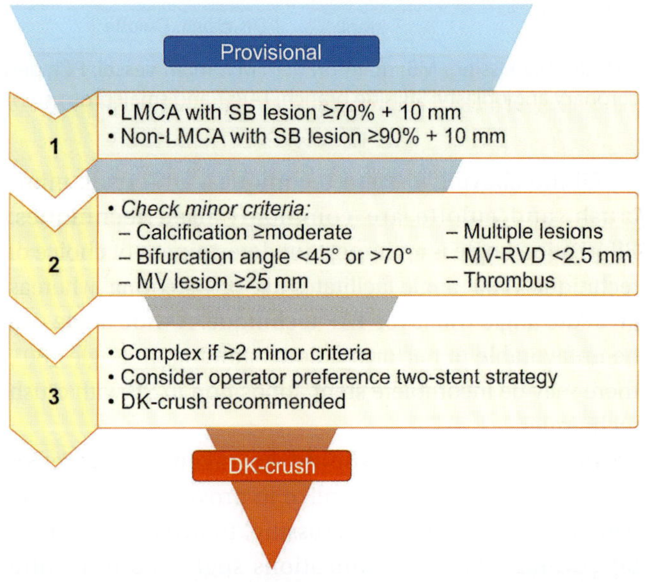

Fig. 5: Definition criteria to guide bifurcation stenting strategy. (DK: double kissing; LMCA: left main coronary artery; MV: main vessel; RVD: reference vessel diameter; SB: side branch)[20]

STUDIES ON LEFT MAIN BIFURCATION

Distal left main (LM) bifurcation is involved in 60–85% of cases,[21] and is associated with inferior outcomes of PCI.[22] Both branches of LM are significant, unless left circumflex (LCX) is very small nondominant artery. The angle of LM bifurcation is usually larger compared to non-left main bifurcation. Meticulous planning, including use of imaging, is preferred for distal LM bifurcation stenting to give optimal result and good long-term outcomes **(Table 3)**.

The preferred two-stent technique, MACE end points used [all-cause mortality and myocardial infarction (MI) were used in European Bifurcation Club (EBC) MAIN rather than cardiac death and target vessel myocardial infarction (TVMI) in DK crush] could have influenced the outcomes in these studies. Patients in DK crush V study had higher SYNTAX (Synergy between Percutaneous Coronary Intervention with Taxus and Cardiac Surgery) scores (31 vs. 23) and longer SB lesion lengths (16 mm vs. 7 mm), which explains more requirement of second stent in PS arm. Conversion of PS to two-stent is also limited to TAP/reverse mini-crush or reverse culotte, which may further compromise result. Also, subanalysis of anatomy

TABLE 3: Trials specifically addressing left main (LM) bifurcation.

Study name	*Study details*	*Procedural details*	*Outcome*
DK crush III[23]	• 419 patients • IVUS used in >70%	DK crush was compared to culotte stenting	• MACE at 1 year was high in culotte group (16.3% vs. 6.2%, $p = 0.001$), driven predominantly by increased TVR (11% vs. 4.3%, $p = 0.016$). • 3-year follow-up also showed increased MACE in culotte group (23.7% vs. 8.2%, $p = <0.001$), driven by increased MI (8.2% vs. 3.4%, $p = 0.037$) in addition to TVR (18.8% vs. 5.8%, $p <0.001$)
DK crush V[24]	• 482 patients • SB lesion length ≥10 mm in 50% of cases	DK crush was compared with PS	• 47% in PS arm required second stent • MACE at 1 year was lower with DK crush 5.0% versus 10.7%, $p = 0.02$ • MACE at 3 years remained worse with PS arm (16.9% vs. 8.3%, $p = 0.005$), with significantly more TVMI, TLR, and stent thrombosis
EBC MAIN[25]	• 467 patients • SB lesion length averaged 7 mm	• PS vs. systematic two-stent strategy • Culotte or T/TAP were most performed	• 22% of PS arm required second stent • MACE at 1 year were similar between 2 groups (14.7% vs. 17.7%, $p = 0.34$)

(DK: double kissing; EBC: European Bifurcation Club; IVUS: intravascular ultrasound; MACE: major adverse cardiovascular event; MI: myocardial infarction; PS: provisional stent; TAP: T and small protrusion; TLR: target lesion revascularization; TVMI: target vessel myocardial infarction; TVR: target vessel revascularization; SB: side branch)

in DK crush as per definition criteria revealed better outcomes with PS in simple bifurcation lesions compared to complex bifurcation lesions, which did better with DK crush. Operator experience also differed as seen by only 5% patients undergoing DK crush in EBC MAIN study.

Though challenging with multiple steps, greater procedural time, and requirement of higher contrast volume, and involves a greater learning curve, DK crush is a preferred technique in distal LM bifurcation technique in experienced hands, especially in complex bifurcation lesions.

CONCLUSION

Though in majority of bifurcation lesions, PS seems to be default strategy; two-stent strategy will be required in select patients, especially in complex bifurcation lesions. Each two-stent technique has advantages and disadvantages, and its application is dictated mainly by specific anatomy, clinical characteristics of patient and operator's experience. FKI and POT should be mandatory in all two-stent techniques (except in V and SKS stenting). As long-term result is more operator-dependent, rather than technique-dependent, we should be familiar with one or two techniques that can be used as per specific anatomy.

REFERENCES

1. Lassen JF, Holm NR, Banning A, Burzotta F, Lefèvre T, Chieffo A, et al. Percutaneous coronary intervention for coronary bifurcation disease: 11th consensus document from the European Bifurcation Club. EuroIntervention. 2016;12(1):38-46.
2. Behan MW, Holm NR, Curzen NP, Erglis A, Stables RH, de Belder AJ, et al. Simple or complex stenting for bifurcation coronary lesions: a patient-level pooled-analysis of the Nordic Bifurcation Study and the British Bifurcation Coronary Study. Circ Cardiovasc Interv. 2011;4(1):57-64.
3. Sirker A, Sohal M, Oldroyd K, Curzen N, Stables R, de Belder A, et al. The impact of coronary bifurcation stenting strategy on health-related functional status: a quality-of-life analysis from the BBC One (British Bifurcation Coronary; Old, New, and Evolving Strategies) study. JACC Cardiovasc Interv. 2013;6(2):139-45.
4. Latib A, Moussa I, Sheiban I, Colombo A. When are two stents needed? Which technique is the best? How to perform? EuroIntervention. 2010;6(Suppl J):J81-7.
5. Ahn JM, Lee JY, Kang SJ, Kim YH, Song HG, Oh JH, et al. Functional assessment of jailed side branches in coronary bifurcation lesions using fractional flow reserve. JACC Cardiovasc Interv. 2012;5:155-61.
6. Steigen TK, Maeng M, Wiseth R, Erglis A, Kumsars I, Narbute I, et al.; Nordic PCI Study Group. Randomized study on simple versus complex stenting of coronary artery bifurcation lesions: the Nordic bifurcation study. Circulation. 2006;114(18):1955-61.

7. Hildick-Smith D, de Belder AJ, Cooter N, Curzen NP, Clayton TC, Oldroyd KG, et al. Randomized trial of simple versus complex drug-eluting stenting for bifurcation lesions: the British Bifurcation Coronary Study: old, new, and evolving strategies. Circulation. 2010;121(10):1235-43.
8. Colombo A, Bramucci E, Saccà S, Violini R, Lettieri C, Zanini R, et al. Randomized study of the crush technique versus provisional side-branch stenting in true coronary bifurcations: the CACTUS (Coronary Bifurcations: Application of the Crushing Technique Using Sirolimus-Eluting Stents) Study. Circulation. 2009;119(1):71-8.
9. Kang SJ, Mintz GS, Kim WJ, Lee JY, Oh JH, Park DW, et al. Changes in left main bifurcation geometry after a single-stent crossover technique: an intravascular ultrasound study using direct imaging of both the left anterior descending and the left circumflex coronary arteries before and after intervention. Circ Cardiovasc Interv. 2011;4(4):355-61.
10. Zhang JJ, Ye F, Xu K, Kan J, Tao L, Santoso T, et al. Multicentre, randomized comparison of two-stent and provisional stenting techniques in patients with complex coronary bifurcation lesions: the DEFINITION II trial. Eur Heart J. 2020;41(27):2523-36.
11. Kumsars I, Holm NR, Niemelä M, Erglis A, Kervinen K, Christiansen EH, et al; Nordic baltic bifurcation study group. Randomised comparison of provisional side branch stenting versus a two-stent strategy for treatment of true coronary bifurcation lesions involving a large side branch: The Nordic-Baltic Bifurcation Study IV. Open Heart. 2020;7(1):e000947.
12. Chen SL, Santoso T, Zhang JJ, Ye F, Xu YW, Fu Q, et al. A randomized clinical study comparing double kissing crush with provisional stenting for treatment of coronary bifurcation lesions: results from the DKCRUSH-II (Double Kissing Crush versus Provisional Stenting Technique for Treatment of Coronary Bifurcation Lesions) trial. J Am Coll Cardiol. 2011;57(8):914-20.
13. Chen SL, Zhang JJ, Ye F, Chen YD, Patel T, Kawajiri K, et al. Study comparing the double kissing (DK) crush with classical crush for the treatment of coronary bifurcation lesions: the DKCRUSH-1 Bifurcation Study with drug-eluting stents. Eur J Clin Invest. 2008;38(6):361-71.
14. Chevalier B, Glatt B, Royer T, Guyon P. Placement of coronary stents in bifurcation lesions by the "culotte" technique. Am J Cardiol. 1998;82(8):943-9.
15. Raphael CE, O'Kane PD. Contemporary approaches to bifurcation stenting. JRSM Cardiovasc Dis. 2021;10:2048004021992190.
16. Raphael CE, O'Kane PD, Johnson TW, Prasad A, Gulati R, Sandoval Y, et al. Evolution of the Crush Technique for Bifurcation Stenting. JACC Cardiovasc Interv. 2021; 14(21):2315-26.
17. Colombo A. Stankovic G. Bifurcations and branch vessel stenting. Textb Interv Cardiol. 2012:270-87.
18. Bifurcations. In: Brilakis E (Ed). Manual of Percutaneous Coronary Interventions: A Step-by-Step Approach, 1st edition. Amsterdam: Elsevier; 2020. pp. 267-301.
19. Hildick-Smith D, Behan MW, Lassen JF, Chieffo A, Lefèvre T, Stankovic G, et al. The EBC TWO Study (European Bifurcation Coronary TWO): A Randomized Comparison of Provisional T-Stenting Versus a Systematic 2 Stent Culotte Strategy in Large Caliber True Bifurcations. Circ Cardiovasc Interv. 2016;9(9):e003643.
20. Hildick-Smith D, Arunothayaraj S, Stankovic G, Chen SL. Percutaneous coronary intervention of bifurcation lesions. EuroIntervention. 2022;18(4):e273-e291.
21. Lefèvre T, Girasis C, Lassen JF. Differences between the left main and other bifurcations. EuroIntervention. 2015; 11:V106-10.
22. Song PS, Song YB, Lee JM, Hahn JY, Choi SH, Choi JH, et al. Major Predictors of Long-Term Clinical Outcomes After Percutaneous Coronary Intervention for Coronary Bifurcation Lesions with 2-Stent Strategy: Patient-Level Analysis of the Korean Bifurcation Pooled Cohorts. JACC Cardiovasc Interv. 2016;9(18):1879-86.
23. Chen SL, Xu B, Han YL, Sheiban I, Zhang JJ, Ye F, et al. Comparison of double kissing crush versus Culotte stenting for unprotected distal left main bifurcation lesions: results from a multicenter, randomized, prospective DKCRUSH-III study. J Am Coll Cardiol. 2013;61(14):1482-8.
24. Chen SL, Zhang JJ, Han Y, Kan J, Chen L, Qiu C, Jiang T, et al. Double Kissing Crush Versus Provisional Stenting for Left Main Distal Bifurcation Lesions: DKCRUSH-V Randomized Trial. J Am Coll Cardiol. 2017;70(21):2605-17.
25. Hildick-Smith D, Egred M, Banning A, Brunel P, Ferenc M, Hovasse T, et al. The European bifurcation club Left Main Coronary Stent study: a randomized comparison of stepwise provisional vs. systematic dual stenting strategies (EBC MAIN). Eur Heart J. 2021;42(37):3829-39.

Comprehensive Coronary Assessment Co-registration of Imaging and Physiology Techniques

Rohit Mody, Debabrata Dash, Bhavya Mody

INTRODUCTION

Coronary artery disease (CAD) is commonly assessed through coronary angiography (CAG). However, CAG's two-dimensional imaging lacks detail on plaque morphology, leading to advancements in intravascular imaging such as intravascular ultrasound (IVUS), optical coherence tomography (OCT), angioscopy, and near-infrared spectroscopy (NIRS).

Intravascular ultrasound and OCT enhance percutaneous coronary intervention (PCI) outcomes by identifying key plaque features. Ischemia-guided revascularization has improved CAD management by assessing stenosis significance, though recent data question using ischemia alone for interventions, as some insignificant lesions may lead to events.[1] Newer IVUS systems allow co-registration with angiography, fractional flow reserve (FFR), and instantaneous wave-free ratio (iFR), providing complete view of diseased arteries.

In summary, co-registration of intravascular imaging and physiology has advanced, PCI CAD diagnosis and management.

INTRAVASCULAR ULTRASOUND TECHNOLOGIES

Intravascular ultrasound and OCT have become crucial tools in interventional diagnostics. IVUS visualizes coronary plaques, lumen, and vessel walls, aiding in lesion length assessment and stent placement. OCT provides high-resolution vessel wall imaging but requires saline flushing, which presents challenges.

Choosing the optimal tool involves weighing benefits and costs. Factors such as lesion characteristics and clinical needs influence decisions. Combining OCT and IVUS enhances plaque composition analysis, though separate pullbacks are needed for co-registration, limiting certain landmark identification.

Intravascular ultrasound co-registration with other imaging, such as angiography, enhances plaque visualization, and improved interventional outcomes.

INTRACORONARY PHYSIOLOGICAL ASSESSMENT

In acute coronary syndrome (ACS), intracoronary physiological assessment is recommended to evaluate flow-limiting stenosis and guide PCI. In catheter laboratories, physiological assessment routinely guides PCI. CAG's limitations in detecting stenosis are mitigated by adjunctive physiology, with strong guideline support **(Figs. 1A to C)**. Clinical trials demonstrate invasive physiology's value in revascularization, increasing its use. **Table 1** shows physiological PCI guidance, with software providing stable FFR, iFR, and resting full-cycle ratio (RFR) to assess stenosis.[2] Longitudinal assessment distinguishes focal from diffuse disease, indicating pressure loss along the vessel **(Fig. 2)**.

Fractional flow reserve is the most common index for coronary stenosis severity, measuring hyperemic pressure directly. iFR evaluates stenosis without adenosine, allowing faster assessment and highlighting individual lesions' hemodynamic effects. Longitudinal vessel analysis helps plan PCI by pinpointing flow-limiting disease, using co-registered physiological data with angiography for precise lesion localization, as shown in **Figure 3**, and identifying regions benefiting from PCI. **Table 2** summarizes challenges in physiological assessment.

In summary, intracoronary physiological assessment is essential in ACS, with indices such as FFR and iFR, integrated with imaging, aiding effective PCI planning.

Planning of periprocedural PCI and simulation
- Clinical indications of PCI setting
- Investigation of pattern of disease—focal, diffuse, and tandem
- Use of PCI various strategies for simulation of functional results

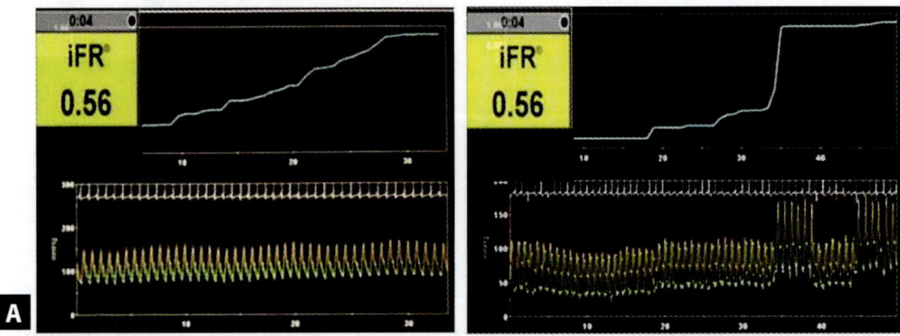

Improvement in PCI precision
- Investigation of location of target flow-limiting disease over PCI by avoiding the geographic mismatch
- Intravascular imaging method use in an accurate manner for the planning and guidance of stenting

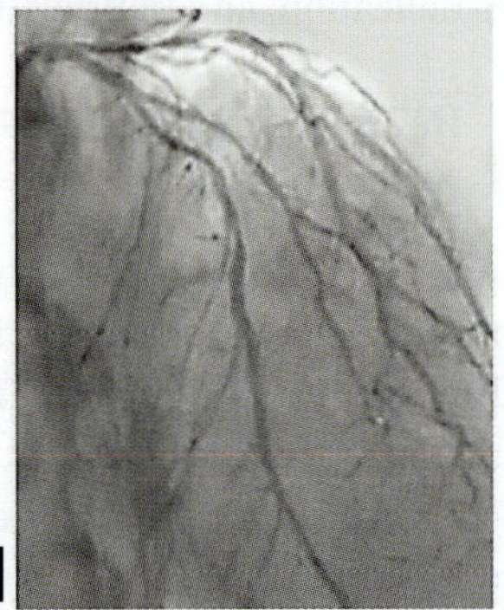

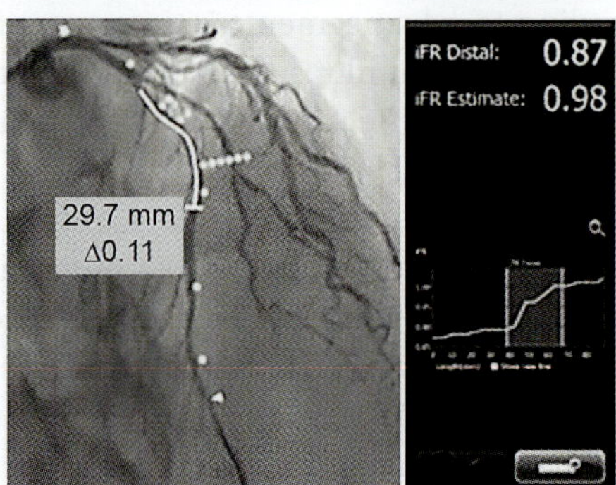

Post-procedural investigation and optimization
- Use of longitudinal physiological analysis to rule out the flow-limiting disease
- Focal patterns use to achieve the post-PCI optimization

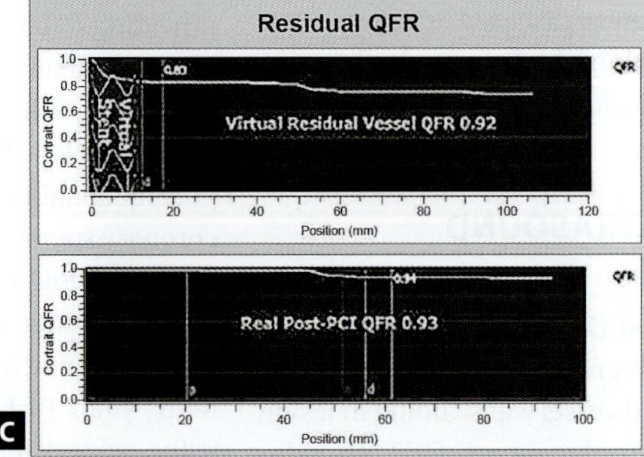

Figs. 1A to C: Physiology applications in guiding and planning percutaneous coronary intervention (PCI) procedures.

FRACTIONAL FLOW RESERVE

Fractional flow reserve is essential for assessing coronary stenosis severity and guiding revascularization. Studies validate FFR's ability to identify ischemia-causing lesions.

The DEFER trial showed FFR can prevent unnecessary PCI by identifying non-significant lesions.[3] The FAME trial confirmed that FFR-guided PCI reduces MI and revascularization compared to angiography guidance.[4] FAME-2 established FFR's predictive value, regardless of anatomy.[5]

New FFR technologies combine functional and anatomical data through invasive CAG or non-invasive

TABLE 1: Objectives of physiology-based planning and guidance for percutaneous coronary intervention (PCI).

Objective	*Technique*	*Advantages*
	Pre-PCI physiological assessment	
PCI clinical indication determination	Determination of flow-limiting disease presence by using the pressure wire or functional coronary angiography (FCA)	Prognostic or symptomatic benefit is achieved by significant stenosis management. Risk of unnecessary PCI is reduced by the deferral of non-flow-limiting disease
Flow-limiting disease patterns investigation	Various patterns of low-limiting disease such as diffuse, tandem, and local identification by using longitudinal physiological vessel analysis	Facilitates the PCI effectiveness. Potentiates the planning of stent length and stent numbers
In specific areas simulating of stenting impact	Simulation of stenosis relief virtually by using imaging-based and NHPR-based functional investigations	Before deployment of stent- PCI planning in an effective manner. Before PCI, facilitates various simulations
Potentiation of precision deployment of stent	Use of co-registration technologies or virtual assessment to correlate angiography and physiology	During stenting, reducing the risk of geographical miss, missing flow-limiting lesions. Balloons and stents sizing in an accurate manner
	Post-PCI physiological assessment	
Ensuring the PCI functional result in an optimum way	After achieving the angiographic results quite satisfactory, PCI target vessel physiological investigations, jailed side-branch interrogation	After the intervention, in the PCI target vessel, residual flow-limiting disease early determination
PCI functional optimization potential targets prediction	Post-PCI longitudinal vessel analysis	Suboptimal functional PCI results cause development. PCI optimization and feasibility method development
PCI optimization impact assessment	After physiology-based optimization, physiological measurements in repeat manner	Directed medical therapy or surgical revascularization is needed in case if residual disease is not amenable to PCI

computed tomography coronary angiography (CTCA). Overall, FFR has redefined coronary assessment and revascularization, inspiring advanced options such as FFR-CT for comprehensive CAD evaluation.

INSTANTANEOUS WAVE-FREE RATIO

Fractional flow reserve adoption is limited by procedure time, cost, and unfamiliarity, leading to iFR as an adenosine-free alternative for coronary stenosis assessment, especially effective for left main coronary artery (LMCA) disease.

Studies show iFR is non-inferior to FFR, with iFR-guided deferral in LMCA lesions associated with lower cardiovascular events.[6] iFR's vessel hemodynamic mapping aids in stenting strategies and outcome prediction, with imaging co-registration enhancing lesion detail. Overall iFR is an efficient alternative to FFR with similar clinical outcomes. **Figures 4A to C** illustrate an iFR pullback curve and simulated stenting.

NOVEL NON-HYPEREMIC PRESSURE RATIOS

Alternative non-hyperemic pressure ratios (NHPRs) such as diastolic hyperemia-free ratio (DFR), diastolic pressure ratio (DPR), and resting full-cycle ratio (RFR) have gained traction due to their simplicity, bypassing the need for adenosine. Software generates smooth FFR, iFR, and RFR pullback curves, eliminating Venturi effect fluctuations **(Fig. 5)**.

As guidewires cross stenoses, dips in ratios such as iFR/FFR occur due to high flow velocity; software corrects these for clearer analysis, shown in **Figure 5**. Studies confirm NHPR-guided revascularization matches FFR outcomes for major adverse cardiovascular events (MACE) at 1- and 5-year follow-ups.

SEVERITY OF LEFT MAIN AND NON-LEFT MAIN LESIONS

Unprotected LMCA intervention, affecting 3–10% of CAG patients, has improved with drug-eluting stents, operator

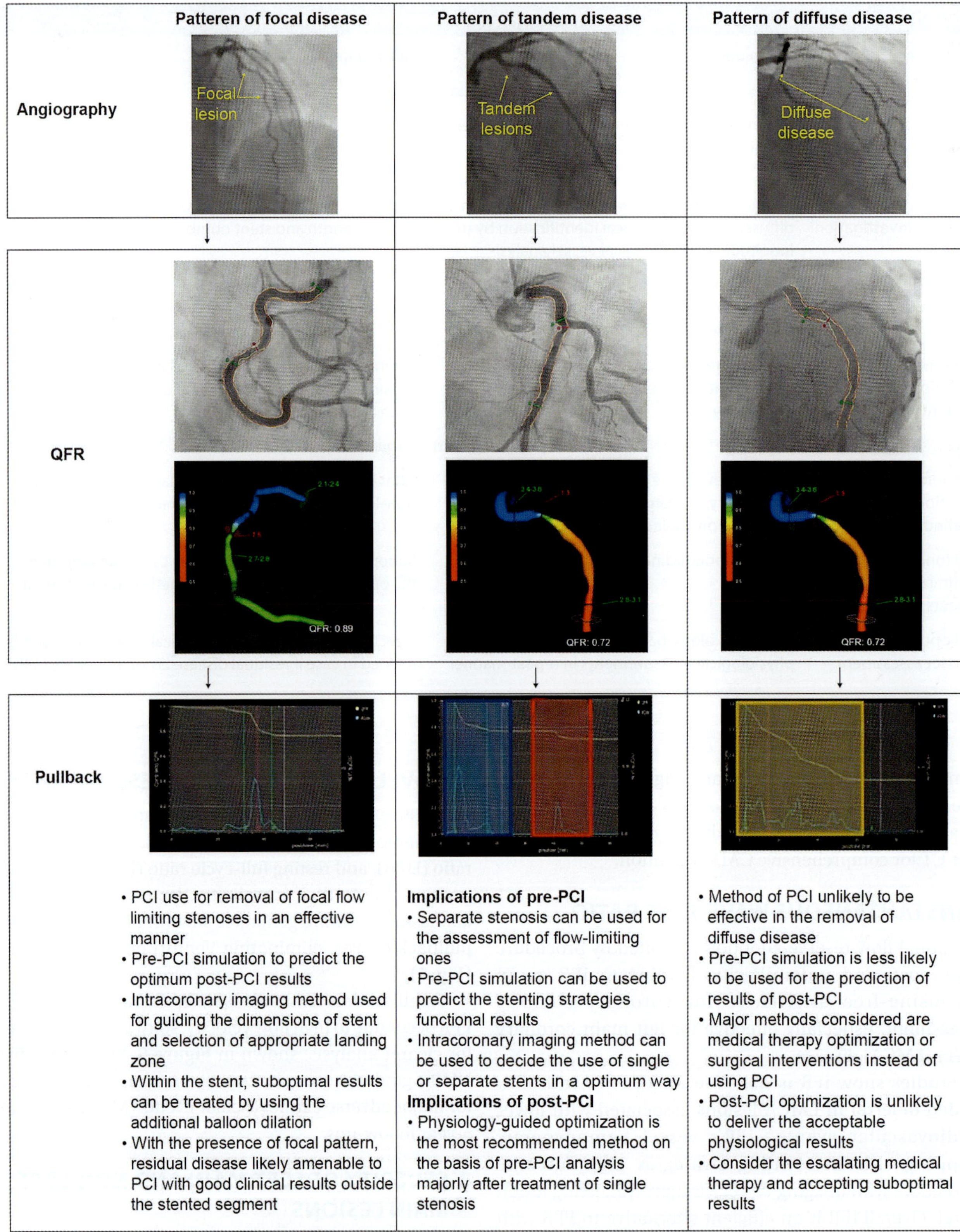

Fig. 2: Longitudinal vessel analysis used pre- and post-percutaneous coronary intervention (PCI) to assess flow-limiting disease patterns.

expertise, and IVUS, leading to guideline updates. FFR is class-I recommended for non-LMCA lesion assessment, supported by DEFER, FAME, and FAME-2, though recent studies (FLOWER-MI, FUTURE, FAME-3) question its universal use. For Angiographically intermediate coronary lesions (AICL), OCT is increasingly considered alongside FFR. In the FORZA trial with 350 AICL patients, OCT-guided intervention showed lower MACE and angina, while FFR guidance led to higher medical management rates and lower costs.[7] FORZA suggests OCT-guided interventions are safe, reducing MACE and angina, with FFR guidance favoring medical management at follow-up.

POST-PERCUTANEOUS CORONARY INTERVENTION, PHYSIOLOGY ASSESSMENT, AND IMAGING

Tools such as IVUS, OCT, and physiological measures (FFR and iFR) aid in post-PCI evaluation, revealing factors behind suboptimal outcomes. Studies suggest that using coronary physiology and imaging for stent optimization improves outcomes, but each tool requires specialized training to assess vessel and stent issues effectively. **Figure 6** shows mechanisms for suboptimal post-PCI results, while **Flowchart 1** illustrates stent malapposition needing correction.

Residual ischemia (FFR ≤0.80) may persist post-PCI, linked to poorer prognosis, though guidelines do not mandate routine post-PCI FFR. iFR has correlated well with non-invasive ischemia tests and matched FFR's efficacy in guiding revascularization. The DEFINE PCI study found residual ischemia in 25% of patients post-stenting, with inapparent focal lesions often as the cause.[8] An algorithm for lesion assessment pre- and post-PCI is in **Figure 7**.

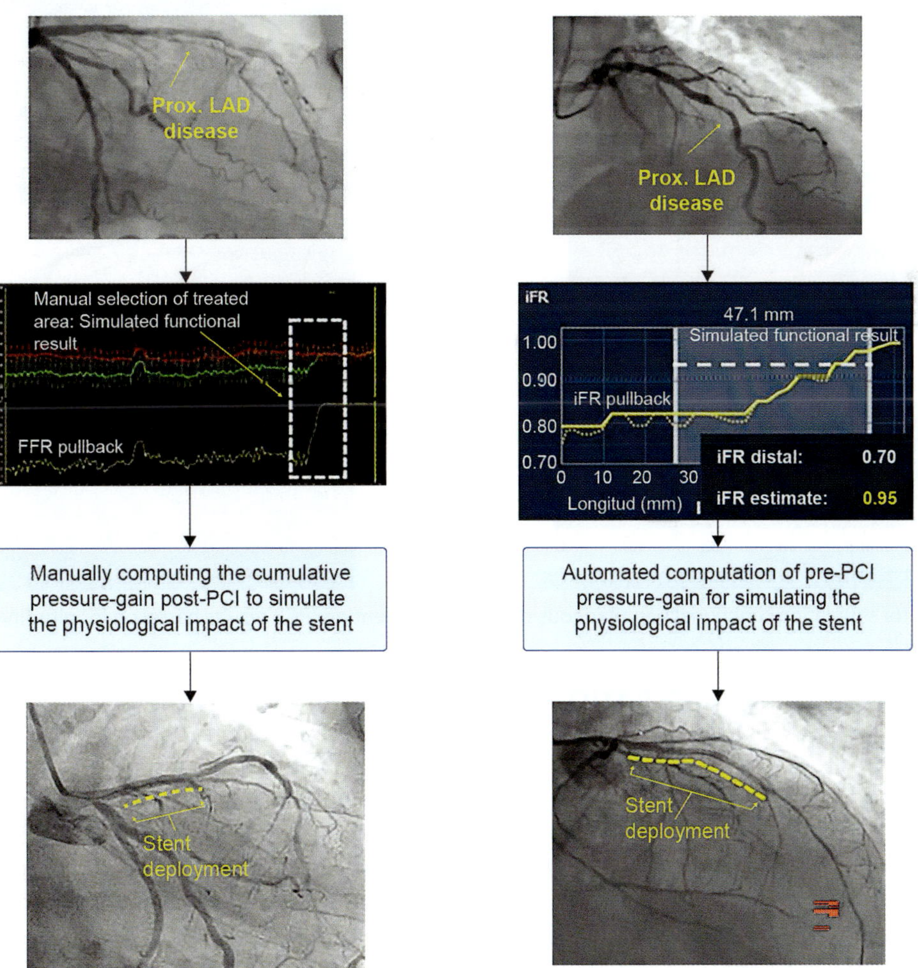

Fig. 3: *Contd...*

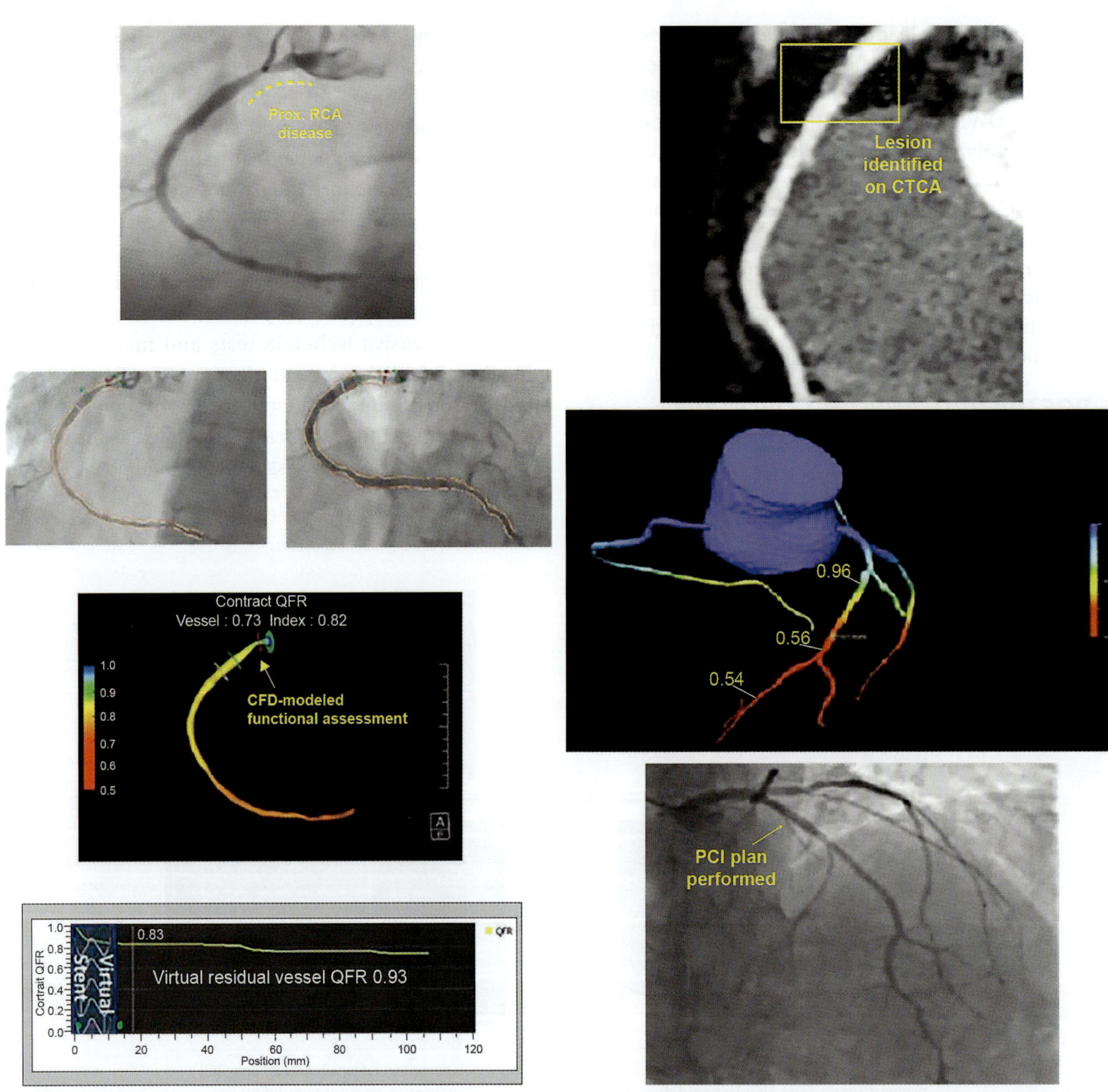

Fig. 3: Methods for simulating functional percutaneous coronary intervention (PCI) results based on longitudinal vessel analysis.

INSTANTANEOUS WAVE-FREE RATIO WITH VIRTUAL STENTING

In many catheter laboratories, FFR is the standard for guiding PCI, but assessing FFR is challenging in serial lesions. Quantitative flow ratio (QFR), developed through angiographic reconstruction and fluid dynamics, avoids the need for pressure wires or hyperemia. Recent QFR software updates, with automatic side branch detection, enhance vessel reconstruction.

A study of 54 patients used the micro-quantitative flow ratio (μQFR) virtual stenting technique for seriallesions, with FFR as the reference. μQFR effectively identified primary flow-limiting lesions for revascularization.[9] **Figure 8** shows virtual stenting to simulate post-stenting outcomes.

TABLE 2: Pitfalls and challenges in physiological assessment.

Objective	*Comment*	*Solution*
Patient factors		
Significant ostial CAD presence	If FCA modalities are not able to assess, using damping pressure or destructuralization to investigate it. Modalities	To a more proximal position, guide catheter repositioning, ensure coaxiality, guide catheter downsizing consideration, controlling catheter tip position by using an additional guidewire or septal wire
In the presence of tandem lesions, hemodynamic crosstalk	Other lesions in the vessel are affected in physiological manner by sequential lesions along a vessel	On the basis of longitudinal vessel analysis obtained with various imaging methods such as NHPR, or FFR, functional coronary angiography, before undertaking PCI on 1 or 2 stenoses, considering simulated planning
Procedural factors		
Pressure wire drift	During the procedure, offset of pressure reading	Repeat procedure by using the imaging-based methods or drift correction/re-normalize
Intracoronary wires-induced pseudo-stenosis	Introsusceptions may be generated by intracoronary wire used for tortuous vessels straightening	As an alternative option to the intracoronary pressure guidewire, functional coronary angiography can be considered
Aortic pressure damping/ventricularization	In significant ostial lesions or during the abutting of vascular lumen, guiding catheter was engaged	Guide catheter repositioning, guide catheter downsizing consideration, pressure guidewire equalization.
Using the guide catheter presence with two holes	At the guiding catheter tip, Pa false estimation	Intracoronary assessment should not be done with using catheter with two side holes. Even after that, it is required for clinical reasons, ensure the usage of IV adenosine and catheter disengagement
Guide catheter extension usage	Pa ventricularization can occur if it is introduced after equalization of pressure	Use extension present within guide catheter with the objective to perform pressure equalization, further during the physiological assessment, withdraw guide extension
Coronary microcatheters usage	Measurements can be affected, and Pa can be modified, if after pressure equalization it is used	Microcatheter within guide catheter can be used to achieve pressure equalization before measurements
Wire whipping	Through the contact with vascular lumen, degradation of pressure wire signal	This issue can be resolved by pressure wire repositioning
Procedure induced transient microvascular dysfunction	Microparticles generated by PCI tools and rotational atherectomy may induce transient microvascular dysfunctioning which further influence pressure indices.	If there is risk of transient microvascular dysfunction, consider FCA as an alternative approach for intracoronary assessment
Without stable hyperemia, investigation of FFR in region	While lowest physiological reporting is demonstrated by software, in stable hyperemia, these might not be stable and therefore severity of lesions overestimation can occur	In stable hyperemia, measure FFR and if required, adopt manual adjustments of points

FRACTIONAL FLOW RESERVE VERSUS ANGIOGRAPHY FOR MULTIVESSEL CORONARY ARTERY DISEASE EVALUATION

For multivessel CAD, coronary bypass surgery is recommended. However, PCI targeting ischemia-causing lesions has shown positive results, though lesion identification is challenging in multiple stenoses. The FAME trial assessed FFR-guided PCI in multivessel disease (1,005 patients: 496 angiography-guided, 509 FFR-guided). At 5 years, FFR-guided PCI reduced MACE, procedure time, costs, and resource use.[10]

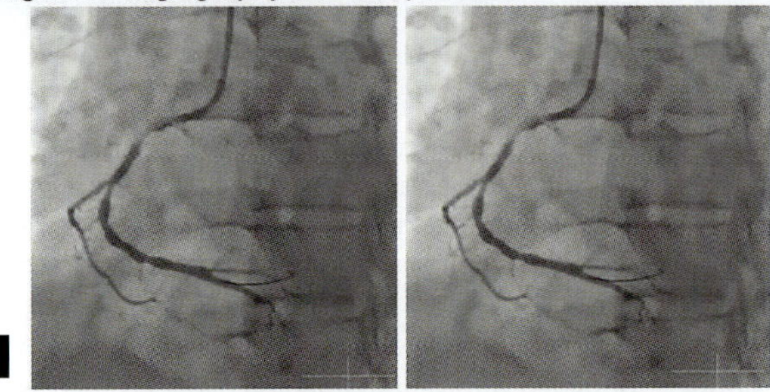

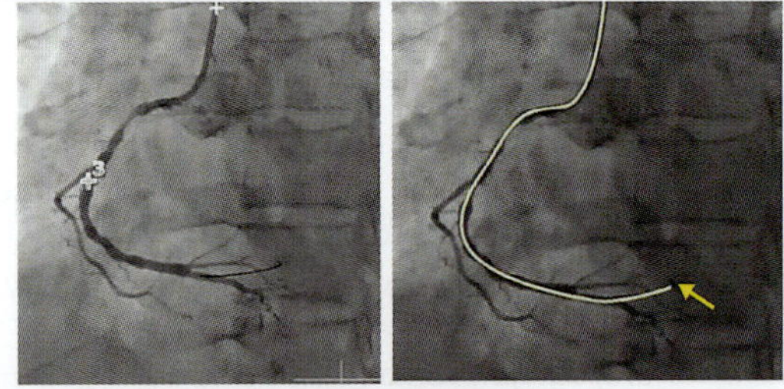

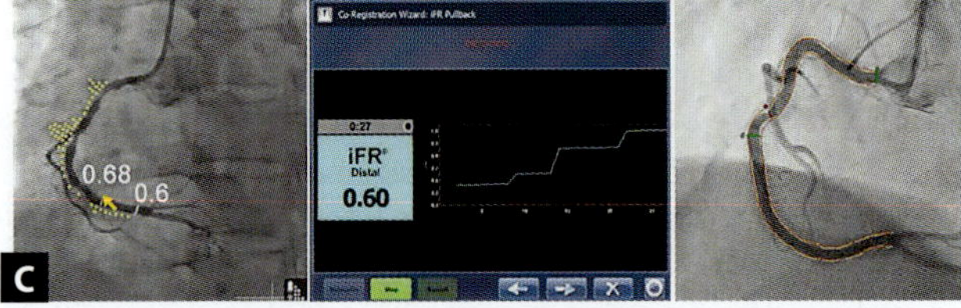

Figs. 4A to C: Simulation of functional percutaneous coronary intervention (PCI) results through coronary angiogram and physiology co-registration; (A) Longitudinal vessel assessment for left circumflex artery angiography; (B) Distal instantaneous wave-free ratio (iFR) of 0.57 indicating flow-limiting disease presence; longitudinal vessel analysis reveals a focal disease phenotype, with iFR co-registration enabling precise localization in the coronary anatomy; (C) Final co-registered angiography-physiology results with a concluding iFR of 0.90.

LEFT MAIN CORONARY ARTERY DISEASE ASSESSMENT BY FRACTIONAL FLOW RESERVE AND INSTANTANEOUS WAVE-FREE RATIO

Coronary angiography limitations in LMCA disease assessment have led to IVUS and FFR as adjunctive methods. iFR's role in LMCA assessment remains under study.

A multicenter study of 314 patients showed that deferring LM revascularization based on iFR was safe, with comparable outcomes to revascularized cases.[11] Another study of 125 patients with intermediate LMCA confirmed iFR's role, correlating IVUS MLA <6 mm^2 with iFR ≤0.89.[12] These findings support iFR as a promising tool for LMCA stenosis assessment.

FRACTIONAL FLOW RESERVE VERSUS ANGIOGRAPHY IN THE SETTING OF ACUTE MYOCARDIAL INFARCTION

To compare outcomes of FFR-guided versus angiography-guided PCI in multivessel STEMI, the FLOWER-MI trial found no significant difference in outcomes such as urgent revascularization, death, or MI at 1-year.[12] Additional studies, such as FAME and FAMOUS-STEMI, also showed no strong evidence of improved outcomes with FFR-guided PCI in ACS.

FRACTIONAL FLOW RESERVE IN ACUTE CORONARY SYNDROME

Fractional flow reserve is a proven technique for assessing intermediate coronary lesions in stable CAD, but its use in ACS is less studied. A pooled analysis of seven studies compared FFR-guided revascularization deferral in ACS versus non-ACS patients, finding no significant differences in target vessel revascularization (TVR) or cardiovascular disease (CVD) mortality between groups. While FFR's prognostic value is limited in ACS, ACS patients showed low mortality but had a higher MI risk and lower TVR rate than stable patients.

FUNCTIONAL PATTERNS OF CORONARY ARTERY DISEASE

Coronary artery disease patterns, including serial lesions, diffuse, and mixed disease, impact coronary physiological assessment. An algorithm aids in using coronary physiology for serial, focal, and diffuse lesions, with intracoronary imaging as needed. **Table 3** outlines criteria for focal, diffuse, and tandem CAD patterns based on physiological assessment.

CO-REGISTRATION OF INTRAVASCULAR IMAGING METHODS WITH ANGIOGRAPHY

Interventional X-ray imaging, such as fluoroscopy and angiography, primarily views coronary lumens, while IVUS details stent expansion and vessel wall composition. Co-registering these methods offers a complete view of coronary arteries. A new device-tracking solution enables efficient co-registration without extra equipment, using coronary branch detection and ECG-triggered imaging,

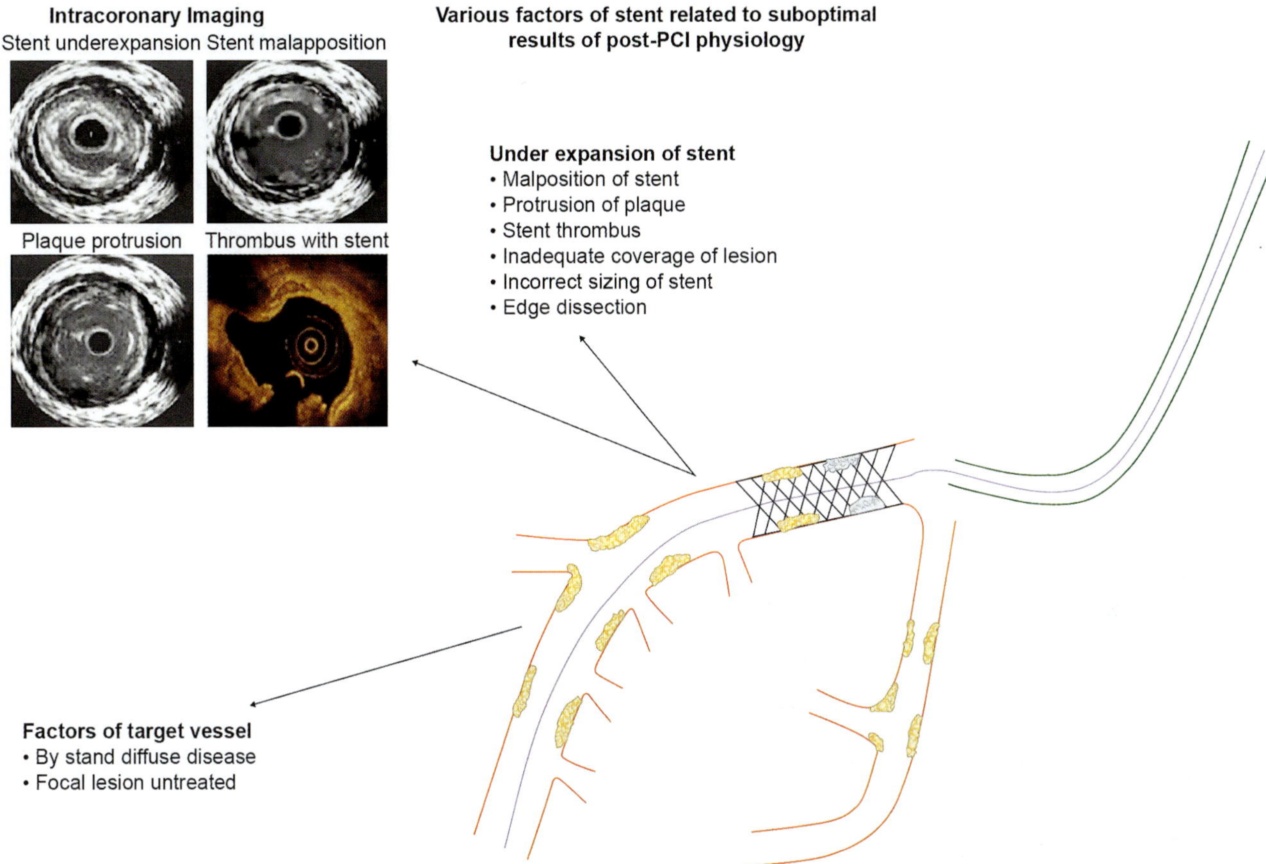

Fig. 5: Software correction of intracoronary pressure pullback curves addressing Venturi effect fluctuations.

easily integrating into workflows. Modified software facilitates IVUS/OCT and angiography co-registration, removing the need for manual landmark identification.

CO-REGISTRATION WITH ANGIOGRAPHY

Mapping angiography with vessel physiology localizes flow-limiting lesions and aids planning, enhancing target lesion identification and pressure loss areas. Used with iFR, it aids therapeutic strategies for tandem and diffuse disease.

CO-REGISTRATION OF INSTANTANEOUS WAVE-FREE RATIO AND INTRAVASCULAR ULTRASOUND

Instantaneous wave-free ratio, validated for CAD severity, can be co-registered with anatomy to improve accuracy. The SyncVision Volcano system integrates iFR and IVUS with angiography, showing each lesion's functional impact. A trial compares SyncVision/iFR-guided and angiography-guided PCI for long, diffuse lesions, with results pending.

TRI-REGISTRATION OF IMAGING, PHYSIOLOGY, AND ANGIOGRAPHY

Tri-registration enables seamless navigation among angiography, physiology, and IVUS. Consistency in IVUS and physiological pullbacks is ensured by keeping zoom, table, and C-arm positions constant.

FUTURE DIRECTIONS

- Coronary artery disease patterns—such as diffuse disease, mixed patterns, focal lesions, and serial lesions—significantly impact coronary lesion physiology assessment.
- These patterns affect the accuracy of both angiography-derived physiology indexes and pressure wire measurements.

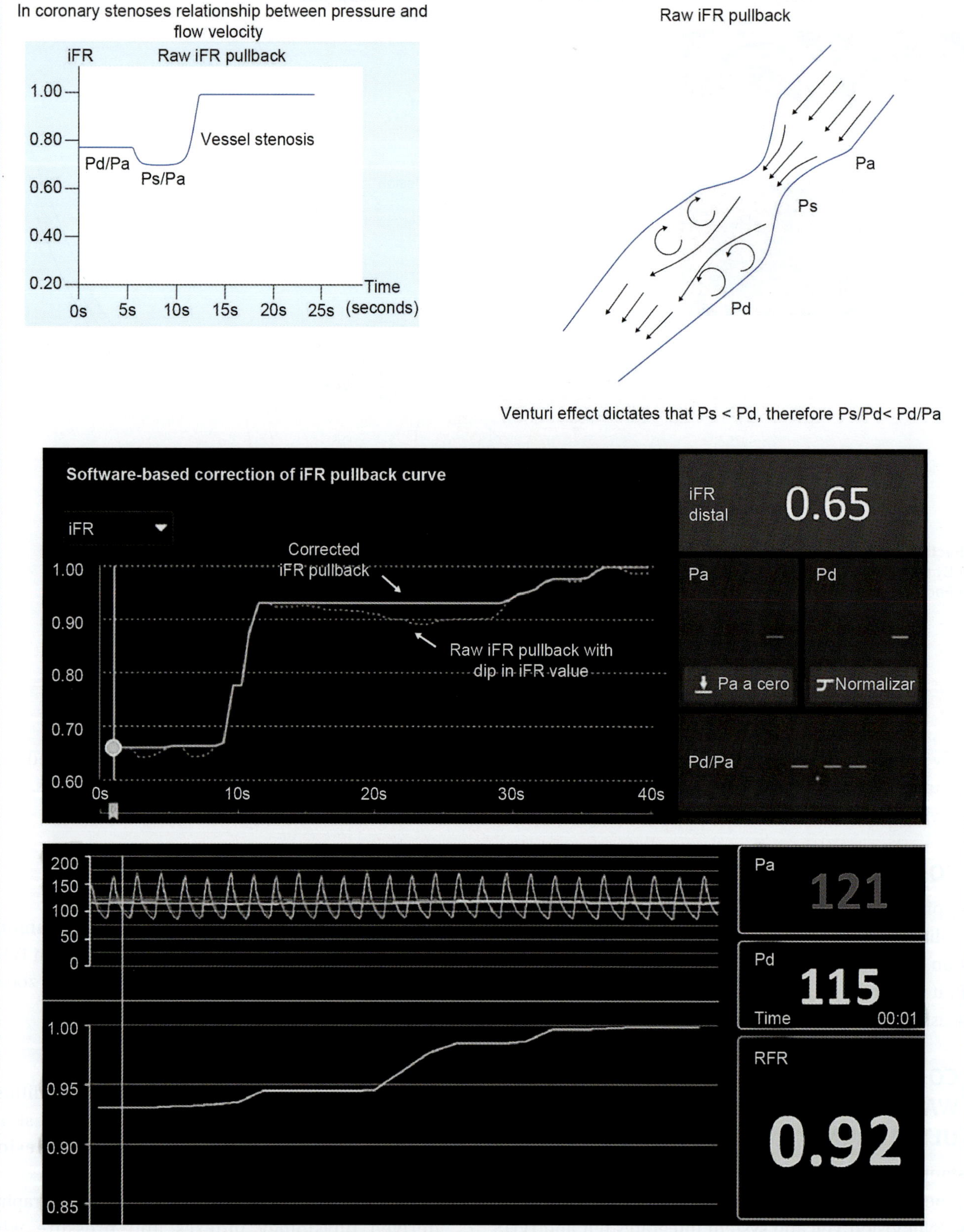

Fig. 6: Mechanisms behind suboptimal physiological results post-percutaneous coronary intervention (PCI).

Flowchart 1: Intravascular ultrasound (IVUS) detection of post-stenting malapposition and subsequent correction.

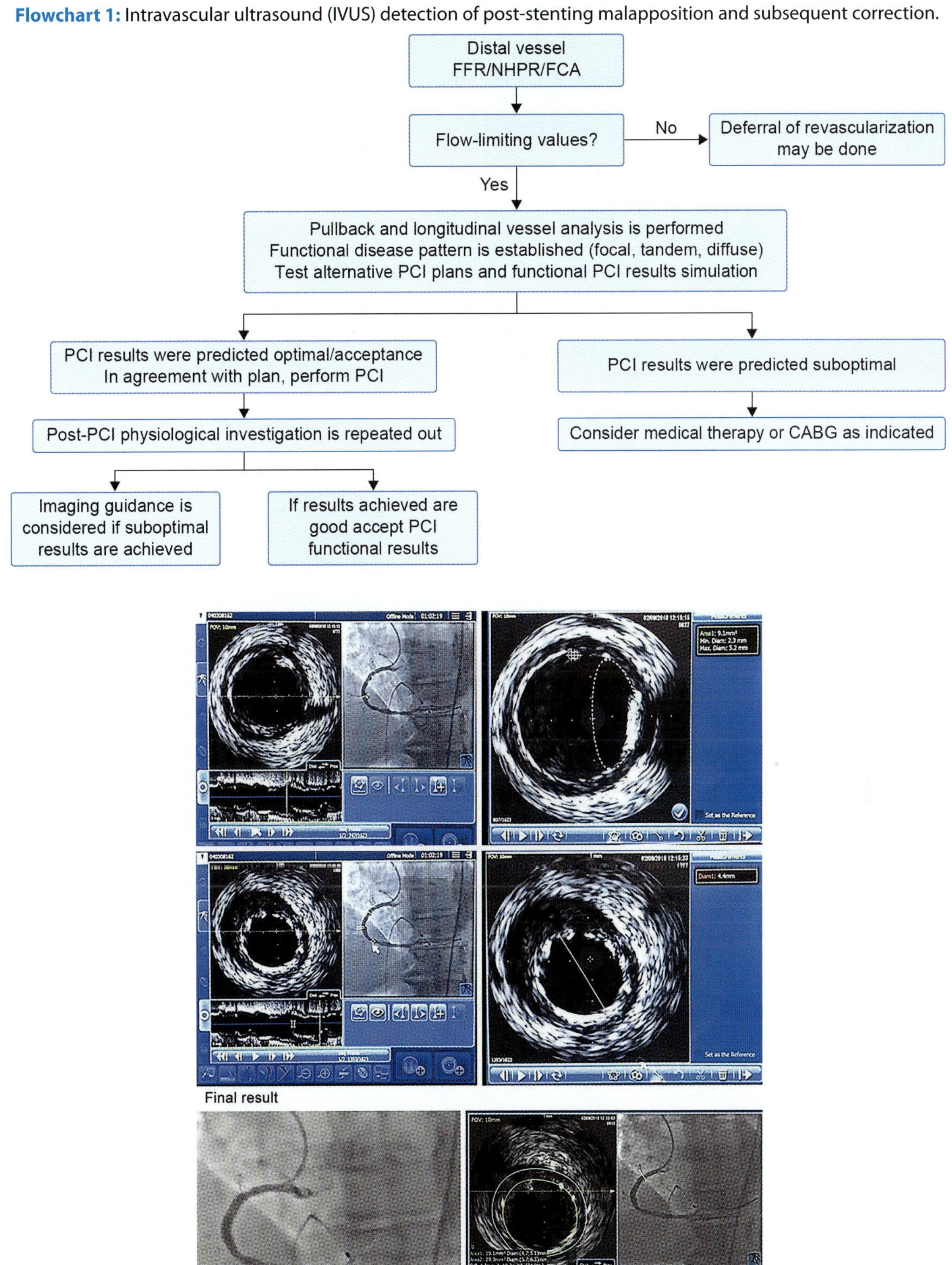

Fig. 7: Proposed algorithm for pre-percutaneous coronary intervention (PCI) planning and assessment based on physiological interrogation.

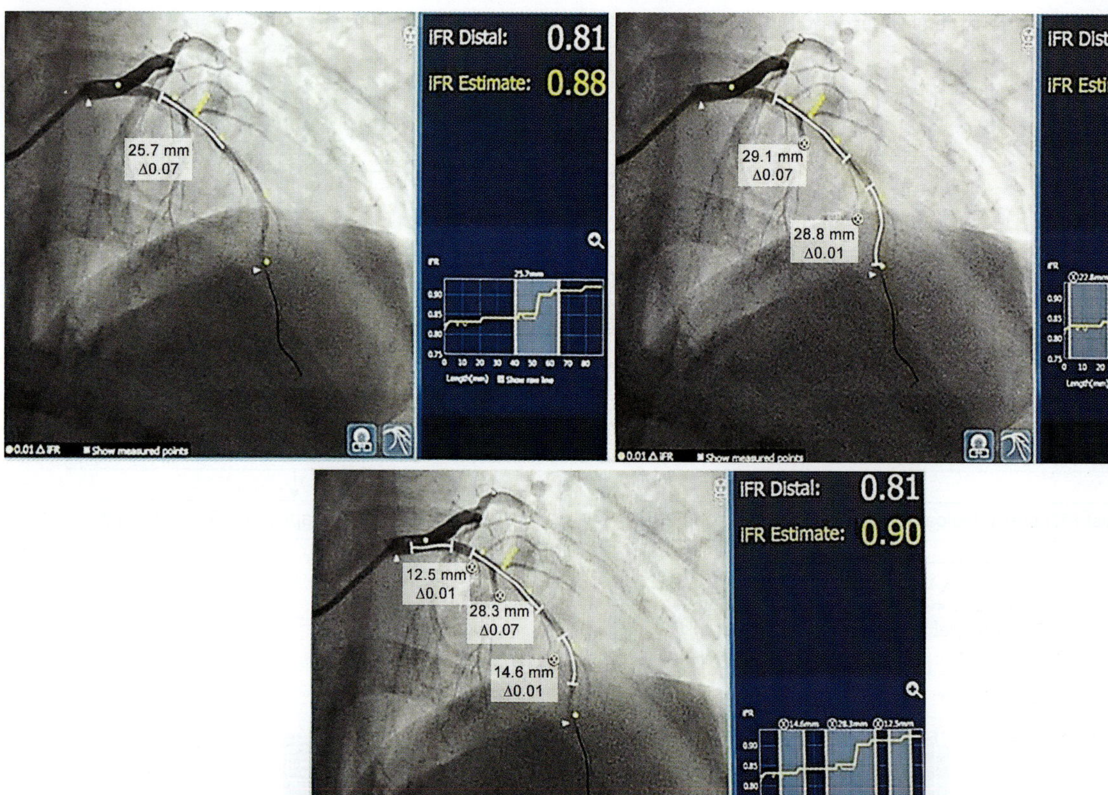

Fig. 8: Virtual stenting showing predicted post-stenting results.

TABLE 3: Criteria for characterizing patterns of obstructive coronary disease, including focal, tandem, and diffuse patterns.

Pattern	*FFR*	*NHPR*	*FCA*
Pre-PCI physiology measurements			
Focal	Abrupt the pressure loss single point, if FFR is ≤0.80 at the distal segment	Over ≤15 mm segment, abrupt single point of ≥0.03 index units if iFR/RFR/DFR is measured ≤0.89 at distal segment	In <10 mm segments pressure loss single region of >0.05 with QFR/vFFR/FFRCT measured ≤0.80 at distal segment
Tandem	FFR ≤0.80 at distal segment, presence of ≥2 abrupt change of FFR values		
Post-PCI physiology measurements			
Focal	At the stented site or at certain other site within the treated vessel, loss of FFR with abrupt pressure	At the stented site or at certain other site within the treated vessel abrupt loss of iFR/RFR/DFR values	At the stented site or at certain other site within the treated vessel abrupt loss of QFR/FFR values
Tandem	At the level of an untreated tandem stenosis, drop of FFR values abruptly	At the level of an untreated tandem stenosis, drop of iFR/RFR/DFR values abruptly	At the level of an untreated tandem stenosis, drop of QFR/FFR values abruptly
Diffuse	During pullback, over length of stented vessel loss in FFR values in progressive and linear manner	During pullback, over length of stented vessel loss in iFR/RFR/DFR values in progressive and linear manner	During pullback, over length of stented vessel loss in QFR/FFR values in progressive and linear manner

- Evaluating disease physiology provides critical insights for CAD management and guides PCI planning.
- A practical algorithm now supports clinical use of angiography-derived and pressure wire indexes in patients with serial, focal, and diffuse CAD.
- Advances in coronary physiology assessment include physiology co-registration in the catheter lab.
- Optical flow ratio (OFR) (OCT-derived FFR) is an innovative tool that improves evaluation of hemodynamically significant lesions compared to OCT alone.
- Philips' "iFR and IVUS tri-registration" co-registers IVUS and iFR with angiography, providing precise measurements in complex cases, such as ostial LMCA in-stent restenosis, where FFR may be misleading.

CONCLUSION

Real-time co-registration of diagnostic modalities enhances precision in coronary interventions by combining functional and imaging techniques. Integrating intracoronary imaging with post-PCI vessel pullback enables accurate assessment of focal pressure loss. As precision PCI advances, routine co-registration of intravascular imaging and physiology with angiography is expected. With ongoing pressure-wire technology improvements, optimized PCI outcomes through detailed physiological assessment will become more accessible to clinicians.

AUTHOR CONTRIBUTIONS

The lead author of the review article is Dr Rohit Mody. Dr Debabrata Dash Dr Bhavya Mody had equal and substantial contributions in the formation of this review article. They were involved in conceptualization, data curation, formal analysis, resources, software, validation, visualization, writing—original draft, writing, review, and editing.

ACKNOWLEDGMENT

I thank Mr Rohit for assisting me to finalize the review article. Figures are edited by Jiwan Singh.

REFERENCES

1. Marin F, Scarsini R, Terentes-Printzios D, Kotronias RA, Ribichini F, Banning AP, et al. The Role of Coronary Physiology in Contemporary Percutaneous Coronary Interventions. Curr Cardiol Rev. 2022;18(1):e080921196264.
2. Pijls NH, De Bruyne B, Peels K, Van Der Voort PH, Bonnier HJ, Bartunek J Koolen JJ, et al. Measurement of fractional flow reserve to assess the functional severity of coronary-artery stenoses. N Engl J Med. 1996;334:1703-8.
3. Bech GJW, De Bruyne B, Pijls NH, de Muinck ED, Hoorntje JC, Escaned J, et al. Fractional flow reserve to determine the appropriateness of angioplasty in moderate coronary stenosis. Circulation. 2001;103:2928-34.
4. Tonino PAL, De Bruyne B, Pijls NH, Siebert U, Ikeno F, van't Veer M, et al. Fractional flow reserve versus angiography for guiding percutaneous coronary intervention. N Engl J Med. 2009;360:213-24.
5. De Bruyne B, Fearon WF, Pijls NH, Barbato E, Tonino P, Piroth Z, et al. Fractional flow reserve-guided PCI for stable coronary artery disease. N Engl J Med. 2014;371:1208-17.
6. Sen S, Ahmad Y, Dehbi HM, Howard JP, Iglesias JF, Al-Lamee R, et al. Clinical Events After Deferral of LAD Revascularization Following Physiological Coronary Assessment. J Am Coll Cardiol. 2019;73(4):444-53.
7. Burzotta F, Leone AM, Aurigemma C, Zambrano A, Zimbardo G, Arioti M, et al. Fractional Flow Reserve or Optical Coherence Tomography to Guide Management of Angiographically Intermediate Coronary Stenosis: A Single-Center Trial. JACC Cardiovasc Interv. 2020;13(1):49-58.
8. Jeremias A, Davies J, Maehara A, Matsumura M, Schneider J, Tang K, et al. Blinded Physiological Assessment of Residual Ischemia After Successful Angiographic Percutaneous Coronary Intervention. J Am Coll Cardiol Intv. 2019;12(20):1991-2001.
9. Guan S, Gan Q, Han W, Zhai X, Wang M, Chen Y, et al. Feasibility of Quantitative Flow Ratio Virtual Stenting for Guidance of Serial Coronary Lesions Intervention. J Am Heart Assoc. 2022;11(19):e025663.
10. Piroth Z, Otsuki H, Zimmermann FM, Ferenci T, Keulards DCJ, Yeung AC, et al. on behalf of the FAME 3 Investigators. Prognostic Value of Measuring Fractional Flow Reserve After Percutaneous Coronary Intervention in Patients with Complex Coronary Artery Disease: Insights From the FAME 3 Trial. Circ Cardiovasc Interv. 2022; 15(11):884-91.
11. Warisawa T, Cook CM, Rajkumar C, Howard JP, Seligman H, Ahmad Y, et al. Safety of Revascularization Deferral of Left Main Stenosis Based on Instantaneous Wave-Free Ratio Evaluation. JACC Cardiovasc Interv. 2020;13(14):1655-64.
12. El Hajj SC, Toya T, Warisawa T, Nan J, Lewis BR, Cook CM. Correlation of Intravascular Ultrasound and Instantaneous Wave-Free Ratio in Patients with Intermediate Left Main Coronary Artery Disease. Circ Cardiovasc Interv. 2021; 14(6):e009830.

CHAPTER 17

Chronic Total Occlusion Retrograde Techniques: Tips and Tricks

Prathap Kumar, Manu Rajendran, Blessvin Jino

INTRODUCTION

The retrograde approach for chronic total occlusion (CTO) percutaneous coronary intervention (PCI) was first introduced in 1990,[1] and it has increased the success rate of CTO PCI.[2] Since the inception, the retrograde approach has evolved significantly with newer techniques and materials. Though antegrade and retrograde approaches have similar mortality rates, complication rates are higher with the retrograde approach. Moreover, the retrograde approach is often attempted in complex morphologies, and it is associated with a higher failure rate.[3] Furthermore, the retrograde approach requires highly skilled operators, and high operator volume is associated with improved success rates.[4] The hybrid approach improves the technical success rate in CTO PCI,[5] and various algorithms have been introduced to increase the success rates.

CASE SELECTION FOR RETROGRADE APPROACH

Most commonly, a retrograde approach is attempted when the antegrade approach fails. However, the retrograde approach can be selected as a primary approach when there is an ambiguous proximal cap, aorto-ostial flush occlusion, CTO in an anomalous vessel where the guide catheter engagement is difficult, and CTOs with a significant side branch origin at the distal cap.[6] The global CTO crossing algorithm suggests a retrograde approach in poor distal vessel quality also.[7]

The JR-CTO score is a tool to identify CTO lesions that will achieve successful retrograde PCI **(Table 1)**. Patients with lower scores have higher guidewire and technical success rates and lower guidewire crossing and procedural times.[8]

TABLE 1: Angiographic parameters in the JR-score that predict procedural success.

Angiographic characteristics	*Score*
Moderate–severe calcification	1
Tortuosity	1
CC grade ≤1	1
Nonseptal channel	1

ARTERIAL ACCESS

Bifemoral arterial access is the most common approach used, though the radial-femoral approach is being increasingly used. Biradial access is uncommonly used. The radial approach has less bleeding and fewer vascular complications compared to the femoral approach. However, catheter backup is less with the radial approach. Even in a radial approach, a ≥7F catheter is preferred to lower-sized catheters. Usage of <7F catheter in radial access is associated with procedural failure. Furthermore, taking a balloon and covered stent simultaneously (block and deliver technique) in case of perforation is not possible with <7F-sized catheters. Similarly, the success rate is lower in the radial approach in complex CTO cases.[9]

HARDWARES

It is preferable to use longer sheaths since they facilitate the guide catheter and wire manipulation by straightening the iliac tortuosity, and reduce the risk of catheter kinking. Sheathless guide catheters offer a larger inner lumen compared to conventional guide catheters (Eaucath, ASAHI), and they allow us to use larger guides through an arterial puncture equivalent to that created by smaller sheaths (Railway, Cordis). A shorter (90 cm) guide catheter helps in easier externalization, particularly when longer collateral channels (CCs) (apical collaterals or bypass grafts) or epicardial channels are selected. If short guide catheters are not available, regular catheters can be manually shortened. However, it may result in poor torque transmission.

Guide extensions are useful in both antegrade and retrograde approaches.[10] In a retrograde approach:

- It increases the retrograde support for equipment delivery.
- It helps in the reverse controlled antegrade and retrograde tracking (CART) technique (guide extension-assisted reverse CART).
- It facilitates the ipsilateral externalization with a single guide catheter.
- It helps in externalization during retrograde CTO PCI via bypass grafts and distal epicardial collaterals. The retrograde microcatheter may not be long enough to reach the antegrade guide catheter. However, the antegrade guide extension catheter can reach and capture the retrograde microcatheter.

Microcatheters commonly used in the retrograde approach are Finecross MG, Corsair Pro, Corsair Pro XS, Turnpike, Turnpike LP, and Caravel. Sasuke, a dual lumen microcatheter, can also be used retrogradely. It helps in retrograde wire crossing when there is a bifurcation at the distal cap of CTO.

SELECTING THE APPROPRIATE COLLATERALS AND CROSSING

Retrograde approach can be done through septal, epicardial collaterals, or through bypass grafts. An interventional collateral is defined as a CC that is considered suitable to deliver an interventional equipment from the donor vessel to the target vessel beyond the CTO segment by an operator experienced in retrograde CTO techniques.[11] Selecting the appropriate is the most crucial part of success in the retrograde approach. Septal collaterals are the most common channels to be attempted. Both septal and saphenous venous grafts are the preferred channels for the retrograde approach due to the lower risk of complications. Epicardial channels are usually long and tortuous and produce more ischemia during the procedure.[12] Hence, they are the least preferred channels. Moreover, the risk of perforation and cardiac tamponade is higher with epicardial collaterals **(Table 2)**.

The CC score and J-channel score are used to predict the successful CC crossing by guidewires.

Collateral channel score:[13]

- Large size—1 point
- Lack of tortuosity—2 points.

When the score is ≥2, the CC tracking and technical success rates are >90%.

TABLE 2: Characteristics of different retrograde channels.

Retrograde channel	*Saphenous vein grafts*	*Septal channels*	*Epicardial channels*
Tortuosity	Less	Less	More
Size	Larger	Variable	Variable
Perforation risk	Less	Less	More
Successful wiring	More	More	Less
Channel dilatation	Not required	Possible	Not possible

TABLE 3: J-Channel score for septal and nonseptal channels.[14]

Collateral	*Septal*	*Nonseptal*
CC vessel size: Small	2	3
Reverse bend: Yes	1	1
Continuous bends: Yes	1	0
Corkscrew: Yes	0	1

J-channel score predicts difficulty in crossing the channel **(Table 3)**.

Category of difficulty (Total score):

- *Easy:* 0
- *Intermediate:* 1–2
- *Difficult:* ≥3

The Werner classification:[15]

- *CC0:* No visible connection between the donor and recipient artery
- *CC1:* Thread-like connections between the donor and recipient artery
- *CC2:* Small vessel-like connections between the donor and recipient artery.

Though the CC assessment is done with multiple grading systems like J-channel score, Rentrop classification, Werner grade, and CC score, for successful CC guidewire, all have limited value in predicting technical CTO PCI success.[16] An ideal CC should have a clear connection with an adequately sized channel (Werner CC2), optimal entry and exit angles (>90°) and no branches or tortuosity **(Figs. 1 and 2)**.

Collaterals may be crossed using two techniques:

1. Contrast-guided approach
2. Surfing

In the "contrast-guided approach," contrast is injected through a microcatheter inside a CC, and the connecting channel is visualized and isolated **(Figs. 3A and B)**. Once the channel is identified, it is crossed with a dedicated wire.

In "surfing technique," the wire is probed across the septal channel by "trial and error" without distal tip injections, and ultimately the wire follows the path of low resistance. Even in small CCs (particularly septal channels), "surfing" technique may be attempted gently if there is distal filling of the collateral bed. Commonly used wires for retrograde collateral crossing are SION (Asahi Intecc), SION black (Asahi Intecc), SUOH 03 (Asahi Intecc), Fielder XT-R (Asahi Intecc), Fielder FC (Asahi Intecc), and Runthrough NS (Terumo Corp).

Tips for crossing epicardial collateral:

- Sion black and Suoh 03 are the wires of choice.
- Always ensure that the guidewire is ahead of the microcatheter at all times.
- Follow the "contrast-guided approach" after back bleeding from the microcatheter.

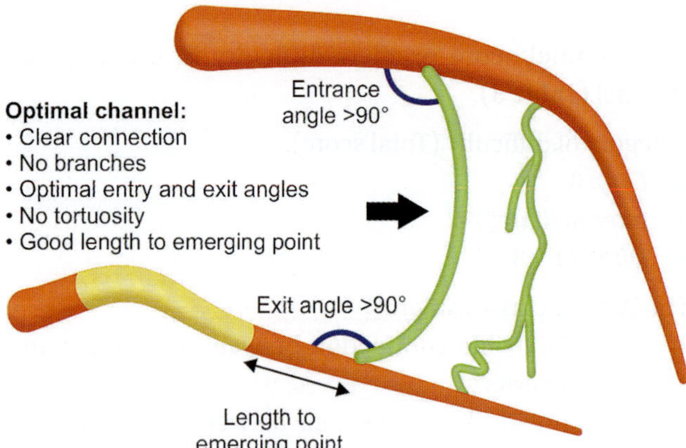

Fig. 1: Angiographic characteristics of an ideal collateral channel.

- Avoid surfing.
- Dilation of an epicardial collateral vessel is strongly discouraged.

The Asia-Pacific retrograde CTO PCI algorithm[17] recommends specific wires and approaches for right-to-left, left-to-right septal channels and epicardial collaterals **(Table 4)**. They suggest selective injection for angiographic visualization of left-to-right septal and epicardial channels and nonselective injections for right-to-left septal channels. Selective injection over right to left septal collaterals may lead to rupture or hematoma due to the back-and-forth movement of the microcatheter in the tortuous PDA. They suggest surfing when the majority of the channels are straight but small and a directional wiring strategy when the channel is larger (CC2) or epicardial. The Asia-Pacific CTO club recommends Sion or Fielder XTR for septal surfing, Sion for directional wiring, and Suoh-03 for epicardial and corkscrew channels.

The Asia-Pacific CTO club advocates Corsair and Turnpike as the initial microcatheters of choice in septal collaterals. If Corsair fails, Turnpike LP is a better alternative. Finecross provides less support for CTO crossing, and it crosses easily after Corsair or Turnpike dilatation of the collateral. In larger epicardial channels, Corsair or Turnpike is preferred, and in smaller channels, Finecross or Turnpike LP is preferred. Corsair is a torquable microcatheter, and it eliminates the need for channel dilatation due to its low profile, soft, and tapered tip. However, when there is an acute angulation in the channel, the joint between the tip and shaft of the corsair makes it difficult to cross. Corsair Pro XS has improved

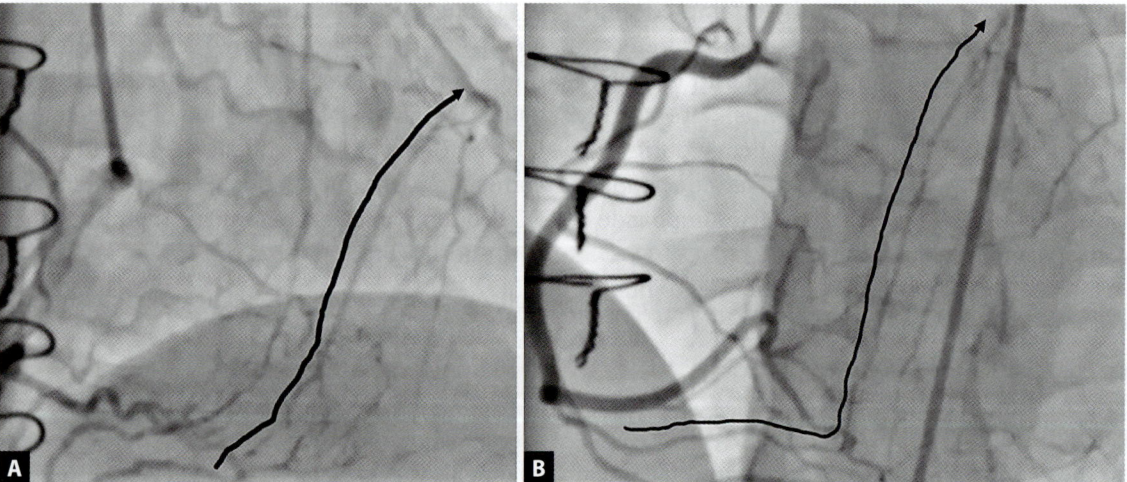

Figs. 2A and B: Angiogram showing ideal septal collateral from RCA for retrograde approach. (RCA: right coronary artery)

pushability due to a balanced shaft stiffness transition. Corsair should not be advanced more than 10 rotations in either direction, and if resistance is felt, further rotation should be stopped to avoid tip damage. After an initial push, the Corsair should be rotated when there is difficulty in the advancement. Rotation of the catheter should be avoided when it is not needed, to reduce the risk for Corsair fatigue. The Corsair catheter can be rotated in either direction, although it has better torque transmission with counterclockwise rotation. Caravel is designed for a forward push, but it can be rotated to cross challenging collaterals. However, the Caravel cannot withstand aggressive rotations.

Even after successful guidewire crossing of collaterals, retrograde microcatheter crossing may be challenging, and it is encountered in 22% of cases.[18] For an easier microcatheter crossing in septal collaterals, the straighter the better; for epicardial collaterals, the bigger the better. Hence, a less tortuous septal channel is chosen irrespective of its size, and a larger-sized epicardial channel is selected irrespective of the tortuosity. Microcatheter switching and support enhancement are effective in managing the microcatheter tracking failure **(Flowchart 1)**. Excessive, forceful pushing may lead to channel perforation.

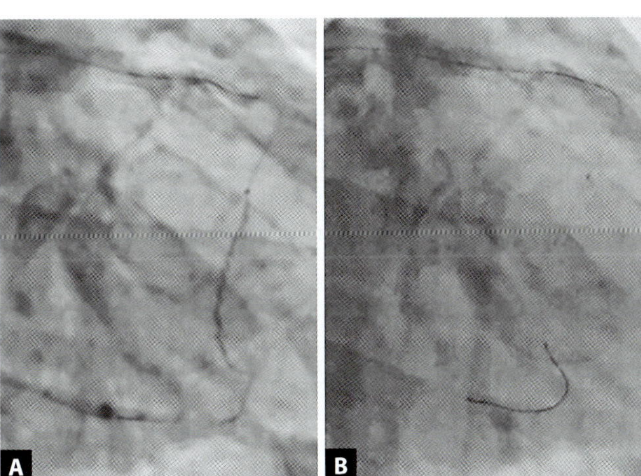

Figs. 3A and B: Contrast injection through a microcatheter showing the connecting channel.

When all the above techniques fail to track the microcatheter, selecting another channel or following the kissing wire technique is an option. Once the microcatheter reaches the distal cap, a medium or high-penetration wire is exchanged to cross the CTO segment.

CROSSING THE CHRONIC TOTAL OCCLUSION

Puncturing the distal cap retrogradely offers less resistance compared to the proximal cap and the distal cap frequently has a favourable morphology. Compared to antegrade wiring, wire control is inferior in the retrograde approach due to the tortuosity in CCs. The CTO segment can be crossed by four methods in the retrograde approach. Reverse CART is the preferred method to connect the retrograde and antegrade spaces, and hence maintaining the intra-plaque position of the wire may not be required always.

- Retrograde wiring
- Controlled antegrade and retrograde subintimal tracking (CART)
- Reverse CART
- Marker wire technique.

The Asia-Pacific CTO algorithm for the retrograde approach **(Flowchart 2)** suggests "antegrade preparation first" before going for the retrograde approach, and that reduces ischemic time of the CTO territory and donor artery risks.[17] It is useful in impenetrable proximal caps, and it facilitates reverse CART.

Retrograde Wiring

Puncturing the distal cap in a retrograde approach is usually easier, and it requires only intermediate or low-penetrating force wires like XTA or UB3. However, when there is a major branch at the distal cap, high penetration

TABLE 4: Wires recommended by the Asia-Pacific CTO club for collateral crossing.

Collateral channel	*First choice*	*Second choice for small channel*	*Second choice for tortuous channel*	*Third choice for tortuous channel*
L to R septals	Sion	Fielder XTR	Suoh 03	Sion black
R to L septals	Sion	Fielder XTR	Suoh 03	Sion black
Epicardial	Suoh 03	Fielder XTR/Sion	Sion XTR	Sion black

(CTO: chronic total occlusion)

force wires like Conquest Pro-12 may be required **(Figs. 4A to F)**. A low-profile dual-lumen microcatheter like Sasuke may be used for better support in such cases. Most of the short segment CTOs can be crossed by loose tissue tracking with XTA or similar wires. However, when there is much resistance in the intraplaque wiring, switching over to the dissection re-entry method (knuckling) helps. Since the reverse CART has a high success rate, there should be a low threshold for switching over to the dissection re-entry method.

Controlled Antegrade and Retrograde Tracking

In the CART technique, a balloon is advanced over the retrograde wire, and it is inflated in the CTO segment to create a localized subintimal dissection. An antegrade guidewire is then tracked into this subintimal space and then finally into the distal true lumen. Reverse CART may be difficult to perform in aorto-ostial CTOs, tortuous collaterals where it is difficult to torque wires, and impenetrable CTO. CART is an alternative technique in those cases.[19] However, CART has many limitations. First, it may be difficult to cross the small and tortuous septal collaterals, and dilating such channels may create perforation. Similarly, tracking a balloon across the epicardial collaterals carries a high risk of perforation. Finally, the retrograde balloon dilatation is done without intravascular ultrasound (IVUS) guidance or any idea on the wire position or vessel size. Hence, it carries a higher risk of complications.[20]

Flowchart 1: Techniques to overcome the microcatheter tracking failure.

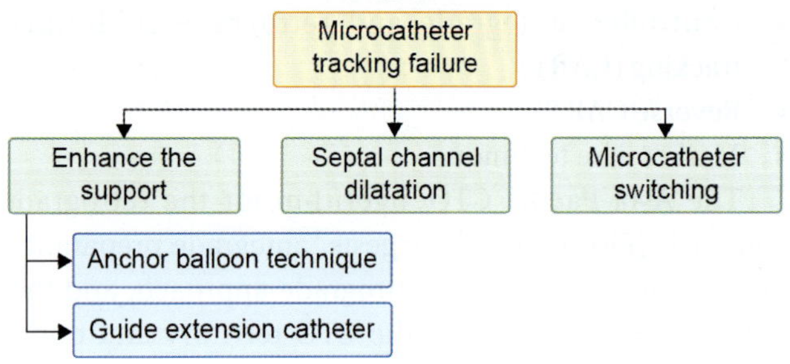

Reverse Controlled Antegrade and Retrograde Tracking

In this technique, an antegrade balloon is inflated over the CTO segment to create a localized subintimal dissection. Then a retrograde wire along with a microcatheter is advanced from the distal lumen into this subintimal space and finally into the proximal true lumen. Compared to CART, the reverse CART is easier, faster, and safer.

Various terminologies are used for the modifications in reverse CART.

- Conventional reverse CART
- Directed reverse CART
- Extended reverse CART

Conventional reverse CART—step by step:

- Both antegrade and retrograde wires should overlap longitudinally (use dissection re-entry techniques if tortuosity or heavy calcium is noticed).

Flowchart 2: Asia-Pacific CTO club recommendation for a retrograde approach.

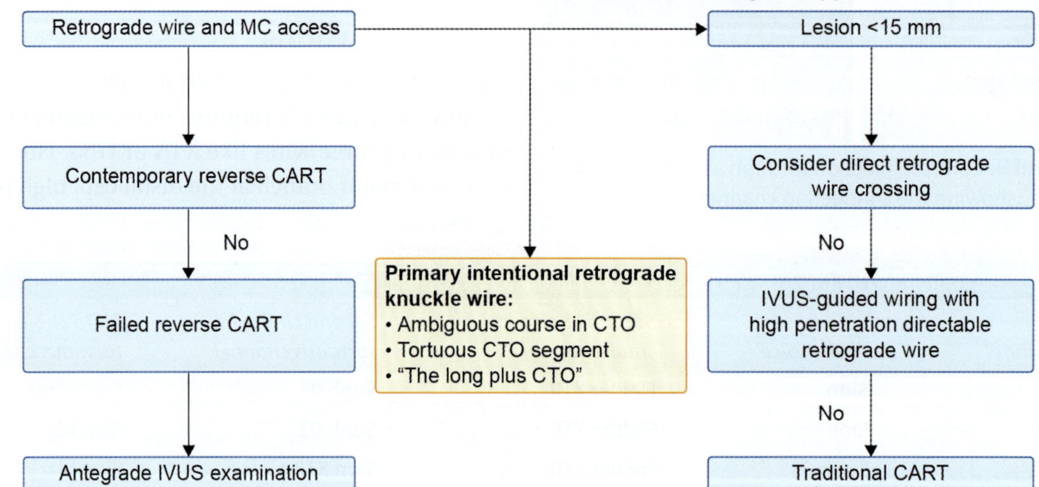

(CART: controlled antegrade and retrograde tracking; CTO: chronic total occlusion; IVUS: intravascular ultrasound)

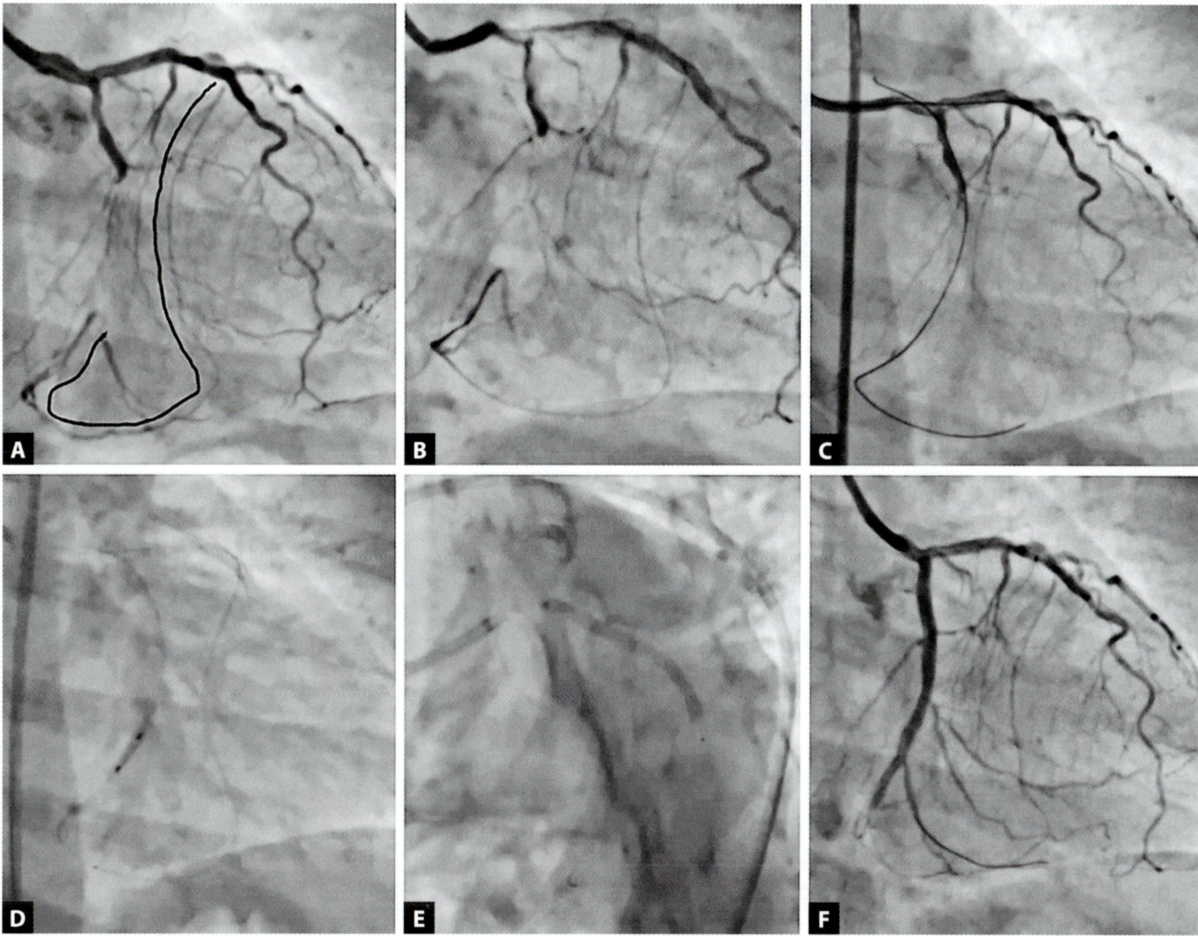

Figs. 4A to F: Case example of retrograde wire crossing. (A) Proximal LCX CTO with a good interventional septal channel; (B) Septal channel was crossed with Sion black and finecross; (C) Gaia next-3 crossed the CTO segment and entered LMCA; (D) RG3 wire was used for externalization and lesion was dilated with 2 × 10-mm balloon through the RG3 wire; (E) Stenting was done with 3 × 36-mm DES; (F) Final angiogram showed well-expanded stent. (CTO: chronic total occlusion; DES: drug-eluting stents; LCX: left circumflex artery; LMCA: left main coronary artery)

- Balloon dilatation through antegrade wire, according to the vessel size.
- The balloon size should be larger in order to maximize the connection space.
- Track the space created by the balloon using retrograde wire to reach the proximal true lumen.
- IVUS through the antegrade wire helps in selecting the balloon size, the location of both guidewires (intimal or subintimal), and the ideal zone for connection.

Directed reverse CART: In the conventional reverse CART, a large space is created by a larger balloon. Hence, there is a risk of perforation. In directed reverse CART, initially antegrade preparation is done using a small balloon (up to 2 mm). Then using a retrograde Gaia guidewire, retrograde puncture is done toward the end of the balloon (end balloon wiring technique).[20] If this attempt fails, retrograde wire is torqued from the lateral side of the balloon, keeping the antegrade balloon and retrograde wire coaxial.

This technique can be attempted when there is no significant tortuosity or calcification since knuckling is not allowed in this technique and intentional intraplaque wire tracking is attempted.

Extended reverse CART: This technique is attempted when the antegrade preparation or retrograde cap penetration is not possible and where there are no significant side branches in the area. Here the antegrade balloon is inflated proximal or distal to the CTO segment, and then the retrograde guidewire is advanced through this connection.

Marker Wire Technique

Retrograde wire is kept as a marker at the distal cap, and the antegrade wire crosses the lesion, keeping the retrograde wire as a marker.

Wire externalization: Once the retrograde wire crosses the lesion, wire externalization is done using dedicated externalization wires (RG3, R350, etc.). Two methods are available for wire externalization.

1. *Wiring the antegrade guide catheter:* It is a simple and preferable method. However, it needs a coaxial guide position and large guide catheters. It can be facilitated by advancing a guide extension through the antegrade guide catheter.
2. *Snaring:* If antegrade guide wiring fails as in aorto-ostial CTO and in noncoaxial guide engagement, snaring the retrograde wire into the antegrade guide catheter is done. Then the retrograde microcatheter is advanced into the antegrade guide directly using the snaring as support, followed by the insertion of an externalization wire.

Step by step approach for wire externalization by wiring the antegrade guide:

- Once the retrograde wire reaches the antegrade guide, a trapping balloon is inflated within the antegrade guide adjacent to the wire to facilitate advancement of the retrograde microcatheter into the antegrade guide catheter **(Figs. 5A to J)**.
- The retrograde guidewire is then removed after deflating the trapping balloon, keeping the retrograde microcatheter within the antegrade guide catheter.
- The externalization wire (RG3 or R350) is then advanced through the retrograde microcatheter.
- Once the externalization wire reaches the Y connector of the antegrade guide, an introducer is inserted through the antegrade Y-connector, and the retrograde guidewire tip is threaded through the introducer.
- Push the retrograde guidewire until 20–30 cm has come out through the Y-connector.

Snaring the retrograde wire into the antegrade guide is preferred in:

- Aorto-ostial CTO
- CTO in vessels with anomalous origin
- Poor retrograde wire control
- Non-coaxial guide engagement
- If the vessel caliber is much larger than the antegrade guide.

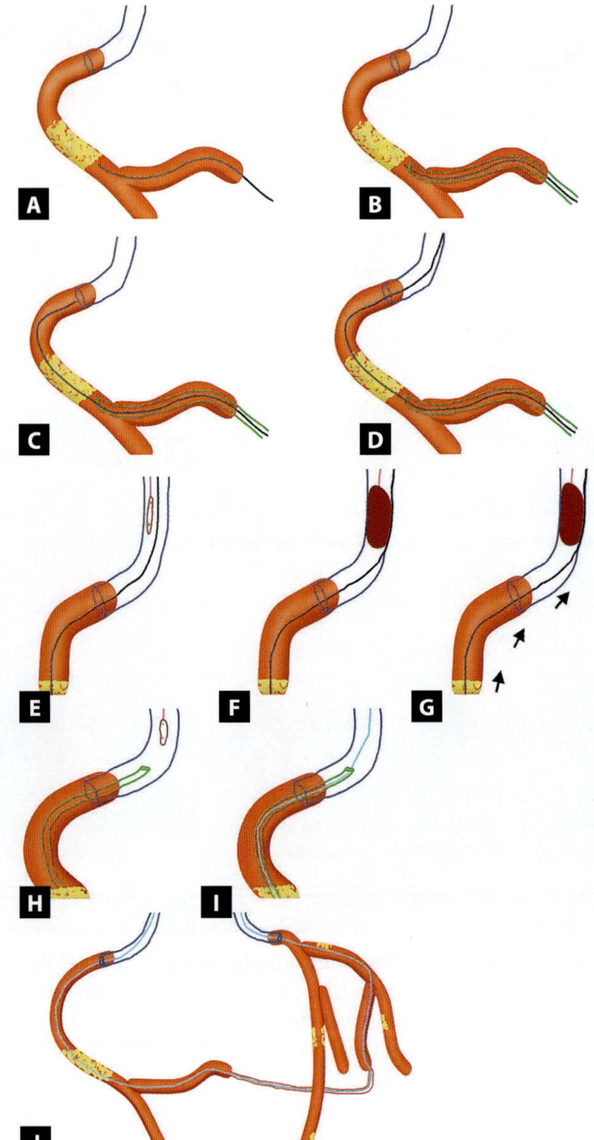

Figs. 5A to J: Step-by-Step approach for retrograde CTO PCI after collateral crossing. (A) After collateral crossing, the wire reaches the distal cap of the CTO segment; (B) The retrograde microcatheter is pushed till the distal cap; (C) A penetration wire is exchanged and lesion is crossed; (D) The retrograde wire enters the antegrade guide catheter; (E) A trapping balloon is advanced into the tip of the antegrade guide catheter; (F) Balloon inflation effectively traps the retrograde wire; (G) The retrograde microcatheter is pushed into the antegrade guide catheter using the trapping balloon support; (H) Trapping balloon is deflated and the retrograde wire is removed; (I) A dedicated externalization wire is pushed from the retrograde guide catheter and it is advanced into the antegrade guide catheter; (J) Final picture showing the fully externalized wire from retrograde guide catheter into the antegrade guide catheter. (CTO PCI: chronic total occlusion percutaneous coronary intervention)

"Ping-Pong" Guide Catheter Technique

The retrograde approach via ipsilateral collaterals is very challenging because of the frequent use of epicardial collaterals. Because of the tortuosity and steep angles of the epicardial collaterals, guidewire and microcatheter manipulations across the collaterals are difficult. Balloon trapping of the retrograde wire inside the guiding catheter, which usually facilitates the advancement of the retrograde microcatheter into the antegrade guide catheter, cannot be done. Using an 8F guide catheter and guide extension into the CTO vessel (recipient vessel), externalization can be done in single catheter retrograde PCI via ipsilateral collaterals. Another option is the "Ping-Pong" technique **(Figs. 6A and B)**. Engagement of the target coronary artery is alternated between the antegrade and retrograde guide catheters in a "Ping-Pong" fashion, enabling the lesion crossing and equipment delivery.

Alternatives to Wire Externalization

In some cases, wire externalization may be impossible or should be avoided. Examples include:

- The retrograde wire or microcatheter may not advance smoothly into the antegrade guide due to tortuosity or calcified retrograde course.
- Presence of a retrograde equipment resulting in a large area of ischemia.

Alternate methods are used in such cases, which include:

- *Rendezvous method:* In the rendezvous technique, an antegrade guidewire is advanced into the retrograde microcatheter, which is positioned within the antegrade guide catheter.
- *Tip-in technique:* In the tip-in technique, an antegrade microcatheter is placed at the outer curvature of the guide catheter, and the retrograde wire is advanced into it. Then the antegrade microcatheter is pushed through the retrograde wire beyond the CTO lesion, followed by removal of the retrograde wire and then insertion of an antegrade guidewire through this microcatheter.

Stenting

Once externalization is done, further balloon dilatations, stenting, and stent optimization using intracoronary imaging are done through the externalized wire.

Externalized Guidewire Removal

Once stenting is finished, the externalized wire should be removed safely, avoiding any damage to the CCs.

- Firstly, the retrograde microcatheter is advanced back into the antegrade guide, and both guide catheters are then disengaged to minimize the risk for deep guide catheter advancement into the coronary ostia.
- The retrograde guidewire is then withdrawn, paying careful attention to the position of the tip of the donor guide catheter. The retrograde microcatheter is then withdrawn into the donor vessel, leaving the retrograde guidewire across the collateral.
- Then, contrast injection via the retrograde guide locates any damage (perforation or rupture) to the CC. If any injury is detected, the microcatheter can

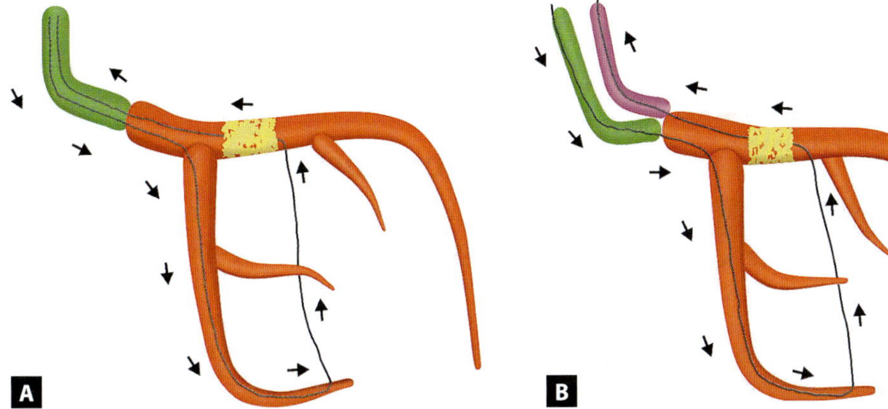

Figs. 6A and B: Single catheter and Ping pong catheters in retrograde CTO PCI through ipsilateral collaterals. (A) Single catheter retrograde CTO PCI in a left dominant system through septal collaterals. Externalization is done using a single large 8F guide catheter; (B) In the Ping-Pong method, one guide catheter acts as an antegrade catheter and another one acts as a retrograde catheter. (CTO PCI: chronic total occlusion percutaneous coronary intervention)

be readvanced over the guidewire to seal the CC perforation and possibly deliver coils or gel foam.

- If no collateral vessel injury is detected, the guidewire is removed after readvancing the microcatheter over the guidewire to lessen the risk for CC damage, particularly in tortuous epicardial collaterals.

Intravascular Ultrasound in Retrograde CTO PCI

Intravascular ultrasound helps in the various steps of retrograde CTO PCI apart from lesion preparation and stent optimization. It helps both in retrograde guidewire crossing and reverse CART technique.

- *IVUS in retrograde wire crossing:* Ostial occlusions and bifurcations with blunt stump: When an IVUS transducer is kept at the ostial segment, it visualizes the exact location of the retrograde guidewire and its re-entry in the true lumen. Without IVUS confirmation, there is a risk of aortic dissection in ostial right coronary artery (RCA) CTO and a risk of subintimal entry in the left main coronary artery (LMCA) in ostial LAD CTO, which may lead to left circumflex artery (LCX) occlusion.
- *IVUS-guided reverse CART:* When the retrograde wire cannot be advanced into the proximal true lumen even after dilatation with a 2.5–3.0 mm antegrade balloon, IVUS helps to identify vessel size, wire position, and plaque morphology **(Table 5)**.

Complications of Retrograde CTO PCI

Collateral channel and donor vessel injury are the two important complications of retrograde PCI apart from the complications of routine PCI.

Tips to avoid CC injury:

- Avoid surfing in an epicardial channel.
- Never dilate an epicardial channel.

TABLE 5: Utility of IVUS in reverse CART.

Vessel size	*Wire position*	*Plaque morphology*
Allows dilatation of the vessel using larger-size balloons	Evaluation of antegrade and retrograde guidewire positions compared with CTO body helps in wire tracking	Where to create connection between antegrade and retrograde guidewires (more proximally or more distally)

(CART: controlled antegrade and retrograde tracking; CTO: chronic total occlusion; IVUS: intravascular ultrasound)

- Manipulate the wires gently while crossing a CC.
- Avoid penetration wires to cross and use dedicated collateral crossing wires.

Septal channel perforation can cause septal hematoma, and usually it is self-limiting and hence managed conservatively. However, it may produce biventricular obstruction, shunt between LV and RV, dry tamponade, or coronary-ventricular fistulas. In such scenarios, occlusion of the septal channel by coils or aspiration through a microcatheter may be required to reduce the septal hematoma. Rarely covered stent over the septal channel origin may be required. Creating a controlled fenestration of the hematoma into the ventricular cavity with a stiff wire followed by balloon dilatation may give rapid relief in compression when there is a hemodynamic compromise. In contrast to septal channel injury, epicardial collateral perforation frequently produces pericardial effusion and tamponade. Hence, sealing both sides of the channel is required.

Donor vessel injury: Donor vessel injury frequently occurs during withdrawal of microcatheters and externalization wire, and it may be life-threatening if flow limitations occur due to dissection. Keeping a wire at the donor vessel may facilitate bail-out stenting when catheter-induced dissection occurs.

Other complications: Rarely, knotting of the guidewire-occurs during retrograde knuckling. Pushing the microcatheter over the knotted wire and slowly withdrawing the wire may help. Rarely, microcatheter tip fracture may occur due to over-torquing and forceful pulling. To avoid this complication, the low-profile microcatheters like Caravel should not be torqued since the connection between the tip and shaft is weak.[21] Guidewire entrapment may occur inside the microcatheter during prolonged manipulations and flushing with saline before insertion may prevent this.

CONCLUSION

Retrograde CTO PCI increases the procedural success rate, albeit with slightly increased risk of complications. However, careful selection of cases, execution of newer techniques and devices, and experienced hands can make the procedure successful without complications.

REFERENCES

1. Kahn JK, Hartzler GO. Retrograde coronary angioplasty of isolated arterial segments through saphenous vein bypass grafts. Cathet Cardiovasc Diagn. 1990;20(2):88-93.

2. Wu EB, Tsuchikane E, Ge L, Harding SA, Lo S, Lim ST, et al. Retrograde Versus Antegrade Approach for Coronary Chronic Total Occlusion in an Algorithm-Driven Contemporary Asia-Pacific Multicentre Registry: Comparison of Outcomes. Heart Lung Circ. 2020;29(6):894-903.
3. Megaly M, Ali A, Saad M, Omer M, Xenogiannis I, Werner GS, et al. Outcomes with retrograde versus antegrade chronic total occlusion revascularization. Catheter Cardiovasc Interv. 2020;96(5):1037-43.
4. Thompson CA, Jayne JE, Robb JF, Friedman BJ, Kaplan AV, Hettleman BD, et al. Retrograde techniques and the impact of operator volume on percutaneous intervention for coronary chronic total occlusions an early U.S. experience. JACC Cardiovasc Interv. 2009;2(9):834-42.
5. Wilson WM, Walsh SJ, Yan AT, Hanratty CG, Bagnall AJ, Egred M, et al. Hybrid approach improves success of chronic total occlusion angioplasty. Heart. 2016;102(18):1486-93.
6. Megaly M, Xenogiannis I, Abi Rafeh N, Karmpaliotis D, Rinfret S, Yamane M, et al. Retrograde Approach to Chronic Total Occlusion Percutaneous Coronary Intervention. Circ Cardiovasc Interv. 2020;13(5):e008900.
7. Wu EB, Brilakis ES, Mashayekhi K, Tsuchikane E, Alaswad K, Araya M, et al. Global Chronic Total Occlusion Crossing Algorithm: JACC State-of-the-Art Review. J Am Coll Cardiol. 2021;78(8):840-53.
8. Tanaka H, Tsuchikane E, Kishi K, Okada H, Oikawa Y, Ito Y, et al. Retrograde Coronary Chronic TotalOcclusion Intervention (JR-CTO) Score- From the Japanese CTO-PCI Expert Registry. J Am Coll Cardiol Intv 2024;17:1374-84.
9. Tanaka Y, Moriyama N, Ochiai T, Takada T, Tobita K, Shishido K, et al. Transradial coronary interventions for complex chronic total occlusions. JACC Cardiovasc Interv. 2017;10:235-43.
10. Garbo R, Iannaccone M, Werner GS, Mashayekhi K, Boudou N, Bufe A, et al. Utility of Guiding Catheter Extensions for Recanalization of Chronic Total Occlusions- A EuroCTO Club Expert Panel Report. J Am Coll Cardiol Intv. 2023;16:1833-44.
11. McEntegart MB, Badar AA, Ahmad FA, Shaukat A, MacPherson M, Irving J, et al. The collateral circulation of coronary chronic total occlusions. EuroIntervention. 2016;11:e1596-603.
12. Allana SS, Kostantinis S, Rempakos A, Simsek B, Karacsonyi J, Alexandrou M, et al. The Retrograde Approach to Chronic Total Occlusion Percutaneous Coronary Interventions. Technical Analysis and Procedural Outcomes. J Am Coll Cardiol Intv. 2023;16:2748-62.
13. Huang CC, Lee CK, Meng SW, Hung CS, Chen YH, Lin MS, et al. Collateral Channel Size and Tortuosity Predict Retrograde Percutaneous Coronary Intervention Success for Chronic Total Occlusion. Circ Cardiovasc Interv. 2018;11:e005124.
14. Nagamatsu W, Tsuchikane E, Oikawa Y, Sumitsuji S, Igarashi Y, Yoshikawa R, et al. Successful guidewire crossing via collateral channel at retrograde percutaneous coronary intervention for chronic total occlusion: the J-Channel score. EuroIntervention. 2020;15:e1624-e1632.
15. Werner GS, Ferrari M, Heinke S, Kuethe F, Surber R, Richartz BM, et al. Angiographic assessment of collateral connections in comparison with invasively determined collateral function in chronic coronary occlusions. Circulation. 2003b;107(15):1972-7.
16. Somsen YBO, de Winter RW, Giunta R, Schumacher SP, van Diemen PA, Jukema RA, et al. Collateral grading systems in retrograde percutaneous coronary intervention of chronic total occlusions. Catheter Cardiovasc Interv. 2023;102(5):844-56.
17. Wu EB, Tsuchikane E, Lo S, Lim ST, Ge L, Chen JY, et al. Retrograde algorithm for chronic total occlusion from the Asia Pacific Chronic Total Occlusion club. AsiaIntervention. 2018;4(2):98-107.
18. Zhong X, Ge L, Ma J, Huang D, Yao K, Zhang F, et al. Microcatheter collateral channel tracking failure in retrograde percutaneous coronary intervention for chronic total occlusion: incidence, predictors, and management. EuroIntervention. 2019;15:e253-60.
19. Moscardelli S, Kearney KE, Lombardi WL, Azzalini L. Controlled antegrade and retrograde subintimal tracking (CART) for recanalisation of chronic total occlusions. EuroIntervention. 2024;20:571-8.
20. Matsuno S, Tsuchikane E, Harding SA, Wu EB, Kao HL, Brilakis ES, et al. Overview and proposed terminology for the reverse controlled antegrade and retrograde tracking (reverse CART) techniques. EuroIntervention. 2018;14:94-101.
21. Megaly M, Sedhom R, Pershad A. Complications and failure modes of coronary microcatheters. EuroIntervention. 2021;17:e436-8.

CHAPTER 18

Drug-coated Balloons: Current and Evolving Indications

Vineet Bhatia, Vidit Bhatia, Parneesh Arora, Upendra Kaul

INTRODUCTION

In 1977, the world witnessed the earliest attempts to revascularize coronary arteries using balloon angioplasty. The success of this ingenious technique was limited by problems such as elastic recoil, abrupt vessel closure, and early restenosis. Abrupt vessel closure often warranted urgent coronary artery bypass surgery. Sigwart et al., in 1984 introduced the bare metal stents (BMS) which as scaffolds took care of elastic recoil and abrupt closure but restenosis remained rampant (20–40% at 6 months).[1] The subsequent introduction of drug-eluting stents (DES) which delivered antiproliferative drug locally into the vessels abluminal side limiting intimal proliferation was seen as a ray of hope but the problem of restenosis and stent thrombosis though lowered persisted. The polymer used to deliver the drug was implicated in inducing inflammation and thrombosis. As drug was only delivered by the struts, there was suboptimal suppression of neointimal hyperplasia at the stent margins and between struts and this was possibly limiting the efficacy of the DES. Metal scaffolds also altered the Vaso motive properties of the stented segment and hampered the adaptive remodeling. The problem seemed to be compounded in small vessels and bifurcation lesions.

With refinements in stent design (thinner struts, polymer free platforms), things improved but restenosis rates today still hover around 7–8%. These improved stent designs along with the newer antiplatelet agents such as Ticagrelor and Prasugrel have lowered rates of stent thrombosis. The search for a scaffold-free drug delivery system was briefly met with the introduction of bioresorbable vascular scaffolds. However, these were later withdrawn due to high thrombosis rates. Thus, restenosis has emerged as the "Achilles heel" of angioplasty. The treatment of restenosis with another DES eluting a different drug is an accepted strategy; however, this adds to the metallic burden and invites higher restenosis. So, the search for alternative strategies which are implant free is ever ongoing. One technique that may hold the key is the drug-coated balloon (DCB).

DEVELOPMENT OF THE DRUG-COATED BALLOON

In 2003, Scheller et al., carried out a novel study wherein after implantation of BMS in pigs, a mixture of an iodinated contrast and paclitaxel was injected into the coronaries.[2] The premise was that the contrast media which is known to adhere to the coronary vessel wall for some seconds after injection would act as the vehicle for antiproliferative drugs to be delivered locally. This technique helped to lower the restenosis rates. A year later, the same group proposed the use of paclitaxel-coated balloons for a more controlled and definite local delivery to treat and prevent restenosis. Paclitaxel was the favoured drug due to its high lipophilicity and unique binding properties but later sirolimus and everolimus ballons also became available. This non-stent-based technique offers several theoretical advantages. It helps to uniformly deliver the drug (360°) to the vessel sections which otherwise are not directly covered by the stent struts limiting intimal proliferation, could be of immense benefit in treating lesions in small and tortuous vessels (where stents fare poorly), treating in stent re-stenotic lesions, bifurcation lesions, and a host of other unique problems in the coronary vasculature[3] (such as high bleeding risk patients where one wants to limit the duration of dual antiplatelet therapy, diabetic patients where disease is often diffuse and invites higher restenosis rates, acute coronary syndrome settings where vessel sizing may be an issue).

The DCBs are rapid exchange semicompliant polyurethane or nylon balloons which carry two components coated on their surface using micropipetting, dipping, spraying, or nanoparticle imprinting techniques.

The nanoparticle technique offers several advantages as it firmly attaches the components to the balloon surface, and ensures the drugs-controlled release only in the fluid environment at the target site. Of the two components, the first is the antiproliferative drug (paclitaxel, sirolimus, biolimus, or everolimus) and second is the delivery vehicle or excipient (iopromide, urea, acetyl tributyl citrate, butylated hydroxy toluolb, n-butyryl tri-n-hexyl citrate, phospholipid, or polylactic-co-glycolic acid). The concentration of the antiproliferative drug varies from 1 to 4 microgram per cubic mm.

The function of the excipient is to augment the drug solubility and aid in its rapid transfer to the vessel wall during the short duration of time when the coated balloon is in contact with the vessel. Despite the fact that of the total drug loaded on the balloon surface only about 15% is delivered to the vessel at inflation, this method of direct delivery helps achieve a concentration several hundred times higher of what would be achieved if the drug was administered parenterally. The excipients also prevent the rapid downstream wash off of the drug from the delivered site.

Meticulous lesion preparation is vital as the drug delivery is pressure and time dependent. The goal is to achieve atherosclerotic plaque and intimal dissection without propagation onto media and adventitia. This may be achieved using noncompliant balloons and if need be, speciality balloons like the scoring and cutting balloons. The latter are especially helpful in dealing with ISR lesions. When necessary, plaque modification may be carried out using intravascular lithotripsy (IVL) or atherectomy.

Once the lesion has been prepared, adequacy may be judged by certain parameters:[3]

- Absence of elastic recoil and adequate luminal gain (<30% residual stenosis)
- Absence of chest pain, ischemic changes on electrocardiography, persistent contrast hang-up or progressive luminal narrowing
- No flow-limiting dissection (evidence of type B National Heart Lung and Blood Institute is an indication for using a stent)
- Thrombolysis in myocardial infarction flow >3.

In this situation, DCB angioplasty will suffice and stent implantation may not be necessary. In case of any ambiguity, research groups have suggested the use of a pressure wire to evaluate the residual gradient across the dissected segment and recognize a threatening dissection [Pd/Pa (distal coronary/aortic pressure ratio)].[4]

The proposed time for which the DCB should be in contact with the vessel wall is 30–60 seconds. The balloon to artery ratio should be 1:1 and the ballon length should exceed the predilated segment at both ends by ≥2 mm. Repeated ballon dilatation does not improve drug delivery. Although low pressure DCB dilatation is unlikely to cause acute problems, they should be looked for and addressed appropriately.[3]

Stenting may be carried out as a bail out strategy in presence of an unsatisfactory result with an aim to cover the entire length of a dissection should it occur. The requirement for such bailout stenting may be needed in 5–15% patients with de novo disease. On the other hand, an up-front, hybrid strategy of stenting in the left main coronary artery/proximal segment and DCB angioplasty distally can be considered when treating long lesions.

SPECIFIC SUBSETS: ROLE OF DRUG-COATED BALLOON

- *DCB in in-stent restenosis (ISR):* An area where DCB use has gained maximal acceptance is in the treatment of ISR. The usual treatment includes strategies such as plain balloon angioplasty, special balloons (cutting balloon), brachytherapy, and repeat stenting with a BMS or DES. The most favoured strategy today is the use of a DES. The arrival of DCBs added a new dimension to the available armamentarium as it obviates the creation of multiple metallic layers.

  The DCBs are superior to plain balloon angioplasty with lower rates of late lumen loss and need for target lesion revascularization. The initial stent type and pattern of restenosis may also influence the success of DCBs.[5] In case of ISR in a BMS, the mechanism of restenosis is usually neointimal hyperplasia and the pattern is diffuse with a homogenous tissue composition. This is perhaps the reason why such type of ISR responds best to treatment with DCBs and results are comparable to DES. DCB is the treatment of choice in BMS–ISR. These recommendations are firmly supported by data from trial such as PACCOCATH-ISR (Treatment of In-Stent Restenosis by Paclitaxel Coated PTCA Balloons),[6] The PEPCAD II (Paclitaxel-Eluting PTCA-Balloon Catheter in Coronary Artery Disease II),[7] and TIS (Treatment of In-Stent Restenosis).[8]

  The DES-ISR is characterized by neointimal proliferation and neoatherosclerosis (with the latter predominating). DCBs are superior to plain balloon angioplasty in DES-ISR management. Scheller et al., reported restenosis and major adverse cardiovascular event (MACE) rates of 43% and 31% at 6 and 12 months respectively in the plain balloon angioplasty group while the comparable rates in the DCB group were 5% and 4%, respectively.[6] Data from trials like the DARE trial[9] showed that the DCB was non inferior to the everolimus eluting DES in terms of 6 months minimal luminal diameter (DEB 1.71 ± 0.51 mm *vs.* DES 1.74 ± 0.61 mm; p for noninferiority <0.0001). The target vessel revascularization rates at 1 year were also similar (DES 7.1% *vs.* DEB 8.8%; $p = 0.65$). Thus, DCB appears to be an attractive option in treating DES-ISR and use of DES restricted to situations as recurrence of disease. DCB use also looks justified where ISR was previously treated with a DES and restenosis recurs. Thus, several guidelines recommend DCB along with DES as the preferred strategies for managing ISR.[10,11] It would also be worthwhile to note that network meta-analysis suggests[12] that repeat stenting with new generation DES (with EES) and DCB are ranked first and second as the highest efficacy treatments. The superior angiographic antirestenotic efficacy of new-generation DES should be weighed against a possible excess of long-term adverse events with repeat stenting during longer-term follow-up of these trials. Also, paclitaxel results of paclitaxel and sirolimus eluting balloons were found to be similar.

- *DCB in de novo lesions:* The use of DCB in treating small vessels or large vessel de novo lesions has been an area of interest.
  - *DCB in small vessel de novo lesions:* The high restenosis rates after small vessel stenting led to initiation of studies in such subsets. One of the first in this series were the PEPCAD[13] and the PICOLETTEO[14] studies.

    The results of the PEPCAD (Paclitaxel Eluting PTCA-Balloon Catheter to Treat Small Vessel Coronary Artery Disease) favoured the use of DCB for de novo small vessel disease. The DCB was associated with favourable safety and efficacy at 12 months which was maintained even at the end of 36 months. These encouraging results were somewhat overshadowed by the PICCOLETO trial data. This angiographic follow up trial compared the use of Dior paclitaxel balloon and Taxus DES in patients with small vessel disease (≤2.75 mm diameter). The study was terminated after enrolment of two third patients due to higher percent diameter stenosis, angiographic restenosis, and MACE in the DCB group. The failure was attributed to faulty DCB design leading to inadequate drug delivery and inadequate lesion preparation (<25% patients assigned to DCB received predilatation).

    The same group in 2020 published the results of the PICCOLETO II trial[15] where newer generation DCB was compared to an everolimus eluting DES in small vessels. This time around the results in the DCB group were gratifying. The in-lesion late lumen loss was lower in the DCB group, while the percentage diameter stenosis and minimal lumen diameter were comparable. At 12 months, the MACE was higher in the DES group (7.5% *vs.* 5.6%; $p=0.55$). There was also a higher rate of spontaneous myocardial infarction (4.7% *vs.* 1.9%; $p = 0.23$) and vessel thrombosis (1.8% vs. 0%; $p = 0.15$) in the DES arm.

    The 3-year clinical follow-up results of the PICOCOLETO II trial[16] were published recently. The cumulative rate of all-cause death, cardiac death, myocardial infarction, and target lesion revascularization did not significantly differ between DCBs and DESs. MACEs and acute vessel occlusion occurred more frequently in the DES group [20.8% *vs.* 10.8% ($p = 0.046$) and 4% *vs.* 0% ($p = 0.042$), respectively].

    However, it is worth noting that though the above data is encouraging, data from other large-scale registries comparing DCBs with second generation DES for the treatment of de novo small-vessel disease have shown contrasting results. The SCAAR (Swedish Coronary and Angioplasty Registry)[17] included more than 14,000 patients with small vessel disease who received treatment with paclitaxel-based DCBs or second-generation DES for the treatment of de novo coronary artery disease. At 3 years, clinically significant restenosis occurred more frequently after DCB angioplasty than DES implantation, while the target lesion thrombosis rates were similar as were the rates of all-cause death and myocardial infarction.

    Further large-scale trials are needed to support the use of DCBs in de novo small vessel lesions.
  - *DCB in large vessel de novo lesions:* In the DEB-AMI trial,[18] DES was found to be superior to BMS or DCB + BMS strategies. The late lumen loss,

binary restenosis, and 3-point MACE rates were lowest in the DES followed by the BMS and then by the DCB + BMS group. Malapposition and endothelial function were also studied using optical coherence tomography and acetylcholine infusion, respectively. The median percentage of uncovered and malapposed stent struts per lesion was lowest in BMS followed by DCB + BMS followed by the DES group. Significant paradoxical vasoconstriction was seen in DES and DCB + BMS groups. A smaller trial for Japan found both approaches to deliver similar results.[19]

The REVELATION trial[20] compared DCB to DES in ST-segment-elevation myocardial infarction patients. Patients with a new, nonseverely calcified culprit lesion in a native coronary artery and a residual stenosis of <50% after predilatation were randomized to treatment with a DCB or DES. The fractional flow reserve was studied at 9 months thereby allowing for a functional measurement of the infarct-related lesion. The fractional flow reserve values were 0.92 ± 0.05 in the DCB group ($n = 35$) and 0.91 ± 0.06 in the DES group ($n = 38$) ($p = 0.27$).

Thus, in coming times, this shall also be an area of active research.

- *Bifurcation lesions:* Pose a challenge for intervention cardiologists and account for up to 15–20% of all interventions. One of the commonly followed strategies is to open the main branch stent struts toward the side branch by performing a plain balloon angioplasty. Side branch stenting is kept provisional. However, this technique is associated with high restenosis rates.[21] Side branch angioplasty with a DCB is an attractive alternative to plain ballon angioplasty or DES for side branch.[22] The associated advantage is that the anatomy of the carina is maintained and this helps deliver the drug evenly across the entire blood vessel surface. As discussed previously, adequate predilatation is the key as suboptimal results at predilatation are an important predictor of subsequent target lesion revascularization. DCBs as a stand-alone treatment for bifurcation lesions following good predilation results appears a very attractive proposition; however, data from only 1 small proof-of-concept German trial with standard balloon angioplasty as a comparator is published.[23]

CONCLUSION

Our knowledge regrading coronary artery disease (CAD) has grown by leaps and bounds. This along with refinement of techniques and availability of cutting-edge technology has helped us treat CAD with great success. The concept of "Leave nothing behind" seems to be gaining momentum more so with thc introduction of DCBs. DCB use may be the answer to a host of problems especially ISR. However, at the present time, there is still ground to be covered before this can be finalised as the destination therapy for this varied scenario.

REFERENCES

1. Scheller B, Speck U, Abramjuk C, Bernhardt U, Böhm M, Nickenig G. Paclitaxel balloon coating, a novel method for prevention and therapy of restenosis. Circulation. 2004;110:810-4.
2. Scheller B, Speck U, Schmitt A, Böhm M, Nickenig G. Addition of paclitaxel to contrast media prevents restenosis after coronary stent implantation. J Am Coll Cardiol. 2003;42:1415-20.
3. Leone PP, Colombo A, Maurina M, Paradies V, Cozzi O, Mangieri A, et al. Optimizing PCI specialty balloon. Cardiac int today. 2024;18(3);53-5.
4. Giacoppo D, Saucedo J, Scheller B. Coronary Drug-coated balloons for de novo and in-stent restenosis indications. J Soc Cardiovasc Angiogr Int. 2023;2:100625.
5. Korijan S, McCarthy KJ, Larnad EA, Cutlip DE, McEntegart MB, Kirtane AJ, et al. Drug-coated balloons in the management of coronary artery disease. Circ Cardiovasc Interv. 2024;17:e013302.
6. Scheller B, Hehrlein C, Bocksch W, Rutsch W, Haghi D, Dietz U, et al. Treatment of coronary in-stent restenosis with a paclitaxel-coated balloon catheter. N Engl J Med. 2006;355(20):2113-24.
7. Unverdorben M, Vallbracht C, Cremers B, Heuer H, Hengstenberg C, Maikowski C, et al. Paclitaxel-coated balloon catheter versus paclitaxel-coated stent for the treatment of coronary in-stent restenosis. Circulation. 2009;119(23):2986-94.
8. Pleva L, Kukla P, Kusnierova P, Zapletalova J, Hlinomaz O. Comparison of the efficacy of paclitaxel-eluting balloon catheters and everolimus-eluting stents in the treatment of coronary in-stent restenosis: the treatment of in-stent restenosis study. Circ Cardiovasc Interv. 2016;9(4):e003316.
9. Baan J, Classen BE, Dijik KB, Vendrik J, van der Schaaf RJ, Meuwissen M, et al. A randomized comparison of paclitaxel-eluting balloon versus everolimus-eluting stent for the treatment of any in-stent restenosis: The DARE Trial. J Am Coll Cardiol Intv. 2018;11(3):275-83.

10. Neumann FJ, Sousa-Uva M, Ahlsson A, ESC Scientific Document Group. 2018 ESC/EACTS Guidelines on myocardial revascularization. Eur Heart J. 2019;40:87-165.
11. Nakamura M, Yaku H, Ako J, Japanese Circulation Society Joint Working Group. JCS/JSCVS 2018 guideline on revascularization of stable coronary artery disease. Circ J. 2022;86:477-588.
12. Siontis GC, Stefanini GG, Mavridis D, Siontis KC, Alfonso F, Pérez-Vizcayno MJ, et al. Percutaneous coronary interventional strategies for treatment of in-stent restenosis: A network meta-analysis. Lancet. 2015;386:655-64.
13. Unverdorben M, Kleber FX, Heuer H, Figulla HR, Vallbracht C, Leschke M, et al. Treatment of small coronary arteries with a paclitaxel-coated balloon catheter. Clin Res Cardiol. 2010;99(3):165-174.
14. Cortese B, Micheli A, Picchi A, Coppolaro A, Bandinelli L, Severi S, et al. Paclitaxel-coated balloon versus drug-eluting stent during PCI of small coronary vessels, a prospective randomised clinical trial. The PICCOLETO study. Heart. 2010;96(16):1291-6.
15. Cortese B, Palma GD, Guimaraes MG. Drug-coated balloon versus drug-eluting stent for small coronary vessel disease. PICCOLETO II Randomized Clinical Trial. J Am Coll Cardiol Intv. 2020;13:2840-9.
16. Cortese B, Testa G, Rivero F, Erriquez A, Alfonso F. Long-Term Outcome of drug-coated Balloon vs Drug-Eluting Stent for Small Coronary Vessels: PICCOLETO-II 3-Year Follow-Up. JACC Cardiovasc Interv. 2023;16(9):1054-61.
17. Silverio A, Buccheri S, Venetsanos D, Alfredsson J, Lagerqvist B, Persson J, et al. Percutaneous treatment, and outcomes of small coronary vessels: a SCAAR report. J Am Coll Cardiol Intv. 2020;13(7):793-804.
18. Belkacemi A, Agostoni P, Nathoe HM, Voskuil M, Shao C, Van Belle E, et al. First results of the DEB-AMI (drug eluting balloon in acute ST-segment elevation myocardial infarction) trial: a multicenter randomized comparison of drug-eluting balloon plus bare-metal stent versus bare-metal stent versus drug-eluting stent in primary percutaneous coronary intervention with 6-month angiographic, intravascular, functional, and clinical outcomes. J Am Coll Cardiol. 2012;59:2327-37.
19. Nishiyama N, Komatsu T, Kuroyanagi T, Fujikake A, Komatsu S, Nakamura H, et al. Clinical value of drug-coated balloon angioplasty for de novo lesions in patients with coronary artery disease. Int J Cardiol. 2016; 222:113-18.
20. Vos NS, Fagel ND, Amoroso G. Paclitaxel-coated balloon angioplasty versus drug-eluting stent in acute myocardial infarction: the REVELA TION randomized trial. JACC Cardiovasc Interv. 2019;12:1691-9.
21. Lassen JF, Burzotta F, Banning A. Percutaneous coronary intervention for the left main stem and other bifurcation lesions: 12th consensus document from the European bifurcation Club. EuroIntervention. 2018;13:1540-53.
22. Herrador JA, Fernandez JC, Guzman M, Aragon V. Drug-eluting vs. convenational balloon for side branch dilation in coronary bifurcations treated by provisional T stenting. J Interv Cardiol. 2013;26:454-62.
23. Kleber FX, Rittger H, Ludwig J, Schulz A, Mathey DG, Boxberger M, et al. Drug eluting balloons as stand-alone procedure for coronary bifurcational lesions: results of the randomized multicenter PEPCAD-BIF trial. Clin Res Cardiol. 2016;105:613-21.

Fractional Flow Reserve versus Intravascular Ultrasound for Percutaneous Coronary Intervention Guidance: A Comprehensive Clinical Analysis

PC Rath, Shabbir Ali Shaik

INTRODUCTION

Percutaneous coronary intervention (PCI) remains a cornerstone of treatment for patients with coronary artery disease (CAD). The success of PCI relies heavily on accurate lesion assessment and optimal stent deployment. Two advanced methodologies for guiding PCI are: (1) Fractional flow reserve (FFR) and (2) intravascular ultrasound (IVUS). FFR offers a physiological assessment by measuring pressure gradients across a coronary stenosis to evaluate its impact on myocardial perfusion.[1] Conversely, IVUS provides detailed anatomical insights through high-resolution cross-sectional images of the vessel lumen and wall.[2] Each modality offers unique advantages, and their use continues to evolve in clinical practice.

This comprehensive analysis explores the comparative utility of FFR and IVUS for PCI guidance. We review their methodologies, clinical evidence, specialized applications, cost-effectiveness, and future directions. The discussion aims to clarify their role in optimizing clinical outcomes and resource utilization in contemporary interventional cardiology.

METHODOLOGIES OF FRACTIONAL FLOW RESERVE AND INTRAVASCULAR ULTRASOUND

Fractional Flow Reserve

Fractional flow reserve is a physiological measurement that quantifies the pressure difference across a coronary artery lesion during maximal hyperemia. It is defined as the ratio of distal coronary pressure (Pd) to proximal aortic pressure (Pa) under conditions of maximal vasodilation, typically induced by adenosine.[3] A value of FFR $\leq$0.80 has been validated as the threshold below which myocardial ischemia is likely, warranting revascularization.[4] FFR offers a real-time, lesion-specific assessment of ischemia, which helps in the decision-making process of whether to proceed with PCI.

Intravascular Ultrasound

Intravascular ultrasound is an imaging modality that uses a miniaturized ultrasound probe mounted on the tip of a coronary catheter. It provides high-resolution, cross-sectional images of the vessel wall, allowing for precise measurements of lumen diameter, plaque burden, and stent expansion.[2] IVUS is particularly valuable in complex or ambiguous lesions, long segments of disease, and left main CAD, where anatomical details significantly influence outcomes.[5]

PHYSIOLOGICAL VERSUS ANATOMICAL GUIDANCE

While FFR focuses on the physiological impact of a lesion, IVUS provides comprehensive anatomical visualization.[6] FFR identifies lesions responsible for ischemia, potentially allowing clinicians to defer unnecessary PCI in cases where stenosis appears severe on angiography but is functionally insignificant.[1] IVUS, on the other hand, enables operators to optimize stent placement, ensuring adequate expansion and apposition, which reduces the risk of restenosis and stent thrombosis.[7]

CLINICAL EVIDENCE: HEAD-TO-HEAD COMPARISONS

Fractional Flow Reserve REACT Trial (2022)

In the FFR REACT (Rapid Early Action for Coronary Treatment) trial, 291 patients who underwent PCI with suboptimal postprocedure FFR (<0.90) were randomized to IVUS-guided optimization versus standard care. IVUS guidance led to significant improvement in post-PCI FFR values (from 0.82 to 0.85, p <0.001).[8] However, this physiological gain did not translate into a reduction in

1-year target vessel failure (TVF) rates (4.2% in IVUS group vs. 4.8% in control, $p = 0.79$). This result was attributed to lower-than-expected event rates in the control group, highlighting the challenge of demonstrating outcome differences when baseline risk is low.

FLAVOUR Trial (2023)

The FLAVOUR (Fractional Flow Reserve and Intravascular Ultrasound for Clinical Outcomes in Patients with Intermediate Stenosis) trial compared FFR- and IVUS-guided PCI strategies for intermediate coronary lesions in a randomized setting. The 2-year follow-up demonstrated similar vessel-oriented composite outcomes [3.8% in IVUS vs. 4.1% in FFR group, hazard ratio (HR): 0.91, $p = 0.77$] and patient-oriented outcomes (6.2% vs. 5.9%, $p = 0.86$).[6] These findings suggest that both modalities are safe and effective for guiding PCI in this patient subset.

Long Lesion Optimization Study (2023)

A single-center study evaluated 154 patients with long coronary lesions (≥30 mm stents), comparing IVUS and FFR for post-PCI optimization. IVUS-guided PCI eliminated post-PCI FFR ≤0.80 and reduced the incidence of ischemia at 1 year (6% vs. 20% with FFR guidance).[9] However, despite these physiological improvements, TVF rates were similar between groups. Notably, IVUS-guided PCI used longer stents (63 mm vs. 49 mm, $p = 0.001$), suggesting that improved lesion coverage may contribute to better physiological outcomes **(Table 1)**.

SPECIALIZED CLINICAL SCENARIOS

Deferred Lesion Management

Deferring PCI in lesions not causing ischemia is a proven strategy to avoid unnecessary procedures and to reduce healthcare costs. In the FLAVOUR trial, deferred lesions guided by IVUS or FFR had comparable outcomes (3.8% vs. 4.1%, respectively), reinforcing the safety of deferral based on either physiological or anatomical assessment.[4] For lesions revascularized, outcomes were again similar (3.5% IVUS vs. 3.6% FFR).

TABLE 1: Comparison of FFR and IVUS optimization in long lesions.

Parameter	*FFR optimization*	*IVUS optimization*
Post-PCI FFR ≤0.8	12%	0%
1-year ischemia	20%	6%
Stent length	49 mm	63 mm ($p = 0.001$)

(FFR: fractional flow reserve; IVUS: intravascular ultrasound; PCI: percutaneous coronary intervention)

Long Lesion Optimization

Long lesions present unique challenges due to increased risk of restenosis and stent failure. IVUS allows precise measurement of lesion length and vessel size, facilitating optimal stent selection and deployment.[9] In the Long Lesion Optimization Study, IVUS eliminated post-PCI FFR values ≤0.80 and significantly reduced ischemia on follow-up. These data support IVUS as the preferred modality in complex, long-segment coronary disease.

Left Main and Bifurcation Lesions

In left main and bifurcation lesions, precise anatomical assessment is crucial. IVUS is particularly beneficial in these cases, allowing visualization of ostial involvement and side-branch dimensions.[10] Studies have shown that IVUS guidance improves long-term outcomes in left main PCI, including reduced rates of restenosis and mortality.[11] While FFR can help assess the functional significance of left main disease, its reliability is limited in certain anatomical configurations and presence of serial lesions.[12]

Chronic Total Occlusions

Fractional flow reserve has limited applicability in chronic total occlusions (CTOs) due to absent antegrade flow pre-revascularization. IVUS, however, plays a significant role in guiding wire crossing and stent deployment.[13] IVUS-guided PCI in CTOs has been associated with higher procedural success and fewer complications, making it the modality of choice in this context.

ECONOMIC IMPLICATIONS

Cost-effectiveness Analysis

Data from the FLAVOUR trial and economic models suggest that FFR-guided PCI is more cost-effective than IVUS guidance. Specifically:

- FFR guidance reduced lifetime healthcare costs by 18%.[14]
- FFR increased quality-adjusted life years (QALYs) by 0.3 years.[14]
- In both Korean and US models, FFR was dominant (i.e., lower cost and better outcomes).[14]

These findings are driven by FFR's ability to safely defer unnecessary PCIs, reducing stent use and procedure duration.

Resource Utilization

Fractional flow reserve requires hyperemic agents like adenosine, which may pose logistical challenges and patient discomfort.[15] IVUS, while offering greater anatomical insight, entails higher equipment costs and procedural complexity.[2] Thus, institutional expertise, resource availability, and patient-specific factors should inform modality selection.

Real-world Utilization Trends

In clinical practice, FFR remains underutilized despite guideline endorsements.[16] Barriers include the need for pharmacologic hyperemia, operator familiarity, and reimbursement policies. IVUS use is more common in complex PCI and East Asian countries, where imaging-guided strategies are favored.[17] Increasing awareness and availability of both modalities may help expand their appropriate use.

HYBRID APPROACHES: THE BEST OF BOTH WORLDS

Emerging data support a hybrid approach that leverages both physiological and anatomical insights.[18] For instance, FFR can guide initial decision-making by identifying functionally significant lesions, while IVUS ensures optimal stent deployment.[19] Hybrid strategies may be particularly useful in complex multivessel disease, where physiological and structural assessments are both crucial.

LIMITATIONS AND CONSIDERATIONS

Each modality has limitations. FFR can be affected by microvascular dysfunction and may yield false-negative results in cases of diffuse atherosclerosis.[20] IVUS, while highly informative, may misinterpret plaque morphology and requires interpretation expertise.[21] No single modality is universally superior, emphasizing the need for tailored approaches based on lesion characteristics and clinical context.

CLINICAL IMPLICATIONS AND FUTURE DIRECTIONS

Current evidence affirms that both FFR and IVUS have essential roles in PCI guidance. FFR is advantageous for intermediate lesions, allowing safe deferral and cost savings.[1] IVUS offers superior anatomical optimization, especially in complex lesions like long segments and left main disease.[9,10] As technology evolves, newer tools such as optical coherence tomography (OCT) and nonhyperemic pressure ratios (NHPRs) are entering the clinical landscape.[15,22]

Future research should focus on:

- Prospective trials comparing hybrid versus single-modality strategies[23]
- Cost-effectiveness studies across diverse healthcare systems[7]
- Integration of artificial intelligence (AI) for automated interpretation and decision support.[24]

CONCLUSION

Fractional flow reserve and IVUS are complementary tools for guiding PCI. FFR provides physiological guidance that helps avoid unnecessary interventions and reduces costs, while IVUS enhances anatomical precision, particularly in complex lesions. Their appropriate use depends on clinical scenario, lesion characteristics, and institutional capabilities. A nuanced, patient-centered approach, potentially integrating both modalities, represents the future of interventional cardiology.

REFERENCES

1. Pijls NH, De Bruyne B, Peels K, Van Der Voort PH, Bonnier HJ, Bartunek J Koolen JJ, et al. Measurement of fractional flow reserve to assess the functional severity of coronary- artery stenoses. N Engl J Med. 1996;334(26):1703-8.
2. Mintz GS, Nissen SE, Anderson WD, Bailey SR, Erbel R, Fitzgerald PJ, et al. American College of Cardiology clinical expert consensus document on standards for acquisition, measurement and reporting of intravascular ultrasound studies (IVUS). A report of the American College of Cardiology Task Force on Clinical Expert Consensus Documents. J Am Coll Cardiol. 2001;37(5):1478-92.
3. Tonino PA, De Bruyne B, Pijls NH, Siebert U, Ikeno F, van' t Veer M, et al.; FAME Study Investigators. Fractional flow reserve versus angiography for guiding percutaneous coronary intervention. N Engl J Med. 2009;360(3):213-24.
4. De Bruyne B, Fearon WF, Pijls NH, Barbato E, Tonino P, Piroth Z, et al.; FAME 2 Trial Investigators. Fractional flow reserve-guided PCI versus medical therapy in stable coronary disease. N Engl J Med. 2014;371(13):1208-17.
5. Ahn JM, Kang SJ, Yoon SH, et al. Meta-analysis of Barlis P, et al. Real-world insights on IVUS-guided stenting. EuroIntervention. 2016;12(7):856-62.

6. Kim BK, Shin DH, Hong SJ, et al. Clinical outcomes of physiologic versus intravascular ultrasound guidance for coronary revascularization: The FLAVOUR trial. J Am Coll Cardiol. 2023;81(8):763-74.
7. Ali ZA, Karimi Galougahi K, Nazif TM, et al. IVUS and OCT imaging in coronary stenting. JACC Cardiovasc Interv. 2014;7(11):1254-63.
8. Choi KH, et al. Outcomes of IVUS-guided stent optimization. Circulation. 2020;141(20):1629-40.
9. Zhang J, Ge J, Chen SL, et al. Functional optimization in long lesion PCI: A head-to-head comparison of FFR vs. IVUS guidance. EuroIntervention. 2023;18(11):916-23.
10. Fujino A, et al. Post-PCI FFR and MACE risk. J Am Coll Cardiol. 2020;75(13):1436-48.
11. Maehara A, et al. Long-term stent outcomes with IVUS guidance. J Am Coll Cardiol. 2015;66(20):2223-33.
12. Kubo T, Akasaka T, Shite J, et al. OCT and IVUS in coronary intervention. Circ Cardiovasc Interv. 2013;6(1):38-45.
13. Barbato E, et al. European consensus on coronary physiology. JACC Cardiovasc Interv. 2016;9(8):848-56.
14. Lee JM, Koo BK, Nam CW, et al. Cost-effectiveness of FFR versus IVUS in coronary revascularization: Insights from the FLAVOUR economic subanalysis. Circulation. 2023;147(1):10-21.
15. Prasad A, et al. Clinical implications of coronary physiology. Mayo Clin Proc. 2004;79(9):1153–1163.
16. IVUSguided versus angiography-guided DES implantation. J Am Coll Cardiol. 2016;68(17):1865-75.
17. Fearon WF, Nishi T, De Bruyne B, et al. Clinical outcomes after FFR-guided vs. angiography-guided stent implantation. J Am Coll Cardiol. 2021;78(20):1865-75.
18. Jeremias A, Davies JE, Maehara A, et al. FFR optimization post-PCI: The REACT trial. J Am Coll Cardiol. 2019; 73(22):2812-22
19. Park SJ, et al. Optimal revascularization strategy in left main disease. N Engl J Med. 2011;364(19):1815-26.
20. Kang SJ, Lee JY, Ahn JM, et al. Impact of IVUS guidance in complex bifurcation lesions. J Am Coll Cardiol. 2011; 58(17):1773-80.
21. FAME Study Investigators. FFR vs angiography in multivessel disease. N Engl J Med. 2009;360(3):213-24.
22. Sgueglia GA, Gaspardone A. Transradial PCI for CTOs: IVUS role. JACC Cardiovasc Interv. 2020;13(8):1100-10.
23. Nishi T, et al. Clinical use of non-hyperemic pressure ratios. JACC Cardiovasc Interv. 2019;12(20):1993-2001.
24. Neumann FJ, Sousa-Uva M, Ahlsson A, Alfonso F, Banning AP, Benedetto U, et al.; ESC Scientific Document Group. ESC/EACTS Guidelines on myocardial revascularization. Eur Heart J. 2019;40(2):87-165.

Echocardiographic Assessment of Left Ventricular Hypertrophy and Left Atrial Volume in Heart Failure

HK Chopra, Manish Bansal, Ravi R Kasliwal

INTRODUCTION

Development of left ventricular hypertrophy (LVH) and left atrial (LA) enlargement are common cardiac structural changes that occur in patients with heart failure. These changes either occur as the primary cardiac abnormality responsible for heart failure or result from the altered loading conditions that the left ventricle and left atrium are chronically exposed to. Their presence, thus, provides important pathophysiological insights into heart failure and has both diagnostic and prognostic implications. For this reason, assessment of LVH and LA size forms an important part of evaluation of patients with heart failure. Echocardiography is the most commonly used modality for this purpose, owing to its easy availability, simplicity, safety, and the ability to permit comprehensive cardiac assessment in virtually no time.

LEFT VENTRICULAR HYPERTROPHY

Left ventricular hypertrophy usually occurs as a response to chronic pressure or volume overload of the left ventricle. In some patients, such as those with cardiomyopathies or infiltrative myocardial disorders, LVH is the direct manifestation of the underlying etiological process. Although LVH can be detected on ECG also, echocardiography is more sensitive and specific than ECG alone for detection of LVH.[1] Additionally, echocardiography also permits quantification of LV mass, characterization of LVH pattern, and recognition of any hemodynamic or functional effects of LVH.

Echocardiographic Assessment of Left Ventricular Hypertrophy

The diagnosis of LVH on echocardiography can be made based on increased left ventricular (LV) wall thickness, or more formally, by estimation of LV mass. Compared with LV wall thickness, LV mass assessment is more accurate and has superior prognostic value.[2] For this reason, LV mass estimation is the preferred method for diagnosis of LVH by echocardiography. There are several echocardiographic methods available for estimation of LV mass,[3] all of which rely on calculating LV myocardial volume by subtracting LV cavity volume from the total LV volume. Multiplying LV myocardial volume with density factor yields LV mass, which is then index to body surface area.

Linear Method

This is the simplest and the most commonly employed method for estimation of LV mass. The following equation is used for calculating LV mass:[4]

$$\text{LV mass (g)} = 1.04 \times [(\text{LVIDd} + \text{IVSd} + \text{PWd})^3 - \text{LVIDd}^3] \times 0.8 + 0.6$$

where 1.04 is the myocardial density, and 0.8 is the correction factor. LVIDd, IVSd, and PWd represent the end-diastolic LV internal diameter, interventricular septal thickness, and posterior wall thickness, respectively **(Fig. 1)**. These chamber dimensions are obtained from the parasternal long-axis view. Traditionally, M-mode imaging has been used for obtaining these measurements. However, two-dimensional echocardiography (2DE) or 2DE-guided M-mode is currently preferred because they allow accurate alignment of measurement plane perpendicular to the long-axis of the left ventricle.

Despite its popularity, the linear method has several limitations because of which it is less preferred nowadays **(Table 1)**. The most important limitation is that it is based only on a single dimension and involves mathematical assumptions about LV geometry, which do not hold true if the LV shape is distorted. Furthermore, the method is error prone as any error in the measurement of LV dimension gets greatly amplified once the dimension is raised to power 3 for converting to volumes. Nonetheless, in uniformly enlarged left ventricles, it remains a reasonably accurate method for assessment of LVH.

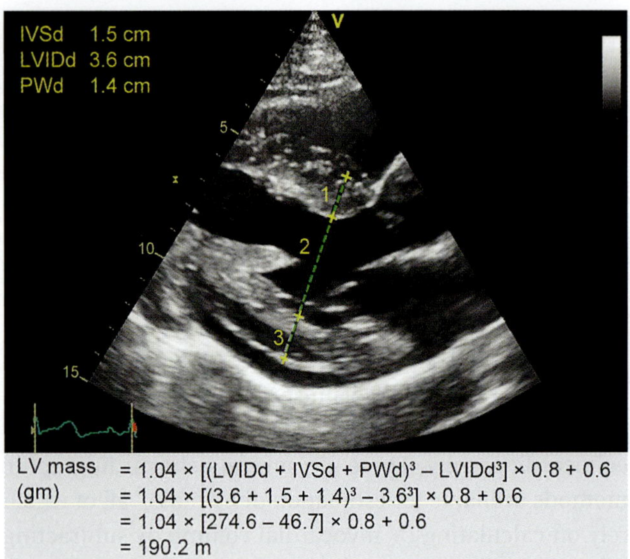

LV mass (gm) = 1.04 × [(LVIDd + IVSd + PWd)³ – LVIDd³] × 0.8 + 0.6
= 1.04 × [(3.6 + 1.5 + 1.4)³ – 3.6³] × 0.8 + 0.6
= 1.04 × [274.6 – 46.7] × 0.8 + 0.6
= 190.2 m

Fig. 1: Estimation of left ventricular mass using the linear method. See text for more details. (IVSd: interventricular septal thickness; LV: left ventricular; LVIDd: LV internal diameter; PWd: posterior wall thickness)

Two-dimensional Methods

Two different 2DE methods are currently available for estimation of LV mass—the area-length method and the truncated ellipsoid method.

For the area-length method, parasternal short-axis view is obtained at the papillary muscle level and the LV epicardial and endocardial cross-sectional areas.

(A_1 and A_2) are measured by tracing the epicardium and the endocardium, respectively **(Figs. 2A and B)**. Care should be taken to include the papillary muscles in the cavity and not in the myocardium. Next, the LV length (L) is measured from the apical four-chamber view, and the LV mass is calculated using the following equation:

$$\text{LV mass} = 1.05 \times (\text{total LV volume} - \text{LV cavity volume}) = 1.05 \times [5/6A_1 (L + t) - 5/6A_2 L]$$

where t is the mean wall thickness derived by subtracting the LV cavity radius from the LV radius as described below:

$$t = \sqrt{(A_1/\pi)} - \sqrt{(A_2/\pi)}$$

TABLE 1: Relative advantages and limitations of different echocardiographic methods for estimation of left atrial (LV) mass.

Method	*Advantages*	*Limitations*
Linear method (M-mode or 2D)	• Simple and quick method • Suitable for screening large populations • Fairly accurate in normally shaped ventricles • Most commonly used method in various studies; hence, it has demonstrated prognostic value with a wealth of published data	• It involves mathematical assumptions about LV shape which may not necessarily be correct • LV dimensions are measured only along one axis; therefore, not accurate in presence of asymmetric hypertrophy, distorted ventricles • Alignment of measurement plane perpendicular to the long-axis of the left ventricle is essential for accurate measurement • Even small measurement errors in dimensions or thickness result in significant error in LV mass as the measurements are cubed • Overestimates LV mass
2D methods (area-length method, truncated ellipsoid method)	• Provides partial correction for LV shape distortions • Less dependent on geometrical assumptions than the linear measurements	• Requires good image quality with good endocardial and epicardial definitions • Proper orientation of parasternal short-axis views (no oblique planes) is crucial • Cumbersome methodology • Higher measurement variability • Few published normative data • Limited prognostic data
3D echocardiography	• Direct measurement without geometrical assumptions about cavity shape and hypertrophy distribution • More accurate than the linear or the 2D measurements • Higher inter-measurement and test/retest reproducibility • Better discriminates small changes within a patient	• Highly dependent on image quality • Patient's cooperation required for acquisition of analysis quality images • Normal values less well established

(2D: two dimensional; 3D: three dimensional; LV: left ventricular)
Source: Modified from Lang et al.[3]

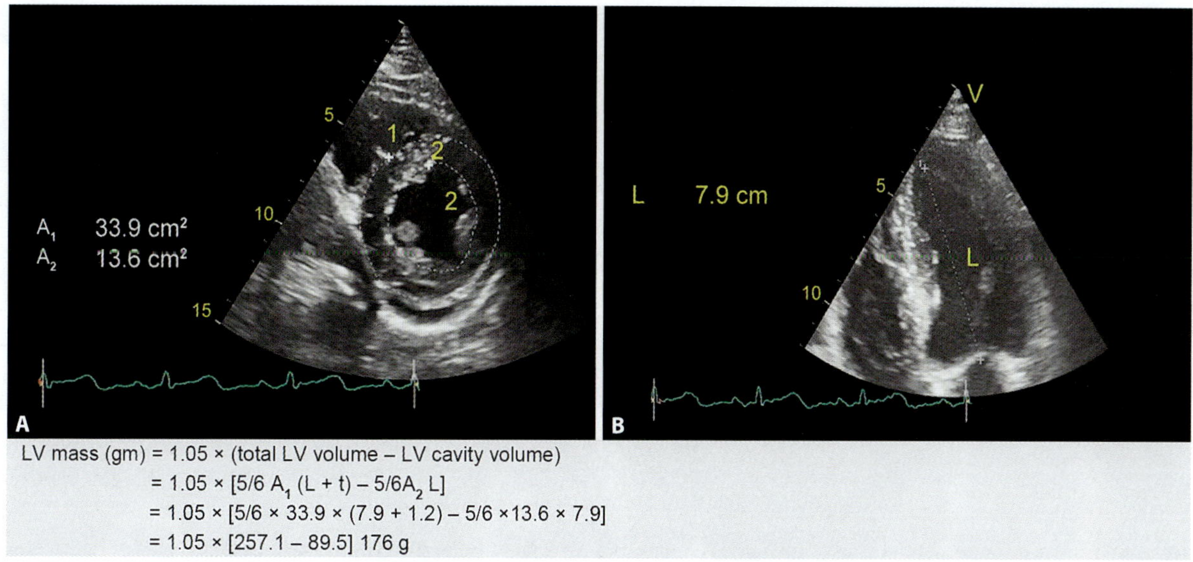

Figs. 2A and B: Estimation of the left ventricular (LV) mass using the area-length method. (A) measurement of LV cross-sectional areas from the parasternal short axis view; (B) LV length measurement from the apical four-chamber view. See text for more details. (A_1: total LV cross-sectional area; A_2: LV cavity area; L: length of the left ventricle; t: mean wall thickness)

The echocardiographer does not have to perform these calculations manually as the analysis package on most of the currently available echocardiography machines includes this calculation. Thus, once the LV short-axis areas and LV length are measured, the inbuilt software automatically calculates LV mass.

The truncated ellipsoid method is somewhat more complex and hence, not discussed here in detail.

Three-dimensional Echocardiography

Three-dimensional (3D) echocardiography (3DE) is currently the most accurate echocardiographic method for estimation of LV. The greater accuracy of 3DE relates to the fact that, unlike the 2D methods, the 3D method includes whole left ventricle in the image and analyzes it in toto, without resorting to any mathematical assumption. For 3DE estimation of LV mass, first a full-volume 3D dataset is acquired from apical position and then LV endocardial and epicardial borders are semiautomatically traced at end-diastole and end-systole in different LV projections. The border tracking is reviewed throughout the cardiac cycle and along different imaging planes and can be manually adjusted as required. Once satisfactory border tracking is achieved, the in-built software automatically calculates LV mass **(Fig. 3)**. Compared with 2DE, 3DE-derived LV mass is more accurate and more reproducible with less interobserver variability.[5-7] Several studies have shown that LV mass measured by 3DE has excellent correlation with the measurements obtained using cardiac myocardial resonance imaging.[5-16] Furthermore, the accuracy is maintained even in the presence of regional wall motion abnormalities or abnormal LV geometry due to other causes.[12,13,17] Keeping with these evidences, the American Society of Echocardiography (ASE) recommends 3DE as the preferred method for LV mass assessment, whenever feasible, and particularly in abnormally shaped ventricles or in patients with asymmetric or localized hypertrophy.[3] However, the practicality, feasibility, or prognostic value of 3DE-derived LV mass estimation in large-scale clinical environments has not been adequately assessed.[18]

Normal Values of Left Ventricular Mass

The normal ranges and the partition values for LV mass using the linear and the 2DE methods are summarized in **Table 2**. However, only limited data are currently available for 3DE-derived LV mass,[19] which is insufficient for recommending normal reference values for healthy subjects at present.

Pattern of Left Ventricular Hypertrophy

Depending on whether the increase in LV wall thickness is proportionate to the LV cavity size or not, the LVH can be categorized as concentric or eccentric. When the wall thickness is increased out of proportion to LV cavity

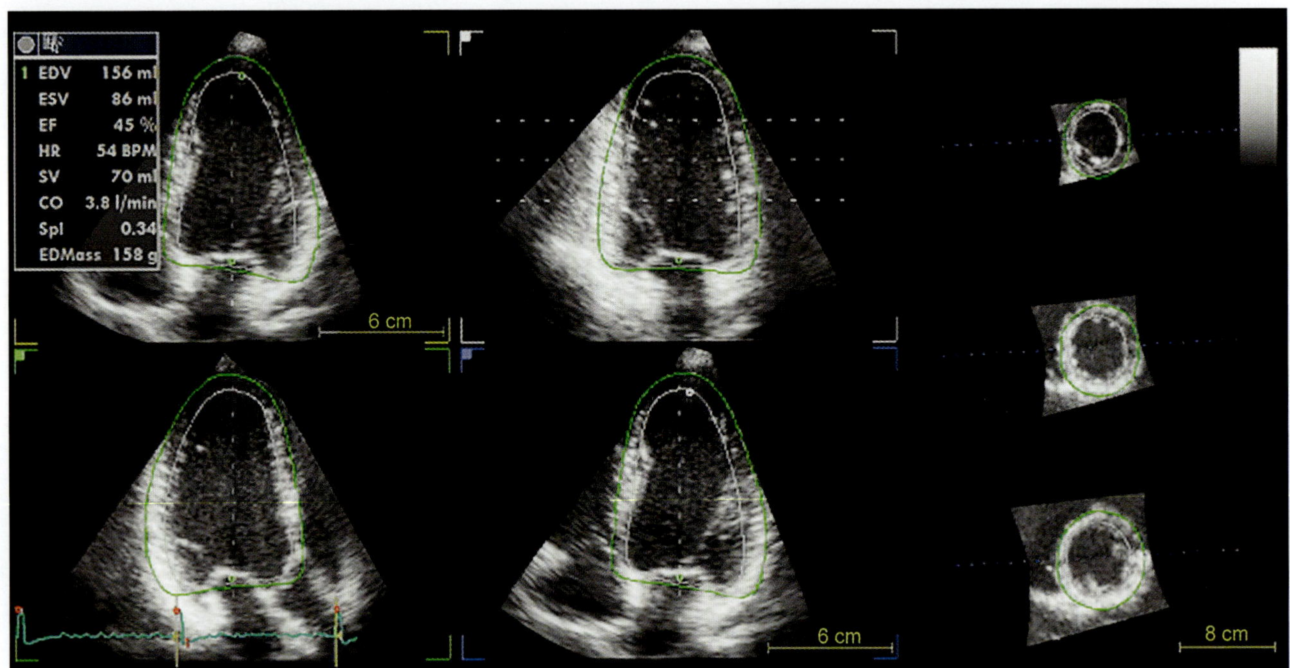

Fig. 3: Estimation of left ventricular mass by three-dimensional echocardiography. See text for more details. (CO: cardiac output; ED mass: end-diastolic mass; EDV: end-diastolic volume; EF: ejection fraction; ESV: end-systolic volume; HR: heart rate; Spl: sphericity index; SV: stroke volume)

TABLE 2: Reference ranges and partition values for left ventricular mass estimated by echocardiography.

	Men				*Women*			
	Reference range	*Mildly abnormal*	*Moderately abnormal*	*Severely abnormal*	*Reference range*	*Mildly abnormal*	*Moderately abnormal*	*Severely abnormal*
Linear method								
LV mass (g)	88–224	225–258	259–292	≥293	67–162	163–186	187–210	≥211
LV mass index* (g/m^2)	49–115	116–131	132–148	≥149	43–95	96–108	109–121	≥122
Two-dimensional method								
LV mass (g)	96–200	201–227	228–254	≥255	66–150	151–171	172–192	≥193
LV mass index* (g/m^2)	50–102	103–116	117–130	≥131	44–88	89–100	101–112	≥112

*Indexed to body surface area.
(LV: left ventricular)
Source: Lang et al.[3]

size, it is called concentric LVH, which typically occurs in response to pressure overload of the left ventricle as seen in longstanding hypertension, aortic stenosis, etc. Conversely, when the LV cavity size is enlarged in proportion to the increase in LV mass, it is known as eccentric LVH. Eccentric LVH usually occurs as a result of LV volume overload as in aortic regurgitation, mitral regurgitation, etc. The distinction between concentric and eccentric LVH is based on relative wall thickness (RWT).[3] RWT is a measure of myocardial thickness relative to the LV cavity size and is calculated using the following equation:

$$RWT = (2 \times PWd)/LVIDd$$

A value of >0.42 indicates increased RWT, supporting a diagnosis of concentric LVH, whereas a value of <0.42 favors a diagnosis of eccentric LVH **(Figs. 4A and B)**. In some individuals, RWT is increased, but the LV mass is

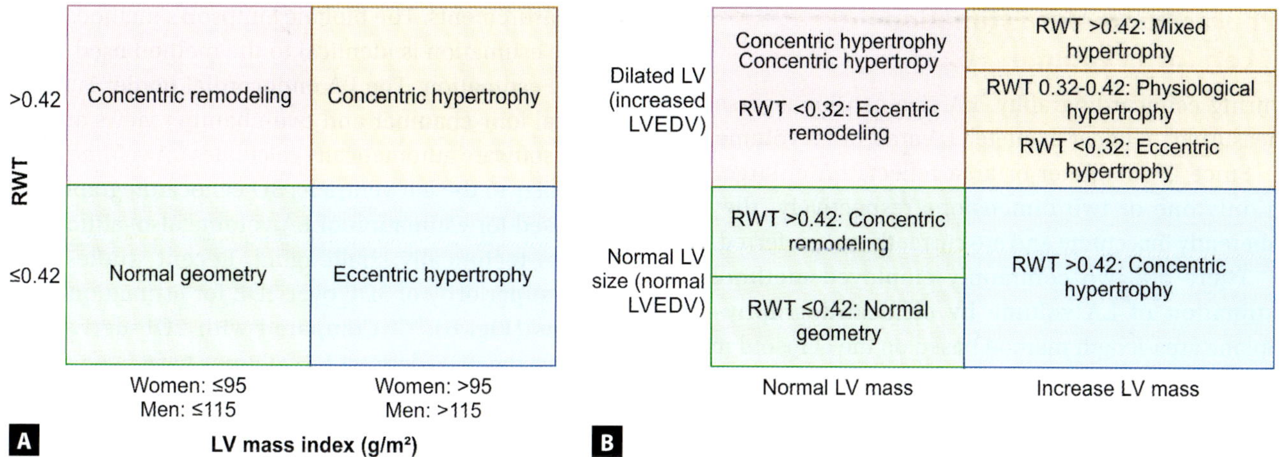

Figs. 4A and B: Classification of patterns of left ventricular geometry. (A) The classification recommended by the American Society of Echocardiography; (B) The alternate classification proposed by Gaasch and Zile.[20] See text for details. (LV: left ventricular; LVEDV: left ventricular end-diastolic volume; RWT: relative wall thickness)

either normal or the increase in LV mass is not sufficient to qualify for LVH. This is known as concentric remodeling, which usually occurs in response to pressure overload. Although concentric LVH is associated with a greater risk of cardiovascular mortality, concentric remodeling too has been shown to be an adverse prognostic marker.[21,22] Gaasch and Zile have proposed an alternative scheme for classification of LVH that takes into account LV cavity size as well.[20] Prognostic value of this classification was assessed in the Cardiovascular Health Study cohort in which it was found to have incremental predictive value for cardiovascular outcomes.[23]

Clinical Significance of Left Ventricular Hypertrophy in Patients with Heart Failure

Concentric LVH or concentric remodeling are common in patients with heart failure with preserved ejection fraction (HFpEF), occurring in 30–35% patients each.[24-28] Eccentric LVH occurs rarely, in 7–9% patients, whereas the remaining 30% patients have normal LV geometry. The high prevalence of concentric LVH/remodeling in HFpEF is due to increased radial thickness of LV myocardial fibers with increased deposition of extracellular collagen, which occur almost ubiquitously in HFpEF.[29-31] The development of concentric LVH leads to LV diastolic dysfunction which is the key pathophysiological abnormality in HFpEF. Hence, the finding of concentric LVH in a patient with HF symptoms with preserved LVEF serves as an important corroborative to support the diagnosis of HFpEF. In contrast, the patients with heart failure with reduced ejection fraction (HFrEF) have an elongation of cardiac myocytes with no increase in the width. There is also myocyte necrosis and degradation of extracellular collagen due to the increased activity of matrix metalloproteinase and other similar enzymes.[29-31] As a result, there is eccentric LV remodeling with an increase in LV cavity size but without any increase in LV wall thickness, or there may even be LV wall thinning. The overall LV mass may remain normal or may be increased. Apart from its diagnostic value in HFpEF, LVH has considerable prognostic significance as well. Being a marker of underlying structural adaptations and a precursor to LV diastolic dysfunction, LVH is associated with increased risk for incident heart failure, arrhythmias, stroke, and sudden death. The adjusted relative risk for cardiovascular mortality is estimated to be 1.5–3.5 in various studies.[32-34] For example, in the MAVI (The MAssa Ventricolare sinistra nell'Ipertensione) study, each 39 g/m^2 increase in LV mass was associated with a 40% rise in the risk of major cardiovascular events and this association was independent of clinical parameters including age, cigarette smoking, and diabetes.[35]

LEFT ATRIAL VOLUME

Left atrial enlargement can occur in a variety of cardiac conditions including LV diastolic dysfunction of any cause, mitral valve diseases, atrial fibrillation, and atrial cardiomyopathy.

Echocardiographic Estimation of Left Atrial Volume

During echocardiography, LA size can be assessed by measuring LA linear diameter, LA area, or LA volume.

Since LA diameter or area reflects LA enlargement in only one or two dimensions respectively, they are inherently inaccurate and are currently not preferred.[36-39]

There are two commonly employed methods for estimation of LA volume by echocardiography—the biplane area-length method based on the ellipsoid model or the Simpson's method. Although most of the data has been derived using the biplane area-length method, the current guidelines recommend Simpson's method owing to its simplicity.[3] For area-length method, the left atrium needs to be planimetered in apical four-chamber and two-chamber views to obtain LA areas (A1 and A2 respectively, **Fig. 5**). The LA length (L) also needs to be measured in both these views, as the perpendicular distance from the mid-point of the mitral annular plane to the superior aspect of the left atrium. Shorter of the two measurements is used for subsequent calculations.

The following equation is used for calculating LA volume:

$$\text{LA volume} = 8/3p\ (A_1 \times A_2/L)$$

Certain precautions need to be taken when planimetering LA area. The confluences of pulmonary veins and LA appendage should be excluded from the area measurement. Additionally, foreshortening of the left atrium should be avoided by ensuring that the base of the left atrium is at its largest size in the views used for the measurements. The biplane Simpson's method for LA volume estimation is identical to the method used for LV volume estimation. The LA endocardial border is traced in apical four-chamber and two-chamber views and the inbuilt software automatically calculates LA volume.

Similar to the left ventricle, 3D echocardiography has been used for estimation of LA volume also, although it remains technically challenging. Recent studies have shown superiority of 3DE over 2DE for estimation of LA volumes **(Fig. 6)**.[40,41] Compared with 2DE-derived LA volumes, the 3DE-derived LA volumes have been shown to be more reproducible and have better correlations with computed tomography and cardiac magnetic resonance imaging.[42-44]

Normal Values

The recommended upper limit of LA volume by 2DE methods is 34 mL/m^2. Compared with 2DE, 3DE generally provides larger values of LA volumes.[44] However, due to paucity of data,[45] reference ranges for 3DE-derived LA volume have not been recommended in the recent guidelines.[3]

Clinical Utility in Heart Failure Patients

Left atrial enlargement is quite common in heart failure, occurring in most patients with HFrEF and nearly 50–66% patients with HFpEF.[24,26] Persistent elevation of LV filling pressure is the main driving force for LA enlargement, though atrial fibrillation and mitral regurgitation also contribute to this.

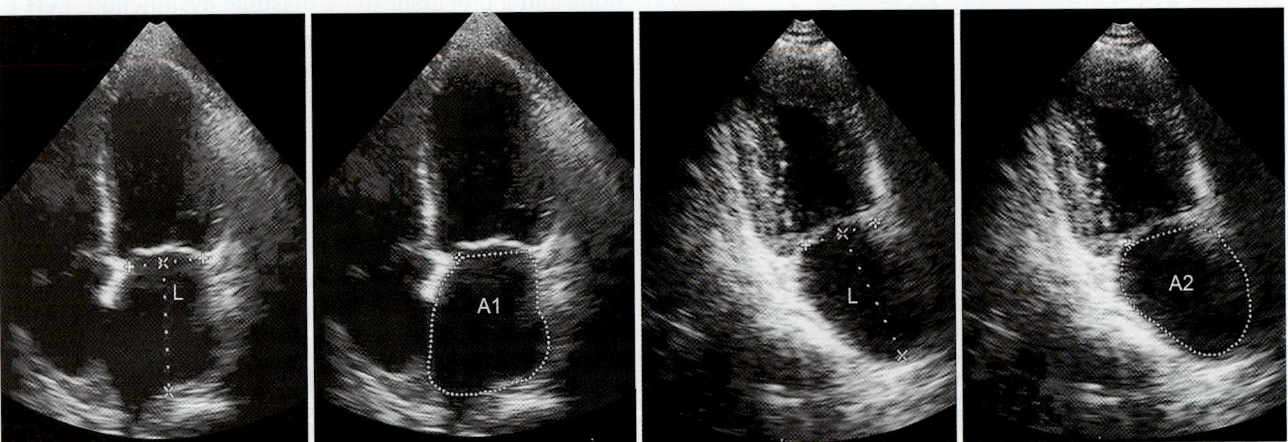

Fig. 5: Estimation of the left atrial volume by the biplane area-length method during transthoracic echocardiography. See text for details. (A1 and A2: left atrial areas obtained by planimetry from the apical four-chamber and two-chamber views; L: left atrial length measured from the apical four-chamber and two-chamber views)

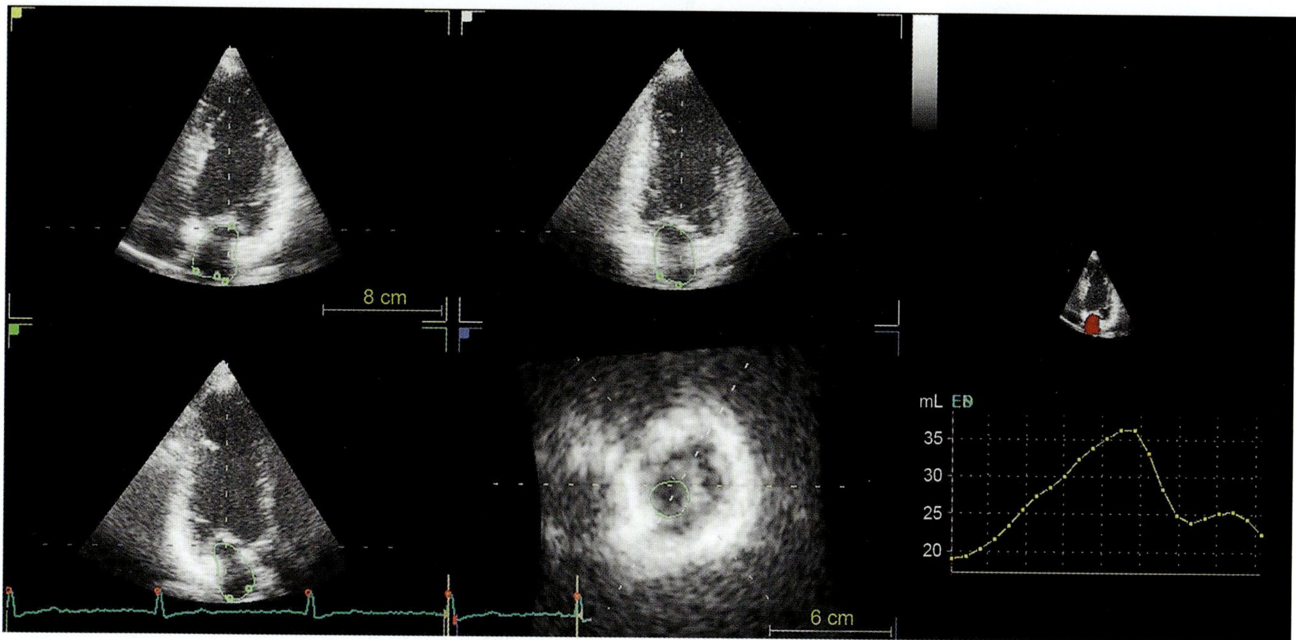

Fig. 6: Three-dimensional echocardiography for estimation of left atrial volume.

Being a marker of chronic LV diastolic dysfunction, LA enlargement is an important supportive evidence for diagnosis of HFpEF. In absence of an alternate cause (such as atrial fibrillation or mitral regurgitation), LA enlargement is virtually diagnostic of LV diastolic dysfunction. Moreover, the size of the left atrium correlates with the severity and the chronicity of LV diastolic dysfunction.[46-48] For this reason, LA size is also considered to be the glycosylated hemoglobin of LV diastolic function.

Left atrial size is a strong predictor of adverse cardiovascular outcomes. It is associated with increased risk of atrial fibrillation, heart failure hospitalizations, stroke, and overall cardiovascular mortality.[24,26,38,46,49-60] In the Framingham Heart Study, prognostic value of LA size was assessed in a subset of 1,924 elderly subjects followed up for 7.2 years.[58] The LA size was found to be a strong independent predictor of the risk of nonrheumatic atrial fibrillation. Similarly, in yet another study involving elderly subjects with no prior atrial fibrillation, LA volume was independently predictive of first ischemic stroke and even death.[56] Several other studies have also reported similar findings.

CONCLUSION

Left ventricular hypertrophy and LA enlargement are common cardiac structural changes occurring in patients with heart failure. Their presence in HFpEF patients provides a confirmation of the underlying LV diastolic dysfunction and is thus helpful in establishing the diagnosis. Their diagnostic utility in HFrEF is relatively limited. Nonetheless, in both HFpEF and HFrEF, LVH and LA enlargement have significant prognostic value. Increase in the LV mass or LA size is strong predictors of adverse cardiovascular outcomes including heart failure hospitalizations, atrial fibrillation, stroke, and overall cardiovascular mortality. Echocardiography is the simplest and widely available diagnostic modality that can easily permit accurate assessment of LV mass and LA size. This further enhances the utility of echocardiography in heart failure.

REFERENCES

1. Victor RG, Kaplan NM. Systemic hypertension: Mechanisms and diagnosis. In: Libby P, Bonow RO, Mann DL, Zipes DP (Eds). Braunwald's Heart Disease: A Text-book of Cardiovascular Medicine, 8th edition. Philadelphia: Saunders; 2008. pp. 1027-48.
2. Cuspidi C, Facchetti R, Bombelli M, Sala C, Grassi G, Mancia G. Differential value of left ventricular mass index and wall thickness in predicting cardiovascular prognosis: Data from the PAMELA population. Am J Hypertens. 2014; 27(8):1079-86.
3. Lang RM, Badano LP, Mor-Avi V, Afilalo J, Armstrong A, Ernande L, et al. Recommendations for cardiac chamber quantification by echocardiography in adults: An update

from the American Society of Echocardiography and the European Association of Cardiovascular Imaging. J Am Soc Echocardiogr. 2015; 28:1-39e14.
4. Devereux RB, Alonso DR, Lutas EM, Gottlieb GJ, Campo E, Sachs I, et al. Echocardiographic assessment of left ventricular hypertrophy: Comparison to necropsy findings. Am J Cardiol. 1986; 57:450-8.
5. Mor-Avi V, Sugeng L, Weinert L, MacEneaney P, Caiani EG, Koch R, et al. Fast measurement of left ventricular mass with real-time three-dimensional echocardiography: Comparison with magnetic resonance imaging. Circulation. 2004;110:1814-8.
6. Yap SC, van Geuns RJ, Nemes A, Meijboom FJ, McGhie JS, Geleijnse ML, et al. Rapid and accurate measurement of LV mass by biplane real-time 3D echocardiography in patients with concentric LV hypertrophy: comparison to CMR. Eur J Echocardiogr. 2008;9:255-60.
7. Pacileo G, Castaldi B, Di Salvo G, Limongelli G, Rea A, D'Andrea A, et al. Assessment of left- ventricular mass and remodeling in obese adolescents: M-mode, 2D or 3D echocardiography? J Cardiovasc Med. (Hagerstown, Md) 2013;14:144-9.
8. Jenkins C, Bricknell K, Hanekom L, Marwick TH. Reproducibility and accuracy of echocardiographic measurements of left ventricular parameters using real-time three-dimensional echocardiography. J Am Coll Cardiol. 2004;44:878-86.
9. Oe H, Hozumi T, Arai K, Matsumura Y, Negishi K, Sugioka K, Ujino K, et al. Comparison of accurate measurement of left ventricular mass in patients with hypertrophied hearts by real-time three-dimensional echocardiography versus magnetic resonance imaging. Am J Cardiol. 2005;95:1263-7.
10. Bicudo LS, Tsutsui JM, Shiozaki A, Rochitte CE, Arteaga E, Mady C, et al. Value of real time three-dimensional echocardiography in patients with hypertrophic cardiomyopathy: Comparison with two-dimensional echocardiography and magnetic resonance imaging. Echocardiography. 2008;25:717-26.
11. Caiani EG, Corsi C, Sugeng L, MacEneaney P, Weinert L, Mor-Avi V, et al. Improved quantification of left ventricular mass based on endocardial and epicardial surface detection with real time three dimensional echocardiography. Heart (British Cardiac Society). 2006;92:213-9.
12. Chang SA, Kim HK, Lee SC, Kim EY, Hahm SH, Kwon OM, et al. Assessment of left ventricular mass in hypertrophic cardiomyopathy by real-time three-dimensional echocardiography using single-beat capture image. J Am Soc Echocardiogr. 2013;26:436-42.
13. van den Bosch AE, Robbers-Visser D, Krenning BJ, McGhie JS, Helbing WA, Meijboom FJ, et al. Comparison of real-time three-dimensional echocardiography to magnetic resonance imaging for assessment of left ventricular mass. Am J Cardiol. 2006;97:113-7.
14. Shimada YJ, Shiota T. A meta-analysis and investigation for the source of bias of left ventricular volumes and function by three-dimensional echocardiography in comparison with magnetic resonance imaging. Am J Cardiol. 2011; 107:126-38.
15. Qin JX, Jones M, Travaglini A, Song JM, Li J, White RD, et al. The accuracy of left ventricular mass determined by real-time three- dimensional echocardiography in chronic animal and clinical studies: A comparison with postmortem examination and magnetic resonance imaging. J Am Soc Echocardiogr. 2005;18:1037-43.
16. Lenstrup M, Kjaergaard J, Petersen CL, Kjaer A, Hassager C. Evaluation of left ventricular mass measured by 3D echocardiography using magnetic resonance imaging as gold standard. Scand J Clin Lab Invest. 2006;66:647-57.
17. Pouleur AC, le Polain de Waroux JB, Pasquet A, Gerber BL, Gérard O, Allain P, et al. Assessment of left ventricular mass and volumes by three-dimensional echocardiography in patients with or without wall motion abnormalities: Comparison against cine magnetic resonance imaging. Heart. 2008;94:1050-7.
18. Marsan NA, Bleeker GB, Ypenburg C, Van Bommel RJ, Ghio S, Van de Veire NR, et al. Real-time three-dimensional echocardiography as a novel approach to assess left ventricular and left atrium reverse remodeling and to predict response to cardiac resynchronization therapy. Heart Rhythm. 2008;5:1257-64.
19. Mizukoshi K, Takeuchi M, Nagata Y, Addetia K, Lang RM, Akashi YJ, et al. Normal values of left ventricular mass index assessed by transthoracic three-dimensional echocardiography. J Am Soc Echocardiogr. 2016;29:51-61.
20. Gaasch WH, Zile MR. Left ventricular structural remodeling in health and disease: With special emphasis on volume, mass, and geometry. J Am Coll Cardiol. 2011;58:1733-40.
21. Berger J, Ren X, Na B, Whooley MA, Schiller NB. Relation of concentric remodeling to adverse outcomes in patients with stable coronary artery disease (from the Heart and Soul Study). Am J Cardiol. 2011;107:1579-84.
22. Verdecchia P, Schillaci G, Borgioni C, Ciucci A, Battistelli M, Bartoccini C, et al. Adverse prognostic significance of concentric remodeling of the left ventricle in hypertensive patients with normal left ventricular mass. J Am Coll Cardiol. 1995;25:871-8.
23. Zile MR, Gaasch WH, Patel K, Aban IB, Ahmed A. Adverse left ventricular remodeling in community-dwelling older adults predicts incident heart failure and mortality. JACC Heart Fail. 2014;2:512-22.
24. Shah AM, Shah SJ, Anand IS, Sweitzer NK, O'Meara E, Heitner JF, et al. Cardiac structure and function in heart failure with preserved ejection fraction: Baseline findings from the echocardiographic study of the Treatment of Preserved Cardiac Function Heart Failure with an Aldosterone Antagonist trial. Circ Heart Fail. 2014; 7:104-15.

25. Katz DH, Beussink L, Sauer AJ, Freed BH, Burke MA, Shah SJ. Prevalence, clinical characteristics, and outcomes associated with eccentric versus concentric left ventricular hypertrophy in heart failure with preserved ejection fraction. Am J Cardiol. 2013;112:1158-64.
26. Zile MR, Gottdiener JS, Hetzel SJ, McMurray JJ, Komajda M, McKelvie R, et al. Prevalence and significance of alterations in cardiac structure and function in patients with heart failure and a preserved ejection fraction. Circulation. 2011;124:2491-501.
27. Gupta DK, Solomon SD. Imaging in heart failure with preserved ejection fraction. Heart Fail Clin. 2014;10:419-34.
28. Kraigher-Krainer E, Shah AM, Gupta DK, Santos A, Claggett B, Pieske B, et al. Impaired systolic function by strain imaging in heart failure with preserved ejection fraction. J Am Coll Cardiol. 2014; 63:447-56.
29. Aurigemma GP, Zile MR, Gaasch WH. Contractile behavior of the left ventricle in diastolic heart failure: With emphasis on regional systolic function. Circulation. 2006;113:296-304.
30. Komajda M, Lam CS. Heart failure with preserved ejection fraction: A clinical dilemma. Eur Heart J. 2014;35:1022-32.
31. van Heerebeek L, Borbely A, Niessen HW, Bronzwaer JG, van der Velden J, Stienen GJ, et al. Myocardial structure and function differ in systolic and diastolic heart failure. Circulation. 2006;113:1966-73.
32. Levy D, Garrison RJ, Savage DD, Kannel WB, Castelli WP. Prognostic implications of echocardiographically determined left ventricular mass in the Framingham Heart Study. N Engl J Med. 1990;322:1561-6.
33. Koren MJ, Devereux RB, Casale PN, Savage DD, Laragh JH. Relation of left ventricular mass and geometry to morbidity and mortality in uncomplicated essential hypertension. Ann Intern Med. 1991;114:345-52.
34. Muiesan ML, Salvetti M, Rizzoni D, Castellano M, Donato F, Agabiti-Rosei E. Association of change in left ventricular mass with prognosis during long- term antihypertensive treatment. J Hypertens. 1995;13: 1091-5.
35. Verdecchia P, Carini G, Circo A, Dovellini E, Giovannini E, Lombardo M, et al. Left ventricular mass and cardiovascular morbidity in essential hypertension: The MAVI study. J Am Coll Cardiol. 2001;38:1829-35.
36. Pritchett AM, Jacobsen SJ, Mahoney DW, Rodeheffer RJ, Bailey KR, Redfield MM. Left atrial volume as an index of left atrial size: A population-based study. J Am Coll Cardiol. 2003;41:1036-43.
37. Tani T, Tanabe K, Ono M, Amaguchi K, Okada M, Sumida T. Left atrial volume and the risk of paroxysmal atrial fibrillation in patients with hypertrophic cardiomyopathy. J Am Soc Echocardiogr. 2004;17:644-8.
38. Tsang TS, Abhayaratna WP, Barnes ME, Miyasaka Y, Gersh BJ, Bailey KR, et al. Prediction of cardiovascular outcomes with left atrial size: is volume superior to area or diameter? J Am Coll Cardiol. 2006;47:1018-23.
39. Lester SJ, Ryan EW, Schiller NB, Foster E. Best method in clinical practice and in research studies to determine left atrial size. Am J Cardiol. 1999;84:829-32.
40. Muller H, Burri H, Shah D, Lerch R. Evaluation of left atrial size in patients with atrial arrhythmias: comparison of standard 2D versus real time 3D echocardiography. Echocardiog. (Mount Kisco, NY) 2007;24:960-6.
41. Anwar AM, Soliman OI, Geleijnse ML, Nemes A, Vletter WB, ten Cate FJ. Assessment of left atrial volume and function by real-time three- dimensional echocardiography. Int J Cardiol. 2008;123: 155-61.
42. Miyasaka Y, Tsujimoto S, Maeba H, Yuasa F, Takehana K, Dote K, et al. Left atrial volume by real-time three-dimensional echocardiography: validation by 64-slice multidetector computed tomography. J Am Soc Echocardiogr. 2011;24:680-6.
43. Rohner A, Brinkert M, Kawel N, Buechel RR, Leibundgut G, Grize L, et al. Functional assessment of the left atrium by real-time three-dimensional echocardiography using a novel dedicated analysis tool: Initial validation studies in comparison with computed tomography. Eur J Echocardiogr. 2011;12:497-505.
44. Mor-Avi V, Yodwut C, Jenkins C, Kühl H, Nesser HJ, Marwick TH, et al. Real-time 3D echocardiographic quantification of left atrial volume: Multicenter study for validation with CMR. JACC Cardiovasc Imaging. 2012;5:769-77.
45. Aune E, Baekkevar M, Roislien J, Rodevand O, Otterstad JE. Normal reference ranges for left and right atrial volume indexes and ejection fractions obtained with real-time three-dimensional echocardiography. Eur J Echocardiogr. 2009;10:738-44.
46. Tsang TSM, Barnes ME, Gersh BJ, Bailey KR, Seward JB. Left atrial volume as a morphophysiologic expression of left ventricular diastolic dysfunction and relation to cardiovascular risk burden. Am J Cardiol. 2002;90:1284-89.
47. Simek CL, Feldman MD, Haber HL, Wu CC, Jayaweera AR, Kaul S. Relationship between left ventricular wall thickness and left atrial size: Comparison with other measures of diastolic function. J Am Soc Echocardiogr. 1995;8:37-47.
48. Appleton CP, Galloway JM, Gonzalez MS, Gaballa M, Basnight MA. Estimation of left ventricular filling pressures using two-dimensional and Doppler echocardiography in adult patients with cardiac disease. Additional value of analyzing left atrial size, left atrial ejection fraction and the difference in duration of pulmonary venous and mitral flow velocity at atrial contraction. J Am Coll Cardiol. 1993;22:1972-82.
49. Benjamin EJ, D'Agostino RB, Belanger AJ, Wolf PA, Levy D. Left atrial size and the risk of stroke and death. The Framingham Heart Study. Circulation. 1995;92:835-41.
50. Moller JE, Hillis GS, Oh JK, Seward JB, Reeder GS, Wright RS, et al. Left atrial volume: A powerful predictor

of survival after acute myocardial infarction. Circulation. 2003;107:2207-12.
51. Meris A, Amigoni M, Uno H, Thune JJ, Verma A, Køber L, et al. Left atrial remodelling in patients with myocardial infarction complicated by heart failure, left ventricular dysfunction, or both: The VALIANT Echo study. Eur Heart J. 2009;30:56-65.
52. Tsang TSM, Barnes ME, Gersh BJ, Takemoto Y, Rosales AG, Bailey KR, et al. Prediction of risk for first age-related cardiovascular events in an elderly population: The incremental value of echocardiography. J Am Coll Cardiol. 2003;42:1199-205.
53. Bolca O, Akdemir O, Eren M, Dagdeviren B, Yildirim A, Tezel T. Left atrial maximum volume is a recurrence predictor in lone atrial fibrillation: An acoustic quantification study. Jpn Heart J. 2002;43:241-8.
54. Di Tullio MR, Sacco RL, Sciacca RR, Homma S. Left atrial size and the risk of ischemic stroke in an ethnically mixed population. Stroke. 1999;30:2019-24.
55. Tsang TS, Barnes ME, Bailey KR, Leibson CL, Montgomery SC, Takemoto Y, et al. Left atrial volume: important risk marker of incident atrial fibrillation in 1655 older men and women. Mayo Clin Proc. 2001;76:467-75.
56. Barnes ME, Miyasaka Y, Seward JB, Gersh BJ, Rosales AG, Bailey KR, et al. Left atrial volume in the prediction of first ischemic stroke in an elderly cohort without atrial fibrillation. Mayo Clin Proc. 2004;79:1008-14.
57. Tsang TS, Barnes ME, Gersh BJ, Bailey KR, Seward JB. Risks for atrial fibrillation and congestive heart failure in patients ≥65 years of age with abnormal left ventricular diastolic relaxation. Am J Cardiol. 2004;93:54-8.
58. Vaziri SM, Larson MG, Benjamin EJ, Levy D. Echocardiographic predictors of nonrheumatic atrial fibrillation. The Framingham Heart Study. Circulation. 1994;89:724-30.
59. Flaker GC, Fletcher KA, Rothbart RM, Halperin JL, Hart RG. Clinical and echocardiographic features of intermittent atrial fibrillation that predict recurrent atrial fibrillation. Stroke Prevention in Atrial Fibrillation (SPAF) Investigators. Am J Cardiol. 1995;76:355-8.
60. Gardin JM, McClelland R, Kitzman D, Lima JA, Bommer W, Klopfenstein HS, et al. M-mode echocardiographic predictors of six- to seven-year incidence of coronary heart disease, stroke, congestive heart failure, and mortality in an elderly cohort (the Cardiovascular Health Study). Am J Cardiol. 2001;87:1051-7.

Metabolic Ill Health: A New Therapeutic Target for Improving Outcome of Cardiometabolic Diseases

PC Manoria, Pankaj Manoria

INTRODUCTION

Metabolic ill health implies that the individual is prone to or has already developed obesity, type 2 diabetes (T2D), metabolic dysfunction associated with fatty liver disease (MAFLD), obstructive sleep apnea (OSA), polycystic ovarian syndrome (PCOS), atherosclerotic cardiovascular disease (ASCVD) such as coronary artery disease (CAD), stroke, kidney disease, etc. **(Fig. 1)**. But the concept of metabolic ill health has not been widely percolated, so if a physician sees a patient with any of the above diseases, he tries to treat himself or tries to refer to the concerned specialist. But the correct approach is that if the patient has one of the manifestations of metabolic ill health, he must look at other components present in the same patient because they tend to conglomerate in the same patient.

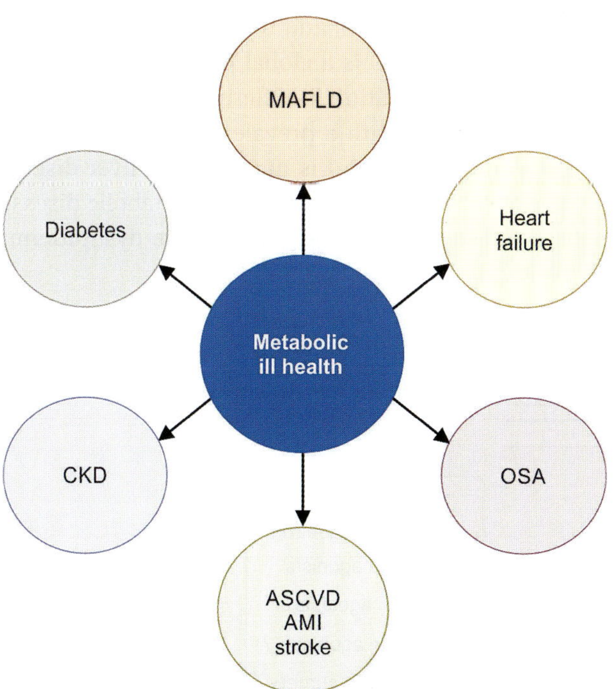

Fig. 1: Components of metabolic ill health. (ASCVD: atherosclerotic cardiovascular disease; CKD: chronic kidney disease; MAFLD: metabolic dysfunction associated with fatty liver disease; OSA: obstructive sleep apnea)

Obesity is central to the pathogenesis of metabolic illness and is the root cause of cardiometabolic diseases. The global prevalence of obesity in 2022 was above 1 billion, whereas in India, the prevalence in 2023 was 224 million. Obesity, on the one hand, is a driver of diabetes, and on the other hand, it is also a driver of cardiovascular disease. If patients develop diabetes, it is also a driver of cardiovascular disease. Therefore, cardiologists and diabetologists are very concerned about obesity. The adipocentric approach has therefore come to the forefront, even ahead of the glucocentric or cardiorenal approach. Any magnitude of weight loss is beneficial, but if the weight loss is more than 15%, it is a predictor of remission of diabetes, improves heart failure with preserved ejection fraction (HFpEF), and also decreases cardiovascular mortality. Lifestyle modification decreases the weight by 5–10%, but its compliance in the long run is difficult. The conventional drugs for obesity also decreased in weight by 5–10%. Endoscopic bariatric procedures decrease weight by about 15–20%, and bariatric surgery decreases weight by above 25% or so.

DRUG REVOLUTION IN OBESITY

During the last couple of years, there has been a drug revolution in obesity. We have a single agonist, a double agonist, and triple agonist.

Single Agonist

Injectable semaglutide 2.4 mg (sc): This is a powerful drug for treating obesity and has shown a reduction in weight in the step trial by about 15–17%. Oral semaglutide 14 mg has shown a decrease in weight of about 5 kg across the pioneer program. Recently, higher oral doses of oral semaglutide 25 and 50 mg have shown incremental benefits. The 50 mg oral dose has shown a reduction in weight of 15%. Interestingly, injectable semaglutide has shown improvement in cardiovascular outcomes in non-diabetic obesity as well. However, injectable semaglutide is not yet available in India.

Dual Agonist

Dual agonist tirzepatide [gastric inhibitory polypeptide (GIP) + glucagon-like peptide-1, (GLP-1) RA] has shown a reduction in weight by 9.5–13 kg.[1] The reduction in HbA1C ranged from 2.07 to 2.59. CagriSema, which is a combination of Sema (2.4 mg) and Cagrilintide (0.16–4.5 mg), has shown a reduction in weight of about 17%.

Triple Agonist

Gastric inhibitory polypeptide + GLP-1 + glucagon receptor agonist (GRA) such as retatrutide in a phase II trial[2] has shown a reduction in weight up to 24.2% in a dose of 12 mg subcutaneous (sc) weekly.

Thus, monotherapy with a single agonist decreases weight by about 15–17%, dual agonists by 20–23%, and triple agonists by 24%, and therefore the gap between pharmacotherapy and bariatric surgery has narrowed down tremendously **(Fig. 2)**.

Weight loss promotes better glycemic control, impacts cardiometabolic risk factors, slows down disease progression, and helps in preventing diabetes microvascular complications.[3-7] If the weight loss is 5%, it starts impacting insulin sensitivity and beta cell function. If the weight loss is 10–11%, the magnitude of the benefit is greater, the spectrum of benefits is wider, and it starts impacting gene expression and adipose tissue. If weight loss is about 15%, there is a greater benefit, and it also starts impacting inflammatory markers. The effect of weight loss on comorbidities is shown in **Figure 3**.

Obesity is also associated with increasing health-care cost[8] **(Table 1)**.

Obesity should be treated upfront so that the development of diabetes can be minimized.

Metabolic dysfunction-associated fatty liver disease (MAFLD), metabolic dysfunction-associated steatohepatitis (MASH), metabolic dysfunction-associated steatotic liver disease (MASLD).

Non-alcoholic fatty liver disease (NAFLD) has been relabeled as MAFLD, and nonalcoholic steatohepatitis (NASH) has been designated as MASH. A new terminology of metabolic dysfunction associated with steatotic liver disease has been added (MASLD). The normal amount of fat in the liver is 5%, when it exceeds 10%, it is termed MAFLD.

The most common cause of death in MAFLD is cardiovascular disease and not liver disease. MAFLD is a gateway for the development of cardiovascular disease. Most of these patients remain symptomatic till late in the course of the disease, and therefore it is also termed a silent killer. MAFLD is a global problem, and roughly 25–30% of the population is suffering from it. India falls into the high zone with a prevalence of >30%. MAFLD is a systemic disease and is not merely a liver disease. It is associated with panoply of cardiometabolic diseases such as obesity, T2D, OSA, atherogenic dyslipidemia,

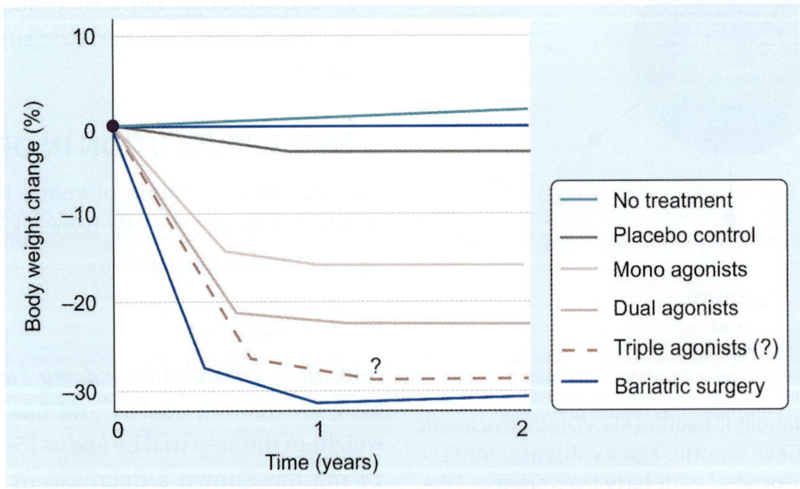

Fig. 2: Effect of drug revolution on change in body weight.

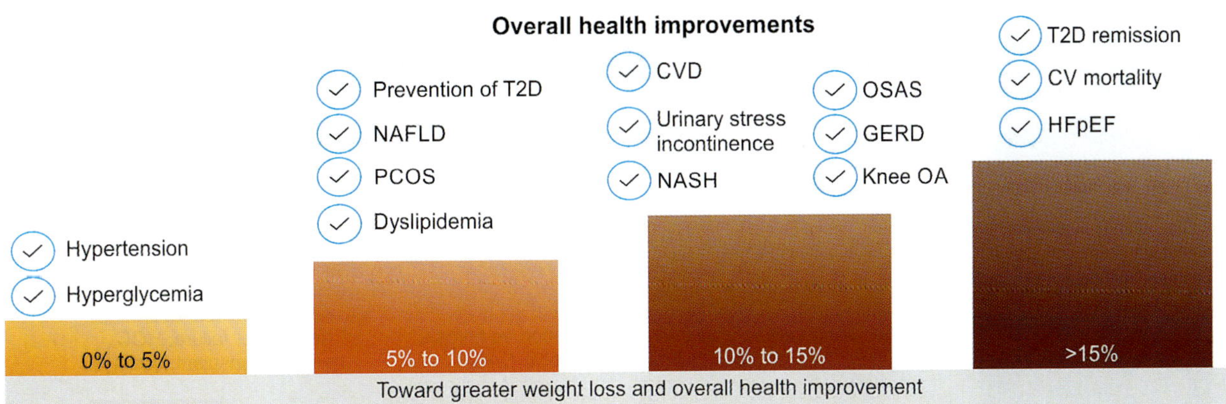

Fig. 3: Effect of weight on comorbidities. (CV: cardiovascular; CVD: cardiovascular disease; GERD: gastroesophageal reflux disease; HFpEF: heart failure with preserved ejection fraction; NAFLD: non-alcoholic fatty liver disease; NASH: nonalcoholic steatohepatitis; PCOS: polycystic ovarian syndrome; OSAS: obstructive sleep apnea syndrome)
Source: Garvey WT, et al. Endo Prac. 2016: 22(Suppl 3)1-203; Look AHEAD Research Group. Lancet Diabetes Endocrine. 2016;4:914-21: Lean ME, et al. Lancet. 2018;391;541-51; Benraoune F, et al. Curr Opin Cardiol. 2011;26:555-61; Sundstrom J, et al. Circulation. 2017;135:1577-85.

TABLE 1: Costs for emergency room, inpatient, and outpatient services, plus pharmacy dispensing in overweight or obese.

Obesity	*Body mass index (BMI)*	*Increased health-care costs*
Overweight	BMI 25.0–29.9 kg/m^2	+ 11% cost
OBESITY (CLASS I)	BMI 30.0–34.9 kg/m^2	+ 17% cost
OBESITY (CLASS II)	BMI 35.0–39.9 kg/m^2	+ 29% cost
OBESITY (CLASS III)	BMI ≥40 kg/m^2	+ 46% cost

hypertension, ASCVD, and PCOS. Diabetic MAFLD may progress to NASH and then to fibrosis. Diabetic patients have faster progression of fibrosis as compared to non-diabetic patients, which leads to compensated cirrhosis and finally decompensated cirrhosis. A small percentage of patients develop hepatocellular carcinoma.

FOLLOW-UP FOR PATIENTS WITH NONALCOHOLIC FATTY LIVER DISEASE

If patients belong to a low-risk group, i.e., the fibrosis-4 (FIB-4) <1.3, liver stiffness measurement (LSM) <8 kPa, or enhanced liver fibrosis (ELF) <7.7, then this can be managed by a primary care physician with a focus on obesity management and cardiovascular disease prevention. If the patient is at intermediate risk, i.e., FIB-4 1.3–2.67, LSM 8–12 kPa, or ELF 7.7–9.8, he should be referred to a hapatologist. If he has a high-risk FIB-4 >2.67, LSM >12 kPa, or ELF >9.8, then he requires a multidisciplinary team to prevent cirrhosis and CVD.

TREATMENT

Lifestyle modification and a low-calorie diet are very important parts of treatment and should be strictly applied.

Drugs

- *Saroglitazar:* This is approved in India by Drugs Controller General of India (DCGI). It is administered in doses of 4 mg per day for treatment of MASH and fibrosis F1 to F3. It also decreases blood glucose due to its dual PPαR action. It decreases triglycerides and decreases fibrosis. It is not effective if the patient has developed cirrhosis.
- *Vitamin E 400 mg* is given once daily in non-diabetic biopsy-proven NASH.
- *Pioglitazone:* This is administered in biopsy-proven NASH in diabetic as well as non-diabetic patients.
- *Glucagon-like peptide-1 receptor agonist (GLP1-RA):* It decreases fat in the liver and histological resolution of MASH, but it is not effective when fibrosis has developed.

Resmetirom: This is a new drug approved by United States Food and Drug Administration (USFDA) on 24th March 2024. It is a liver-directed oral thyroid hormone receptor beta (THR-β) agonist therapy targeting the underlying cause of NASH. The drug was approved after the Maestro-Nash trial,[9] which showed positive results. It showed NASH resolution without worsening of fibrosis at week 52 ($p < 0.001$) and improvement in fibrosis by >1 stage with no worsening of NAFLD activity score ($p < 0.001$). The drug is

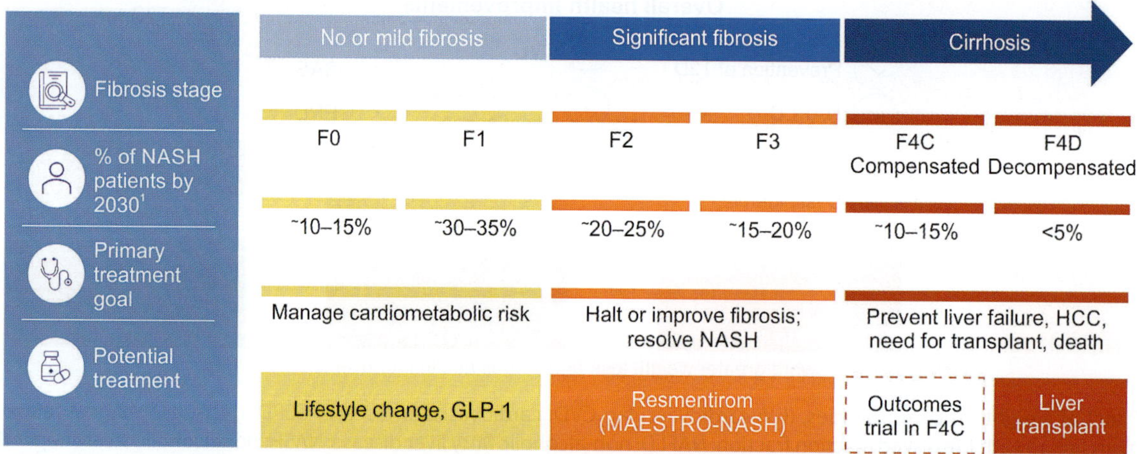

Fig. 4: Progression of metabolic dysfunction associated with fatty liver disease (MAFLD) and its effect on therapies. (GLP-1: glucagon-like peptide-1; HCC: hepatocellular carcinoma; NASH: nonalcoholic steatohepatitis)

administered in doses of 80 mg or 100 mg per day in a single dose. The drug is well tolerated. A small number of patients may develop diarrhea and nausea. The place lifestyle modification and various drugs are outlined in **Figure 4**.

OBSTRUCTIVE SLEEP APNEA

This is another component of metabolic ill health. OSA is diagnosed by polysomnography by apnea hypopnea index, i.e., AHI, which is calculated by dividing the number of apnea (pauses in breathing) + the number of hypopneas (periods of shallow breathing) events by the number of hours of sleep. The AHI limits per hour of sleep for adults are mentioned below:

- *Normal:* <5
- *Mild sleep apnea:* 5–15
- *Moderate sleep apnea:* 15–30
- *Severe sleep apnea:* ≥30

Obstructive sleep apnea increases risk of recurrent heart attack, stroke, atrial fibrillation, sudden cardiac death.

Obstructive sleep apnea associated with a reduced mean nocturnal oxygen saturation <93% and a lowest nocturnal oxygen saturation <78% were independent risk factors for sudden cardiac death (SCD) ($p = 0.0001$). A circadian pattern of ventricular arrhythmia and a higher rate of SCD during sleep time (midnight to 6 am) have been demonstrated. Osa is commonly with cardiovascular diseases (CVDS) **(Box 1)**.

POLYCYSTIC OVARY SYNDROME

Its main features can include cysts in the ovaries, high levels of male hormones, and irregular periods.

BOX 1: Concomitant diseases with obstructive sleep apnea (OSA).

- Arterial hypertension 30–60
- Drug-resistant hypertension 80–90%
- Coronary heart disease 30–60%
- Heart failure (HFrEF) 10–50%
- Heart failure (HFpEF) 20–60%
- Stroke 40–90%

Heart Failure

Heart failure is an important complication of diabetes. In diabetes, HFpEF is more common. Sodium-glucose cotransporter-2 inhibitor (SGLT2i) has a class one recommendation from HFpEF. Recently, injectable semaglutide 2.4 mg weekly has shown positive results in STEP-HFpEF trial and STEP-HFpEF DM trial. The drug is suitable for the obese phenotype of HFpEF. Angiotensin receptor-neprilysin inhibitor (ARNI) and mineralocorticoid receptor antagonist (MRAs) have class 2B recommendations. Diuretics are, of course, used to decrease congestion in HFpEF. For HFrEF, besides diuretics, which are utilized to decrease congestion, the four foundational, i.e., SGLT2i, beta-blockers ARNI, and MRAs, have kicked off a drug revolution in heart failure. For worsening heart failure, vericiguat is used.

CHRONIC KIDNEY DISEASE

Chronic kidney disease (CKD) is a progressive disease; there is no available treatment that can reverse it to normal. However, we have three guideline-recommended pillars of CKD that slow down the trajectory of CKD by slowing

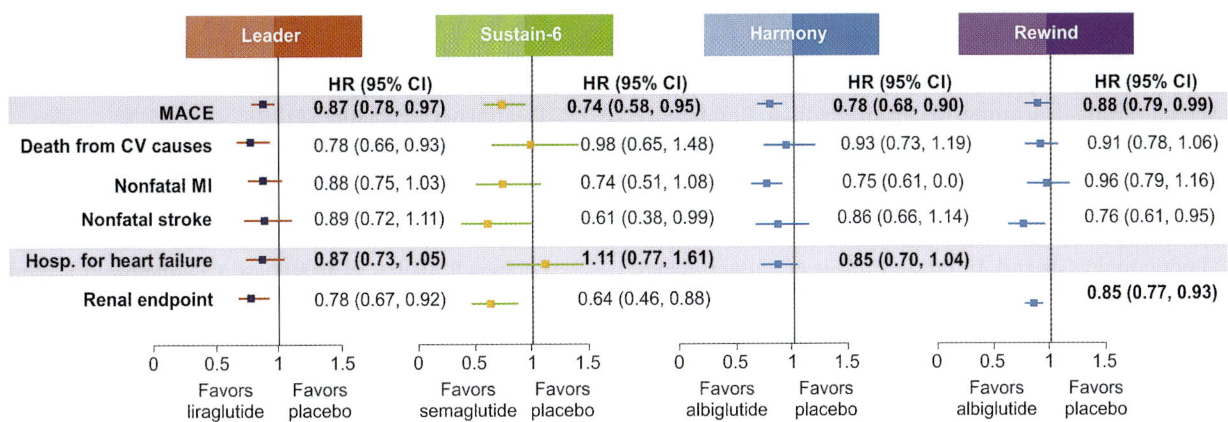

Fig. 5: Positive cardiovascular (CV) outcome trials with glucagon-like peptide-1 receptor agonist (GLP-1RA).

down the decline in estimated glomerular filtration rate (eGFR) and postpone dialysis by 10–15 years.

These include renin-angiotensin system (RAS) blockers, SGLT2i, and non-steroidal MRAs, i.e., finerenone.[10] In the recent past, the flow trial[11] with injectable semaglutide 1 mg weekly has shown positive results, and in the future, this is lightly to become the fourth pillar of CKD management.

CORONARY ARTERY DISEASE

Diabetes is a leading cause of death in people with T2D. About 70% of diabetics die from acute myocardial infarction. Cardiovascular disease in India occurs a decade earlier and is two times more common than non-diabetics. The mere presence of diabetes cuts short the life span by 6 years, and if myocardial infarction gets superimposed, the life span is cut short by 12 years. Besides conventional therapies for the prevention of CAD of diabetes, GLP-1 receptor agonists have shown a reduction in ASCVD events both for primary and secondary prevention and are the standard of care for primary prevention for high-risk diabetics and for secondary prevention of diabetes **(Fig. 5)**.

Oral semaglutide 14 mg has shown good glycemic control and weight reduction in the pioneer program, but the CV outcome is ongoing[12] to evaluate its cardiovascular effects.

STROKE

People with diabetes are at a higher risk for both ischemic and hemorrhagic strokes. The risk of stroke is two to four times higher in individuals with diabetes compared to those without.

Diabetes accelerates atherosclerosis, leading to a greater likelihood of ischemic strokes. Hypertension is more common in diabetes, and these result in an increase incidence of hemorrhagic stroke. Diabetes, particularly in association with hypertension, also involves small arteries producing lacunar infarcts. After a stroke, diabetics are at higher risk of complications such as delayed recovery and poor functional outcomes. Lytic therapy is the standard of care for a large artery stroke if the patient is present within the window period. Endovascular therapy for extraction of the clot is also utilized in advanced centers. Besides this, good glycemic control, control of BP, lipids, and antiplatelet therapy are also useful. A dual pathway inhibitor, i.e., aspirin 100 mg plus rivaroxaban 2.5 mg twice daily, is also utilized to decrease the incidence of ischemic stroke in the future.

CONCLUSION

Cardiometabolic diseases due to metabolic ill health are rocking the entire universe and are the leading cause of cardiovascular morbidity and mortality. Obesity is central to the pathogenesis of metabolic ill health and its further consequences. Due to this obesity has come in forefront of therapeutics. If this can be minimized, most of the components of metabolic ill health will become a rarity. For those who have already developed metabolic ill health panoply of diagnostic and therapeutic strategy are available to improve their outcome.

REFERENCES

1. Qin W, Yang J, Ni Y, Deng C, Ruan Q, Ruan J, et al. Efficacy and safety of once-weekly tirzepatide for weight management compared to placebo: An updated systematic review and

meta-analysis including the latest SURMOUNT-2 trial. Endocrine. 2024;86(1):70-84.
2. Jastreboff AM, Kaplan LM, Frías JP, Wu Q, Du Y, Gurbuz S, et al. Triple–Hormone-Receptor Agonist Retatrutide for Obesity — A Phase 2 Trial. N Engl J Med. 2023;389: 514-26.
3. Garvey WT, Mechanick JI, Brett EM, Garber AJ, Hurley DL, Jastreboff AM, et al. American Association of Clinical Endocrinologists and American College of Endocrinology Comprehensive Clinical Practice Guidelines for Medical Care of Patients with Obesity. Endocr pract. 2016; 22(Suppl 3):1-203.
4. Look AHEAD Research Group; Gregg EW, Jakicic JM, Blackburn G, Bloomquist P, Bray GA, et al. Association of the magnitude of weight loss and changes in physical fitness with long-term cardiovascular disease outcomes in overweight or obese people with type 2 diabetes: a post-hoc analysis of the Look AHEAD randomised clinical trial. Look ahead research group. Lancet diabetes Endocrinol. 2016;4:913-21.
5. Lean ME, Leslie WS, Barnes AC, Brosnahan N, Thom G, McCombie L, Peters C, et al. Primary care-led weight management for remission of type 2 diabetes (DiRECT): an open-label, cluster-randomised trial. Lancet. 2018; 391:541-51.
6. Benraouane F, Litwin SE. Reductions in cardiovascular risk after bariatric surgery. Curr Opin Cardiol. 2011;26:555-61.
7. Sundström J, Bruze G, Ottosson J, Marcus C, Näslund I, Neovius M. Weight Loss and Heart Failure: A Nationwide Study of Gastric Bypass Surgery Versus Intensive Lifestyle Treatment Circulation. 2017;135:1577-85.
8. Li Q, Blume SW, Huang JC, Hammer M, Graf TR. The Economic Burden of Obesity by Glycemic Stage in the United States. Pharmacoeconomics. 2015;33(7):735-48.
9. Harrison SA, Bedossa P, Guy CD, Schattenberg JM, Loomba R, Taub R, et al. A Phase 3, Randomized, Controlled Trial of Resmetirom in NASH with Liver Fibrosis. N Engl J Med. 2024;390:497-509.
10. Agarwal R, Filippatos G, Pitt B, Anker SD, Rossing P, Joseph A, et al. Cardiovascular and kidney outcomes with finerenone in patients with type 2 diabetes and chronic kidney disease: the FIDELITY pooled analysis. Eur Heart J. 2022;43(6):474-84.
11. Perkovic V, Tuttle KR, Rossing P, Mahaffey KW, Mann JFE, Bakris G, et al. Effects of Semaglutide on Chronic Kidney Disease in Patients with Type 2 Diabetes. N Engl J Med. 2024;391:109-21.
12. McGuire DK, Busui RP, Deanfield J, Inzucchi SE, Mann JFE, Marx N, et al. Effects of oral semaglutide on cardiovascular outcomes in individuals with type 2 diabetes and established atherosclerotic cardiovascular disease and/or chronic kidney disease: Design and baseline characteristics of SOUL, a randomized trial. Diabetes Obes Metab. 2023;25(7):1932-41.

CHAPTER 22

Stage B Heart Failure in Clinical Practice

Rakesh Gupta

INTRODUCTION

Stage B heart failure (HF) is an asymptomatic heart failure where structural heart changes (like LA dilation, reduced GLS, LV hypertrophy, raised LA pressure) exist and are detected by tests (echo, biomarkers) but without symptoms. This emphasizes that it's a crucial pre-clinical stage for early intervention to prevent its progression to stage C (Symptomatic) heart failure. This condition highlights its significance as an early opportunity for preventive treatment like lifestyle modification, blood pressure and blood sugar control, and medication (ACE inhibitors, diuretics, antidiabetic medications) to slow down the progression to symptomatic disease.

WHAT IS HEART FAILURE?

Heart failure is a complex clinical syndrome where the heart is unable to pump sufficiently to maintain blood flow to meet the body's needs. It can be either acute and can come on suddenly, or can be a progressive, long-term condition.

In HF, the heart's ventricles may become too stiff, or the heart muscle may become damaged and weakened. Over time, the heart can no longer keep up with the normal demands placed on it to pump blood to the rest of the body.[1]

INCIDENCE OF HEART FAILURE

The prevalence of HF in the United States (US) is estimated at over 6 million adults, with the incidence continuing to increase.[2]

A large portion of the US population is at risk of HF due to the high prevalence of established HF risk factors. Approximately 115 million people in the US have hypertension, 100 million have obesity, 26 million have diabetes, 92 million have prediabetes, and 125 million have atherosclerotic cardiovascular disease (ASCVD), all of which are associated with increased risk of developing HF.[3] Furthermore, many individuals have more than one of these modifiable HF risk factors, which further increases the risk.[4] In addition, these risk factors disproportionately impact various racial and ethnic groups.[2]

Heart Failure Incidence in India

The prevalence of HF in India in 2025 is estimated to be between 1.3 and 4.6 million cases, with an annual incidence ranging from 491,600 to 1.8 million cases. These figures highlight the significant burden of HF, a leading cause of death and disability in both urban and rural India. While HF is a concern across all age groups, it is particularly prevalent in older adults, with 5–10% of those aged 65–79 years and 10–20% of those over 80 years experiencing HF-related hospitalizations. Hypertension, diabetes, and unhealthy lifestyles (including sedentary habits, poor diet, and high salt intake) are major contributors to the increasing prevalence of HF in India. In urban areas and high-income states, ischemic heart disease is a leading cause of HF. However, in rural areas, other factors such as *rheumatic heart disease, nonischemic cardiomyopathies*, and congenital anomalies play a more significant role. India also faces the challenge of HF in a younger population, with studies reporting that 21% of HF cases occur in individuals below 50 years of age, *according to the Indian Journal of Medical Research.* HF is a serious condition with a high mortality rate, particularly in India, where first-time heart attack mortality is significantly higher than in developed countries.[5]

COMMON CAUSES OF HEART FAILURE

Patients with hypertension, cardiovascular disease (CVD), diabetes, obesity, exposure to cardiotoxic agents, a genetic variant for cardiomyopathy, or a family history of cardiomyopathy are at more risk of HF.

CLASSIFICATION OF HEART FAILURE BASED ON EJECTION FRACTION

Left ventricular ejection fraction (LVEF) is clinically considered a key parameter in the evaluation of patients with HF.[6] International guidelines categorized HF on the basis of LVEF, classifying patients into three groups: Those with (1) preserved [heart failure with preserved ejection fraction (HFpEF), LVEF ≥50%], (2) mildly reduced [heart failure with mildly reduced ejection fraction (HFmrEF), LVEF 41–49%], and (3) reduced LVEF [heart failure with reduced ejection fraction (HFrEF), LVEF ≤40%] **(Tables 1 and 2)**.[7]

This HF categorization is based on inclusion criteria of clinical trials and registers and is used by the current European Society of Cardiology (ESC) Guidelines when defining recommended treatments in clinical practice.[8]

Stage B/pre-HF is a condition where the patient has no symptoms and signs of HF but has evidence of one of the following features:

- *Structural heart disease*
  - Reduced left ventricular (LV) or right ventricular (RV) systolic function
  - Reduced ejection fraction, reduced strain
  - Ventricular hypertrophy
  - Chamber enlargement
  - Wall motion abnormalities
  - Valvular heart disease
- *Evidence for increased filling pressures*
  - By invasive hemodynamic measurements
  - By noninvasive imaging, suggesting elevated filling pressures (e.g., Doppler echocardiography)

TABLE 1: Classification of HF: Based on LVEF.

Type of HF according to LVEF	*Criteria*
HFrEF	LVEF ≤40%
HFimpEF	Previous LVEF ≤40% and a follow-up measurement of LVEF >40%
HFmrEF	• *LVEF*: 41–49% • Evidence of spontaneous or provokable increased LV filling pressures (e.g., elevated natriuretic peptide, noninvasive and invasive hemodynamic measurement)
HFpEF	• *LVEF*: ≥50% • Evidence of spontaneous or provokable increased LV filling pressures (e.g., elevated natriuretic peptide, noninvasive and invasive hemodynamic measurement)

(HF: heart failure; HFimpEF: heart failure with improved ejection fraction; HFmrEF: heart failure with mildly reduced ejection fraction; HFpEF: heart failure with preserved ejection fraction; HFrEF: heart failure with reduced ejection fraction; LV: left ventricular; LVEF: left ventricular ejection fraction)

TABLE 2: Classification of heart failure: Stages of heart failure.[9]

Stage A: At risk for heart failure	*Stage B: Pre-heart failure*	*Stage C: Symptomatic heart failure*	*Stage D: Advanced heart failure*
• Patients at risk for HF but without current or previous symptoms/ signs of HF and without structural/ functional heart disease or abnormal biomarkers • Patients with hypertension, CVD, diabetes, obesity, exposure to cardiotoxic agents, genetic variant for cardiomyopathy, or family history of cardiomyopathy	Patients without current or previous symptoms/signs of HF but evidence of one of the following: • Structural heart disease • Evidence of increased filling pressures • Risk factors and: – Increased natriuretic peptide levels or – Persistently elevated cardiac troponin in the absence of competing diagnoses	Patients with current or previous symptoms/signs of HF	Marked HF symptoms that interfere with daily life and with recurrent hospitalizations despite attempts to optimize GDMT

Note: The ACC/AHA stages of HF are shown.

(ACC: American College of Cardiology; AHA: American Heart Association; CVD: cardiovascular disease; GDMT: guideline-directed medical therapy; HF: heart failure)

- Patients with risk factors and increased levels of B-type natriuretic peptides (BNPs) or persistently elevated cardiac troponin

All this is present in the absence of competing diagnoses, resulting in such biomarker elevations as acute coronary syndrome, chronic kidney disease (CKD), pulmonary embolus, or myopericarditis.

If these subjects are not taken care of, these people slip into stage C HF. This stage B heart failure (SBHF) is also very common in the normal population suffering from hypertension, diabetes mellitus, hypothyroidism, obesity, and sleep apnea syndrome, and an ageing population.

DIAGNOSIS

The following modalities of echocardiography are used for diagnosis of SBHF:

- LVEF was measured from the apical four- and two-chamber views using the modified biplane Simpson's method.
- Left atrial (LA) volume was also estimated using the biplane Simpson's method and was indexed to body surface area. Left atrial volume index (LAVI) >34 mL/m^2 was considered abnormal.[10]
- Conventional pulsed wave and *tissue Doppler* were used for measuring the mitral inflow and mitral annular tissue velocities, respectively. The ratio of the early diastolic mitral inflow velocity (E) to the average of the medial and lateral early diastolic mitral annular velocities (e') was calculated and a value >14 was considered abnormal.[11]

Flowchart 1: Treatment of SBHF.

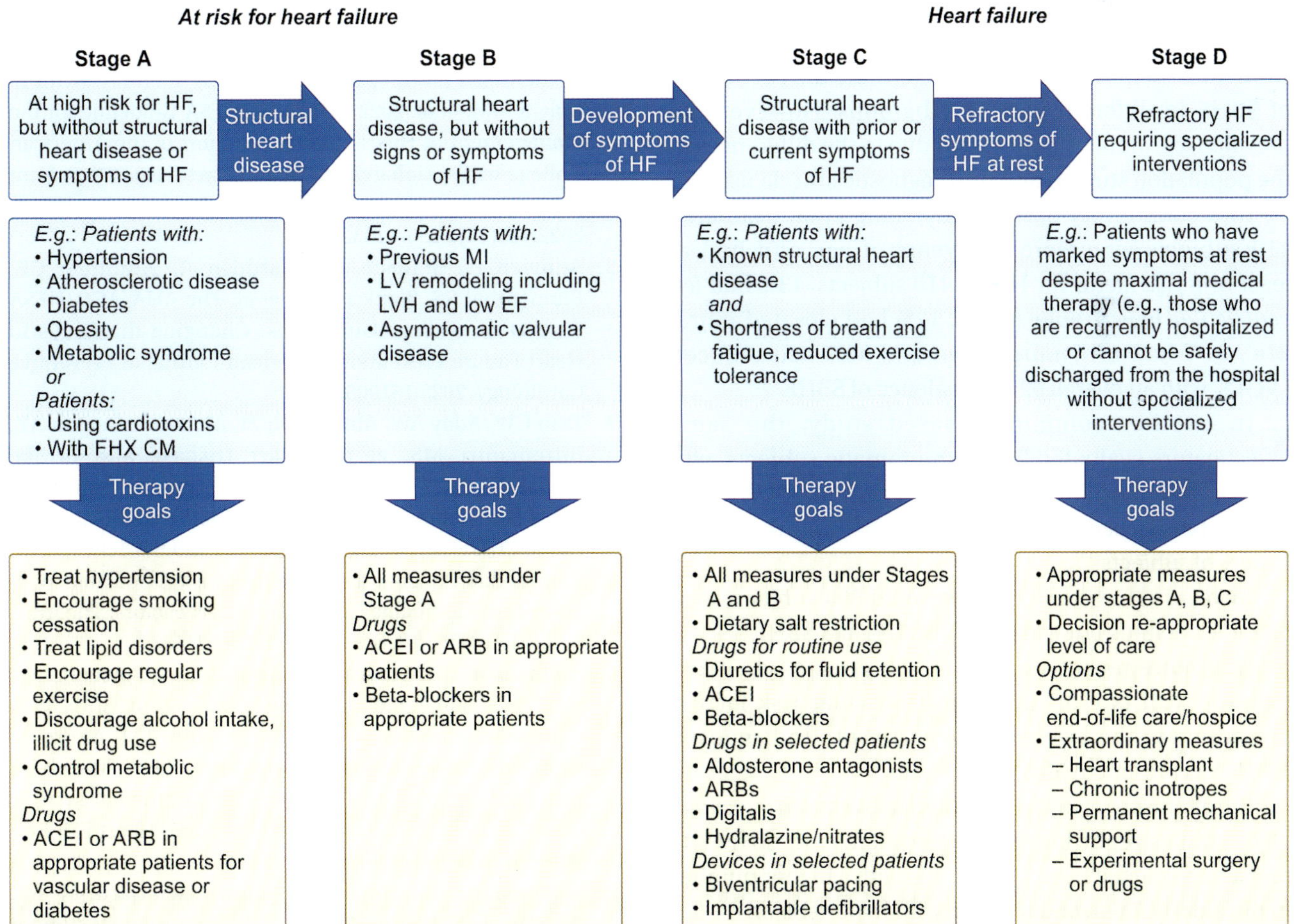

(ACEI: angiotensin-converting enzyme inhibitor; ARB: angiotensin receptor blocker; EF: ejection fraction; FHx CM: family history of cardiomyopathy; HF: heart failure; LV: left ventricular; LVH: left ventricular hypertrophy; MI: myocardial infarction; SBHF: Stage B heart failure)

- The RV *systolic function* was assessed using tricuspid annular plane systolic excursion (TAPSE) and the tricuspid annular systolic velocity (TASV).
- *Speckle tracking echocardiography* was performed for measuring left ventricular global longitudinal strain (LVGLS), left atrial reservoir strain (LARS), and right ventricular free wall longitudinal strain (RVFLS), following the standard techniques and protocols.[12] LVGLS less negative than –16% was considered abnormal.[13]

Stage B HF was diagnosed if any of the following abnormalities were present:
- LAVI >34 mL/m^2
- Mitral E/e′ >14
- LVGLS is less negative than –16%.
- LV mass in parasternal short-axis view
- Natriuretic peptides

DISCUSSION

Numerous studies have tried to determine the prevalence of SBHF in different patient subgroups. However, the prevalence estimates have varied due to the differences in the population studied and the diagnostic criteria used.

In a community-based study, Yang et al. evaluated 410 subjects who were ≥65 years of age and had at least one risk factor for HF. Of 410 subjects, 13% had *left ventricular hypertrophy* (LVH), 12% had elevated mitral E/e′, 31% had *LA enlargement*, and 33% had reduced LVGLS, with an overall 62% prevalence of SBHF.[14]

In another community-based study, the same investigators evaluated 290 asymptomatic subjects with *type 2 diabetes mellitus*, age ≥65 years, preserved LVEF, and no previous *ischemic heart disease*. SBHF was diagnosed in 58% of subjects.[15]

In yet another study that recruited 305 subjects with diabetes mellitus but without CVD, 57% had SBHF.[16]

In a more recent study, Gottlieb et al. studied 209 patients with one or more cardiovascular risk factors presenting to the *emergency department*. Undiagnosed SBHF was present in 59.8% of patients.[17]

Bergamasco et al. performed a *systematic review* of 10 studies reporting on the prevalence of SBHF. The prevalence ranged from 11 to 42.7%, with a higher number in the elderly, men, and in those with hypertension.[18]

In a recent study published from India, SBHF was identified in 52.4% of patients. This prevalence is similar to that reported in previous studies, although a direct comparison is not possible due to differences in patient profiles and clinical settings.[19]

TREATMENT

The treatment of SBHF is directed toward its cause, as shown in **Flowchart 1**.

CONCLUSION

India appears to be the diabetic capital of the world, with almost every third person suffering from it. This, along with other comorbid conditions such as hypertension, obesity, sedentary lifestyle, hypothyroidism, and sleep apnea syndrome, contributes to the high incidence of SBHF. This apparent condition must be identified at the proper time; otherwise, these subjects will develop into stage C HF, necessitating a more corrective role rather than a preventive one.

REFERENCES

1. Heidenreich PA, Bozkurt B, Aguilar D, Allen LA, Byun JJ, Colvin MM, et al. 2022 AHA/ACC/HFSA Guideline for the Management of Heart Failure: A Report of the American College of Cardiology/American Heart Association Joint Committee on Clinical Practice Guidelines. Circulation. 2022;145(18):e895-e1032.
2. Abovich A, Matasic DS, Cardoso R, Ndumele CE, Blumenthal RS, Blankstein R, et al. The AHA/ACC/HFSA 2022 Heart Failure Guidelines: Changing the Focus to Heart Failure Prevention, American Journal of Preventive Cardiology. 2023;15100527.
3. Tsao CW, Aday AW, Almarzooq ZI, Alonso A, Beaton AZ, Bittencourt MS, et al. Heart Disease and Stroke Statistics—2022 Update: A Report From the American Heart Association. Circulation 2022;145(8):e153-639.
4. Hamo CE, Kwak L, Wang D, Florido R, Echouffo-Tcheugui JB, Blumenthal RS, et al. Heart Failure Risk Associated With Severity of Modifiable Heart Failure Risk Factors: The ARIC Study. J Am Heart Assoc. 2022;11(4):e021583.
5. Huffman MD, Prabhakaran D. Heart Failure: Epidemiology and Prevention in India. Natl Med J India. 2010;23(5):283-8.
6. Cameli M, Mondillo S, Solari M, Righini FM, Andrei V, Contaldi C, et al.; Authors/Task Force Members Echocardiographic assessment of left ventricular systolic function: from ejection fraction to torsion. Heart Fail Rev. 2016;21(1):77-94.
7. McDonagh TA, Metra M, Adamo M, Gardner RS, Baumbach A, Böhm M, et al.; ESC Scientific Document Group. 2021 ESC Guidelines for the diagnosis and treatment of acute and chronic heart failure: developed by the task force for the diagnosis and treatment of acute

and chronic heart failure of the European Society of Cardiology (ESC). With the special contribution of the Heart Failure Association (HFA) of the ESC. Eur J Heart Fail. 2022;24(1):4-131.

8. Bozkurt B, Coats AJ, Tsutsui H, Abdelhamid M, Adamopoulos S, Albert N, et al. Universal definition and classification of heart failure: a report of the Heart Failure Society of America, Heart Failure Association of the European Society of Cardiology, Japanese Heart Failure Society and Writing Committee of the Universal Definition of Heart Failure. J Card Fail. 2021;27(4):387-413.
9. Heidenreich PA, Bozkurt B, Aguilar D, Allen LA, Byun JJ, Colvin MM, et al.; ACC/AHA Joint Committee Members. 2022 AHA/ACC/HFSA Guideline for the Management of Heart Failure: A Report of the American College of Cardiology/American Heart Association Joint Committee on Clinical Practice Guidelines. Circulation. 2022;145(18):e895-e1032.
10. Lang RM, Badano LP, Mor-Avi V, Afilalo J, Armstrong A, Ernande L, et al. Recommendations for cardiac chamber quantification by echocardiography in adults: an update from the American Society of Echocardiography and the European Association of Cardiovascular Imaging. J Am Soc Echocardiogr. 2015;28(1):1-39.e14.
11. Nagueh SF, Smiseth OA, Appleton CP, Byrd BF 3rd, Dokainish H, Edvardsen T, et al. Recommendations for the evaluation of left ventricular diastolic function by echocardiography: an update from the American society of echocardiography and the European association of cardiovascular imaging. J Am Soc Echocardiogr. 2016; 29(4):277-314.
12. Mor-Avi V, Lang RM, Badano LP, Belohlavek M, Cardim NM, Derumeaux G, et al. Current and evolving echocardiographic techniques for the quantitative evaluation of cardiac mechanics: ASE/EAE consensus statement on methodology and indications endorsed by the Japanese Society of Echocardiography. J Am Soc Echocardiogr. 2011;24(3):277-313.
13. D'Elia N, Caselli S, Kosmala W, Lancellotti P, Morris D, Muraru D, et al. Normal global longitudinal strain: an individual patient meta-analysis. JACC Cardiovasc Imaging. 2020;13(1 Pt 1):167-9.
14. Yang H, Negishi K, Wang Y, Nolan M, Saito M, Marwick TH. Echocardiographic screening for non-ischaemic stage B heart failure in the community. Eur J Heart Fail. 2016; 18:1331-9.
15. Wang Y, Yang H, Huynh Q, Nolan M, Negishi K, Marwick TH. Diagnosis of Nonischemic stage B heart failure in type 2 diabetes mellitus: optimal parameters for prediction of heart failure. JACC Cardiovasc Imaging. 2018;11:1390-400.
16. Oo MM, Tan Chung Zhen I, Ng KS, Tan KL, Tan ATB, Vethakkan SR, et al. Observational study investigating the prevalence of asymptomatic stage B heart failure in patients with type 2 diabetes who are not known to have coronary artery disease. BMJ Open. 2021;11(1):e039869.
17. Gottlieb M, Schraft E, O'Brien J, Patel D, Peksa GD. Prevalence of undiagnosed stage B heart failure among emergency department patients. Am J Emerg Med. 2024; 85:153-7.
18. Bergamasco A, Luyet-D´eruaz A, Gollop ND, Moride Y, Qiao Q. Epidemiology of asymptomatic pre-heart failure: a systematic review. Curr Heart Fail Rep. 2022;19:146-56.
19. Gupta R, Das T, Suchak MK, Suraj Kudalkar S, Pandey P, Shrivastava S, et al. Prevalence of stage B heart failure in patients undergoing echocardiography during regular clinical practice. Indian Heart J. 2025. [Online ahead of print]

CHAPTER 23

Lipoprotein (A) and Cardiovascular Disease

Amrish Agrawal, Thair Khuziem, Vishal Agrawal

INTRODUCTION

Since its discovery in 1963 of "Lipoprotein (a)" by geneticist Kåre Berg and the discovery of its strong genetic control, "Lp(a)" has emerged as a strong, independent, and genetically determined risk factor for cardiovascular disease (CVD). Though lowering low-density lipoprotein cholesterol (LDL-C) has been the traditional and predominant focus for atherosclerotic cardiovascular disease (ASCVD) risk reduction, several studies have underscored that residual cardiovascular risk remains despite its adequate control. The recent emergence of potential therapeutics targeting Lp(a) has brought this biomarker into the limelight.[1]

STRUCTURE AND BIOCHEMISTRY OF LIPOPROTEIN (A)

Similar to LDL-C, Lp(a) particles contain a core made of triglycerides and cholesterol esters, encased by a membrane of phospholipids.[2] This LDL-like particle is bound to a unique glycoprotein, apolipoprotein(a) [apo(a)], via a disulfide bond and is structurally homologous to plasminogen but lacks the fibrinolytic activity. This structural mimicry is responsible for many of the prothrombotic and atherogenic properties of Lp(a) **(Fig. 1)**.

GENETIC REGULATION AND EPIDEMIOLOGY

Approximately 20–30% of the global population have elevated Lp(a) >50 mg/dL (~125 nmol/L) levels. The alleles encoding for LPA are codominant and responsible for determining 90% of the plasma concentration of Lp(a). Most individuals possess two identifiable circulating Lp(a) isoforms, each generated from an apo(a) of varying size; typically, the smaller isoform exists at greater concentrations in plasma.[3,4] The tail-like attachment of apo(a) in Lp(a) is comprised of repeating Kringle domains with a variable number of repeats in the Kringle IV type 2 (KIV-2) domain. The variation in KIV2 repeats leads to substantial size heterogeneity and is inversely correlated with plasma Lp(a) levels: fewer repeats result in higher levels. Individuals with small isoforms (up to

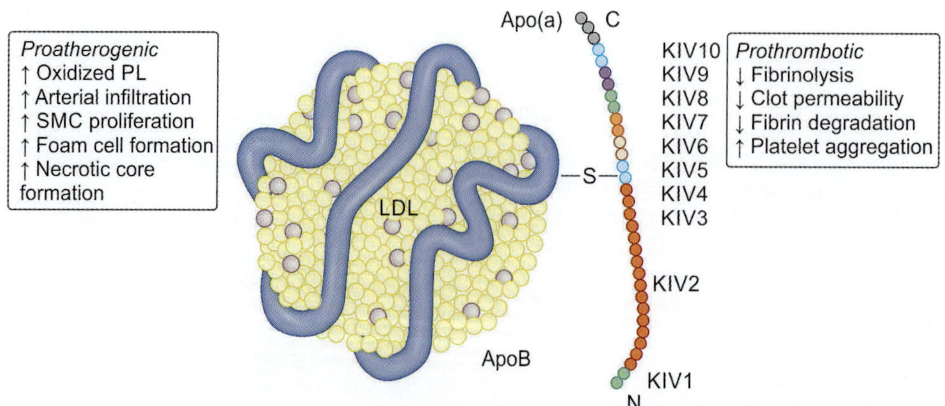

Fig. 1: Lipoprotein (a) [Lp(a)] components: dual mechanisms of harm.
[Apo(a): apolipoprotein (a); KIV: Kringle IV type; LDL: low-density lipoprotein; PL: phospholipids; SMC: smooth muscle cell]

22 KIV repeats) have 4–5 times higher Lp(a) concentrations compared to those who carry only large isoforms (>22 KIV repeats).[5]

In addition, numerous single nucleotide polymorphisms (SNPs) have been identified at the LPA locus, which strongly associate with Lp(a) levels.[3,4] Though some of them are in linkage disequilibrium with the KIV2 variant, however, SNPs associated with both high and low levels of Lp(a) have been reported. Among them, two SNPs *rs10455872* and *rs3798220* show a pronounced association with high Lp(a) concentrations as they "tag" small apo(a) isoforms.[6,7]

Lipoprotein (a) as a Risk-enhancing Factor for Atherosclerotic Cardiovascular Disease

After its initial discovery of Lp(a) in 1963, it took nearly 10 years for the first observations that high Lp(a) concentrations might be linked to cardiovascular disease.[8] Further advancements were hampered by a lack of a good animal model for Lp(a) research.

In 1992, two studies conducted by Sandholzer et al. employing the principles of Mendelian randomization, provided strong evidence supporting a causal relationship between Lp(a) levels and cardiovascular outcomes. Both studies examined apo(a) phenotypes, with the first study focusing on the general population of Chinese individuals living in Singapore, and the second involving participants from diverse ethnic backgrounds. In each ethnic group, smaller apo(a) isoforms were linked not only to elevated Lp(a) concentrations but also to a higher prevalence of coronary heart disease (CHD) among each ethnic group. This study demonstrated that alleles at the apo(a) locus influence the risk for CHD by affecting Lp(a) levels in various populations with significant variations in CHD incidence and risk factor characteristics.

An updated meta-analysis released in 2008 encompassing 31 prospective studies, which included a total of 9,870 cases of CHD, indicated a combined relative risk of 1.5 (1.3–1.8).[9] In the Framingham Offspring study, which comprised 2,000 participants[10] with LDL-C levels of 135 mg/dL or higher, the presence of Lp(a) at concentrations of 100 nmol/L or greater was linked to a 43% rise in cardiovascular risk after accounting for other significant cardiovascular risk factors.

Number of other studies including the analysis in 2021, of >400,000 participants from the United Kingdom (UK) Biobank,[11] showed over a median follow-up of 11.2 years the relationship between Lp(a) and ASCVD was linear, with a hazard ratio (HR) of 1.11 (95% CI: 1.10–1.12) per 50 nmol/L increment. The risk increase was consistent across the Lp(a) distribution and was similar across racial groups. Overall, a threshold of ≥150 nmol/L (~70 mg/dL) was clinically significant, identifying individuals at markedly higher ASCVD risk.

In the context of pronounced atherosclerosis, as evidenced by the coronary artery calcium (CAC) score, elevated levels of Lp(a) may represent a significant indicator of risk enhancement. A comprehensive analysis of the Multi-Ethnic Study of Atherosclerosis (MESA) and the Dallas Heart Study[12] revealed a synergistic association, wherein participants exhibiting heightened Lp(a) levels and CAC scores of ≥100 demonstrated the highest risk for ASCVD (HR: 4.71; 95% CI: 3.01–7.40).[12] These findings underscore the critical importance of implementing proactive modifications in risk factors and lifestyle interventions aimed at mitigating ASCVD risk among individuals with both elevated Lp(a) and CAC. The extent to which Lp(a) influences CAC remains an area of ongoing uncertainty.

The evaluation of advanced plaque composition in individuals with advanced stable coronary artery disease (CAD), utilizing coronary computed tomography angiography (CCTA), has indicated that Lp(a) is correlated with the expedited development of low-attenuation plaque, which serves as a quantitative indicator of necrotic core and signifies a vulnerable plaque.[13] This transformation in plaque phenotypes may elucidate the persistent risk of atherosclerotic incidents among individuals exhibiting elevated levels of Lp(a), thereby reinforcing the significance of Lp(a) as a potential target for therapeutic intervention.

CAUSAL ASSOCIATION WITH AORTIC VALVE STENOSIS: A SURPRISE

In 2013, George Thanassoulis and colleagues in a landmark study discovered the *LPA* gene to be significantly associated with aortic valve calcification [calcific aortic valve disease (CAVD)]. Number of other studies followed and in 2020, same authors analyzed data from the CHARGE consortium,[14] involving >100,000 participants and showed Lp(a) levels >90 mg/dL were associated with a two- to threefold increased risk of incident AS (HR: ~2.6). The association was stronger in younger individuals and those without CAD.

This is of special interest since aortic valve stenosis prevalence is projected to increase dramatically in coming decades as population is aging, and longevity is increasing and there is lack of any medical therapy for slowing disease progression.

PATHOPHYSIOLOGY: ATHEROGENIC AND THROMBOGENIC EFFECTS

Due to its similarity to LDL, the apoB moiety of Lp(a) is anticipated to be atherogenic. Certainly, even in the presence of very high Lp(a) levels, the number of circulating plasma Lp(a) is expected to be fewer than LDL particles. Enhanced atherogenecity is postulated through binding of apo(a) to extracellular matrix proteins and their selective retention in the arterial wall.[15]

Whether Lp(a) contributes to atherothrombotic disease by directly inhibiting fibrinolysis, promoting thrombosis, or because of its role in atherogenesis remains the subject of investigation.[16] Apo(a) inhibits plasmin-mediated fibrinolysis in vitro, and the antifibrinolytic properties of apo(a) may be masked when covalently associated with apoB in the Lp(a) particle. Further, OxPLs which are covalently bound to apo(a) are recognized by the innate immune system,[17] triggering sterile inflammation and calcification with relevance to ASCVD and CAVD pathogenesis.

Progression of the CAVD is primarily dependent on aortic valve mineralization and ossification. The main postulated mechanism by which elevated Lp(a) can affect the accelerate transformation is through its associated proinflammatory oxidized phospholipids (OxPL), which start osteogenic differentiation and mineralization of valve interstitial cells. This, in turn, causes the valve tissue to stiffen, accelerates the progression of aortic valve calcification on serial computed tomography scans, and has a negative impact on clinical outcomes.[18] OxPL can cause upregulation of procalcific and osteogenic genes by Lp(a) and apo(a) in human valvular interstitial cells. Additionally, hydroxyapatite mineral deposition was observed in valvular interstitial cells treated with Lp(a).

LIPOPROTEIN (A) LEVELS AND CUTOFF

As mentioned before up to 90% of variation in Lp(a) concentrations is genetically determined, and there are considerable ethnic differences in Lp(a) concentrations. The highest Lp(a) concentrations are found in those with Black anchestory, followed by South Asians, White, Hispanic, and East Asian people.

The precise measurement of Lp(a) is challenging due to the distinctive structure of the Lp(a) particle, which contains numerous repetitive KIV repeats in apo(a) that affect its molecular weight. As a result, measuring it in mg/dL is complicated by differences in the size of Lp(a) stemming from variations in its isoforms. The use of the older, commonly used unit of mg/dL assumes that the mass of individual Lp(a) components remains constant across all individuals. This assumption is, in fact, unacceptable, particularly given the well-documented significant variability in the size of apo(a). Therefore, the gold standard enzyme-linked immunosorbent assay (ELISA) method has been calibrated in nanomoles per liter (nmol/L), accurately reflecting the quantity of Lp(a) particles, which is recommended by the National Heart, Lung, and Blood Institute. Various Lp(a) guidelines and statements have suggested that Lp(a) values should be reported in nmol/L [2018 American College of Cardiology/the American Heart Association (ACC/AHA), 2019 European Society of Cardiology (ESC), and 2019 National Lipid Association (NLA)]. The current ACC/AHA guideline recommends reporting Lp(a) levels as concentration (nmol/L) and a universal cutpoint of ≥100 nmol/L (approximately ≥50 mg/dL), which approximates the 80th percentile in the Caucasian US population.

Details on measuring Lp(a) are provided in **Box 1**, while **Box 2** presents a collective agreement on Lp(a) risk thresholds as outlined by various guidelines.

What can be done in the Case of High Lp(a) Concentrations?

Guidelines recommendations for when to measure Lp(a) are outlined in **Box 3**.

Although there is evidence of causality between Lp(a) and cardiovascular events, we currently do not possess

BOX 1: How should one measure lipoprotein (a) [Lp(a)]?

Lp(a) should be measured with:
- An isoform-insensitive assay
- Assay that is traceable to the internationally accepted calibrator (World Health Organization/International Federation of Clinical Chemistry Reference Material SRM-2B)
- Assay that is reported in nanomoles per liter (nmol/L).

Note: If measurements are not uniformly calibrated, one cannot compare measurements generated by different assays.

BOX 2: Generalized consensus on lipoprotein (a) Lp(a) risk thresholds by guidelines

- More than or equal to 50 mg/dL (or ≥125 nmol/L) is an accepted target in the American College of Cardiology/the American Heart Association (ACC/AHA) guidelines
- More than or equal to 50 mg/dL (or ≥100 nmol/L) is an accepted target in the 2021 Canadian Cardiovascular Society (CCS) guidelines
- Less than 30 mg/dL (or <75 nmol/L) is considered normal, 30–50 mg/dL (or 50–125 nmol/L) intermediate, and >50 mg/dL (or >125 nmol/L) abnormal in the 2022 European Atherosclerotic Society (EAS) consensus statement
- More than 50 mg/dL (or >100 nmol/L) is accepted as a risk-enhancing cutoff in the 2019 National Lipid Association (NLA) scientific statement

BOX 3: When to measure Lp(a) ?

- *2022 EAS consensus statement:* Lp(a) level measured at least once in all adults and in youth with a history of ischemic stroke or a family history of premature ASCVD or elevated Lp(a) level and no other known risk factors
- *2021 CCS dyslipidemia guideline:* Measure once in a person's lifetime as part of initial lipid screening
- *2019 NLA scientific statement on Lp(a):* Measure in individuals with premature ASCVD, LDL-C level ≥190 mg/dL, men <55 years of age, and women <65 years of age. Use Lp(a) level >50 mg/dL (or >100 nmol/L) as increased risk; less-than-expected LDL-C–lowering response, despite good adherence; recurrent or progressive ASCVD despite optimal lipid-lowering therapy; calcific valvular aortic stenosis; and family history of elevated Lp(a) levels
- *2019 ESC/EAS dyslipidemia guideline:* A relative indication for Lp(a) level measurement is family history of premature ASCVD; favors statin initiation in primary prevention in patients with intermediate or borderline ASCVD
- *2018 multisociety cholesterol guideline:* Recommends measurement in individuals with a family history of premature ASCVD

conclusive evidence that targeted pharmacological reduction of Lp(a) leads to improved cardiovascular outcomes, and secondly, there are no approved Lp(a)-lowering medications available.

While statins are highly effective at lowering LDL-C, they paradoxically minimally increase Lp(a) levels. Monoclonal antibodies that target the PCSK9 protein inhibitor (PCSK9i), such as evolocumab and alirocumab have shown only a modest reduction in Lp(a) of about 25–30% **(Table 1)**. Niacin may reduce Lp(a) levels in a dose-dependent manner by 25–40%, although its adverse side effects, particularly when used in combination with statins, might be a concern. Currently, lipoprotein apheresis stands as the most effective intervention for Lp(a) that is clinically available. It is approved for familial hypercholesterolemia, with each treatment session typically resulting in a 60–85% reduction in both LDL and Lp(a) levels,[19] along with similar decreases in oxidized phospholipids.

To achieve a clinically significant outcome, Lp(a) needs be reduced by 80%. Novel therapies aimed at Lp(a) mRNA have been created and demonstrate promise, currently progressing through clinical trials.[20]

The first approach involves the utilization of antisense oligonucleotides (ASOs) to inhibit mRNA expression. ASOs, which range from 13 to 20 nucleotides in length, attach directly to the mRNA of apo(a). This interaction creates a complex with the intracellularly available RNAse H1, leading to mRNA degradation and thus preventing the synthesis of the targeted protein. *Pelacarsen* is an improved, second-generation antisense oligonucleotide that is linked to a triantennary N-acetylgalactosamine (GalNAc) moiety, facilitating targeted delivery to hepatocytes with a higher potency in reducing Lp(a) levels by 80% with a subcutaneous dose of 60–80 mg administered once every 4 weeks. The Phase 3 HORIZON trial has successfully recruited 7,682 participants and assigned them to receive either pelacarsan or a placebo. Results are anticipated by the end of this year and will determine if the reduction of Lp(a) with this medication positively influences cardiovascular outcomes in individuals with elevated Lp(a) (>70 mg/dL) in a secondary prevention context.

The second method utilizes small interfering, double-stranded RNA (siRNAs). These enter the hepatocyte and are released from the endosome, where the two RNA strands separate into the sense and antisense strands. The antisense strand then creates a highly stable interaction with the RNA-induced silencing complex (RISC), which leads to the cleavage of the target mRNA, degradation by exonucleases, and a decrease in the synthesis of apo(a). Because the siRNA-RISC complex is very stable, this results in prolonged cleavage of the targeted transcripts, leading to a suppression of protein production that lasts over 6 months.

Several molecules utilizing this methodology are currently undergoing trials. Olpasiran demonstrated a reduction in Lp(a) levels exceeding 95% in the OCEAN(a)-DOSE Phase 2 study.[21] Remarkably, nearly a year following the last dose, participants sustained a

TABLE 1: Effect of lipid-lowering therapies on lipoprotein (a) [Lp(a)] levels.[27]

Lipid-lowering therapy		*Effect on Lp(a) levels*	*Key Consideration*	*References*
Current therapies associated with increase in Lp(a)				
Bile acid sequestrants		0.2		
Fibric acid derivatives		1.6–20%		
Statins		8.5–19.6%		
Bempedoic acid		0.024		
Ezetimibe		Minimal effect		
Current therapies associated with decrease in Lp(a)				
Niacin		–20 to –40%	Significant side effects	
Mab for *PCSK9*	Evolocumab	–26.9%		
	Alirocumab	–23%	Not primarily indicated for Lp(a); requires injections	
siRNA targeting *PCSK9*	Inclisiran	–18.6 to –26%		
Newer therapies in the pipeline associated with decrease in Lp(a)				
siRNA; silences *LPA* gene expression	Zerlasiran	–98%		20
	Lepodisiran	–97%		22
	Olpasiran	–71 to –98%	High efficacy; not yet approved, Trials ongoing	21
ASO; inhibits *LPA* gene mRNA	Pelacarsen	–66 to –92%	Promising; targets Lp(a) specifically, Phase 3 [Lp(a)] HORIZON results expected 2025	25
ASO; inhibits ApoB100 mRNA	Mipomersen	–26.4%		26
MTP inhibitor for VLDL	Lomitapide	–17%		
Mab for *ANGPTL3*	Evinacumab	–5.5%		

ASO: antisense oligonucleotide; *VLDL:* very low-density lipoprotein)
Source: Greco A, Di Minno A, Di Minno MND, et al. Lipoprotein(a) as a Pharmacological Target: Premises, Promises, and Prospects. Circulation. 2024;150(21):1605-19.

40–50% placebo-adjusted decrease in Lp(a). Recruitment for the Phase 3 OCEAN(a) cardiovascular Outcomes trial has been completed, with the study anticipated to conclude by the end of 2026 (NCT05581303). Zerlasiran (SNL360) represents another siRNA therapy that achieved a 98% reduction in Lp(a) levels after a single 600 mg subcutaneous administration in its Phase 1 study. Lastly, lepodisiran, which also employs an siRNA strategy, reported in a Phase 1 study median dose-dependent reductions in Lp(a) levels exceeding 90% for the three highest doses examined. The treatment effect was maintained at approximately –94% after 337 days of observation.[22]

Muvalaplin (LY3473329) utilizes a different strategy as it is an orally taken small molecule that inhibits the formation of Lp(a). By interacting with apo(a) KIV type 7 and KIV type 8, it prevents the creation of the disulfide bond, thereby halting Lp(a) formation. A Phase 1 trial with multiple ascending doses assessed the effects of administering daily doses of muvalaplin (ranging from 30 to 800 mg) or a placebo over 14 days in individuals with Lp(a) levels of 30 mg/dL or greater. The medication was well tolerated, leading to a maximum placebo-adjusted reduction in Lp(a) of 63–65%. Interestingly, similar results were seen with daily doses of 100, 300, 500, and 800 mg. A Phase 2 randomized, double-blind, placebo-controlled study known as KRAKEN indicated significantly lower Lp(a) levels after 12 weeks, with an 85.7% reduction in the group receiving 240 mg daily, and it was well-tolerated.[23] The effect on cardiovascular events necessitates further exploration in Phase 3 trials.

FUTURE DEVELOPMENTS ON LP (A)—LOWERING STRATEGIES

Somatic gene-editing therapies hold the promise of enduring and potentially irreversible effects by modifying DNA. The *CRISPR/Cas9* system[24] is highly efficient, and its use for *LPA* gene modification has already garnered the interest of several companies. Given its ability to induce permanent alterations in an individual's somatic genome, considerations regarding long-term safety and ethics are of critical importance.

CONCLUSION

Mendelian randomization research conducted in the early 1990s strongly indicated that Lp(a) is a causal factor in cardiovascular diseases. Since that time, there has been significant progress in understanding Lp(a), leading to the development of several targeted therapies aimed at lowering its levels. Currently, mRNA-targeting treatments are undergoing clinical trials, demonstrating a potential reduction of Lp(a) by nearly 80–100%. These innovative therapies offer promise not only in reducing this novel cardiovascular risk but also in potentially mitigating degenerative changes in the aortic valve. It remains to be determined whether these reductions will translate into actual clinical benefits, specifically regarding the decrease in cardiovascular events, and clinical trials are in progress to investigate this.

REFERENCES

1. Berman A, Blankstein R. Current and future role of Lipoprotein(a) in preventive cardiology. Curr Opin Cardiol. 2019;34:514-8.
2. Schmidt K, Noureen A, Kronenberg F, Utermann G. Structure, function, and genetics of lipoprotein (a). J Lipid Res. 2016;57:1339-59.
3. Kaur G, Abdelrahman K, Berman AN, Biery DW, Shiyovich A, Huck D, et al. Lipoprotein(a): Emerging insights and therapeutics. Am J Prev Cardiol. 2024;18:100641.
4. Reyes-Soffer G, Ginsberg HN, Berglund L, Duell PB, Heffron SP, Kamstrup PR, et al. Lipoprotein(a): A Genetically Determined, Causal, and Prevalent Risk Factor for Atherosclerotic Cardiovascular Disease: A Scientific Statement from the American Heart Association. Arterioscler Thromb Vasc Biol. 2022;42:e48-e60.
5. Tsimikas S, Fazio S, Viney NJ, Xia S, Witztum JL, Marcovina SM. Relationship of lipoprotein(a) molar concentrations and mass according to lipoprotein(a) thresholds and apolipoprotein(a) isoform size. J Clin Lipidol. 2018;12:1313-23.
6. Kronenberg F. Lipoprotein(a): from Causality to Treatment. Curr Atheroscler Rep. 2024;26:75-82.
7. Clarke R, Peden JF, Hopewell JC, Kyriakou T, Goel A, Heath SC, et al. Genetic variants associated with Lp(a) lipoprotein level and coronary disease. N Engl J Med. 2009; 361:2518-28.
8. Dahlen G. The pre-beta-1 lipoprotein phenomenon in relation to serum cholesterol and triglyceride levels, the Lp(a) lipoprotein and coronary heart disease. Acta Med Scand. 1974;570:1-45.
9. Bennet A, Di Angelantonio E, Erqou S, Eiriksdottir G, Sigurdsson G, Woodward M, et al. Lipoprotein(a) levels and risk of future coronary heart disease: large-scale prospective data. Arch Intern Med. 2008;168:598-608.
10. Afshar M, Rong J, Zhan Y, Chen HY, Engert JC, Sniderman AD, et al. Risks of incident cardiovascular disease associated with concomitant elevations in Lipoprotein(a) and low-density lipoprotein cholesterol-The Framingham Heart Study. J Am Heart Assoc. 2020;18:e014711.
11. Patel AP, Wang M, Pirruccello JP, Ellinor PT, Ng K, Kathiresan S, et al. Lp(a) (Lipoprotein[a]) Concentrations and Incident Atherosclerotic Cardiovascular Disease: New Insights From a Large National Biobank. Arterioscler Thromb Vasc Biol. 2021;41:465-74.
12. Mehta A, Vasquez N, Ayers CR, Patel J, Hooda A, Khera A, et al. Independent association of Lipoprotein(a) and coronary artery calcification with atherosclerotic cardio-vascular risk. J Am Coll Cardiol. 2022;79:757-68.
13. Kaiser Y, Daghem M, Tzolos E, Meah MN, Doris MK, Moss AJ, et al. Association of Lipoprotein(a) with atherosclerotic plaque progression. J Am Coll Cardiol. 2022;79:223-33.
14. Kronenberg F, Mora S, Stroes ESG, Ference BA, Arsenault BJ, Berglund L, et al. Lipoprotein(a) and the risk of aortic valve stenosis in the general population. JAMA Cardiol. 2020; 5:1113-20.
15. Kamstrup PR. Lipoprotein(a) and cardiovascular disease. Clin Chem. 2021;67:154-66.
16. Boffa MB, Koschinsky ML. Lipoprotein (a): truly a direct prothrombotic factor in cardiovascular disease? J Lipid Res. 2016;57:745-57.
17. Binder CJ, Papac-Milicevic N, Witztum JL. Innate sensing of oxidation-specific epitopes in health and disease. Nat Rev Immunol. 2016;16:485-97.
18. Zheng KH, Tsimikas S, Pawade T, Kroon J, Jenkins WSA, Doris MK, et al. Lipoprotein(a) and oxidized phospholipids promote valve calcification in patients with aortic stenosis. J Am Coll Cardiol. 2019;73:2150-62.
19. Tsimikas S, Karwatowska-Prokopczuk E, Gouni-Berthold I, Tardif JC, Baum SJ, Steinhagen-Thiessen E, et al. Lipoprotein(a) reduction in persons with cardiovascular disease. N Engl J Med. 2020;382:244-55.
20. Landmesser U, Poller W, Tsimikas S, Most P, Paneni F, Lüscher TF. From traditional pharmacological towards nucleic acid-based therapies for cardiovascular diseases. Eur Heart J. 2020;41(40):3884-99.
21. Rosenson RS, López JAG, Gaudet D, Baum SJ, Stout E, Lepor NE, et al. Olpasiran, Oxidized Phospholipids, and

Systemic Inflammatory Biomarkers: Results From the OCEAN(a)-DOSE Trial. JAMA Cardiol. 2025;10(5):482-6.

22. Nissen SE, Linnebjerg H, Shen X, Wolski K, Ma X, Lim S, et al. Lepodisiran, an extended-duration short interfering RNA targeting lipoprotein(a): a randomized dose-ascending clinical trial. JAMA. 2023;330(21):2075-83.
23. Nicholls SJ, Ni W, Rhodes GM, Nissen SE, Navar AM, Michael LF, et al. Oral Muvalaplin for Lowering of Lipoprotein(a): A Randomized Clinical Trial. JAMA. 2025;333:222-31.
24. Stankov S, Cuchel M. Gene editing for dyslipidemias: new tools to "cut" lipids. Atherosclerosis. 2023;368:14-24.
25. Assessing the Impact of Lipoprotein (a) Lowering With Pelacarsen (TQJ230) on Major Cardiovascular Events in Patients With CVD (Lp(a)HORIZON) https://clinicaltrials.gov/study/NCT04023552
26. Randomized, Placebo-Controlled Trial of Mipomersen in Patients with Severe Hypercholesterolemia Receiving Maximally Tolerated Lipid-Lowering Therapy https://doi.org/10.1371/journal.pone.0049006
27. Greco A, Di Minno A, Di Minno MND, et al. Lipoprotein(a) as a Pharmacological Target: Premises, Promises, and Prospects. Circulation. 2024;150(21):1605-19.

Imaging—Echocardiography

Reimagining Coronary Artery Disease Evaluation: The Expanding Frontier of Echocardiography and Global Longitudinal Strain

Sanjay Mittal, Abhishek Kumar Tiwari, Chris Alvls Shaji

INTRODUCTION

Coronary artery disease (CAD) continues to cast a long shadow over global health, afflicting an estimated 126 million individuals—approximately 1.76% of the world's population—and accounting for greater than 9 million deaths each year, as documented by the World Health Organization and the Global Burden of Disease (GBD) Study 2019. Despite the evolution of diagnostic paradigms and therapeutic strategies, CAD remains the preeminent cause of mortality worldwide.[1]

The clinical evaluation of CAD necessitates a multidimensional strategy, integrating bedside assessment with a spectrum of noninvasive and invasive modalities. Among the noninvasive tools, echocardiography stands as a cornerstone—uniquely positioned at the intersection of diagnostic precision, accessibility, and cost-effectiveness. Although conventional two-dimensional (2D) echocardiography does not directly visualize atherosclerotic plaque or luminal stenosis, its unparalleled ability to assess myocardial performance in real time renders it indispensable in the functional appraisal of ischemia.

At the heart of CAD pathophysiology lies a mismatch between myocardial oxygen supply and demand, culminating in ischemia and, ultimately, myocardial dysfunction. This ischemic burden manifests as regional wall motion abnormalities (RWMAs), which are readily detectable by 2D echocardiography **(Fig. 1)**. Nevertheless, the inherent operator dependency of standard echocardiographic interpretation poses limitations to reproducibility and interobserver variability.[2]

Myocardial strain rate imaging, most notably the global longitudinal strain (GLS), is a transformative advancement in the echocardiographic arsenal. GLS quantifies myocardial deformation with exquisite sensitivity, enabling the detection of subtle impairments in myocardial contractility that may elude conventional visual assessment. Its semiautomated methodology not only enhances diagnostic precision but also mitigates observer variability, thus addressing a critical limitation of traditional 2D echocardiography.[2]

As the field of cardiovascular imaging continues to evolve, the integration of GLS into routine clinical practice represents a paradigm shift—enabling earlier detection of ischemia, refined risk stratification, and more individualized patient care. This chapter delves into the in-depth role of echocardiography in CAD and burgeoning role of GLS in the contemporary evaluation of CAD, illuminating its potential to redefine how we detect, characterize, and ultimately confront this global epidemic.

ECHOCARDIOGRAPHIC EVALUATION OF CORONARY ARTERY DISEASE

Echocardiography provides a host of information regarding cardiac hemodynamic and structural abnormalities associated with a case of CAD. Moreover, its universal availability and accessibility make it an extension of clinical examination rather than a specialized test in many cardiac centers. Echo provides various information in a patient with CAD, as follows:

- RWMAs
- Global left ventricular (LV) systolic functions
- Hemodynamic information on ventricular systolic and diastolic functions
- GLS
- Extent of inducible ischemia
- Degree of myocardial viability
- Myocardial Infarction and its complications
- Concomitant cardiac defects

The information is important not only for establishing or suspecting the diagnosis of CAD but also in assessment of prognosis besides serving as a tool to monitor the effect of therapy and progression of disease. Various echo modalities could be used to provide these inputs.

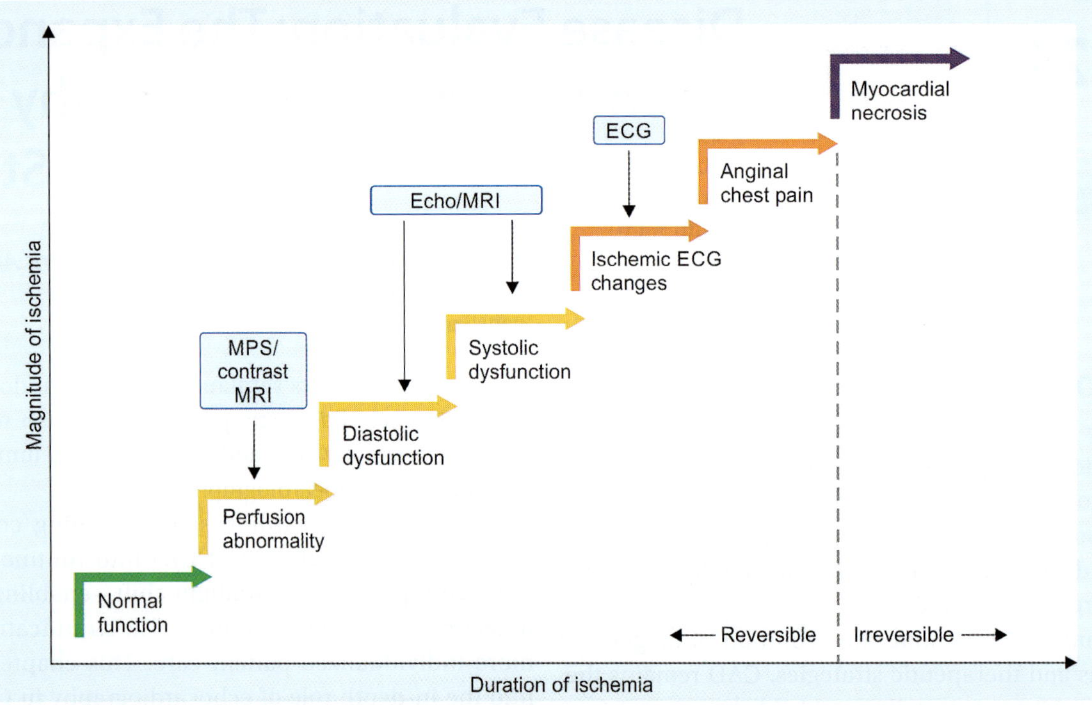

Fig. 1: Ischemia cascade.
Source: Research Gate. The assessment of coronary artery disease in patients with end-stage renal disease—Scientific Figure on ResearchGate. [online] Available from https://www.researchgate.net/figure/schaemic-cascade-Sequence-of-pathophysiological-events-after-a-coronary-artery_fig1_335396201 [Last accessed September, 2025].

These may be the simple 2D echo, Doppler, color Doppler, tissue Doppler, strain imaging, contrast echo, 3D echo/strain, stress echo, etc.

Unlike tomographic modalities such as cardiac computed tomography (CT) or cardiac magnetic resonance (CMR), 2D echocardiography is operator-dependent. The quality and diagnostic accuracy of the study are heavily reliant on the skill and experience of the sonographer or physician performing and interpreting the exam. For this reason, echocardiography is best regarded not merely as a "test" but as a comprehensive and nuanced "examination" **(Fig. 2)**.

Regional/Segmental Wall Motion Abnormalities

Whenever there is impediment of flow in an epicardial coronary artery due to occlusion, the myocardium segments supplied by the artery become ischemic and eventually show impairment of contractility (see the ischemic cascade—**Fig. 1**), while the remaining segments maintain their contractility or at times show a compensatory increase in contractility. Segmental wall motion abnormalities or RWMAs are thus sine qua non for CAD, though sometimes patchy myocarditis also may produce RWMAs.

Careful interpretation of wall motion patterns allows clinicians to diagnose and localize CAD, evaluate the extent of myocardial injury, and guide therapeutic decisions.

Imaging Protocol

- Standard 2D transthoracic echocardiography (TTE) is performed in multiple views: Parasternal long-axis, parasternal short-axis (at basal, mid, and apical levels), and apical two-, three-, and four-chamber views.
- The *American Society of Echocardiography (ASE) 17-segment model* is typically used to ensure comprehensive coverage of the LV myocardium.[3]
- Wall motion analysis requires at least 70% of endocardium to be visualized.
- Poor acoustic window renders RWMA analysis impossible in 10% of people.
- Adjunctive techniques can help improve endocardial border delineation in difficult situations, such as harmonic imaging, contrast echo, etc.

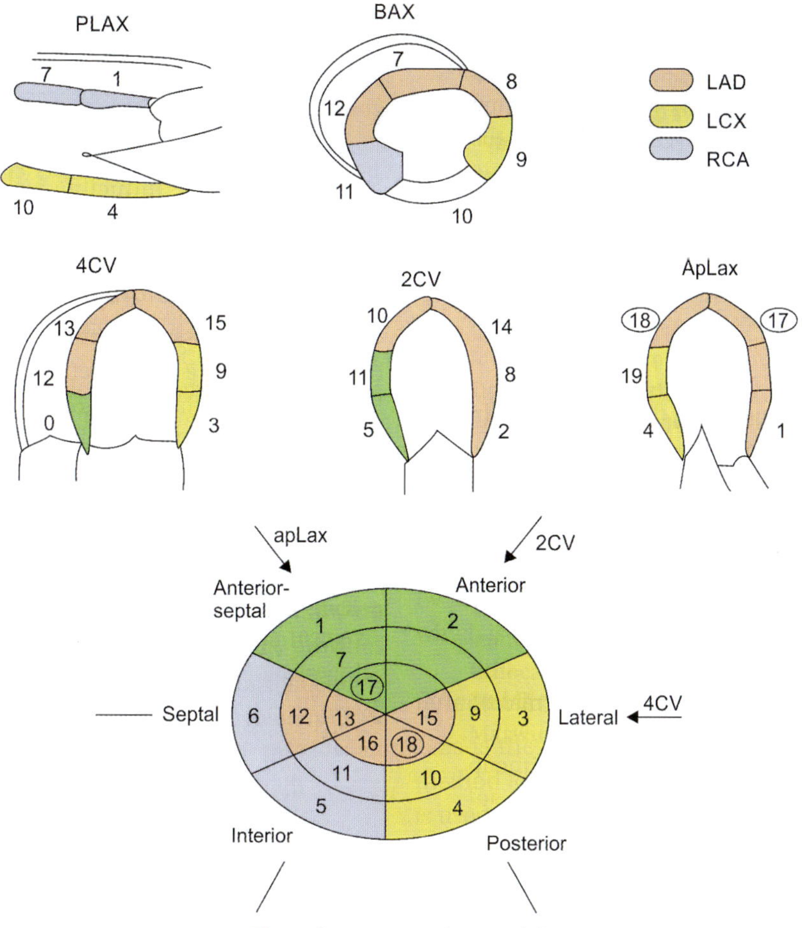

Fig. 2: Segment cardiac model.

- Confirm the RWMA in multiple views to avoid errors.
- Focus on myocardial thickening rather than motion alone.

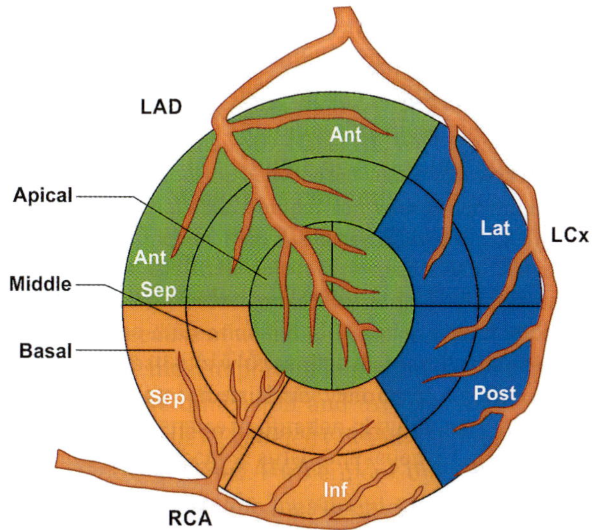

Fig. 3: Common coronary artery distribution pattern and the related segments on a bull's eye plot. (Ant: anterior; Inf: inferior; Lat: lateral; LCx: left circumflex artery; Post: posterior; RCA: right coronary artery; Sep: septal)

Correlation of RWMA with Coronary Anatomy

Regional wall motion abnormality may occasionally occur in patchy myocarditis but does not correlate with coronary distribution. Assessment of RWMA is incomplete without an understanding of coronary anatomy. Though there is variability in coronary artery anatomy from person to person, the common distribution is shown in **Figure 3**.

Severity of RWMA

While evaluating the RWMA on echo, there should always be an attempt to grade the severity of defect for each segment. Commonly, we use the term kinesis to depict contractility and the RWMA could be normokinetic, hypokinetic, akinetic, dyskinetic, or aneurysmal.

TABLE 1: Segmental scoring system.

Score	RWMA	Definition
1	Normokinetic	Normal thickening and inward motion
2	Hypokinetic	Reduced thickening and inward motion
3	Akinetic	Absent thickening/motion
4	Dyskinetic	Paradoxical outward motion
5	Aneurysm	Persistent deformation with systolic expansion

As the severity of RWMA increases, the proportion of viable myocardium decreases and consequently the prognosis is adversely impacted.

Segmental scoring system: Each myocardial segment is visually assessed for systolic endocardial excursion and wall thickening **(Table 1)**.

Wall Motion Score Index

Wall motion score index (WMSI) can be calculated after analysis of all segments as below:

$$\text{WMSI} = \frac{\text{Sum of segmental scores}}{\text{Number of segments analyzed}}$$

A WMSI of 1 indicates normal LV function; higher values suggest worse systolic dysfunction.

Benefits

A comprehensive RWMA report should be able to answer all of the following questions:

- Are RWMAs present or absent?
- What is the severity of RWMA?
- Is there viability or scarring?
- Which coronary artery is involved?
- How many vessels are involved?

Proper assessment of RWMA is paramount in enabling the cardiologist in:

- *Early detection of ischemia:* RWMA can appear within seconds of coronary occlusion, often preceding electrocardiographic or biomarker changes.
- *Localization of CAD:* RWMA patterns correspond to coronary artery territories, aiding in diagnosis and interventional planning.
- *Assessment of infarct size and viability:* Differentiating stunned, hibernating, or scarred myocardium informs revascularization strategies.
- *Prognosis:* WMSI correlates strongly with overall LV function and long-term outcomes in ischemic heart disease.
- *Evaluating stress-induced ischemia:* Dynamic wall motion assessment during stress echocardiography helps diagnose inducible ischemia and risk stratify patients.

Pitfalls and Limitations

Though RWMA assessment is essential for all evaluations of CAD, there are some definite limitations, which may lead to inappropriate diagnosis **(Table 2)**.

- *Operator dependence and subjectivity:* Visual interpretation varies significantly with experience, leading to interobserver variability. In subtle wall motion abnormalities, even experienced observers can make errors.
- *Poor image quality:* In patients with obesity, lung disease, or poor acoustic windows, segment visualization may be suboptimal.
- *Physiological and nonischemic mimics:*
  - Left bundle branch block (LBBB) and paced rhythms cause abnormal septal motion mimicking ischemia.
  - Right ventricular (RV) overload or pulmonary embolism can produce septal flattening and paradoxical motion.
  - Pericardial disease or postsurgical changes may distort regional motion.
- *Limited differentiation of acute versus chronic abnormalities:* Akinesia may reflect acute stunning or chronic scar, requiring additional modalities such as cardiac MRI, nuclear imaging, or dobutamine stress echo (DSE) for viability assessment.
- *Interpretation in complex pathologies:* Cardiomyopathies, myocarditis, and infiltrative disorders may also produce regional dysfunction, underscoring the need for clinical correlation.

Global Longitudinal Strain in Coronary Artery Disease

Principles of GLS

Strain refers to the percentage of deformation between two myocardial regions, such as the shortening of myocardial fibers during systole or their lengthening during diastole. Strain was initially derived from Doppler-based tissue imaging, which measured the relative displacement

TABLE 2: Common pitfalls and challenges related to echocardiographic evaluation of coronary artery disease (CAD).

Pitfall/challenge	*Explanation*	*Outcomes*
Suboptimal endocardial border visualization	Poor acoustic windows or imaging quality impair ability to accurately assess wall motion	Leads to false-positive or false-negative interpretation
Transducer angulation (superior angulation)	May cause nonmuscular membranous septum to appear as akinetic myocardium	False-positive for wall motion abnormality
External compression of inferior wall (pseudodyskinesis)	Ascites/abdominal contents compress inferior wall, mimicking wall motion abnormality	False-positive
Paradoxical septal motion/ dyssynchrony	Seen in bundle branch block or postcardiac surgery	May be misinterpreted as myocardial abnormality
Poor acoustic window/off-axis imaging	Suboptimal probe position or patient habitus limit visualization	*False negatives:* True wall motion abnormalities may be missed
Limited sensitivity for subendocardial/ microvascular ischemia	Resting echocardiography may not detect small or subtle ischemic changes	*False-negatives:* Small infarcts or microvascular disease undetected
Asymptomatic status at imaging	Transient ischemia, reperfusion, or symptom resolution at time of echo may normalize wall motion	Resting echo may miss dynamic or recent ischemia

between adjacent myocardial points. However, 2D speckle-tracking echocardiography (STE) has become the more widely adopted method due to its superior robustness, reproducibility, and angle independence. This technique has been rigorously validated using sonomicrometry and takes advantage of speckle patterns—unique interference patterns generated by the interaction of ultrasound waves with myocardial tissue. These speckles serve as distinct digital markers, allowing for the tracking of myocardial motion throughout the cardiac cycle and differentiating actively contracting segments from those moving passively.

Strain can be assessed in longitudinal, circumferential, and radial directions depending on the imaging plane. Longitudinal and circumferential strain values are typically negative, reflecting myocardial shortening, while radial strain is expressed as a positive value due to wall thickening during contraction **(Figs. 4A to C)**.

Modern echocardiographic systems compute GLS by averaging the regional strain values or by calculating the percentage change in the endocardial contour between systole and diastole. Longitudinal deformation primarily reflects the function of subendocardial myocardial fibers, whereas circumferential strain, which is best assessed in short-axis views, represents the function of more epicardial layers. Since strain during systole is a measure of compression, values closer to 0 indicate worse myocardial function. Regional strain analysis provides further insight by identifying localized areas of dysfunction.[4,5]

GLS in the Detection of CAD

Global longitudinal strain has emerged as a valuable tool for the early detection of CAD. Studies have shown that GLS is reduced in patients with CAD, even in the absence of overt wall motion abnormalities or a reduced left ventricular ejection fraction (LVEF). This is particularly relevant in patients with non-ST-segment elevation myocardial infarction (NSTEMI) or chronic coronary syndromes, where traditional echocardiographic findings may be subtle.

- *Acute coronary syndromes (ACS):* In patients with ACS, GLS is significantly reduced in the ischemic territory. GLS can also differentiate between ischemic and nonischemic causes of acute chest pain, with higher sensitivity and specificity than conventional echocardiography.
- *Chronic coronary syndromes:* In patients with chronic CAD, GLS is often reduced even in the absence of symptoms or significant coronary stenosis. This suggests that GLS may detect subclinical myocardial dysfunction, potentially identifying patients at higher risk for future events.
- *Postrevascularization assessment:* GLS can evaluate the effectiveness of revascularization procedures, such as percutaneous coronary intervention (PCI) and coronary artery bypass grafting (CABG). Improvement in GLS after revascularization is associated with better clinical outcomes.

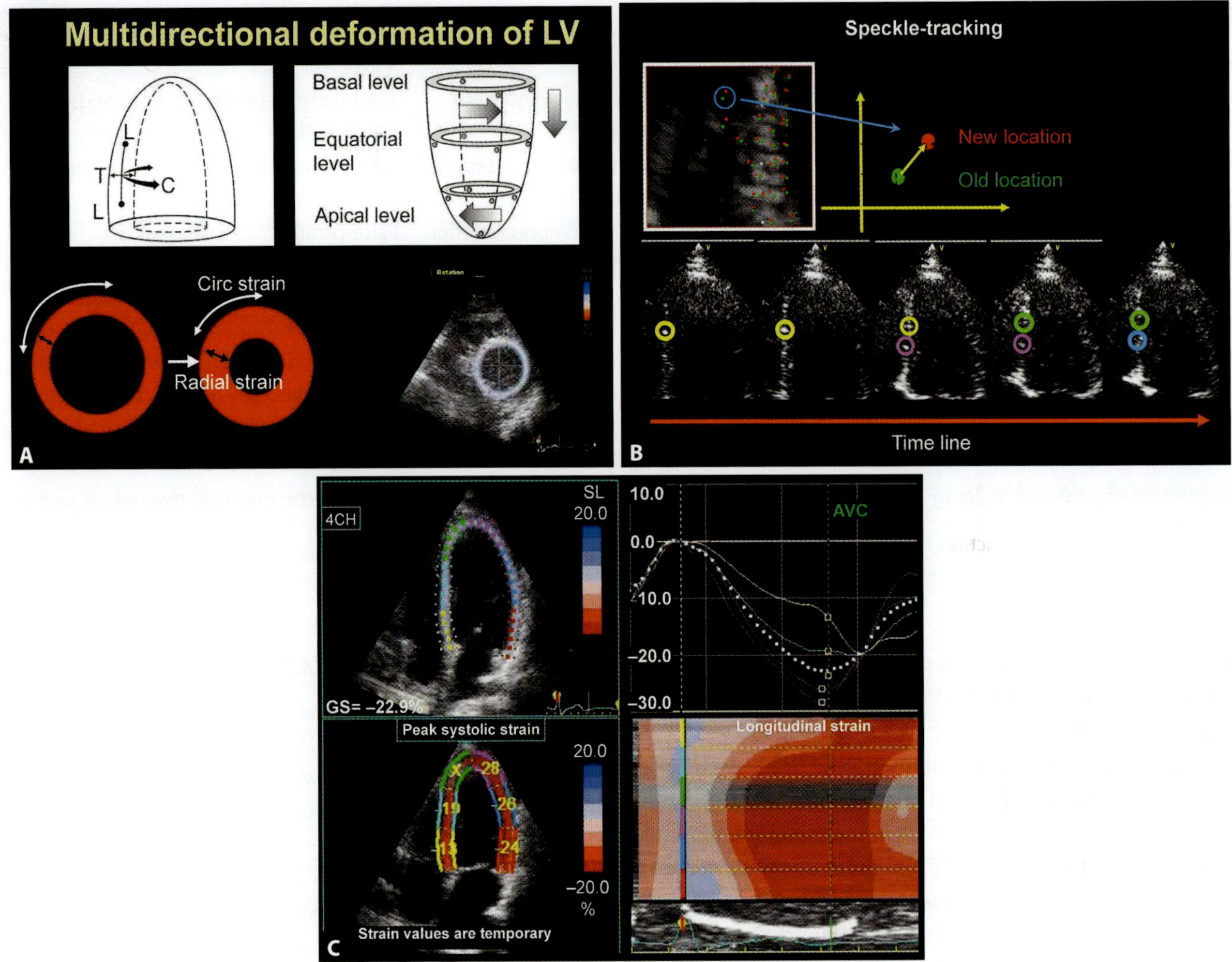

Figs. 4A to C: Principle of speckle tracking. (T: thickness (radial strain); L: length (longitudinal strain); C: circumference (circumferential strain)

- *Microvascular dysfunction:* GLS can assist in the evaluation of coronary microvascular dysfunction, which is common in patients with CAD and is associated with adverse outcomes.[6]

GLS in Risk Stratification and Prognosis

Global longitudinal strain has important prognostic implications in patients with CAD. A reduced GLS is associated with adverse outcomes, including increased mortality, heart failure, and recurrent MI. This is independent of LVEF, highlighting the added value of GLS in risk stratification.

- *Post-MI risk stratification:* In patients post-MI, GLS is a strong predictor of adverse LV remodeling, myocardial fibrosis, heart failure, and mortality. It can identify patients who may benefit from more aggressive medical therapy or revascularization **(Figs. 5A and B)**.
- *Assessment of viability:* GLS can also assess myocardial viability in patients with ischemic cardiomyopathy. A higher GLS in the infarcted territory suggests viable myocardium, which may respond favorably to revascularization.

GLS in the Evaluation of Ischemic Burden

Global longitudinal strain can quantify the extent of myocardial ischemia in patients with CAD. The degree of GLS reduction correlates with the severity of coronary stenosis and the extent of ischemic burden on MPI. This makes GLS a useful tool for guiding revascularization decisions, particularly in patients with multivessel disease.

Cohort studies have confirmed that impaired baseline GLS independently predicts adverse clinical endpoints, even after adjusting for confounding variables such as age, comorbidities, and baseline LVEF levels.

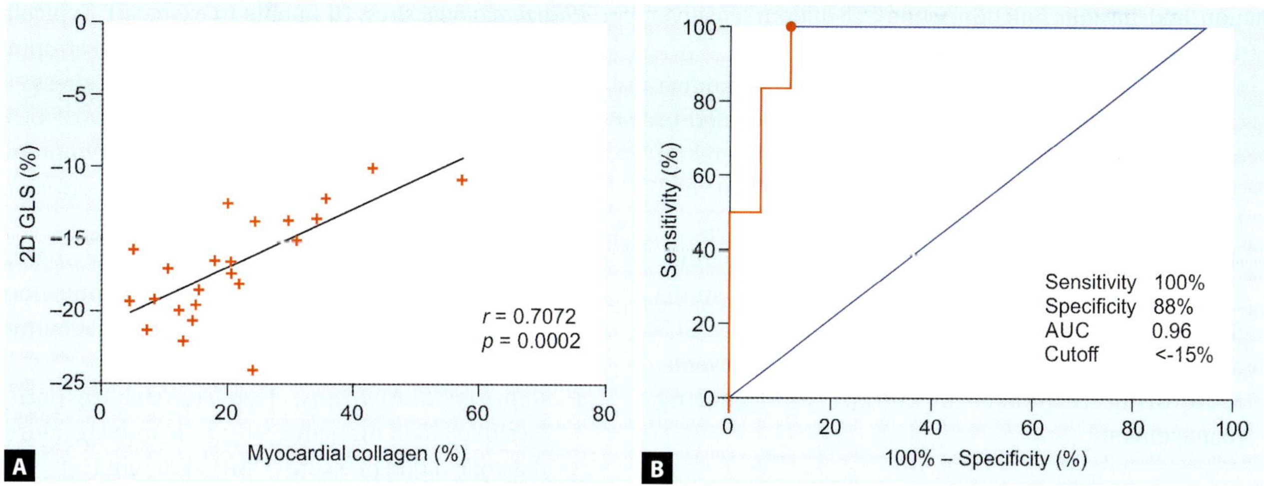

Figs. 5A and B: GLS and its relation in predicting myocardial fibrosis. (AUC: area under curve; GLS: global longitudinal strain)
Source: Kočková, Radka et al. Correlation of Left Ventricular Strain and Myocardial Fibrosis in Patients with Severe Aortic Valve Disease and Preserved Ejection FBaction: A Magnetic Resonance and Histology Study Journal of Cardiovascular Magnetic Resonance, Volume 26, 100761.

The predictive capacity of GLS extends to major adverse cardiac events (MACE), including recurrent ischemic episodes and hospitalization due to heart failure exacerbations. Serial assessment of GLS provides valuable insights into the progression or improvement of myocardial function following revascularization procedures or pharmacological treatment, serving as a dynamic marker for guiding personalized management strategies.

Sensitivity and Specificity of GLS

Global longitudinal strain consistently demonstrates higher sensitivity than traditional markers such as LVEF in detecting subtle myocardial impairment. In a meta-analysis of resting echocardiography studies, pooled GLS sensitivity for predicting obstructive CAD was calculated to be 79% [95% confidence interval (CI) 74–83%), with a specificity of 77% (95% CI 72–82%). When considering dobutamine stress echocardiograms alone, the sensitivity of GLS was 77% (95% CI 59–89%) and specificity was 78% (95% CI 53–92%). These values appear comparable to other diagnostic stress testing methods, but STE offers the advantage of no additional radiation exposure or extensive postprocessing.[7]

A study investigating the additional diagnostic accuracy of GLS at peak dobutamine stress in patients with intermediate pretest probability for CAD found that standard DSE had 79.6% sensitivity and 92.3% specificity. However, GLS (with a cutoff value ≤ −20.5%) alone achieved 89.8% sensitivity and 84.6% specificity. Critically, combining GLS with DSE significantly improved diagnostic accuracy, yielding 95.9% sensitivity and 84.6% specificity.

Subgroup analyses suggest that patients with preserved LVEF but impaired GLS represent a high-risk phenotype often missed by conventional evaluation methods. The ability of GLS to detect myocardial dysfunction at an earlier, subclinical stage, even when LVEF is preserved, is a significant advancement. This is because the longitudinally arranged subendocardial fibers, which are particularly vulnerable to ischemia, are the first to show impairment, and GLS directly assesses this longitudinal function. This early detection capacity allows for earlier intervention strategies, potentially improving patient outcomes.[8-11]

Limitations of GLS

Despite its advantages, GLS is highly dependent on image quality, and accurate measurement requires expertise in STE. Additionally, GLS values can be influenced by loading conditions, heart rate, and age, which should be considered when interpreting results.

INTEGRATING 2D ECHOCARDIOGRAPHY AND GLOBAL LONGITUDINAL STRAIN IN CLINICAL PRACTICE

The combined use of 2D echocardiography and GLS provides a comprehensive assessment of cardiac structure and function in patients with CAD. 2D echocardiography provides valuable information on RWMAs, ejection fraction, and diastolic function, while GLS offers a sensitive marker of subclinical myocardial dysfunction.

- *Clinical workflow:* In patients with suspected or known CAD, 2D echocardiography should be performed to assess cardiac structure and function. GLS should be measured in all patients, especially those with normal LVEF or those undergoing stress echocardiography
- *Risk stratification:* The combination of 2D echocardiographic parameters and GLS can improve risk stratification in patients with CAD. Reduced LVEF and GLS are associated with an increased risk of adverse events.
- Monitoring response to therapy and guiding management

STRESS ECHOCARDIOGRAPHY

- It is particularly valuable as a first-line diagnostic tool in patients with baseline electrocardiographic abnormalities—such as LBBB, pre-excitation, or paced rhythms—that limit the interpretability of exercise ECG testing.
- In terms of diagnostic accuracy, stress echocardiography is comparable to stress radionuclide perfusion imaging.
- For the detection of significant CAD—typically defined as >50% luminal stenosis by coronary angiography—stress echocardiography yields a sensitivity of approximately 88% and a specificity of around 83%.
- Notably, the specificity of stress echocardiography appears to exceed that of nuclear imaging in the detection of left main or triple-vessel CAD, likely due to its superior spatial resolution and direct assessment of RWMA.

Stress Echocardiographic Protocol

- *Pretest preparation:* Conduct baseline echocardiogram to assess heart structure and LVEF (should be ≥50%), ensure image quality, and rule out contraindications like significant structural disease or pericardial effusion.
- *Stress modality selection:* Choose between:
  Exercise stress:
  - Treadmill (Bruce protocol)—standard staged increases every 3 minutes
  - Stationary bicycle (upright/supine)—workload increases by 25 W every 2–3 minutes; allows real-time imaging at peak stress (American Society of Echocardiography)

  Pharmacologic stress (if unable to exercise): Typically graded dobutamine up to 40 μg/kg/min, with atropine as needed; allows controlled imaging at peak stress
- *Monitoring during test:* Continuously record ECG (12-lead), blood pressure, and monitor for symptoms such as chest pain, dyspnea, or signs of poor perfusion.
- *Termination criteria:*
  - *Absolute indications:* Moderate to severe angina, ST-elevation, sustained VT, near-syncope/poor perfusion, BP drop >10 mm Hg with ischemia, intolerable symptoms
  - *Relative indications:* Hypertensive response [systolic blood pressure (SBP) >220 mm Hg and/or diastolic blood pressure (DBP) >120 mm Hg]
- *Image acquisition:*
  - *Treadmill:* Perform immediate postexercise imaging (within ~90 seconds), ideally using quad-screen format comparing rest versus stress.
  - *Bicycle:* Capture images at real-time peak stress and compare with rest.
- *Interpretation of results:*
  - *A normal response:* Hyperdynamic LV, decreased cavity size, no new RWMAs (WMSI = 1.0), LVEF ≥50%
  - *Fixed RWMAs:* Suggest prior infarction (no change with stress)
  - *New or worsening RWMA:* Indicates inducible ischemia and likely CAD
  - *Extensive ischemia:* May present transient LV dilation and reduced global LVEF in multivessel or left main disease
- *Post-test follow-up:* Monitor for adverse events (rare): Incidence approximately 0.015% for exercise and 0.18% for dobutamine stress, with most common complications being arrhythmias or myocardial infarction.
- *Limitations of stress echocardiography* **(Table 3)**.

Risk Stratification with Stress Echocardiography and Assessment of Myocardial Viability

- In patients who achieve adequate exercise capacity or reach the target heart rate during exercise or pharmacologic stress testing, the subsequent annual risk of major cardiac events is <1% per year following a normal exercise stress echocardiogram and <2% per year following a pharmacologic study.

TABLE 3: Limitations of stress echocardiography.

Limitation	*Specific causes*	*Explanation*
False-negative results	Submaximal stress	Inadequate exercise capacity or use of negative chronotropic agents (e.g., beta-blockers) prevents the heart from reaching its target stress level, potentially masking signs of ischemia
	Poor image quality	Blurry or low-resolution images make it difficult to define the endocardial border, hindering the accurate assessment of wall motion
	Small or localized ischemic territories	Small areas of ischemia, particularly in single-vessel disease or the left circumflex artery, may be too small or poorly visualized to be detected
	Preexisting cardiac conditions	Conditions like marked left ventricular hypertrophy (LVH) or hyperdynamic circulatory states can hide regional dysfunction that would otherwise be visible
False-positive results	Low pretest probability of CAD	Patients with a low likelihood of coronary artery disease are more susceptible to false-positive readings
	Left bundle branch block (LBBB) or septal dyssynchrony	LBBB or septal dyssynchrony (caused by ventricular pacing or surgery) can lead to abnormal septal motion that is exaggerated by exercise, mimicking ischemia

- A significant increase in WMSI during stress, involvement of >3 LV segments, and no improvement or a reduction in exercise-induced LVEF is each associated with a greater than fourfold increased risk of cardiac death or myocardial infarction.
- DSE is also a valuable tool for assessing myocardial viability—specifically, contractile reserve—and for predicting the potential for functional recovery following reperfusion. Although the overall sensitivity of DSE is slightly lower compared to nuclear imaging or CMR, it offers superior specificity in identifying viable myocardial segments that are likely to regain systolic function.[12,13]

The most specific indicator of viability on DSE is a biphasic response: An initial improvement in wall thickening at low doses of dobutamine, followed by a decline at higher doses. This pattern reflects the presence of viable but jeopardized myocardium with inducible ischemia. Nevertheless, any observable improvement in wall motion by at least one grade in two or more segments during dobutamine infusion is considered a reliable sign of myocardial viability, whether the tissue is stunned or hibernating.

MECHANICAL COMPLICATIONS AFTER MYOCARDIAL INFARCTION

Myocardial infarction (MI) can lead to grave collateral damage from tissue necrosis and bleeding, which is often heralded by cardiogenic shock. These events may appear within days of the initial infarct or may be delayed by years **(Table 4)**.

Other Causes of Cardiogenic Shock in Myocardial Infarction

Beyond the mechanical complications previously discussed, several other factors can contribute to hypotension in the setting of acute MI:

- Loss of effective pump function due to extensive myocardial damage (most common)
- RV infarction, often associated with inferoposterior MI, may also present as an isolated event, particularly in patients with occlusion of a nondominant right coronary artery (RCA) **(Table 5)**
- Reocclusion of a previously treated coronary artery, resulting in infarct extension
- Effusive pericarditis (Dressler syndrome), which may cause pericardial effusion and impaired diastolic filling
- Acute dynamic left ventricular outflow tract (LVOT) obstruction with systolic anterior motion (SAM) of the mitral valve, particularly in patients with basal hyperkinesis compensating for apical hypokinesis—often seen in those with preexisting upper septal hypertrophy.

Recognition of these diverse mechanisms is essential for timely diagnosis and appropriate hemodynamic management in the acute MI setting.

TABLE 4: Clinical description and echocardiographic findings of complications post myocardial infarction.

Complication	*Clinical description and echocardiographic findings*
MR	Caused by papillary muscle rupture leading to a flail mitral leaflet. A flail posterior leaflet results in an anteriorly and septally directed mitral regurgitation (MR) jet, whereas flail anterior leaflet causes the jet to be directed posterolaterally. This results in significant valvular incompetence with an eccentric jet directed away from the affected leaflet. *Transthoracic echocardiography (TTE)* may be inconclusive, and *transesophageal echocardiography (TEE)* is often needed for confirmation **(Fig. 6)** 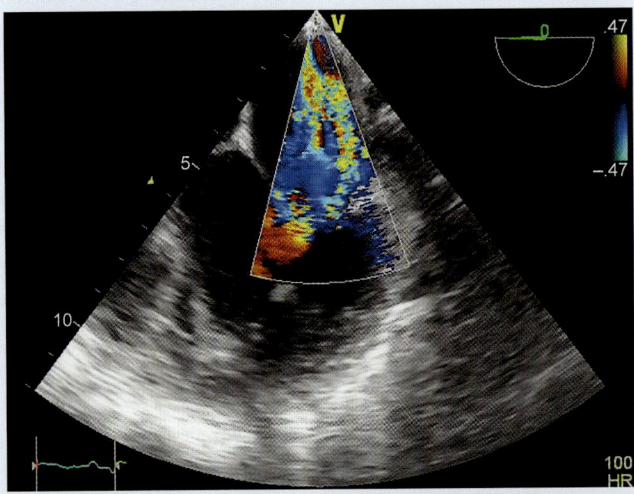 **Fig. 6:** Severe MR due to papillary muscle rupture.
Ventricular septal defect (VSD)	An abnormal left-to-right flow across the interventricular septum, visualized as echogenic dropout on 2D imaging and with color Doppler. Defects can be simple (anteroseptal infarctions) or complex (inferior infarctions). *Color Doppler* is crucial for confirming the presence, location, and size of the shunt. The hemodynamic significance is assessed by the pressure gradient, with a high gradient indicating a small, restrictive VSD **(Fig. 7)** 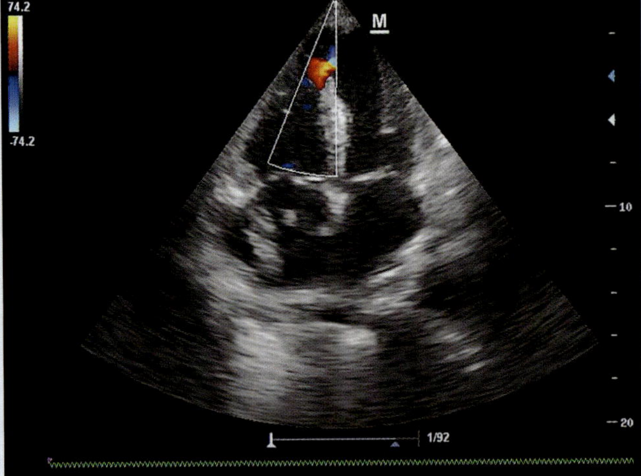 **Fig. 7:** Apical VSR with RA clot. (RA: right atrium; VSR: ruptured ventricular septum)
Pseudoaneurysm	A contained rupture of the left ventricular free wall sealed by the pericardium. It appears as an additional echo-free cavity with a *narrow neck*, irregular margins, and turbulent bidirectional flow. It can be distinguished from a true aneurysm (which has a wide neck) using echocardiography, sometimes with the aid of *ultrasound contrast agents*. While it carries a risk of rupture, it can also remain stable for long periods.

Contd...

Contd...

Complication	*Clinical Description and Echocardiographic Findings*
Free wall rupture	When visualized, it presents as a new *pericardial effusion* with signs of cardiac tamponade. The pericardial fluid may show echogenic swirling (active hemorrhage) or organized clot formation. *Color Doppler* can confirm the rupture by showing flow from the ventricle into the pericardial space **(Fig. 8)** 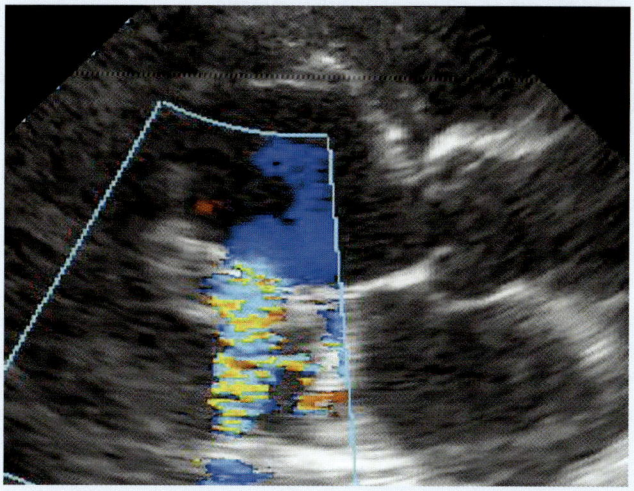 **Fig. 8:** Free wall rupture.
Tamponade	Occurs when hemorrhage from complications like pseudoaneurysm, free wall rupture, or aortic dissection fills the pericardial sac. On echocardiography, *hemopericardium* is characterized by a distinctive gel-like echogenic appearance of the pericardial fluid. Organized thrombus within the effusion may suggest a prior, spontaneously sealed rupture.

TABLE 5: Assessment of right ventricular (RV) function (ASE-2025).

Parameter	*Measurement technique/ description*	*Normal value*	*Mild dysfunction*	*Moderate dysfunction*	*Severe dysfunction*
Fractional area change (FAC)	Percentage change in RV area from end-diastole to end-systole, traced from apical four-chamber view	>35%	≤35 to >29%	≤29 to >22%	≤22%
TAPSE (tricuspid annular plane systolic excursion)	M-mode measurement of longitudinal motion of lateral tricuspid annulus in apical four-chamber view	>1.7 cm	≤1.7 to >1.3 cm	≤1.3 to >1.0 cm	≤1.0 cm
Tissue Doppler S′ velocity	Peak systolic velocity of basal RV free wall segment measured at lateral tricuspid annulus by pulsed tissue Doppler	>9.5 cm/s	≤9.5 to >7.2 cm/s	≤7.2 to >5.0 cm/s	≤5.0 cm/s
RV myocardial performance index (MPI)—tissue Doppler	Sum of isovolumic contraction time and isovolumic relaxation time divided by ejection time, derived from tissue Doppler at tricuspid annulus	<0.55	≥0.55 to <0.62	≥0.62 to <0.70	≥0.70
RV myocardial performance index (MPI)—pulsed Doppler	Derived from pulsed Doppler of RVOT and tricuspid inflow	<0.40	≥0.40 to <0.49	≥0.49 to <0.57	≥0.57

Contd...

Contd...

Parameter	*Measurement Technique/ Description*	*Normal Value*	*Mild Dysfunction*	*Moderate Dysfunction*	*Severe Dysfunction*
3D RVEF (right ventricular ejection fraction)	Volumetric assessment of RV ejection fraction using 3D echocardiography (disk summation method)	>45%	≤45 to >39%	≤39 to ≥32%	<32%
RV longitudinal free wall strain (3-segment)	2D speckle-tracking measurement of longitudinal deformation of RV free wall (absolute value)	>20%	≤20 to ≥15%	<15 to ≥11%	<11%
RV longitudinal global strain (6-segment)	2D speckle-tracking measurement of longitudinal deformation of entire RV (absolute value)	>17%	≤17 to >13%	≤13 to >9%	≤9%

TABLE 6: Summary of post-MI complications detected by echocardiographic evaluation.

Complication	*Key pathophysiology and features*	*Diagnostic echocardiography findings*
Left ventricular aneurysm	Dyskinetic outpouching of the LV wall with preserved layers. Leads to blood stasis and predisposes to thrombus formation	• Discrete, dyskinetic outpouching, often at the apex • Spontaneous echocardiographic contrast may be visible
Left ventricular thrombus	Stagnant blood flow in aneurysms or akinetic regions, leading to thrombus formation. Mobile thrombi carry a high risk of embolization	• Discrete, homogeneously echogenic, and deformable mass contiguous with the endocardium • Enhanced detection with intravenous contrast agents.
Left ventricular (LV) remodeling	Increase in LV volume and a change in ventricular geometry from elliptical to spherical	*Sphericity Index* (long-axis/short-axis ratio): Normal ≥1.5; values approaching 1.0 indicate a globular, remodeled ventricle
Ischemic mitral regurgitation	• Secondary to LV ischemia, not intrinsic valve disease • An imbalance between closing and tethering forces prevents proper coaptation of the mitral leaflets	Appears as a failure of mitral valve leaflets to coapt fully, resulting in a regurgitant jet, in the absence of primary valve pathology

LATE COMPLICATIONS OF MYOCARDIAL INFARCTION

See **Table 6**.

CONCLUSION

The evaluation of CAD is a complex process that requires a combination of clinical assessment, noninvasive imaging, and invasive procedures. Echocardiography, particularly with the use of advanced techniques such as GLS, plays a central role in the diagnosis, risk stratification, and management of CAD. GLS has emerged as a sensitive and prognostic marker of myocardial function, providing valuable information that complements traditional imaging methods. The combined use of these techniques can improve diagnostic accuracy, risk stratification, and management of patients with CAD. As technology continues to advance, the integration of multimodality imaging and artificial intelligence (AI) is expected to further improve our ability to detect and treat CAD, ultimately leading to better patient outcomes.

REFERENCES

1. Regmi M, Siccardi MA. Coronary Artery Disease Prevention. [Updated 2023 Aug 7]. In: StatPearls [Internet]. Treasure Island (FL): StatPearls Publishing; 2025 Jan-. Available from: https://www.ncbi.nlm.nih.gov/books/NBK547760/
2. Aziz AA, AbouShokka RD, Abdelsamie MM. Myocardial longitudinal strain reserve is a marker of coronary artery disease severity during dobutamine stress echocardiography. J Med Sci Res. 2020;3(1):74.
3. Ko SM, Kim TH, Chun EJ, Kim JY, Hwang SH. Assessment of Left Ventricular Myocardial Diseases with Cardiac

Computed Tomography. Korean J Radiol. 2019;20(3): 333-51.

4. Giger ML, Suzuki K. Computer-aided diagnosis. In: Biomedical Information Technology. Oxford: Academic Press; 2008. pp. 359-74.
5. Kočková R, Hlubocká Z, Línková H, Mědílek K, Skalsky I, Sedmera Det al. Correlation of Left Ventricular Strain and Myocardial Fibrosis in Patients with Severe Aortic Valve Disease and Preserved Ejection Fraction: A Magnetic Resonance and Histology Study. J Cardiovasc Magn Reson. 2024;26:100761.
6. Bhuyan S, Satapathy C, Mohanty N. To determine how beneficial global longitudinal strain (GLS) at rest is for detecting substantial coronary artery disease. J Cardiovasc Dis Res. 2023;14(11):289-99.
7. Zuo HJ, Yang XT, Liu QG, Zhang Y, Zeng HS, Yan JT, et al. Global longitudinal strain at rest for detection of coronary artery disease in patients without diabetes mellitus. Curr Med Sci. 2018;38:413-21.
8. Kosaraju A, Muppidi V, Makaryus AN. Stress Echocardiography. [Updated 2023 Jul 25]. In: StatPearls [Internet]. Treasure Island (FL): StatPearls Publishing; 2025 Jan-. Available from: https://www.ncbi.nlm.nih.gov/books/NBK448062/
9. Abdelrazek G, Yassin A, Elkhashab K. Correlation between global longitudinal strain and SYNTAX score in coronary artery disease evaluation. Egypt Heart J. 2020;72:1-7.
10. Ionac I, Lazăr MA, Șoșdean R, Văcărescu C, Simonescu M, Luca CT, et al. Considering Both GLS and MD for a Prognostic Value in Non-ST-Segment Elevated Acute Coronary Artery Syndrome. Diagnostics. 2023;13(4):745.
11. Pararajasingam G, Heinsen LJ, Larsson J, Andersen TR, Løgstrup BB, Auscher S, et al. Diabetic microvascular complications are associated with reduced global longitudinal strain independent of atherosclerotic coronary artery disease in asymptomatic patients with diabetes mellitus: a cross- sectional study. BMC Cardiovasc Disorders. 2021;21(1):269.
12. Geleijnse ML, Elhendy A, Van Domburg RT, Cornel JH, Rambaldi R, Salustri A, et al. Cardiac imaging for risk stratification with dobutamine atropine stress testing in patients with chest pain. Circulation. 1997;96:137-47.
13. Olmos LI, Dakik H, Cordon R, Dunn JK, Verani MS, Quiñones MA, et al. Long-term prognostic value of exercise echocardiography compared with exercise 201TL, ECG, and clinical variables in patients evaluated for coronary artery disease. Circulation. 1998;98:2679-86.

Role of Echocardiography in the Assessment of Cardiac Amyloidosis

Simranpreet Singh Daid, Nitesh Raj Dulal, Ravindra Bhardwaj, Raj Wasan, Navin C Nanda

INTRODUCTION

Cardiac amyloidosis (CA) is a condition that affects the heart and often leads to heart failure with preserved ejection fraction (HFpEF). It is primarily caused by the deposition of misfolded amyloid proteins, notably transthyretin (ATTR) and light chain (AL) proteins. Emerging forms, including those involving apolipoprotein AI (AApoAI) and apolipoprotein AIV (AApoAIV), are now being identified.[1,2] In ATTR CA, the tetrameric plasma protein transthyretin dissociates abnormally into oligomers and monomers, which misfold and ultimately form pathological fibrils. This process can occur in two main forms: (1) Wild-type ATTR (wtATTR) CA, associated with age-related protein misfolding and now recognized as the highly prevalent form in adults over 65 years of age[3,4] and (2) hereditary ATTR (hATTR) CA, a less common form caused by autosomal dominant mutations in the TTR gene.

In contrast, AL CA results from abnormal clonal proliferation that produces misfolded monoclonal immunoglobulins which deposit in the heart, leading to more aggressive disease course due to the cardiotoxic effects of the amyloidogenic light chains.[4-6] Additionally, while amyloid deposition in ATTR-CA is typically transmural, AL CA more commonly exhibits a subendocardial pattern.[7] AL amyloid (AL-CA) remains the predominant variant of CA, with prevalence of about 50% of cases, and generally follows a more aggressive disease course compared to transthyretin amyloidosis (ATTR-CA). In contrast, wild-type ATTR (wtATTR) CA is the most prevalent form of ATTR-CA in the elderly, with an average survival of 3.6 years after diagnosis. Moreover, wtATTR CA in elderly individuals may be noted in patients with low-flow and low-gradient aortic stenosis.[6]

CLINICAL FEATURES AND DIAGNOSIS

Table 1 demonstrates in brief the clinical features of AL and ATTR types of amyloidosis.

Since symptoms alone are nonspecific, additional tests are essential. An ECG may show low QRS voltage,

TABLE 1: Clinical manifestations of AL and ATTR amyloidosis.[4,8-13]

AL amyloidosis	*wT ATTR amyloidosis*	*hATTR amyloidosis*
Cardiomyopathy	Cardiomyopathy	Cardiomyopathy
Neuropathy	Neuropathy	Neuropathy
Orthostatic dizziness	Orthostatic dizziness	Orthostatic dizziness
Severe spinal stenosis	Severe spinal stenosis	Severe spinal stenosis
Carpal tunnel syndrome	Carpal tunnel syndrome	Carpal tunnel syndrome
Atraumatic biceps rupture	Atraumatic biceps rupture	–
Ophthalmopathy	–	–
Enteropathy	–	–
Macroglossia	–	–
Hepatopathy	–	–
Nephropathy	–	–
Goiter	–	–

(AL: light chain amyloidosis; wTATTR: wild type transthyretin amyloidosis; hATTR: hereditary transthyretin amyloidosis)

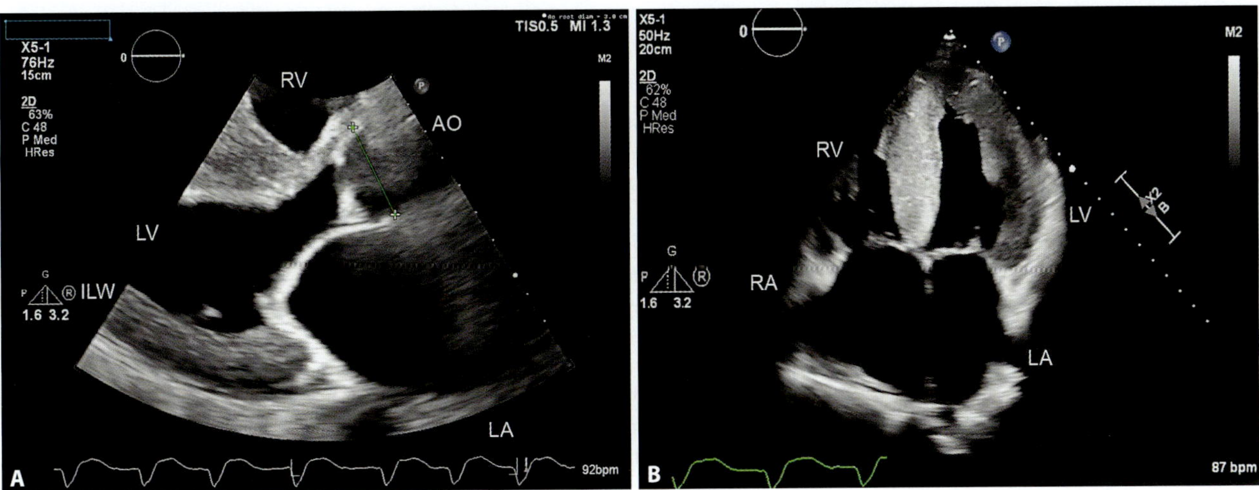

Figs. 1A and B: Cardiac amyloidosis. Two-dimensional transthoracic echocardiography shows thickening and hyperechogenicity of left ventricular walls in (A) parasternal long axis and (B) apical four-chamber views. (AO: aorta; ILW: inferolateral wall; LA: left atrium; LV: left ventricle; RA: right atrium; RV: right ventricle)

pseudoinfarction patterns, or conduction delays. Elevated NT-pro-BNP (N < 300 pg/mL) and chronically low troponin levels (N < 0.04 ng/mL) can hint at CA, while abnormal free light chains or positive immunofixation tests may confirm AL amyloidosis. Biopsy continues to be the definitive method for confirming both AL and ATTR amyloidosis.

ECHOCARDIOGRAPHIC FINDINGS AND THEIR USEFULNESS (FIGS. 1 AND 2)

We decided to summarize the echocardiographic findings and scoring systems useful for the diagnosis, prognostication and management of CA in tabular form **(Tables 2 and 3)** rather than in a detailed narrative format for ease and convenience of the readers and to keep the chapter within a reasonable length.

The following echocardiographic scoring systems have been developed for diagnosing CA using echocardiographic parameters alone or in combination with other findings. These scoring systems, reproduced with permission from Comprehensive Textbook of Echocardiography (3rd edition) edited by Dr Navin C Nanda (2025) and published by Jaypee Brothers Medical Publisher, New Delhi, India, are listed in **Tables 3A to D**.[3]

This IWT score was shown to have good accuracy for diagnosing CA in patients who were noted to have increased LV wall thickness on 2DTTE. A score <2 virtually ruled out the presence of CA whereas a score ≥8 strongly indicated the disease. The study did not specify which form of CA was diagnosed more accurately using this score.

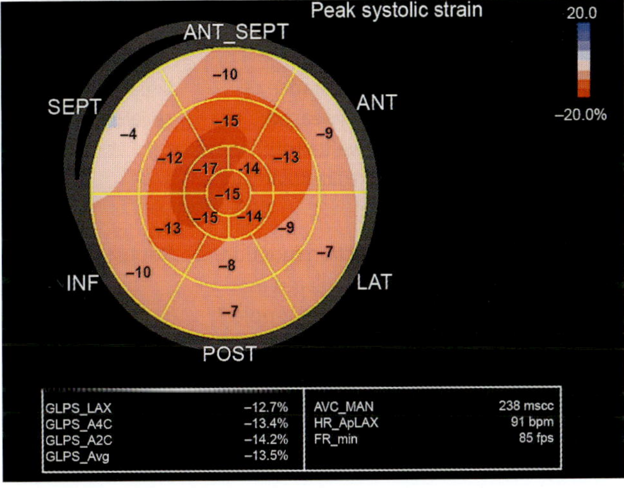

Fig. 2: Bull's eye view of cardiac amyloidosis with decreased longitudinal strain in the basal and middle portions of the left ventricle with apical sparing, the so-called "cherry on top" sign. *Source:* Reproduced with permission from Reference 3.

However, considering that the other multiparametric score shown in **Table 3B** evaluated patients with AL CA, it is presumed that the IWT score was useful for accurately diagnosing TTR CA.

This AL score was shown to have good accuracy for diagnosing AL CA in patients who had systemic AL amyloidosis. A score <1 virtually ruled out cardiac AL amyloidosis whereas a score ≥5 essentially clinched the diagnosis.

Based on the score given in **Table 3C**, in a population where TTR CA is prevalent in ≥10% of HFpEF cases, a score of ≥6 indicates a high risk that a patient may have TTR CA.

TABLE 2A: Left ventricular (LV) echocardiographic parameters.

Parameter and abnormal findings	*Accuracy/Prognostic and therapeutic implications*	*Limitations*
• LV wall thickness >12 mm by 2DTTE. Due to amyloid deposition (AD)[14] • AL CA displays concentric thickening and TTR CA asymmetric thickening[15,16]	• When coupled with low ECG voltage increases suspicion for CA, AD increases myocardial mass without proportional increase in electrical activity. Increased LV wall thickness is often an early finding in CA[17] • *Tafamidis:* Only medication approved for TTR CA significantly reduces all-cause mortality and functional decline. Mitigates progressive AD[16] • *Patisiran:* (*TTR* gene silencer) associated with reductions in both mean and LV relative wall thickness and increase in LV average peak global longitudinal strain (GLS), and cardiac output[15]	Other causes such as systemic hypertension and HCM need to be excluded
LV relative wall thickness (RWT) by 2DTTE >0.42 (calculated as either 2 × inferolateral LV wall dimension/LVIDd or ventricular septum + inferolateral LV wall dimension)/ LVIDd; the latter preferred by British Society of Echocardiography, especially in TTR-CA with asymmetric septal thickening)[16]		Same as above
"Speckled" or "sparkling" appearance of LV/RV walls on 2DTTE with increased echogenicity (hyperreflective texture). Due to AD laid as sheets extracellularly in myocardium[17,18]	Greater diagnostic value when in conjunction with severely reduced LV GLS by 2D-STE	Need to exclude other causes such as CKD, Fabry's disease, glycogen storage disorders, etc.
Reduced myocardial contraction function (MCF) (typically 20–30%), calculated as stroke volume (SV) measured by Doppler/ LV end-diastolic volume measured by 2DTTE. AD increases myocardial mass while reducing LV cavity size, thereby lowering SV[16,19]	Robust validation in TTR CA[19]	• Utility in other types of CA is less established • Needs accurate measurement of LV and stroke volumes and measurement may be affected by coexisting valvular regurgitation
LV ejection fraction (EF): Preserved or only mildly reduced in early CA. Significant decrease in advanced stages with greater AD[17]	A normal or near-normal LVEF, when accompanied by other abnormal LV findings described above helpful in diagnosis[17]	Need to exclude other causes of decreased LVEF
LV GLS by 2DTTE STE < −16% (Normal > −16%)[17,20-22]	• Detects early subclinical LV dysfunction before LVEF declines due to early AD in subendocardial fibers. Distinguishes CA from other conditions with thickened LV walls, e.g., HCM, HFpEF, where LV GLS may not decrease before LVEF[17] • One study found that diminished LV basal strain, measured by 2DTTE STE, independently predicted both cardiac and overall mortality.[23] Another study showed reduced LV early diastolic strain rate by 2DTTE STE (cutoff value of 0.85) was associated with four times risk of death even with normal LVEF[24]	Need to exclude other causes of decreased LV GLS such as ischemic heart disease and other cardiomyopathies

Contd...

Contd...

Parameter and abnormal findings	*Accuracy/Prognostic and therapeutic implications*	*Limitations*
• LV GLS apical sparing pattern (by 2DTTE STE) in contrast to significant reduction in other regions ("cherry-on-top" bull's eye pattern) • Due to preferential AD in LV basal and mid-segments[25-28]	One study achieved sensitivity and specificity of 93 and 82%, respectively in distinguishing CA from other etiologies of LV wall thickening.[25-28] However, further studies have shown only moderate accuracy	Similar patterns can be observed occasionally in some other conditions such as severe chronic kidney disease, aortic stenosis, and systemic hypertension[25-28]
LV apical septum to basal septum GLS ratio (by 2DTTE STE) >2.1[17,27]	One study found that using this ratio in combination with reduced mitral E wave deceleration time effectively distinguished CA from other etiologies of concentric LV hypertrophy[17,27]	Moderate accuracy in clinical settings
LVEF/LV GLS ratio (by STE) >4.1. Highlights preserved LVEF despite reduced LV GLS[16,29]	In one study, high sensitivity (~89.7%) and specificity (~91.7%)[16,29]	Moderate accuracy in everyday practice
LV diastolic dysfunction and atrial changes. Grade 2 or greater LV diastolic dysfunction. Elevated mitral early diastolic pulsed Doppler E wave velocity (E)/tissue Doppler early diastolic (e') wave velocity ratio >15. Also, pulsed Doppler E wave velocity/mitral atrial systolic velocity (A) >2. Shortened mitral Doppler E wave deceleration time (<150 ms). Markedly reduced tissue Doppler e' wave velocity <6 cm/s. Biatrial enlargement ("owl's eyes" appearance) by 2DTTE. These findings reflect increased left-sided filling pressure due to AD[30-33]	• Mitral E/e' ratio (commonly >14–15) often noted[30-33] • In AL amyloidosis, pre-ejection period of ≤240 ms predicts 1-year cardiac mortality (specificity almost 90%)[34,35] • 3DTTE left atrial total emptying fraction below 34%, particularly when paired with lower 3DTTE STE peak left atrial LS, is linked to a notably poorer 2-year survival outcome[36]	Need to exclude other causes of LV diastolic dysfunction and biatrial enlargement such as other cardiomyopathies
Low tissue Doppler velocities: Reduction in lateral mitral annulus velocities: s' (normally 8–9 cm/s), e' (normally 10–12 cm/s), and a' (normally 7–12 cm/s). Findings due to AD[17,30]	The "5-5-5" sign—where each of the three tissue Doppler velocities is under 5 cm/s—is typically indicative of advanced CA[17,30]	Similar reductions can occur in other forms of myocardial dysfunction, limiting stand-alone diagnostic specificity

(AD: amyloid deposition; CA: cardiac amyloidosis; CKD: chronic kidney disease; HCM: hypertrophic cardiomyopathy; HFpEF: heart failure with preserved ejection fraction; LVIDd: left ventricular internal diameter in diastole; LS: longitudinal strain; 2D: two-dimensional; 3D: three-dimensional)

TABLE 2B: Right ventricular (RV) echocardiographic parameters.

Parameter and abnormal findings	*Accuracy/Prognostic and therapeutic implications*	*Limitations*
RV free wall (FW) thickness >7 mm by 2DTTE (normal <5 mm). Owing to preferential AD in the apex[22,30]	RV involvement can occur early in CA[22,30]	Need to exclude other causes such as pulmonary-hypertension. Early changes may be subtle and require careful assessment
RV dilation: RV end-diastolic diameter (RVEDD >31 mm) and end-diastolic area (RVEDA >13 cm^2) in AL CA are increased[38]	In AL CA, RV cavity area/LV cavity are ratio of ≤2 is associated with better survival outcomes[37]	Same as above
• *RV function:* Reduced lateral tricuspid annulus plane systolic excursion (TAPSE) by M-mode <16 mm • Reduced RV systolic velocity using tissue Doppler interrogation of the lateral tricuspid annulus (s') <10 cm/s[22,30]	• When combined with LV abnormalities, these findings support a diagnosis of biventricular involvement in CA[22,30] • In patients with both AL CA and TTR CA, TAPSE measurement below 14 mm has been linked with heightened risk of major adverse cardiovascular events over a 6-month period[38]	Same as above

Contd...

Contd...

Parameter and abnormal findings	*Accuracy/Prognostic and therapeutic implications*	*Limitations*
RV GLS apical sparing pattern (by STE). Relative preservation of RV apical strain versus impaired in other more peripheral regions[39,40]	Early RV GLS abnormalities serve as independent predictor of mortality[41]	Validation of this finding is less extensive compared to LV parameters
RV FW strain by 2DTTE STE was impaired compared to healthy controls (≈ −23% vs. ≈ −30% in controls)[40,42]	• Lower RV FW strain significantly and independently predicted of survival in CA[40,42] • Some studies suggest that RV dysfunction might occur even before LV involvement, thus facilitating early diagnosis. Additionally, reduced TAPSE together with diminished RV FW strain is linked to a poorer prognosis[40,42]	Need to exclude other conditions

(AD: amyloid deposition; AL CA: light chain cardiac amyloidosis; GLS: global longitudinal strain; LV: left ventricle; 2DTTE: two-dimensional transthoracic echocardiography)

TABLE 2C: Other echocardiographic parameters.

Parameter and abnormal findings	*Accuracy/Prognostic and therapeutic implication*	*Limitations*
Interatrial septum and valve abnormalities: Thickened interatrial septum (>5 mm during atrial diastole). Valvular thickening with a "sparkling" appearance (affecting aortic, mitral, and tricuspid valves). Due to amyloid deposition[22,33]	These findings alongside LV and RV abnormalities, further raise suspicion for CA.[22,33]	Need to exclude other causes of interatrial septum and valve thickening

(CA: cardiac amyloidosis; LV: left ventricle; RV: right ventricle;)

TABLE 3A: Multiparametric echocardiography score for patients with increased LV wall thickness (IWT).[3]

Parameter	*Score*
Relative LV wall thickness >0.6	3
"Cherry on top" sign with a systolic LV GLS apex to base ratio >2.9	3
TAPSE ≤19 mm	2
LV GLS absolute value ≤ −13%	1
Doppler mitral E/e′ wave velocities >11	1

Note: Abbreviations as in Table 2.

TABLE 3B: Multiparametric echocardiography score for patients with light chain Amyloidosis (AL)[3]

Finding	*Score*
Relative LV wall thickness >0.52	2
Doppler mitral E/tissue Doppler e′ wave velocities >10	2
TAPSE ≤19 mm	1
LV GLS absolute value ≤ −14%	1

Note: Abbreviations as in Table 2.

TABLE 3C: Multiparametric ATTR score.[3]

Parameter	*Score*
Age: 60–69 years	2
Age: 70–79 years	3
Age: ≥80 years	4
Male sex	2
Relative LV wall thickness >0.57	2
LV inferolateral wall thickness ≥12 mm	1
LVEF <60%	1
Diagnosis of systemic hypertension	−1

(ATTR: amyloid proteins, notably transthyretin; LVEF: left ventricular ejection fraction)
Note: No score is given for an absent parameter.

This study aimed to develop a simpler scoring system based on the multiparametric scores presented in **Tables 1 and 2**, using only two parameters. The authors found that, in patients being evaluated for CA, a product of RWT and E/e′ <2.22 excluded the diagnosis of CA. In patients with increased relative LV wall thickness and AL CA, a value <2.22 and <2.36 excluded the diagnosis of TTR CA and AL CA, respectively.

TABLE 3D: The AMYLI score.[3]

Echocardiographic parameter	*Value*
RWT * E/e′	<2.22
RWT * E/e′	<2.22
RWT * E/e′	<2.36

[AMYLI: amyloidosis index; RWT: relative wall thickness; E/e′: pulsed Doppler mitral early diastolic wave (E)/Tissue Doppler early diastolic wave (e′)]

CONCLUSION

2D-TTE is performed in most patients referred for cardiac consultation and can provide valuable clues for detecting CA when used in conjunction with clinical and ECG findings. However, in most cases, further testing with other noninvasive modalities is required for a more comprehensive assessment. Tissue biopsy remains the definitive standard for diagnosis.

REFERENCES

1. Fontana M, Ioannou A, Cuddy S, Dorbala S, Masri A, Moon JC, et al. The last decade in cardiac amyloidosis: Advances in understanding pathophysiology, diagnosis and quantification, prognosis, treatment strategies, and monitoring response. JACC Cardiovasc Imaging. 2025; 18(4):478-99.
2. Ioannou A, Porcari A, Patel RK, Razvi Y, Sinigiani G, Martinez-Naharro A, et al. Rare forms of cardiac amyloidosis: Diagnostic clues and phenotype in Apo AI and AIV amyloidosis. Circ Cardiovasc Imaging. 2023;16(7):523-35.
3. Shirwany HAK, Espinola-Zavaleta N, Nanda NC. Using echocardiography to assess for cardiac amyloidosis. In: Nanda NC (Ed). Comprehensive Textbook of Echocardiography, 3rd edition. New Delhi: Jaypee Brothers Medical Publishers (P Ltd.); 2025.
4. Grogan M, Scott CG, Kyle RA, Zeldenrust SR, Gertz MA, Lin G, et al. Natural history of wild-type transthyretin cardiac amyloidosis and risk stratification using a novel staging system. J Am Coll Cardiol. 2016;68:1014-20.
5. Triposkiadis F, Briasoulis A, Xanthopoulos A. Amyloids and the Heart: An Update. J Clin Med. 2024;13(23):7210.
6. Bukhari S. Cardiac amyloidosis: State-of-the-art review. J Geriat Cardiol. 2023;20(5):361-75.
7. Dungu JN, Valencia O, Pinney JH, Gibbs SD, Rowczenio D, Gilbertson JA, et al. CMR-based differentiation of AL and ATTR cardiac amyloidosis. JACC: Cardiovas Imaging. 2014;7(2):133-42.
8. Aus dem Siepen F, Hein S, Prestel S, Baumgärtner C, Schönland S, Hegenbart U, et al. Carpal tunnel syndrome and spinal canal stenosis: Harbingers of transthyretin amyloid cardiomyopathy? Clin Res Cardiol. 2019; 108(12):1324-30.
9. Nakagawa M, Sekijima Y, Yazaki M, Tojo K, Yoshinaga T, Doden T, et al. Carpal tunnel syndrome: A common initial symptom of systemic wild-type ATTR (ATTRwt) amyloidosis. Amyloid. 2016;23(1):58-63.
10. Sperry BW, Reyes BA, Ikram A, Donnelly JP, Phelan D, Jaber WA, et al. Tenosynovial and cardiac amyloidosis in patients undergoing carpal tunnel release. J Am Coll Cardiol. 2018;72(17):2040-50.
11. Zegri-Reiriz I, de Haro-Del Moral FJ, Dominguez F, Salas C, de la Cuadra P, Plaza A, et al. Prevalence of cardiac amyloidosis in patients with carpal tunnel syndrome. J Cardiovasc Transl Res. 2019;12(6):507-13.
12. Aus dem Siepen F, Hansen T. Diagnosing AL and ATTR amyloid cardiomyopathy: A multidisciplinary approach. J Clin Med. 2024;13(19):5873.
13. Mohanty S, Torlapati PG, La Fazia VM, Kurt M, Gianni C, MacDonald B, et al. Best anticoagulation strategy with and without appendage occlusion for stroke prophylaxis in postablation atrial fibrillation patients with cardiac amyloidosis. J Cardiovasc Electrophysiol. 2024;35(7):1422-8.
14. Garcia-Pavia P, Rapezzi C, Adler Y, Arad M, Basso C, Brucato A, et al. Diagnosis and treatment of cardiac amyloidosis: A position statement of the ESC Working Group on Myocardial and Pericardial Diseases. Eur Heart J. 2021; 42(16):1554-68.
15. Solomon SD, Adams D, Kristen A, Grogan M, González-Duarte A, Maurer MS, et al. Effects of patisiran, an RNA interference therapeutic, on cardiac parameters in patients with hereditary transthyretin-mediated amyloidosis: Analysis of the APOLLO study. Circulation. 2019;139(4):431-3.
16. Maurer MS, Schwartz JH, Gundapaneni B, Elliott PM, Merlini G, Waddington-Cruz M, et al. Tafamidis treatment for patients with transthyretin amyloid cardiomyopathy. N Engl J Med. 2018;379(11):1007-16.
17. Bhandari AK, Nanda NC. Myocardial texture characterization by two-dimensional echocardiography. Am J Cardiol. 1983;51(5):817-25.
18. Bhandari AK, Nanda NC. Two-dimensional echocardiographic recognition of abnormal changes in the myocardium. Ultrasound Med Biol. 1982;8(6):663-71.
19. Moody WE, Turvey-Haigh L, Knight D, Coats CJ, Cooper RM, Schofield R, et al. British Society of Echocardiography guideline for the transthoracic echocardiographic assessment of cardiac amyloidosis. Echo Res Pract. 2023;10(1):13.
20. Chacko L, Martone R, Bandera F, Lane T, Martinez-Naharro A, Boldrini M, et al. Echocardiographic phenotype and prognosis in transthyretin cardiac amyloidosis. Eur Heart J. 2020;41(14):1439-47.
21. Almeida ALC, Melo MDT, Bihan DCSL, Vieira MLC, Pena JLB, Del Castillo JM, et al. Position statement on the use of myocardial strain in cardiology routines by

the Brazilian Society of Cardiology's Department of Cardiovascular Imaging - 2023. Arquivos Brasileiros de Cardiologia. 2023;120(12):e20230646.

22. Pagourelias ED, Mirea O, Vovas G, Duchenne J, Michalski B, Van Cleemput J, et al. Relation of regional myocardial structure and function in hypertrophic cardiomyopathy and amyloidosis: A combined two-dimensional speckle tracking and cardiovascular magnetic resonance analysis. Eur Heart J Cardiovasc Imaging. 2019;20(4):426-37.
23. Koyama J, Falk RH. Prognostic significance of strain Doppler imaging in light-chain amyloidosis. JACC Cardiovasc Imaging. 2010;3(4):333-42.
24. Liu D, Hu K, Störk S, Herrmann S, Kramer B, Cikes M, et al. Predictive value of assessing diastolic strain rate on survival in cardiac amyloidosis patients with preserved ejection fraction. PLoS One. 2014;9(12):e115910.
25. Moura B, Aimo A, Al-Mohammad A, Keramida K, Ben Gal T, Dorbala S, et al. Diagnosis and management of patients with left ventricular hypertrophy: Role of multimodality cardiac imaging. Eur J Heart Fail. 2023;25(9):1493-506.
26. Kiotsekoglou A, Saha SK, Nanda NC, Lindqvist P. Echocardiographic diagnosis of cardiac amyloidosis: Does the masquerader require only a cherry on top? Echocardiography. 2020;37:1713-5.
27. Phelan D, Collier P, Thavendiranathan P, Popović ZB, Hanna M, Plana JC, et al. Relative apical sparing of longitudinal strain using two-dimensional speckle-tracking echocardiography is both sensitive and specific for the diagnosis of cardiac amyloidosis. Heart. 2012;98(19):1442-8.
28. Liu D, Hu K, Niemann M, Herrmann S, Cikes M, Störk S, et al. Effect of combined systolic and diastolic functional parameter assessment for differentiation of cardiac amyloidosis from other causes of concentric left ventricular hypertrophy. Circ Cardiovasc Imaging. 2013;6(6):1066-72.
29. Pagourelias ED, Duchenne J, Mirea O, Vovas G, Van Cleemput J, Delforge M, et al. The relation of ejection fraction and global longitudinal strain in amyloidosis: Implications for differential diagnosis. JACC Cardiovasc Imaging. 2016;9(11):1358-9.
30. Martinez-Naharro A, Treibel TA, Abdel-Gadir A, Bulluck H, Zumbo G, Knight DS, et al. Magnetic resonance in transthyretin cardiac amyloidosis. J Am Coll Cardiol. 2017; 70(4):466-77.
31. Dorbala S, Cuddy S, Falk RH. How to image cardiac amyloidosis: A practical approach. JACC Cardiovasc Imaging. 2020;13(6):1368-83.
32. Knight DS, Zumbo G, Barcella W, Steeden JA, Muthurangu V, Martinez-Naharro A, et al. Cardiac structural and functional consequences of amyloid deposition by cardiac magnetic resonance and echocardiography and their prognostic roles. JACC Cardiovasc Imaging. 2019;12(5):823-33.
33. Dorbala S, Ando Y, Bokhari S, Dispenzieri A, Falk RH, Ferrari VA, et al. ASNC/AHA/ASE/EANM/HFSA/ISA/SCMR/SNMMI expert consensus recommendations for multimodality imaging in cardiac amyloidosis: Part 1 of 2—Evidence base and standardized methods of imaging. J Nucl Cardiol. 2019;26(6):2065-123.
34. Migrino RQ, Mareedu RK, Eastwood D, Bowers M, Harmann L, Hari P. Left ventricular ejection time on echocardiography predicts long-term mortality in light chain amyloidosis. J Am Soc Echocardiography, 2009; 22:1396-402.
35. Bellavia D, Pellikka PA, Al-Zahrani GB, Abraham TP, Dispenzieri A, Miyazaki C, et al. Independent predictors of survival in primary systemic (AL) amyloidosis, including cardiac biomarkers and left ventricular strain imaging: An observational cohort study. J Am Soc Echocardiography. 2010;23:643-52.
36. Mohty D, Petitalot V, Magne J, Fadel BM, Boulogne C, Rouabhia D, et al. Left atrial function in patients with light chain amyloidosis: A transthoracic 3D speckle tracking imaging study. J Cardiol. 2018;71:419-27.
37. Patel AR, Dubrey SW, Mendes LA, Skinner M, Cupples A, Falk RH, et al. Right ventricular dilation in primary amyloidosis: An independent predictor of survival. Am J Cardiol. 1997;80:486-92.
38. Bodez D, Ternacle J, Guellich A, Galat A, Lim P, Radu C, et al. Prognostic value of right ventricular systolic function in cardiac amyloidosis. Amyloid. 2016;23:158-67.
39. Arvidsson S, Henein MY, Wikström G, Suhr OB, Lindqvist P. Right ventricular involvement in transthyretin amyloidosis. Amyloid. 2018;25(3):160-6.
40. Huntjens P, Zhang K, Soyama Y, Karmpalioti M, Zhang R, Lenihan D, et al. Right ventricular free wall strain predicts mortality in patients with cardiac amyloidosis. J Am Coll Cardiol. 2020;75(11_Supplement_1):693.
41. Miller F Jr, Bellavia D. Comparison of right ventricular longitudinal strain imaging, tricuspid annular plane systolic excursion, and cardiac biomarkers for early diagnosis of cardiac involvement and risk stratification in primary systemic (AL) amyloidosis: Reply. Eur Heart J Cardiovasc Imaging. 2013;14(1):91-2.
42. Arvidsson S, Henein, MY, Wikström G, Suhr OB, Lindqvist P. Right ventricular involvement in transthyretin amyloidosis. Amyloid. 2018;25(3):160-6.

Echocardiographic Assessment of Right Ventricular Systolic and Diastolic Function

Satish Kumar Parashar

INTRODUCTION

Echocardiography (echo) is an established tool for the evaluation of cardiac structure and function and can be used for diagnosis, monitoring, and treatment guidance. Its widespread availability, versatility, and relative ease of use make it a fundamental investigation tool. However, most of the parameters derived from cardiac ultrasound examination mainly focused on the left chamber function, and less attention was paid to the study and interpretation of right ventricular (RV) systolic function. However, it has now been appreciated that RV function assessment plays a significant role in morbidity and mortality in large number of diseases. RV function is dependent on *preload*, afterload, *contractility*, pericardial constraint, interaction with the left ventricle, and cardiac rhythm. Hence, RV functions can be affected by RV volume overload, pressure overload, and intrinsic myocardial disease. Right ventricle responds better to volume overloading compared to pressure load being a thin-walled structure, with favorable loading conditions. Though cardiac magnetic resonance imaging (cMRI) is the gold standard for evaluation of RV systolic functions, together with computed tomography (CT) and nuclear imaging, but both older and new echo techniques are rapidly catching up to provide significant diagnostic and prognostic information. For clarity on RV systolic functions, the chapter will be covered in the following headings:

- Why is it important to evaluate?
- Problems in evaluating
- Imaging planes for evaluation
- Principles in evaluation, RV dimensions
- The basic and advanced parameters for evaluation

WHY IS IT IMPORTANT TO EVALUATE?

The importance of evaluation was felt because of its unfavorable impact on prognosis in various cardiac disorders. In a study of 416 patients with myocardial infarction with left ventricular ejection fraction (LVEF) of <40%, RV function remained an independent predictor of total mortality, cardiovascular mortality, and heart failure (HF). Each 5% decrease in the right ventricular fractional area change (RVFAC) was associated with 16% increased odds of cardiovascular mortality.[1] In pulmonary hypertension (PH), morbidity and mortality are more related to RV adaptation rather than absolute value of PH. Prognosis is strongly related to RV function.[2,3]

PROGNOSTIC ROLE OF RIGHT VENTRICULAR FUNCTIONS IN CARDIAC SURGERY

It is well recognized that right ventricular dysfunction (RVD) has an adverse short- and long-term impact in various interventional or surgical procedures.[4-7] Preoperative RVD assessed by a composite of echocardiographic variables was independently associated with 3.5-fold increased risk of 30-day mortality after left-sided heart valve surgery. In addition, it is associated with 4.2-fold increased risk of multiple postoperative adverse events. Preoperative RVD is present in approximately 20% of subjects undergoing left-sided valve surgery. As such a strong consideration should be given to incorporation of RVD in preoperative surgical risk scores. Right heart dysfunction in patients with left HF also increases mortality. Right heart function and functional reserve have also gained attention in patients with valvular heart disease.

PROBLEMS IN EVALUATING

- Some of the problems in evaluating RV function have been few limitations in its anatomy and physiology. The right ventricle is located behind the sternum, which limits echo image quality. It has an unusual shape, which is crescentic to triangular. It has an irregular endocardial surface with pronounced apical trabeculations, which leads to difficulty in tracing endocardium. The right ventricle is divided into three major components: (1) The inflow tract which consists of the tricuspid valve (TV), tendinous chords, and three or more papillary muscles; (2) the trabeculated apex; and (3) the infundibulum or RV outflow tract, All the three cannot be seen at the same time by 2D echo.

- The right ventricle has a distinct myocardial structure compared with the left ventricle. The RV wall is mainly composed of superficial and deep muscle layers, where the fibers of the superficial layer are arranged more or less circumferentially and the deep muscle fibers are longitudinally aligned from the base to the apex. The deep muscle layers account for about 80% of RV contraction, RV contraction relies more on longitudinal shortening than twisting and rotational movements as in the left ventricle.
- *Imaging planes:* As per the usual echocardiographic protocol, all views in which right ventricle is visualized should be scanned. However, acquisition of right ventricle-focused apical four-chamber view is vital for full delineation of the right ventricular free wall (RVFW). The right ventricle-focused view has been shown to provide more reproducible measurements of RV size and function than the conventional apical four-chamber view, especially for the evaluation of some functional parameters as described further. Moreover, whole right ventricle is seen in this view with no foreshortening **(Fig. 1)**.

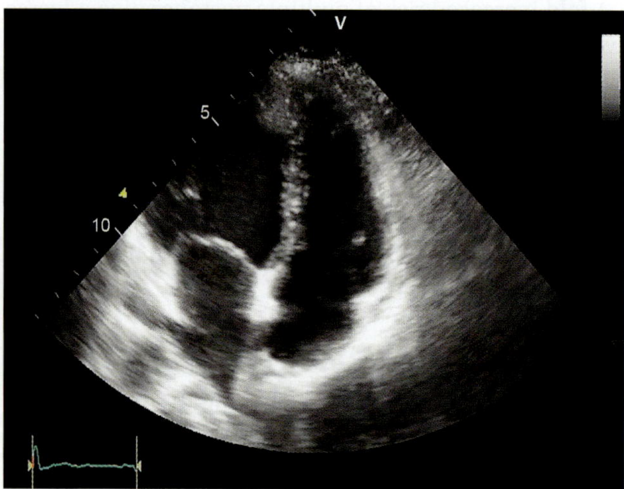

Fig. 1: Focused view of right ventricle which is seen on the right side of image.

EVALUATION OF BASIC, BUT IMPORTANT, PARAMETERS BEYOND RIGHT VENTRICULAR FUNCTION

Prior to evaluation of RV functions, certain right-sided dimensions and other hemodynamic parameters need to be evaluated by qualitative and quantitative methods. These include: Right atrial (RA) and RV dimensions, evaluation of RA pressure by inferior vena cava (IVC) evaluation of its size and degree of inspiratory collapse, 2D and Doppler evaluation of peak and mean pulmonary artery (PA) pressure, and evaluation of PA early and late end-diastolic pressure by interrogating pulmonary regurgitation jet. Due to the constraint of space, these are not discussed here. For RV size, **Figure 2 and Box 1** show a rough estimate of RV size in relation to left ventricle. **Figure 3** shows a dilated right ventricle in relation to left ventricle.

Parameters for evaluation of right ventricular systolic functions: These are usually divided into basic and advanced parameters **(Boxes 2 and 3)**.

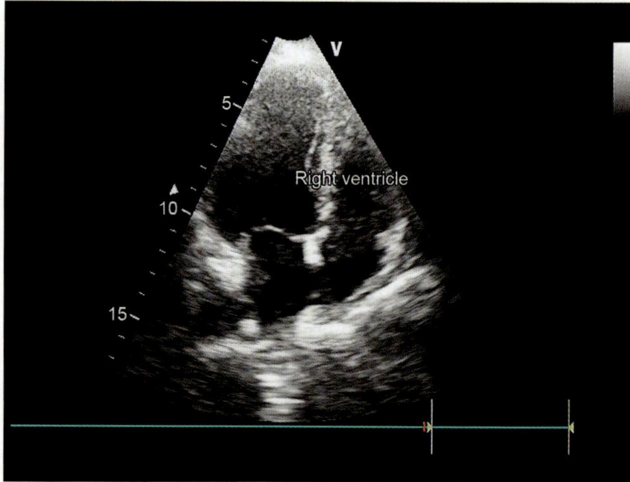

Fig. 2: Qualitative idea of right ventricle dimension in relation to left ventricle.

BOX 1: Rough estimate of RV size in comparison to left ventricle.

- *Normal:* <2/3rds of left ventricle
- *Mildly enlarged:* >2/3rds but inferior to left ventricle
- *Moderately enlarged:* Roughly equal to left ventricle
- *Severely enlarged:* More than left ventricle
- *Rule of thumb:* Normal EDDr < 1.0: Any value >1.0 indicates right ventricle +, >1.5: Severe

(EDDr: end-diastolic dimension ratio; RV: right ventricle)

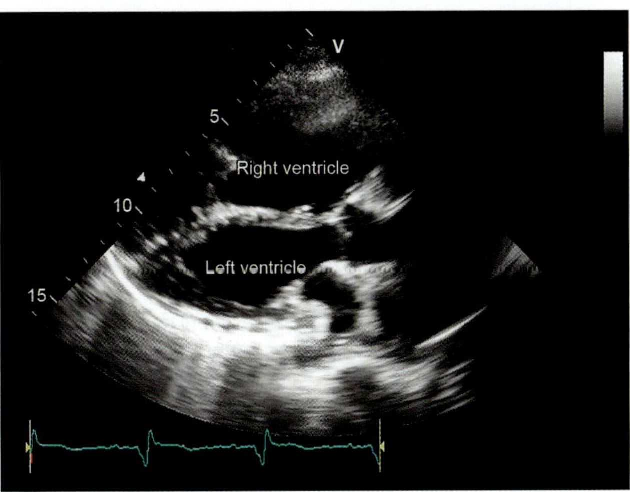

Fig. 3: Parasternal long-axis (PLAX) view showing a large right ventricle in relation to left ventricle.

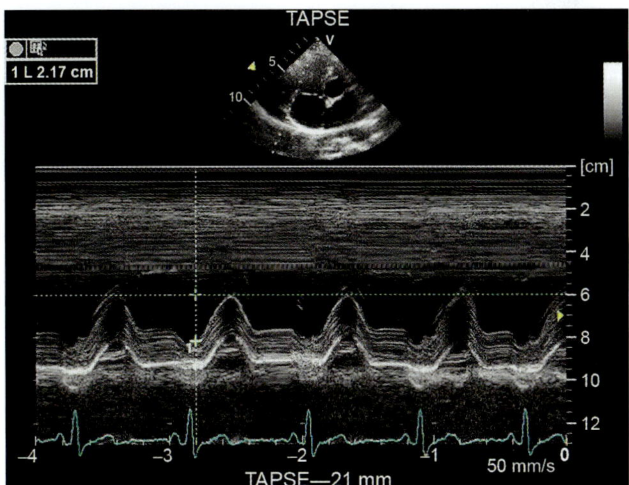

Fig. 4: Normal RV function with TAPSE of 21 mm. (RV: right ventricular; TAPSE: tricuspid annular plane systolic excursion)

BOX 2: Basic parameters employed in daily clinical practice.

Basic parameters
- *RV, RA dimensions:*
  - *Global functions:*
    - Pulsed Doppler—MPI
    - TDI-derived MPI
  - *Global systolic functions:* Fractional area change
  - *Longitudinal systolic functions:*
    - TAPSE
    - TDI—S′ velocity

(MPI: myocardial performance index; RA: right atrial; RV: right ventricular; S′ velocity: systolic velocity; TAPSE: tricuspid annular plane systolic excursion; TDI: tissue Doppler imaging)

BOX 3: Advanced parameters available in high-end equipment.

RV systolic functions:
- *Advanced parameters:*
  - 3D echocardiography
  - RVEF
  - Myocardial deformation echocardiography
  - Free-wall longitudinal strain

(RV: right ventricular; RVEF: right ventricular ejection fraction)

Basic Parameters for Evaluation of Right Ventricular Systolic Function

Under normal preload and afterload conditions, the longitudinally oriented myofibers predominantly generate RV stroke volume. Thus, imaging parameters that reflect longitudinal function such as tricuspid annular plane systolic excursion (TAPSE), tissue Doppler imaging (TDI) systolic (S′) velocities, and free-wall longitudinal strain (FWLS) may be ideal measures of RV function.

Tricuspid Annular Plane Systolic Excursion

It is one of the most frequently used parameters because of the ease and rapidity in obtaining it. Like left ventricle, it is based on the principle that right ventricle contracts like a piston, with annulus showing a prominent motion in comparison to apical motion. Greater the movement of the annular plane the better is the RV function. To obtain, it is ensured that the M-mode cursor intersects the lateral tricuspid annulus and RV apex throughout the cardiac cycle and maintains parallel alignment with annular motion from the right ventricle-focused view and patient is asked to hold breath. Excursion of the annulus is measured from end diastole to peak systole **(Figs. 4 and 5)**. Focusing on the TV annulus, using the zoom feature, and increasing the sweep speed will improve TAPSE accuracy The normal value is about 20–24 mm. Abnormal threshold is <17 mm. It is an indicator of RV longitudinal function and a good indicator of right ventricular ejection fraction (RVEF). TAPSE has been shown to correlate closely with RVEF determined by radionucleotide ventriculography and magnetic resonance imaging (MRI), and it is a strong prognostic marker in PH and other cardiovascular diseases.

Sato et al.[8] in a study of 53 patients with PH reported that TAPSE ≥2.0 cm had a sensitivity 84.6%, specificity 88.9%, positive predictive value (PPV) 88%, and negative

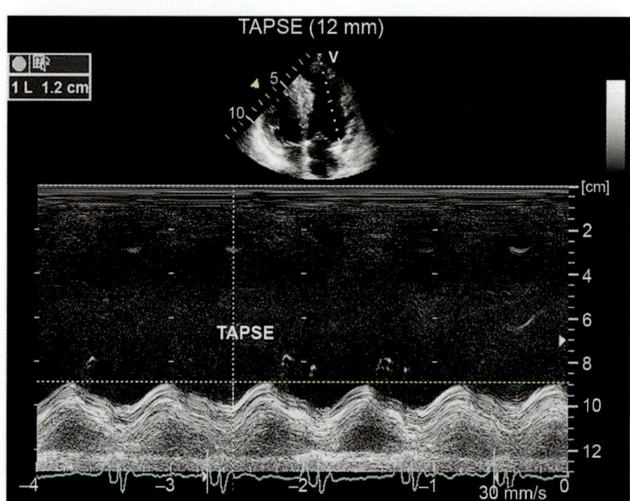

Fig. 5: A case of RV dysfunction with TAPSE of 12 mm. (RV: right ventricular; TAPSE: tricuspid annular plane systolic excursion)

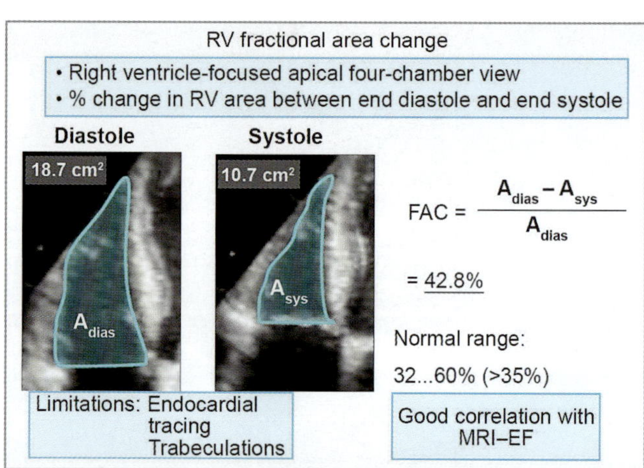

Fig. 6: Diagrammatic representation for calculation of FAC. (A_{dias}: end-diastolic area; A_{sys}: end-systolic area; EF: ejection fraction; FAC: fractional area change; MRI: magnetic resonance imaging; RV: right ventricle)

predictive value (NPV) 85.7% *to predict* cardiac magnetic resonance (CMR) RVEF >40%, while TAPSE ≤15 mm had a PPV of 100% *to predict* RVEF <40%.

Limitations of tricuspid annular plane systolic excursion

- Angle- and load-dependent
- Underestimation in suboptimal image quality, misalignment of the M-mode cursor with tricuspid annular motion, interference from indwelling pacemakers or catheters, and the postoperative state, following cardiothoracic surgery
- Reflects primarily longitudinal function and interrogates only one small segment of right ventricle
- Should not be reported in isolation
- Increased with severe tricuspid regurgitation (TR)

Right Ventricular Fractional Shortening

Together with TAPSE it is one of the most frequently used routine study employed in daily practice. Fractional area change (FAC) is an echocardiographic measure of RV systolic function that correlates well with cMRI-derived RVEF.[9] From a right ventricle-focused view, the RV endocardium is traced in end systole and end diastole from the lateral tricuspid annulus along the RVFW to the apex, then back along the interventricular septum (IVS) to the medial tricuspid annulus, including papillary muscles, trabeculations, and the moderator band. If need be, ultrasound-enhancing agents can be used to enhance RV endocardial border definition for FAC quantification. FAC is the area difference between the RV end-diastolic and end-systolic areas measured through ideally right ventricle-focused apical view **(Figs. 6 and 7)**. FAC, unlike TAPSE and TDI S′ velocity, reflects both RVFW longitudinal shortening and radial thickening. FAC has been validated with cMRI[10] and shown to be an independent predictor for sudden death, mortality after pulmonary embolism, heart failure, stroke, and myocardial infarction. Normal range is 49% ± 7%. An FAC < 35% is considered abnormal. FAC is especially useful in assessing RV systolic function when TDI S′ velocity and/or TAPSE are underestimated in the immediate postoperative period or influenced by loading conditions and geometric remodeling.

Limitations of right ventricular fractional area change

- Technically difficult and heavily depends on image quality, especially good, focused view
- Load dependency
- Uncertainty of correct tracing due to trabeculations
- Only fair interobserver reproducibility, especially in RV enlargement, hence poor reproducibility
- Not useful in atrial fibrillation and tachycardia (~110 beats/min)

Tissue Doppler Systolic Excursion Velocity (TDI-S′)

Tissue Doppler imaging S′ velocity measures how fast the basal RVFW segment moves during peak systole as a surrogate of RV longitudinal systolic function. To measure this parameter, right ventricle-focused view is used with tissue Doppler region of interest placed at the lateral corner of the tricuspid annulus acquired at high

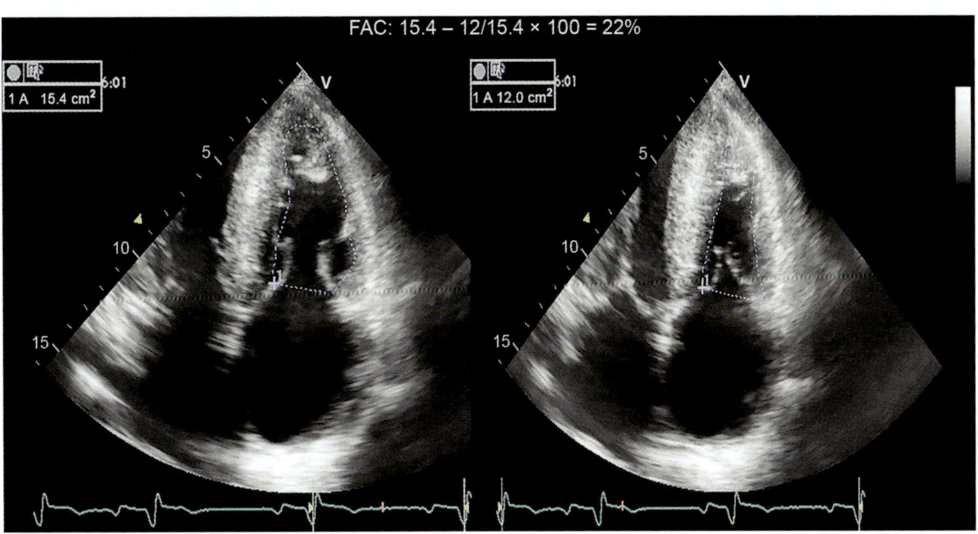

Fig. 7: RV-FAC in a patient with RV dysfunction. Right ventricle is on the right side of the image. The FAC is 22%. (FAC: fractional area change; RV: right ventricle)

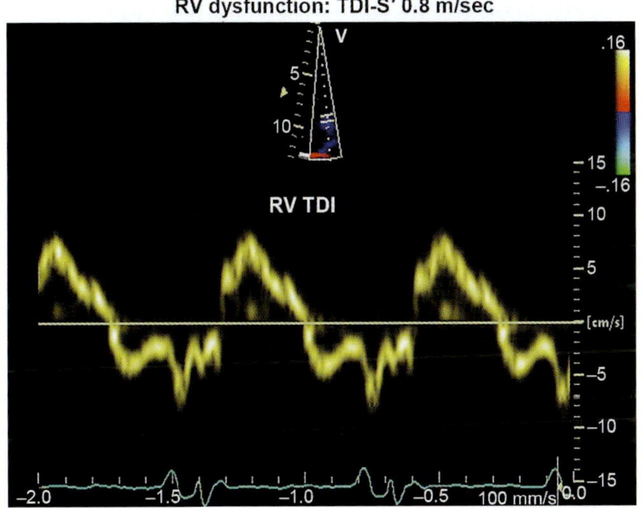

Fig. 8: An RV-TDI systolic velocity of 0.8 m/s in a case of RV cardiomyopathy. (RV: right ventricle; TDI: tissue Doppler imaging)

frame rate. As this measurement is angle dependent, a maximum angle between the axis of contraction and ultrasound beam should be <20°. The velocity S is read as the highest systolic velocity above the baseline. A number of validation studies have been performed which showed moderate correlations to radionuclide angiography and cMRI-determined RVEF. An abnormal value suggestive of RVD is <9.5 cm/s **(Fig. 8)**.

Limitations of tissue Doppler systolic excursion velocity

- Underestimated with poor image quality, inadequate optimization of the Doppler gain or filter settings, and misalignment of the Doppler beam with the plane of motion
- Measures only a small subsection of right ventricle, hence should not be used in isolation but rather in conjunction with other supportive findings
- Values vary with overall heart motion
- Does not parallel TAPSE in all cases

Myocardial Performance Index

Myocardial performance index (MPI), also known as Tei index, is a parameter of global RV systolic and diastolic functions. It is inversely related to RVEF. Following RV diastolic filling, isovolumic contraction begins. Isovolumetric contraction time (IVCT; milliseconds) reflects the interval between TV closure and pulmonary valve (PV) opening. The next interval is RV ejection, corresponding to ventricular systole (b). RV ejection time (ET; milliseconds) measures the interval during which blood is ejected across the PV **(Figs. 9 and 10)**. The next interval reflects the time between PV closure and TV opening, termed as the isovolumetric relaxation time (IVRT; milliseconds). RV-MPI can be calculated using two formulas:

(1) RV-MPI = [(IVRT + IVCT)/ET]

or

(2) RV-MPI = [(TCO – ET)/ET]

where TCO is the tricuspid closure-open interval (a), comprising of IVCT, ET, and IVRT. RV-MPI is acquired through either pulsed wave (PW) Doppler or TDI methods and is dimensionless.

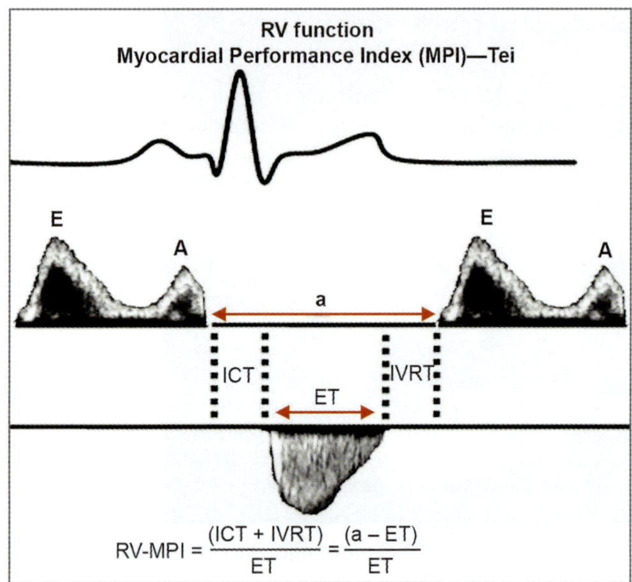

Fig. 9: Variables required to evaluate MPI. (ET: ejection time; ICT: isovolumic contraction time; IVRT: isovolumic relaxation time; RV: right ventricular)

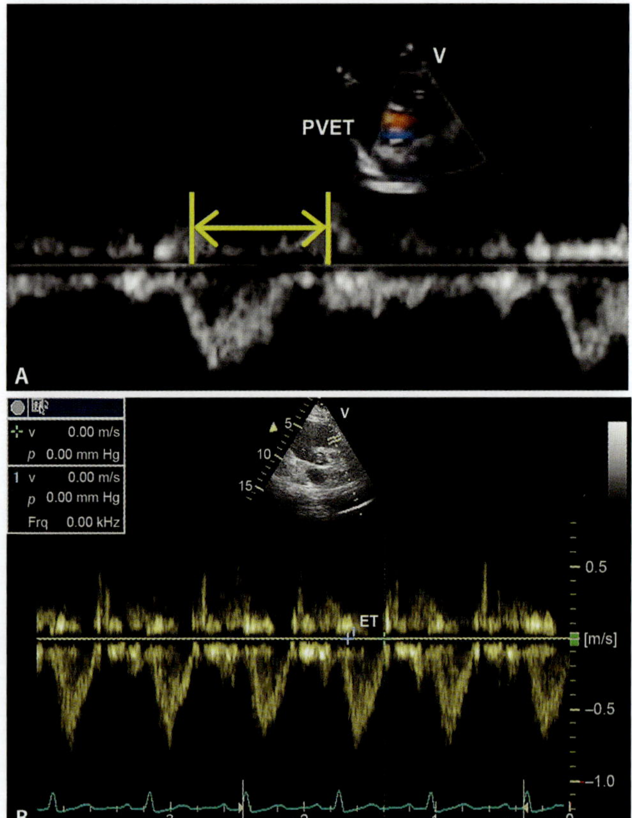

Figs. 10A and B: Ejection time (ET) is measured from onset to termination of RVOT flow. (PVET: pulmonary valve ejection time; RVOT: right ventricular outflow tract)

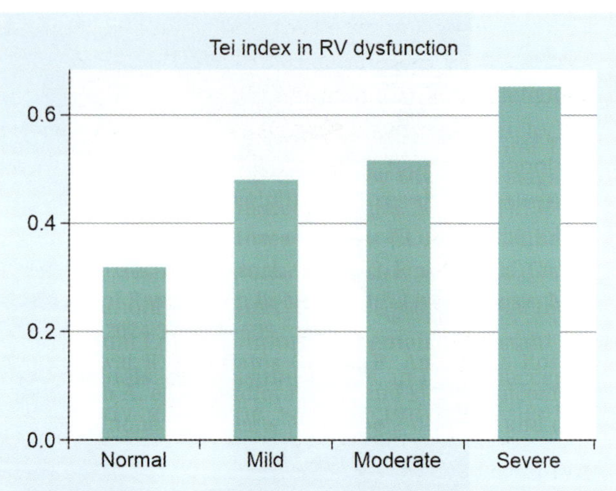

Fig. 11: Progressive increase in Tei index values with deteriorating right ventricular (RV) function.

Three variables need to be recorded by pulsed Doppler. The MPI is calculated as a-b/b. The normal upper value is about 0.40. This can also be calculated from TDI whose upper value is about 0.54. A higher RV-MPI value typically indicates impaired RV function, while a lower value suggests better function. The reason for increase in MPI value is that in RVD, the isovolumic contraction time (ICT) increases and ET decreases, thereby increasing the ratio **(Fig. 11)**. MPI has shown to have predictive values in future events in patients with PH, congenital heart disease, RV infarction, hypertrophic cardiomyopathy, coronary artery disease, etc. However, currently it is not a favored test, except in some institutions.

Limitations of myocardial performance index

- Needs two different cardiac beats for determining the time periods
- Inability to obtain crisp tracing of tricuspid Doppler
- Elevated RA pressure
- Influenced by arrhythmias and R–R interval variability
- Not recommended as the sole quantitative method for evaluating RV function because of load dependency
- Increased preload and right heart congestion, such as fluid overload, can prolong IVCT and IVRT, leading to an increased RV-MPI
- Increased afterload can also prolong IVCT and IVRT, resulting in a higher RV-MPI

Myocardial Deformation: Strain

- Myocardial deformation, or strain [right ventricular longitudinal strain (RVLS)], is defined as deformation of an object compared with its initial shape and is expressed as a percentage. RVLS is the longitudinal shortening of fibers between the base and apex of the right ventricle in systole and is expressed as a negative percentage. RVLS is currently measured by 2D echo speckle tracking analysis, rather than TDI. It depends heavily on the imaging quality of the endocardial/myocardial borders and should be measured in the right ventricle-focused view with a high frame rate. Nomenclature is important when reporting strain. Right ventricular global longitudinal strain (RVGLS) refers to the average strain of six segments, including the basal, midventricular, and apical segments of the RVFW and IVS. In contrast, right ventricular free-wall strain (RVFWS) refers to the average strain of the three segments of the basal, midventricular, and apex. RVFW alone is a more reliable and accurate way to measure RV systolic function, which is not load-dependent and has been validated in various studies including with CMR for several human cardiovascular diseases. The normal value for free wall is about –25% to –30%. Values of RVFWS > –20% is regarded as abnormal with values > –15% identifying those with severe reduction with a strong adverse prognostic factor in a large number of diseases **(Figs. 12A and B)**. It is strongly correlated with RV ejection fraction. It can be a good indicator of RVD, especially at early stages.[10]

Limitations of strain imaging

- Intervendor variability in strain estimates[11]
- *Limited acoustic window:* Unlike LV strain which can be measured from three apical views, the RV strain is only limited to preferably right ventricle-focused view. Hence three-dimensional speckle tracking echocardiography (3DSTE) analysis is the best method for measuring RV strain and is being increasingly employed only in limited canters.
- Increased preload may result in higher strain measurements. Conversely, increased afterload may depress strain measurements.
- Tachycardia decreases temporal resolution.
- Limited availability
- Cost-effectiveness and training

Three Dimension Echocardiography

Over the past decade, improvements in 3D echocardiography (3DE) have led to its incorporation in the assessment of the left heart. This has also led to a growing dataset establishing 3DE as a promising novel way of RV imaging. 3DE can circumvent most of the limitations of 2D parameters and calculate RVEF which is the best measure of global RV function. 3DE has the unique advantages of simultaneously allowing assessment of several parameters of the right heart, including volumes, function, ejection fraction, TAPSE, etc. **(Fig. 13)**. The normal range is 50–60% with abnormal threshold <45%. Several studies have shown 3DE-determined RV volumes and function correlated well with cMRI. This has been made possible with improvement of image quality of 3DE and more user-friendly RV quantification software and fast acquisition. *RVEF* is the most important predictor of clinical outcomes and response to therapy in almost every case of RVD.[12]

Limitations of three dimension echocardiography

- Right ventricular anatomy is not a "friend".
- Dependency on image quality, leading to exclusion of 20–25% of cases
- Severely dilated ventricle, in which whole RV cannot be imaged
- Need for training and expertise
- Specific expensive hardware and software, time, and expertise

Recent update on discordant findings

Máté et al.,[13] in a landmark study, were the first to assess the disagreement between the conventional parameters and 3D RVEF and their clinical significance. The important summary of their study were: (1) RVD assessment based on the guideline-recommended cutoff values of TAPSE, FAC, and FWLS is only modestly concordant with the results of RVEF-based assessment; (2) Among normal RVEF, significant proportions exhibited impaired TAPSE (21%), FAC (33%), or FWLS (8%). Conversely, numerous patients with reduced RVEF had normal TAPSE (46%), FAC (26%), or FWLS (41%). (3) RVD indicated by FWLS shows the best agreement with RVD diagnosed based on RVEF; (4) Combining impaired conventional parameters showed that outcomes were the worst if at least two parameters are impaired and relatively better if only one or none of them are abnormal; (5) As such, a multiparametric approach is needed in the assessment of RV function, especially if 3DE is not available.

Right Ventricle–Pulmonary Artery Coupling (Tricuspid Annular Plane Systolic Excursion: Pulmonary Artery Systolic Pressure Ratio)

The coupling between the right ventricle and the PA reflects the ability of the right ventricle to adapt to the pulmonary

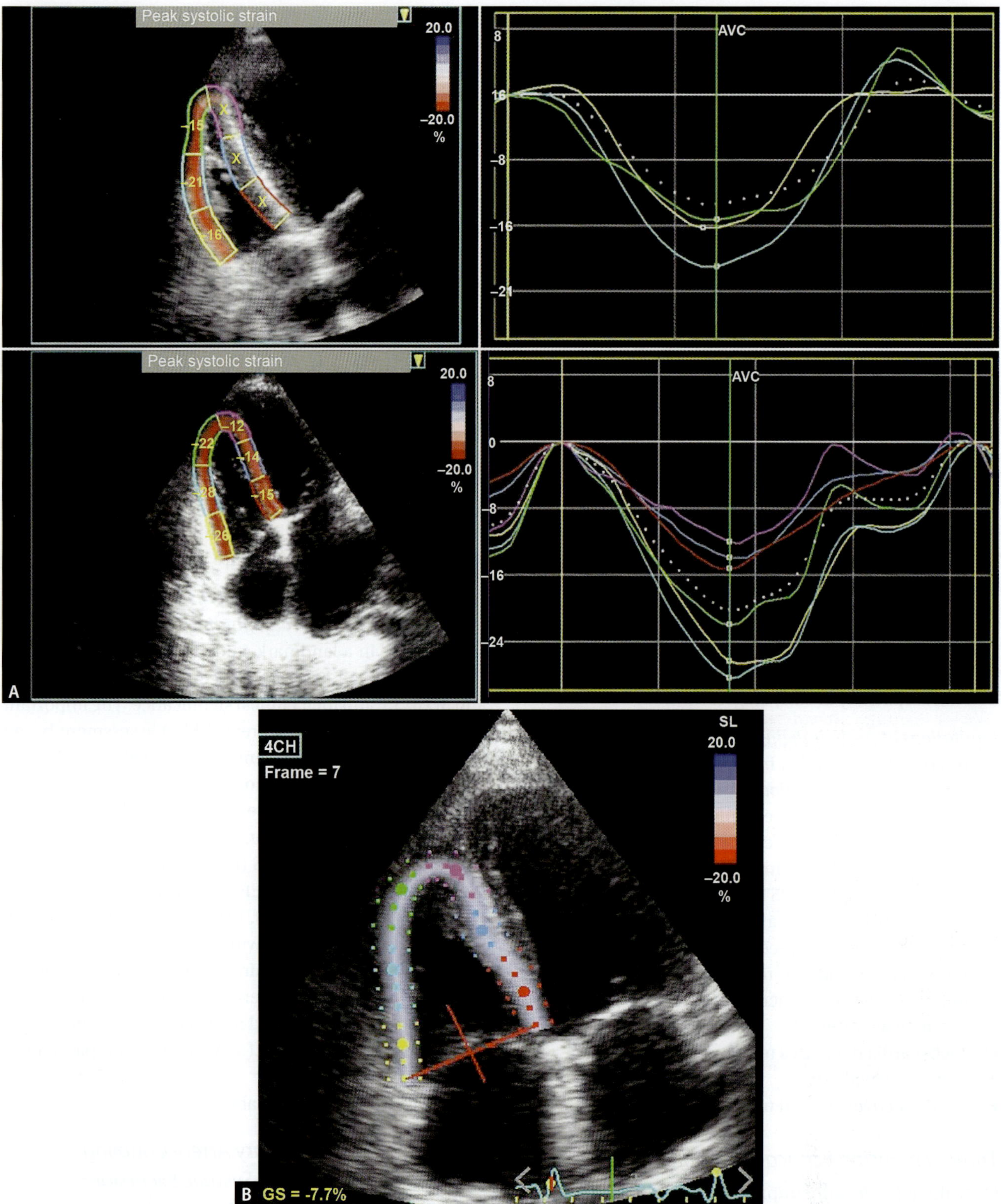

Figs. 12A and B: (A) Upper panel shows average peak systolic strain of three segments of RV free wall, while lower panel shows average global longitudinal strain of all six segments; (B) Shows significantly deranged RV function with average global strain (GS) of -7.7%. (AVC: aortic valve closure)

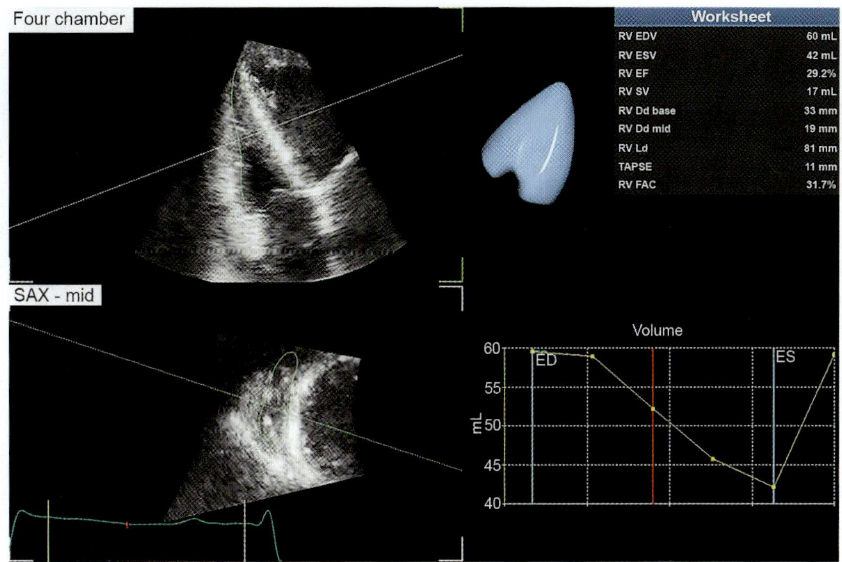

Fig. 13: 3D image for RV function showing multiple parameters being simultaneously evaluated. (ED: end diastole; EDV: end-diastolic volume; EF: ejection fraction; ES: end systole; ESV: end-systolic volume; Dd: diastolic dysfunction; FAC: fractional area change; SAX: short-axis view; SV: stroke volume; TAPSE: tricuspid annular plane systolic excursion)

vascular load and maintain sufficient RV cardiac output. Under normal physiological conditions, the PA system regulates blood flow, which it receives from right ventricle, through its elasticity and resistance to ensure the smooth entry of blood into the pulmonary circulation. This right ventricle-pulmonary artery (RV–PA) coupling is typically assessed through invasive right heart catheterization (RHC). Lately, several novel echocardiographic indices have been tested as noninvasive surrogates of RV–PA coupling, one of which is TAPSE/pulmonary artery systolic pressure (PASP) ratio. Its significance and independent prognostic value has been reported in various studies. Guazzi et al.[14] and Bok et al.[15] reported that TAPSE/PASP ratio serves as a strong and independent predictor of mortality and is negatively correlated with New York Heart Association (NYHA) functional classification. Normal value of TAPSE/PASP is >0.40–0.50 mm/mm Hg. For patients with uncoupled RV–PA coupling, TAPSE/PASP ≤ 0.32 mm/mm Hg is regarded as an indication of severe uncoupling of RV–PA with poor prognosis **(Figs. 14 and 15)**. TAPSE/PASP has been validated with invasive RV pressure–volume (P–V) analysis in a small group of patients with severe pulmonary arterial hypertension (PAH). Consequently, TAPSE:PASP ratio has been incorporated into the risk assessment algorithm of the 2022 European Society of Cardiology (ESC)/European Respiratory Society (ERS) PH Guidelines.[16]

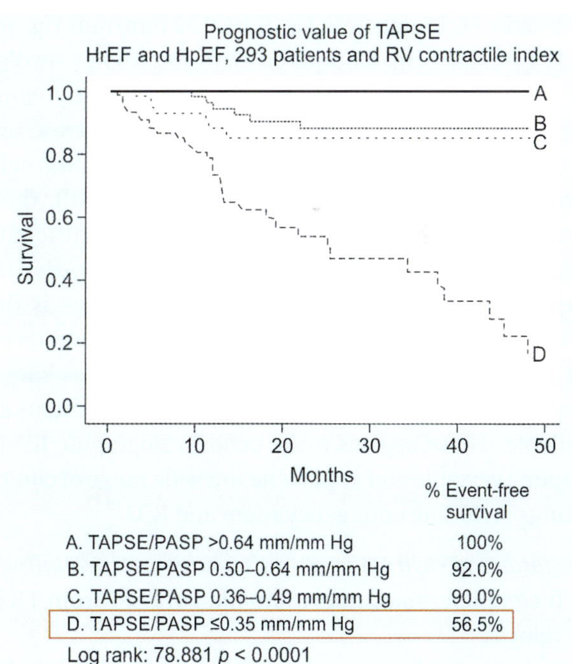

Fig. 14: Outcome of adverse TAPSE:PASP ratio. (HFpEF: heart failure with preserved ejection fraction; HFrEF: heart failure with reduced ejection fraction; PASP: pulmonary artery systolic pressure; TAPSE: tricuspid annular plane systolic excursion)
Source: Adapted from Guazzi M, et al.[14]

Various studies have reported that a TAPSE/PASP ratio <0.33 mm/mm Hg is an independent poor prognostic marker and indicates poor survival. Tello et al.[17] divided

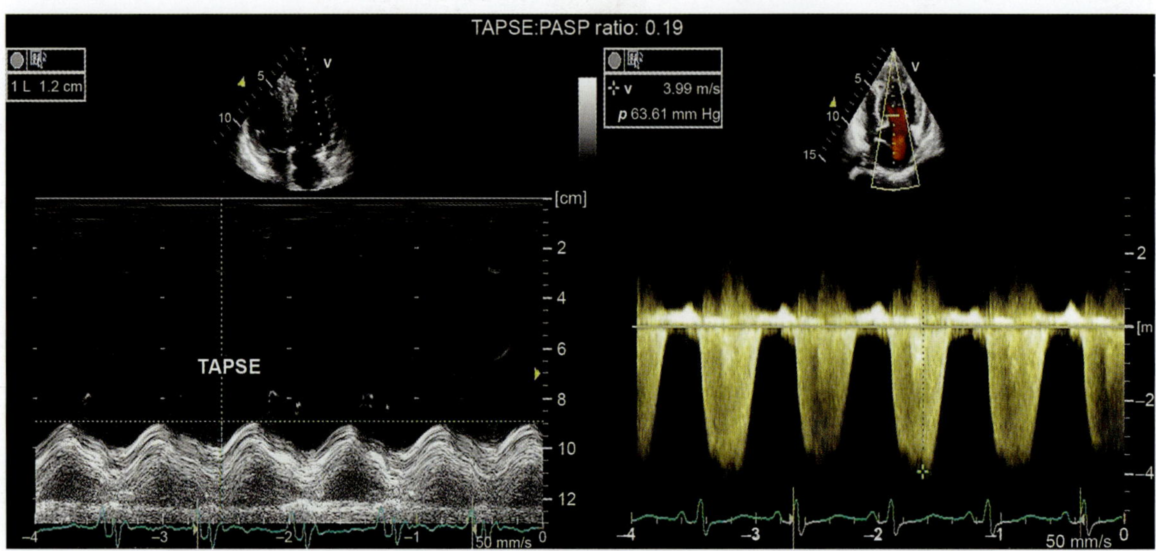

Fig. 15: Ratio of 0.19 indicates an adverse prognosis. (PASP: pulmonary artery systolic pressure; TAPSE: tricuspid annular plane systolic excursion)

patients with PAH into the following tertiles of the TAPSE/PASP ratio: <0.19 mm/mm Hg, 0.19–0.32 mm/mm Hg, and >0.32 mm/mm Hg. Compared with the higher tertiles, the lowest tertile TAPSE/PASP had significantly worse hemodynamics, echocardiographic characteristics, and worse overall survival.[18] These RV–PA coupling echo parameters have several advantages. First of all, these parameters have been demonstrated to significantly correlate with the invasive parameter. Secondly, the notable difference with other novel parameters is that specific software or advanced measurement methods are not required. Its value can be readily calculated as long as M-mode and continuous wave Doppler measurements are available. These aspects make echocardiographic RV–PA coupling versatile and applicable to a wide range of clinical settings including emergency room and ICU.[19]

Limitations of right ventricle–pulmonary artery coupling

- Incomplete/inaccurate estimation of PASP from TR jet velocity
- Incorrect evaluation of inferior vena cava (IVC) profile
- Limitations of TAPSE as mentioned earlier

Myocardial Work

In recent years, noninvasive myocardial work (MW) quantification of the left ventricle has emerged as an innovative tool for assessing myocardial function. This method integrates measurements of strain and LV pressure, providing a comprehensive evaluation of the heart's performance. As for left ventricular myocardial work (LVMW), significant progress has been made in its application to clinical practice. However, data on right ventricular myocardial work (RVMW) remains limited, and its measurement method has yet to be established. Limited studies have explored RVMW using a standard algorithm. These studies utilized software initially designed for LVMW, emphasizing the need for dedicated RVMW software and validation. The review articles by Nonaka et al.[18] and Trimarchi et al.[20] will give a detailed information of MW.[21]

Right Ventricular Diastolic Functions

Compared to left ventricle, the RV diastolic functions have been less studied, because initially it involved hemodynamic studies and limitations of providing good Doppler parameters. RV diastolic function is of crucial importance for both symptoms and survival not only in patients with right-sided HF but also in patients with left-sided HF.

Tricuspid Inflow and Tissue Doppler Imaging Myocardial Velocities

Two major determinants of RV diastolic dysfunction are: (1) Impaired relaxation and (2) decreased compliance or increased stiffness. RV diastole starts with closure of PV and ends with closure of TV. An apical right ventricle-focused view is highly desirable. The early, rapid filling phase of diastole is represented by the tricuspid E wave. The E-wave deceleration time reflects RV relaxation (*n* 150–230 msec). Atrial contraction occurs in late diastole and is represented by the tricuspid A wave. Doppler assessments are integrated with standard morphologic evaluations of the right atrium, right ventricle, and IVC for size and collapsibility **(Fig. 16)**. The early diastolic tissue Doppler velocity, commonly denoted as e′, represents RV relaxation **(Fig. 17)**. The basic rule of diastolic dysfunction is shown in **(Fig. 18)**. Increased E/A and E/e′ ratios represent increased RV filling pressures due to decreased compliance. In adults, E/e′ ratio of <6:1 is considered normal. With normal diastolic function, the early filling velocity is higher than the atrial contraction velocity; therefore, reversal of the E/A ratio (<0.8) with increased deceleration time represents impaired

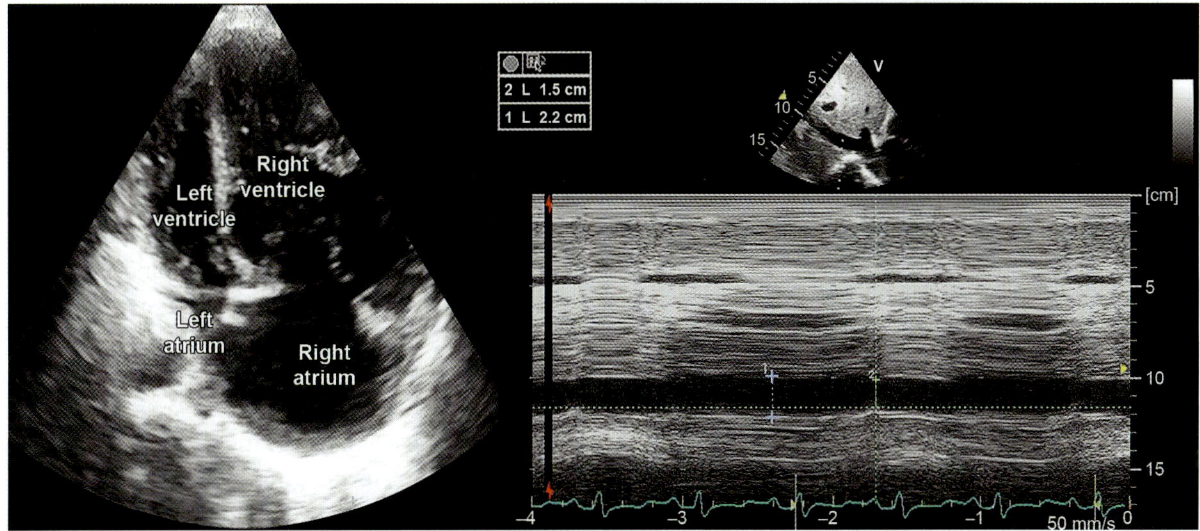

Fig. 16: Dilated right ventricle and right atrium. On the tight side, there is enlargement of inferior vena cava (IVC) with decreased inspiratory collapse (2.2 cm/1.5 cm).

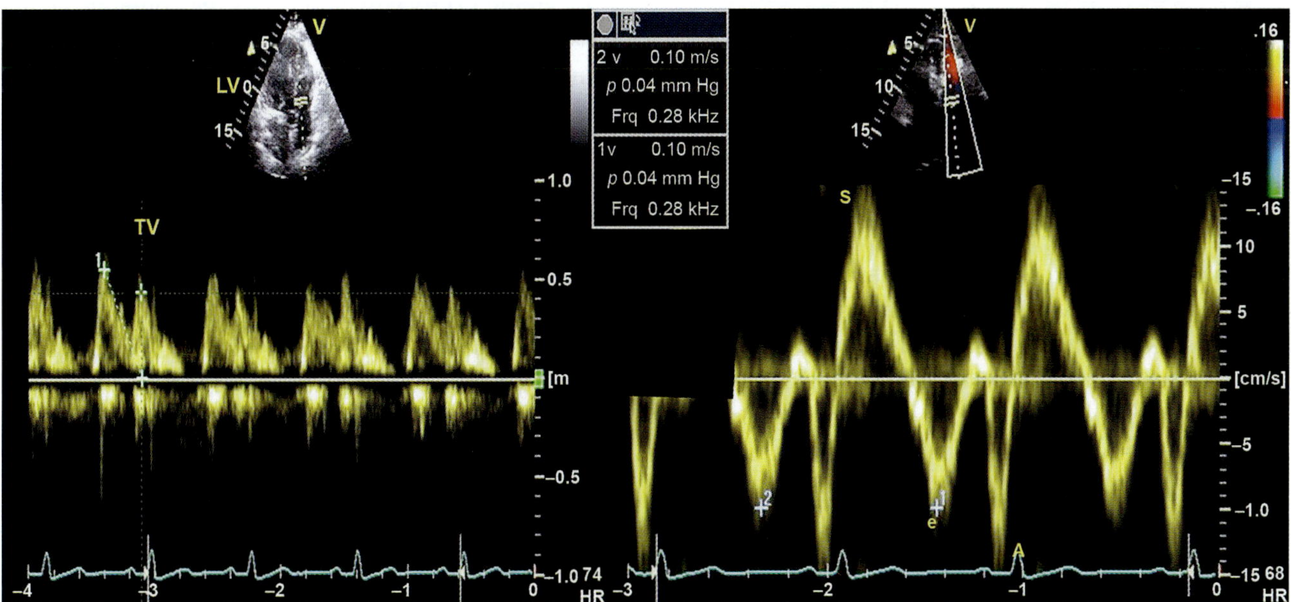

Fig. 17: Shows tricuspid valve (TV) Doppler on left side and TDI at lateral tricuspid annulus on right side. ‘s’: TDI systolic wave, é′: early diastolic wave, Á′: atrial contraction wave. The TV E/A ratio is normal at 1.27.

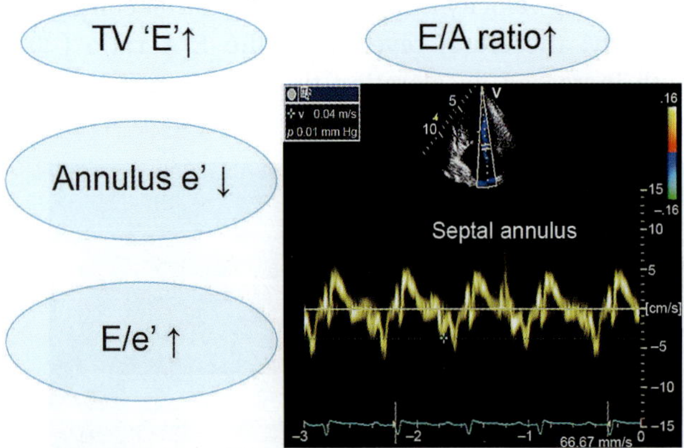

Fig. 18: Algorithm showing rule of diastolic dysfunction. (RVFP: right ventricular filling pressure)

ventricular relaxation. An accentuated relationship of the rapid filling and the atrial contraction velocities (E/A > 2.1) with decreased deceleration time (<120 ms) represents restrictive physiology—a late phase of diastolic dysfunction. Tricuspid inflow is very sensitive to preload, afterload, and respiration, hence Doppler signals should be obtained at end expiration/held respiration/during quiet breathing. Alternatively, five to seven beats should be acquired to account for the effect of respiration on the inflow velocities. Hemodynamically significant TV disease and atrial arrhythmias can also confound diastolic parameters. Age and sex-specific differences in E/A ratio and TDI tricuspid e′ velocities have been described, with higher inflow velocities seen in older healthy women. In summary, the echocardiographic assessment of RV diastolic function is challenging due to limitations inherent to the right ventricle. Nevertheless, quantification of RV diastolic function is possible and should be routinely performed using a combination of different parameters.

CONCLUSION

The evaluation of RV systolic function should be an integral part of all echo examinations due to its prognostic impact in various diseases. Good clinical assessment is imperative before echo studies. A systematic evaluation of RV size and function requires the use of several parameters derived from different noninvasive modalities. 2D echo is the clinical workhorse of RV evaluation and provides simple, reproducible, and meaningful single-plane surrogates of RV function. Visual impression of RV size, contractility, and thickness is a starting point: Starts or ends there? Simple and reproducible methods for routine studies such as TAPSE, TDI-S′, and FAC have gained popularity because of the ease in obtaining these parameters. With the advancement in imaging technology, 3DE is being increasingly utilized for evaluation of RVEF, though cMRI is the gold standard.

In this chapter, three new echocardiographic indices for RV function assessment have been briefly outlined: (1) RV strain, (2) RVMW, and (3) RV–PA coupling. Of the three parameters, RV strain has already accumulated the most clinical data. All these have the potential to become key parameters in RV function assessment in the near future, and larger-scale studies and further preclinical fundamental investigations will enhance their prospects. As each basic and advanced technique has its own limitations, a combination of approaches is still suggested for the overall evaluation of RV function in a complementary fashion only. Machine learning and AI methods may, in the future, help to overcome the obstacles of RV complex shape and physiology and offer a more accurate and reproducible assessment of its global function. Right ventricular diastolic dysfunction (RVDD) is a piece of the puzzle that describes right and left heart functions and their interactions, and its early occurrence should be used to alter management and preempt further deterioration of normal heart function and adverse outcome. **Box 4** shows ideal numbers to remember for normal RV functions.

BOX 4: Preferred values for normal RV functions.

Ideal numbers to remember—right ventricle

- TAPSE > 17 mm
- FAC > 35%
- TDI-S′ > 10 cm/s
- MPI < 0.43
- TDI–MPI: < 0.54
- RV free-wall strain > -25%
- 3D RVEF > 45%
  - RV–PA coupling: TAPSE/PASP: >0.40 mm/mm Hg
- RA area: <18.0 cm^2

(FAC: fractional area change; MPI: myocardial performance index; PA: pulmonary artery; PASP: pulmonary artery systolic pressure; RA: right atrial; RV: right ventricular; RVEF: right ventricular ejection fraction; TDI: tissue Doppler imaging; TDI-S′: tissue Doppler systolic excursion velocity; TAPSE: tricuspid annular plane systolic excursion)

REFERENCES

1. Zornoff LA, Skali H, Pfeffer MA, St John Sutton M, Rouleau JL, Lamas GA, et al.; SAVE Investigators. Right ventricular dysfunction and risk of heart failure and mortality after myocardial infarction. J Am Coll Cardiol. 2002;39(9):1450-5.
2. Labrada L, Vaidy A, Vaidya A. Right ventricular assessment in pulmonary hypertension. Curr Opin Pulm Med. 2023;29(5):348-54.
3. El-Kersh K, Zhao C, Elliott G, Farber HW, Gomberg-Maitland M, Selej M, et al. Derivation of a risk score (REVEAL-ECHO) based on echocardiographic parameters of patients with pulmonary arterial hypertension. Chest. 2023;163(5):1232-44.
4. Towheed A, Sabbagh E, Gupta R, Assiri S, Chowdhury MA, Moukarbel GV, et al. Right ventricular dysfunction and short-term outcomes following left-sided valvular surgery: An echocardiographic study. J Am Heart Assoc. 2021;10(4):e016283.
5. Davlouros PA, Niwa K, Webb G, Gatzoulis MA The right ventricle in congenital heart disease. Heart. 2006;92 (Suppl 1):i27-i38.
6. Merlo A, Cirelli C, Vizzardi E, Fiorendi L, Roncali F, Marino M, et al. Right Ventricular dysfunction before and after cardiac surgery. Prognostic Implications. J Clin Med. 2024;11:13(6):1609.
7. Owyang CG, Kim J. Moving beyond right ventricular ejection fraction: Incremental prognostic role of right ventricular strain on postcardiac transplant outcomes. Circ Cardiovasc Imaging. 2024;17(4):e016789.
8. Sato T, Tsujino I, Oyama-Manabe N, Ohira H, Ito YM, Sugimori H, et al. Simple prediction of right ventricular ejection fraction using tricuspid annular plane systolic excursion in pulmonary hypertension. Int J Cardiovasc Imaging. 2013;29(8):1799-805.
9. Anavekar NS, Gerson D, Skali H, Kwong RY, Yucel EK, Solomon SD, et al. Two-dimensional assessment of right ventricular function: an echocardiographic-MRI correlative study. Echocardiography. 2007;24(5):452-6.
10. Lee JH, Park JH. Strain analysis of the right ventricle using two-dimensional echocardiography. J Cardiovasc Imaging. 2018;26(3):111-24.
11. Yang H, Marwick TH, Fukuda N, Oe H, Saito M, Thomas JD, et al. Improvement in strain concordance between two major vendors after the strain standardization initiative. J Am Soc Echocardiogr. 2015;28(6):642-8.e7.
12. Badano LP, Kolias TJ, Muraru D, Abraham TP, Aurigemma G, Edvardsen T, et al; Industry representatives; Reviewers: This document was reviewed by members of the 2016–2018 EACVI Scientific Documents Committee. Standardization of left atrial, right ventricular, and right atrial deformation imaging using two-dimensional speckle tracking echocardiography: a consensus document of the EACVI/ASE/Industry Task Force to standardize deformation imaging. Eur Heart J Cardiovasc Imaging. 2018;19(6):591-600.
13. Máté T, Attila K, Noela R. Significant disagreement between conventional parameters and 3D echocardiography-derived ejection fraction in the detection of right ventricular systolic dysfunction and Its association with outcomes. J Am Soc Echocardiogr. 2024;37(7):677-86.
14. Guazzi M, Bandera F, Pelissero G, Castelvecchio S, Menicanti L, Ghio S, et al. Tricuspid annular plane systolic excursion and pulmonary arterial systolic pressure relationship in heart failure: an index of right ventricular contractile function and prognosis. Am J Physiol Heart Circ Physiol. 2013;305(9):H1373-81.
15. Bok Y, Kim JY, Park JH. Prognostic role of right ventricular-pulmonary artery coupling assessed by TAPSE/PASP ratio in patients with acute heart failure. J Cardiovasc Imaging. 2023;31(4):200-6.
16. Humbert M, Kovacs G, Hoeper MM, Badagliacca R, Berger RMF, Brida M, et al.; ESC/ERS Scientific Document Group. 2022 ESC/ERS Guidelines for the diagnosis and treatment of pulmonary hypertension. Eur Heart J. 2022; 43(38):3618-731.
17. Tello K, Wan J, Dalmer A, Vanderpool R, Ghofrani HA, Naeije R, et al. Validation of the tricuspid annular plane systolic excursion/systolic pulmonary artery pressure ratio for the assessment of right ventricular-arterial coupling in severe pulmonary hypertension. Circ Cardiovasc Imaging. 2019;12(9):e009047.
18. Nonaka H, Rätsep I, Obonyo NG, Suen JY, Fraser JF, Chan J. Current trends and latest developments in echocardiographic assessment of right ventricular function: load dependency perspective. Front Cardiovasc Med. 2024;11:1365798.
19. Wang X, Chen A, Yang L, Chen Y, Li Z, Li Z, et al. Evaluation methods and progress of right ventricular-pulmonary artery coupling. Adv Ultrasound Diagn Ther. 2024;8(4):205-16.
20. Trimarchi G, Carerj S, Di Bella G, Manganaro R, Pizzino F, Restelli D, et al. Clinical applications of myocardial work in echocardiography: A comprehensive review. J Cardiovasc Echogr. 2024;34(3):99-113.
21. Hameed A, Condliffe R, Swift AJ, Alabed S, Kiely DG, Charalampopoulos A. Assessment of right ventricular function—a state of the art. Curr Heart Fail Rep. 2023; 20(3):194-207.

SUGGESTED READING

1. Mukherjee M, Rudski LG, Addetia K, Afilalo J, D'Alto M, Freed BH, et al. Guidelines for the Echocardiographic Assessment of the Right Heart in Adults and Special Considerations in Pulmonary Hypertension: Recommendations from the American Society of Echocardiography. J Am Soc Echocardiogr. 2025;38(3):141-86.

An Update on Stress Echocardiography and Contrast

Shreya Ohri, Roxy Senior

INTRODUCTION

Over the years the role of stress echocardiography (SE) has evolved significantly, since the 2009 and then 2016 publications of the SE expert consensus by the European Association of Echocardiography, and the American Society of Echocardiography. Its application for the assessment of coronary artery disease has gone beyond simply looking at inducible new or worsening regional wall motion abnormalities (RWMA). This has now come to include perfusion using ultrasound-enhancing contrast agents (UCA), contractile reserve—global left ventricle (LV) function and use of strain, diastolic function, lung ultrasound (LUS), and Doppler-based assessment of the left anterior descending coronary artery (LAD) for coronary flow velocity reserve (CFVR). The most recent consensus statement on the clinical use of SE in chronic coronary artery disease—from the European Association of Cardiovascular Imaging, published in 2023 has converged these biomarkers into the ABCDE protocol.[1] This protocol allows for a more extensive evaluation and risk stratification of patients with coronary artery disease. Additionally, doing a carotid ultrasound scan (CUS)in the same visit allows estimating the atherosclerotic risk and plays a role in primary prevention.

Use of AI and UCA, for chamber quantification and assessment had markedly improved reproducibility and accuracy. It can help to reduce analysis time and increase workflow efficiency.

PATHOPHYSIOLOGY

Stress echocardiography can provoke clinical symptoms like angina or dyspnea, and ST segment changes on ECG by two pathologic mechanisms: (1) obstructive epicardial coronary artery disease (CAD) and (2) ischemia in nonobstructive coronary arteries (INOCA) due to microvascular disease.

The sequence of stress-induced ischemic events in both these scenarios differs. In the first, as is well known, first a reduction in the CFVR and perfusion defects occur, followed by early diastolic dysfunction, occurrence of RWMA, global reduction in LV function and later, ECG changes and chest pain. However, in case of INOCA patients there is first a reduction in CFVR and perfusion abnormalities, then an early presentation of typical chest pain, ECG changes followed by diastolic dysfunction, reduction in global LV longitudinal function (GLS) and rarely RWMA.

This can be used for risk stratification of patients with INOCA **(Table 1)**.

METHODOLOGY

All SE should have continuous 12-lead ECG monitoring, blood pressure response, and symptom evaluation. This adds valuable prognostic and diagnostic information. A resting TTE study should be performed prior to the test to rule out other causes of chest pain and contraindications to the test. The image acquisition should ideally be at rest, intermediate, peak stress and during recovery and displayed in a quad-screen format for easy comparison.

The indications, contraindications, diagnostic, and nondiagnostic endpoints have not changed and please refer to the latest guidelines for them.

TABLE 1: Risk stratification of patients with ischemia in nonobstructive coronary arteries (INOCA).

RWMA/perfusion abnormalities	*CFVR*	*Event risk*
Present	<2	High
Absent	<2	Intermediate
Absent	Absent	Low (likely noncardiac)

(CFVR: coronary flow velocity reserve; RWMA: regional wall motion abnormalities)
Source: Modified and adapted from Picano E., 2024.[1]

The *ABCDE protocol* for SE allows for the simultaneous assessment of five reserves:

A: Looking for RWMA/perfusion abnormalities by two-dimensional (2D) echocardiography, assessing epicardial coronary artery obstruction. Use of UCAs improves visualization and allows simultaneous assessment of perfusion.

B: Lung ultrasound to measure B-lines, assessing diastolic function and presence of pulmonary edema—a sign of left heart failure

C: Contractile reserve, measuring LV volumes, GLS, three-dimensional (3D) LVEF

D: Pulse wave Doppler based assessment of CFVR in mid-distal LAD, evaluating the coronary microvasculature

E: ECG-based calculation of heart rate reserve (HRR), an indicator of cardiac autonomic function and chronotropic response.

Step A: Left Ventricle Regional Wall Motion Abnormalities

The 2D LV RWMA can be assessed using standard apical two-, three-, and four-chamber views, parasternal long axis (PLAX) and short axis (SAX). The focused apical views are essential for longitudinal strain analysis. A standard 16 or 17 segment model is used and a wall motion score index (WMSI) is calculated with the same segmental scoring system: normal/hyperkinesia = 1; hypokinesia = 2; akinesia = 3; dyskinesia = 4. Presence of inducible RWMA in two or more contiguous segments indicates an abnormal result. Simultaneous perfusion assessment gives additive information improving the accuracy and sensitivity of the test. According to the European Society of Cardiology (ESC) 2024 guidelines for management of chronic coronary syndromes, the use of UCA during SE for LV global, regional chamber quantification and myocardial perfusion evaluation is a class I indication.[2]

Step B: B-lines on Lung Ultrasound

To assess presence of pulmonary congestion, a sign of left heart failure and diastolic dysfunction, LUS looking for B-lines (lung comets) is well validated. They are usually absent at rest and their presence during stress in the early recovery phase implies extravascular fluid accumulation in the lungs. By focusing only on the 'wet-spot' it can be assessed using a small transducer and harmonics imaging at a depth of 18 cm; both in the left and right third intercoastal space, starting at the mid-axillary to anterior axillary and then mid-clavicular line. At each point, the scoring ranges from 0 to 10, the sum of the B-lines at each point is calculated. The interpretation of the total is: 0–1—absent, 2–4—mild, 5–9—moderate, and >10—severe. Their presence and number are strong independent predictor of death in patients with chronic coronary syndromes (CCS), heart failure, and ischemic mitral regurgitation.

Step C: Chamber Quantification

Precise chamber quantification using the Biplane Simpson method or real-time 3D (without a foreshortened apex or geometric assumptions) accurately assess the preload (end-diastolic volume) and contractile reserve (end-systolic volume, ESV). During stress, normally ESV should decrease, an increase by 10% or more, indicates abnormal LV dilatation. In the presence of inducible RWMA, this is a sign of triple vessel disease and, in its absence, indicates myocardial dysfunction. Longitudinal strain analysis complements LVEF and is an early marker of myocardial abnormality.

Step D: Doppler of Left Anterior Descending Coronary Artery for Coronary Flow Velocity Reserve

Color-Doppler flow guidance is used to locate coronary blood flow in the mid-distal portion of the LAD in the modified three-chamber view. It is seen as a biphasic flow, higher during diastole and is assessed with pulsed-wave Doppler. The flow signal is best measured using a vasodilator stressor where it becomes clearer and higher at peak. CFVR is the ratio of the maximal diastolic flow velocity at peak to rest and a value >2.0 is normal. An abnormal response is a strong predictor of all-cause mortality in CCS, independent and incremental over resting GLS and RWMA.

Step E: Heart Rate Response

This is an imaging independent parameter assessing the sympathetic reserve of the heart, normal values for exercise and dobutamine >1.8 and for vasodilators >1.22. A blunted response is an indicator of chronotropic incompetence.

Table 2 describes the ABCDE protocol.

CAROTID ULTRASOUND SCAN[3]

Performing an ultrasound scan of the carotid arteries during rest can be beneficial to determine the atherosclerotic plaque burden which has been shown to increase risk of hard cardiac events beyond myocardial ischemia during stress echocardiography[3] and identify vulnerable lesions.[4]

TABLE 2: Description of ABCDE protocol.

	RWM	*B-lines*	*LVCR*	*CFVR*	*HRR*
Step	*A*	*B*	*C*	*D*	*E*
Variable	Ischemia	Water	Function	Reserve	ANS
Reserve	Epicardial	Diastolic	Contractile	Coronary	Sympathetic
Imaging time	Minutes	Seconds	Seconds	Minutes	None
Analysis time	Seconds	Seconds	Minutes	Seconds	Seconds
Feasibility	>95%	100%	>95%	>90%	100%
UCA	+ Perfusion	Neutral	+ Precision	+ Feasibility	Neutral
Normal	Nonischemic	Dry	Strong	Warm	Fast
Abnormal	Ischemic	Wet	Weak	Cold	Slow

(ANS: autonomic nervous system; CFVR: coronary flow velocity reserve; HRR: heart rate reserve; LVCR: left ventricle cardiac contractile reserve; RWM: regional wall motion; UCA: ultrasound-enhancing contrast agents)

Source: Modified and adapted from Picano E, 2020. http://creativecommons.org/licenses/by/4.0/

Identification is particularly useful in patients with normal stress echocardiography as it has implications for primary preventive therapy.

CONTRAST IN STRESS ECHOCARDIOGRAPHY

Ultrasound-enhancing contrast agents are small lipid encased microbubbles, 1–4 µm in size, administered intravenously as a bolus or infusion. They give out nonlinear signals which are received by the probe while suppressing the linear signals of the myocardial tissue allowing for better visualization of the endocardial borders. It should be used whenever two or more contiguous segments are not seen at rest or during deep breathing mimicking conditions during exercise SE.[5] It is also useful for imaging of the LAD for Doppler-based assessment of CFVR. This improves the precision and reproducibility of the results.

A more advanced use is for perfusion assessment using the "flash-replenishment" method as a continuous infusion, ideally with pharmacological stressors. Albeit off-label, but an European Association of Cardiovascular Imaging (EACVI) class I recommendation,[2] it adds important prognostic and diagnostic information and needs special software. The machine should be set at a low mechanical index which allows for simultaneous visualization of inducible RWMA and subendocardial or transmural perfusion defects at peak stress. Once both LV cavity and myocardium are well-opacified, the contrast is cleared transiently by a high mechanical index flash (lasting a few cycles-based on flash frames) destroying the contrast in the myocardial capillaries. If there is good perfusion, then the myocardium should refill with contrast within 5 seconds (at rest) and about 2 seconds at peak stress. Assessment is done during end-systole when the microvasculature is full of blood and the myocardium is the thickest.

There are no contradictions to using these contrast agents except a previous allergy to these contrast agents. Life-threatening reactions are about 1 in 10,000.

CHOICE OF STRESSORS

All stressor agents, exercise—bike or treadmill, pharmacological—dobutamine or vasodilator (regadenoson/adenosine/dipyridamole), or electrical (external pacing), have comparable specificity and sensitivity. Tailoring the appropriate stressor according to the indications and patient circumstances is advisable. Exercise is the safest and only physiological modality, where important prognostic indicators of symptoms, hemodynamics and exercise capacity can be assessed and should be the first-line modality.

It is advisable to stop anti-ischemia medications (particularly β-blockers) prior to testing, as they compromise sensitivity.

Certain scenarios and indications may make one more favorable than the other **(Table 3)**.

In exercise and dobutamine, ischemia is induced by increasing the myocardial oxygen demand, while with vasodilators it is the reduction of the myocardial oxygen supply through horizontal steal (in the presence of coronary collateral circulation) and vertical steal (with critical epicardial coronary stenosis).

TABLE 3: Different scenarios and selection of preferred stressor.

Scenario	*Preferred stressor*
First-line-safest, physiological	Exercise
Limited exercise capacity	Pharmacological (dobutamine)
Myocardial viability	Dobutamine
Contractile reserve	Low dose exercise or low dose dobutamine
Permanent pacemaker	External pacing
Assessment of CFVR	Vasodilator (regadenoson/ adenosine/dipyridamole)
Assessment of perfusion	Pharmacological
Significant arrhythmias (sustained VT and AF)	Vasodilator or exercise (regadenoson/adenosine/ dipyridamole)
Asthma or phylline therapy	Exercise or dobutamine
Bradyarrhythmia	Exercise or dobutamine
SBP <80 mm Hg	Exercise or dobutamine
LVOTO >30 mm Hg	Exercise
High risk of viral contagion	Pharmacological

(AF: atrial fibrillation; CFVR: coronary flow velocity reserve; LVOTO: left ventricular outflow tract obstruction; SBP: systolic blood pressure; VT: ventricular tachycardia)
Source: Modified and adapted from Picano E., 2024.[1]

It is recommended to use standard protocols for exercise with treadmill (Bruce/modified Bruce), bike and semisupine bike (WHO) and pharmacological stressors (dobutamine + atropine, dipyridamole, and regadenoson), which remain unchanged.

REPORTING

When reporting, it is important to mention the stress protocol and type of stressor used informing whether the test was maximal/submaximal or inadequate. Separately, information on the patient's symptoms, exercise capacity (if applicable), ECG findings, and blood pressure response should be given. All the findings from the *ABCDE* protocol should be described. Ideally, the RWM should be shown graphically using the scoring index (described above). The observed phenotype of CAD (normal/ischemic/viable/scar) should be mentioned. Presence or absence of pulmonary congestion (B-lines), LV contractile reserve, CFVR (>2) and autonomic reserve (HRR). The global risk and annual all-cause mortality ranges from 0.4% (score 0—normal) to 2.7% (score 5—abnormal).

CONCLUSION

The comprehensive assessment using the *ABCDE* protocol and CUS allows for better identification of the varied patient phenotypes and accordingly tailoring for specific therapeutic targets such as ischemia, diastolic dysfunction, abnormal myocardial microcirculation, and lack of sympathetic reserve.

Stress echocardiography has comparable prognostic and diagnostic accuracy to other imaging modalities. For patients with moderate or high pretest likelihood of obstructive CAD, it helps to rule out hemodynamically significant CAD[2] with high sensitivity, specificity, and better temporal resolution than other modalities.

Stress echocardiography continues to remain highly cost effective, readily available, with no radiation exposure and near zero carbon footprint. Making it a very sustainable functional imaging modality.

Use of advanced software for artificial intelligence (AI) generated quantification, 3D real-time LVEF and auto-LV strain, the pitfalls of inter- and intraobserver variability, lack of expertise, and time efficiency have been overcome.

Contrast echocardiography increases accuracy and feasibility by improving endocardial border delineation, better visualization of the LAD for Doppler assessment and evaluation of myocardial microcirculation simultaneously using the "flash-replenishment" technique.

REFERENCES

1. Picano E, Pierard L, Peteiro J, Djordjevic-Dikic A, Sade LE, Cortigiani L, et al. The clinical use of stress echocardiography in chronic coronary syndromes and beyond coronary artery disease: a clinical consensus statement from the EACVI. Eur Heart J Cardiovasc Imaging. 2024;25;e65-90.
2. Vrints C, Andreotti F, Koskinas KC, Rossello X, Adamo M, Ainslie J, et al.; ESC Scientific Document Group. 2024 ESC Guidelines for the management of chronic coronary syndromes. Eur Heart J. 2024;45(36);3415-537.
3. Ahmadvazir S, Shah BN, Zacharias K, Senior R. Incremental Prognostic Value of Stress Echocardiography With Carotid Ultrasound for Suspected CAD. JACC Cardiovasc Imaging. 2018;11(2, Part 1):e173-80.
4. Khattar RS, Senior R. Stress Echocardiography and Carotid Ultrasound:Combined Use for the Assessment of Coronary Artery Disease? J Am Soc Echocardiogr. 2021;34(6):625-8.
5. Senior R, Becher H, Monaghan M, Agati L, Zamorano J, Vanoverschelde JL, et al. Clinical practice of contrast echocardiography: recommendation by the EACVI 2017. Eur Heart J Cardiovasc Imaging. 2017;18:1205-af.

Role of Artificial Intelligence in Echocardiography, Where do We Stand?*

Nitesh Raj Dulal, John LaForge, Simranpreet Singh Daid, Ravindra Bhardwaj, Navin C Nanda

INTRODUCTION

Echocardiography (echo) is the most common noninvasive imaging modality used in the day-to-day clinical practice of cardiology.[1] However, its accuracy depends on the skill level of the operator and the quality of images obtained.[2] Integration of artificial intelligence (AI) in echo may enhance diagnostic accuracy, minimize human error, and improve workflow efficiency.[3,4] In this chapter, we review the current role of AI in echo highlighting its usefulness and limitations **(Tables 1 to 4)**. This is done in a tabular format avoiding detailed narration for ease and convenience of the readers and to keep the chapter within a reasonable length. The tables below show various studies done on the use of AI in echo. Earlier studies focused more on the identification of planes and image segmentation. More recently, AI has been used to assess various heart functions, identify cardiovascular diseases, and predict prognosis. Each study has its benefits and limitations. Some of the older studies which have been superseded by newer similar studies have not been included in the tables.

LIMITATIONS OF ARTIFICIAL INTELLIGENCE

Despite the numerous benefits AI brings to echocardiography, it is not without significant limitations. One of the most prominent concerns is the "black box" phenomenon, where the internal workings of AI algorithms remain opaque. These systems are trained

TABLE 1: Use of artificial intelligence (AI) models for classifying echocardiographic views and segmenting* images.

Reference	*Aim*	*Results*	*Limitation*
Østvik et al.[5] 2018	Neural networks** (NN) used to identify up to 7 standard 2DTTE views	High accuracy in both single frame and sequence identification: 98.3 ± 0.6% and 98.9 ± 0.6%, respectively	Motion artifacts, common in 2DTTE, not reviewed
Madani et al.[6] 2018	NN used for still and video image classification by 2DTTE, M mode, pulsed and continuous wave Doppler	• High accuracy in video and still image classification, 97.8% overall • 91.7% average still image accuracy compared to 79.4% for board certified echocardiographers • Algorithm able to accurately classify all TTE views in various modes	Problem with "Black Box"[+] as outcome process not clear
Narang et al.[7] 2021	Assess ability of 8 novice nurses to obtain 10 2DTTE views with deep learning[++] (DL) software. Compared to trained sonographers	Novices acquired interpretive images not significantly different than blinded sonographers. Left ventricular (LV) size and function, existence of pericardial effusion: accuracy 98.8%. Right ventricle (RV) size: accuracy 92.5%	Small number of patients and novices
Kusunose et al.[8] 2020	Used NN to classify images from mislabeled data set	Accuracy: 98.1%. View mislabel rate: 1.9%. LV ejection fraction (EF) prediction: 1.9% error rate	Relatively small cohort of patients, single-center dataset limits generalizability. Method used to predict LVEF not mentioned

Contd...

Contd...

Reference	Aim	Results	Limitation
Hasan et al.[9] 2025	• DL image registration focused on matching warped moving images to fixed images • Algorithm used to improve image quality to better assess parameters like LVEF, LV global longitudinal strain (LVGLS), and stroke volume in difficult studies, such as fetal TTEs	• Strong association between shape-encoded constraint and good anatomical topology. Strong correlation among data-driven texture constraint and image textures. • Algorithm applied to warped images can improve image quality and aid in obtaining crucial clinical measurements	Algorithm tested on only two TTE data sets, need further testing on other data sets
Du et al.[10] 2024	CNN used to automate quality control of 2DTTE videos for cardiac cycle integrity, anatomical structures, depth and gain	High accuracy with mean average precision 0.962 for anatomic structure detection and gain classification model. Area under curve (AUC) >0.98. Kappa coefficient 0.79 for consistency rating compared to expert evaluation	Algorithm trained on apical four chamber (A4C) view only
Cheng et al.[11] 2025	DL algorithm used for nine 2DTTE views classification from eight different echo equipment by three different manufacturers	High overall accuracy of 0.9881	• Limited dataset with unequal distribution of videos through different TTE views • Single center study lacks generalizability. View classification did not include subcostal planes

(2DTTE: two-dimensional transthoracic echocardiography; 3DTTE: three-dimensional transthoracic echocardiography; POCUS: point-of-care ultrasound; ROC: receiver operating characteristic)

*Segmentation/segmenting: Classifying an image into distinct regions with the help of echo properties.

**Neural network/convolutional neural network: Specialized deep learning architecture designed to process visual data.

+Black box: AI systems with opaque internal mechanisms, where inputs and outputs are visible, but the decision-making process remains unclear, pose challenges in clinical environments that require transparency and explainability.

++Deep learning: A type of "machine learning" that uses many layers of neural network akin to human brain.

TABLE 2: Use of artificial intelligence (AI) models for calculating cardiac chamber dimensions and function.

Reference	Aim	Results	Limitation
Asch et al.[12] 2021	Machine learning+ (ML) algorithm trained to estimate LVEF.	High accuracy of automated LVEF calculation with expert cardiologist reference values: $r = 0.95$, mean absolute deviation = 2.9%. Detection of LVEF ≤35% (Simpson biplane method): sensitivity = 0.90, specificity = 0.92.	Small test group of 99 patients with limited generalizability. In absence of endocardial boundaries, users may have difficulty validating accuracy of automated LVEF estimates
Hirata et al.[13] 2024	• Automated software evaluation of clinically significant TTE variables such as LV, RV, LA, and RA size and function of LV and RV, aortic stenosis (AS), pulmonary arterial hypertension (PAH) • Measurement and report production time were correlated with Simpson's biplane method for volume measurements. Compared in A4C and apical two chamber (A2C) views	Time taken for measurement and report generation versus manual method markedly reduced (159 ± 66 s versus 325 ± 94 s, $p < 0.01$). Report creation time (71 ± 39 s versus 429 ± 128 s, $p < 0.01$)	Low sample size (n : 23). Single center study. Study carried out by one technologist. Some poor image quality due to arrhythmias

Contd...

Contd...

Reference	*Aim*	*Results*	*Limitation*
Tsang et al.[14] 2016	Automated algorithm used to measure LA volume, LV volume, and LVEF on 3DTTE. 3DTTE and cardiac MRI images used for comparison	Strong association among automated AI and manual 3D TTE values (*r*: 0.87–0.96). Strong association among automated AI and CMR values (*r*: 0.84–0.95)	• Only assessed patients in sinus rhythm. Select patients required adjustment of endocardial borders by manual method after automation. Excluded were those in whom LV endocardial borders were not visualized • Algorithm accuracy in patients with poor image quality unknown
He et al.[15] 2023	LVEF by AI compared with sonographer. Studies reviewed by board certified cardiologists after initial assessment. Primary endpoint was change in LVEF measurements from initial assessments to final cardiologist measurements	AI derived LVEF more accurate to sonographer. Change in LVEF: AI group = 16.8%, sonographer group = 27.2%. Mean absolute difference between preliminary and final evaluations: AI group = 2.79%, sonographer group = 3.77%	Single-center study lacks generalizability. Study does not evaluate long-term outcomes attributed to variations in LVEF measurements. Used previously acquired echo studies, which could lead to bias if an interpreting sonographer is different than the one who obtained the images
Ali et al.[16] 2025	Convolutional NN used for LVEF estimation from 2DTTEs. Algorithm compared to other established AI techniques	• LVEF by AI comparable to other established techniques • LVEF mean absolute error 3.7. R2 0.82. Algorithm outperformed other AI state-of-the-art techniques for LVEF assessment	Algorithm effectiveness dependent on the quality and consistency of input videos; poor image quality may impact precision of the model. Design restricted by set number of frames which may limit utility for extended frame sequences. Only four-chamber views included in the dataset
MacKay et al.[17] 2024	DL algorithm used to estimate LVEF on POCUS system from one manufacturer in those undergoing some types of cardiac surgery. Compared to manual estimation by Simpson biplane method	AI auto LVEF bias (10.17% similar to expert reader EF (9.82%). Association was less for auto EF (*r* = 0.56) than expert echocardiographer measured EF (*r* = 0.80). Secondary analyses: association between EF measured by Simpson's method and auto EF grew when implemented on 27 acquisitions categorized as sufficient (*r* = 0.86) but diminished when applied to 27 attainments categorized as insufficient (*r* = 0.46)	Small data sample size (54 clips and 30 patients). Video clips obtained by single operator, not generalizable. Used only A4C 2DTTE clips. Small data set used to compare EF estimates. Only two patients had an EF <30%, lacks generalizability. No true gold standard EF calculation was made for comparison. Reference EF was estimated by one sonographer using Simpson's method in two instances separated by 1 month

(2DTTE: two-dimensional transthoracic echocardiography; 3DTTE: three-dimensional transthoracic echocardiography; POCUS: point-of-care ultrasound)

[+]Machine learning: A subset of AI that enables computers to improve their task performance by learning from data patterns, without needing explicit programming for each task.

TABLE 3: Use of AI models for calculating cardiac chamber dimensions and function.

Reference	*Aim*	*Results*	*Limitation*
Zhang et al.[18] 2018	• Fully automated interpretation: view classification, image selection, evaluation of structure and function, disease recognition (5 views) • Measurement: LVEF and LVGLS. Compared to manual segmentation and estimations from standard clinical workflow • Disease detection: hypertrophic cardiomyopathy (HCM), PAH, and cardiac amyloid (CA)	Good AI accuracy for parasternal long axis view identification: 96%. Structure measurements versus report values (15–17% deviation). LVEF and LVGLS median deviation: 9.7% and 7.5%, respectively. HCM, CA, and PAH statistics accuracy: 0.93, 0.87, 0.85, respectively	• Outliers with large deviations. 25% of outliers had clear problem with automated segmentation. • Did not discriminate between HCM, CA, and other hypertrophic diseases
Knackstead et al.[19] 2015	• ML software used to assess LV volumes, LVEF, and LVGLS. A2C and A4C views used in patients in sinus rhythm • EF assessment: Automated software versus visual estimation and manual tracing using Simpson biplane method by cardiologists	• AI EF and LVGLS automated measurements were similar to manual tracking. The AI-automated image evaluation produces information past LV volumes and EF, like LVGLS, and does not include any variability • Average AI analysis time, 8 ± 1s (not compared to manual method)	• Patients with arrhythmia excluded • Interstudy variability not addressed • Visual EF assessment possibly biased by manual assessment
Ouyang et al.[20] 2020	• Video-based DL^{+} algorithm used to segment LV, estimate LVEF, and assess cardiomyopathies. LVEF calculation obtained via frame level segmentation and beat-to-beat evaluation. Classification of heart failure with reduced ejection fraction (HFrEF) • Compared with assessment from cardiologists using Simpson biplane and LVGLS by various methods	• AI accurately predicted LVEF with mean error 4.1–6.0%, and accurately classified HFrEF: AUC 0.96–0.97 • AI variance comparable to or less than human intraobserver variability which can be as high as 13.9%	• Comparison can vary with expertise of sonographer and cardiologist • Variation in beat-to-beat evaluation in patients with arrhythmias or ectopy • Subjectivity in selecting beat for LVEF calculation
Holste et al.[21] 2024	• DL model trained to perform 39 diagnostic reporting assignments from multi-view 2DTTE B-mode and color Doppler videos • Algorithm reported 18 classification and 21 continuous regression assignments across an array of structural, functional, and valvular criteria	• High AI accuracy in several tasks: AUC 0.91 across 18 diagnostic classification assignments • Mean absolute error 0.13 across 21 measurement assignments covering chamber size and function, vascular dimensions, and valvular evaluation. • LV dilation: AUC 0.95 • LV systolic dysfunction: AUC 0.98 • LV hypertrophy: AUC 0.91 • RV systolic dysfunction: AUC 0.93 • Severe AS: AUC 0.99 • Mitral stenosis: AUC 0.96 • Moderate or greater aortic regurgitation: AUC 0.93 • Moderate or more mitral regurgitation (MR): AUC 0.96 • LVEF mean absolute error 4.4%	• Model educated on distinct TTEs and averaged estimations from every video-obtained throughout each study, model unable to adaptively learn which views and videos are relevant for a specific task • Model does not integrate segmentation step for TTE estimations • Algorithm has not been validated in real-world clinical workflow

Contd...

Contd...

Reference	Aim	Results	Limitation
Olaisen et al.[22] 2023	• Processing speed and reproducibility of convolutional NN-based AI measurements of 2DTTE LVEF and LV volumes compared to manual measurements, in real time, in 50 consecutive patients. 40 patients with repeated TTEs and manual measurements by four experts • Manual measurements obtained from Simpson's biplane method • LVEF and LV volumes assessed using A4C and A2C views	• AI quantifications significantly decreased total attainment and processing time: median 1.9 min per patient for AI group, 7.5 min per patient in manual group. Median reduction time of 5.3 min per patient, 77% time saved using AI method. Averaged disparities concerning AI and manual measurements varied from −11.6 to 6.5 mL for LV end-diastolic volumes, −4.0 to 2.7 mL for LV endsystolic volumes, and −5.5 to 0.3% points for EF • Test-retest reproducibility of AI estimation was greater in interobserver situations and noninferior in intraobserver situations. AI estimations exhibited strong consensus with manual assessments in real time and data base scenarios	• Small percentage of patients with low EF or abnormal anatomy • One of the three involved experts may have been biased, lack of interoperator agreement • AI quantifications regarding CMR imaging not validated
Salte et al.[23] 2023	• DL algorithm used to evaluate patient test-retest reproducibility of LVGLS estimated by AI means compared to manual measurements by expert echocardiographers in repeated echos • Two data sets acquired at separate centers • Repeat imaging obtained in immediate sequence by two separate sonographers • Four expert readers assessed LVGLS in both recordings using a semiautomatic commercially available speckle-tracking software to create test-retest, inter-reader and intra-reader scenarios	• AI test-retest irregularity was reduced compared with inter-reader settings. Data set 1: Minimal detectable change, 3.7 vs. 5.5; mean absolute difference, 1.4 vs. 2.1 • Data set 2: Minimal detectable change, 3.9 vs. 5.2; mean absolute difference, 1.6 vs. 1.9 • Bias in LVGLS assessments in 13 out of 24 test-retest inter-reader settings (greatest bias, 3.2 strain units). No bias observed in AI measurements • Beat-to-beat minimal detectable changes were 1.5, 2.1 for AI method; 2.3 for the manual method • AI processing time for LVGLS analysis was 7.96 ± 2.8 s (not compared to manual method)	• Small data sets (40 and 32 patients, respectively) • Studies of data set one were attained in previous generation echo machine than used on data set two. Older ultrasound system possibly generated poorer image quality than the newer system • The readers were expert in echo but with different experience in imaging training • Identical vendor used for each image attainment and reference estimation, lacks generalizability

[+]Deep learning: A type of "machine learning" that uses many layers of neural network akin to human brain.

TABLE 4: Artificial intelligence (AI)-based assessment of various cardiac pathologies.

Reference	Aim	Results	Limitation
Cassiani et al.[24] 2024	Convolutional NN model used to detect patients with heart failure with preserved ejection fraction (HFpEF) using A4C videos	AI: Sensitivity 89.8% • Specificity 86.3% • Positive predicted value (PPV) 87.2% • Negative predicted value (NPV) 89% AI positive output linked with greater risk for HF hospitalization [Hazard ratio, (HR): 3.76; $p < 0.001$] and mortality (HR: 5.55; $p < 0.001$) compared to negative output	Need for prospective studies to validate these findings and assess the model's generalizability

Contd...

Contd...

Reference	Aim	Results	Limitation
Liu et al.[25] 2024	DL method for segmenting MR regions and classifying MR severity	• *Segmentation:* Jaccard index, 84.37%; mean precision array, 92.39%; recall, 90.91%; and precision, 91.9% • *Classification:* accuracy, 95.27%; precision, 88.52%; recall, 91.13%; and F1-score, 90.30%	• Relatively small test dataset of only 75 echocardiograms • Data collected from only two brands of ultrasound machines
Sadeghpour et al.[26] 2025	ML algorithm to improve workflow for grading MR severity	• AI accuracy (MR severity grading): 0.80 • Accuracy (detection of significant MR): 0.97	• Retrospective study of 38 patients cohort, only included echocardiograms from heart failure patients • Study not aimed to analyze clinical outcomes associated with AI-guided assessment of MR severity
Oikonomou et al.[27] 2025	• AI-enabled POCUS method to identify HCM and transthyretin amyloid cardiomyopathy (ATTR-CM) across two health systems • Examined prognostic consequences of positive screen without known HCM or ATTR-CM	• AUROC (HCM): 0.90 and 0.89 • AUROC (ATTR): 0.92 and 0.99 • Diagnosis of HCM and ATTR-CM compared with confirmation by CMR for HCM and technetium pyrophosphate scan for ATTR-CM	• Retrospective analysis of patients presenting with acute symptoms to an emergency department • Acknowledged underdiagnosis of HCM and ATTR-CM, concern for false positives. Several individuals flagged years prior to clinical diagnosis with increased mortality risk. Both could lead a level of ascertainment bias, may imply lesser than reported model performance • Diagnoses established via International Classification of Diseases codes, may create suboptimal precision for flagging specific diseases
Julakanti et al.[28] 2025	Use of ML algorithm to calculate risks of disease worsening and death in patients with mild AS	AS progression model using AI distinguished those with development of severe AS within 2 and 5 years with an AUC of 0.86 for both. Mortality model recognized those with death within 2 and 5 years with an AUC of 0.84 and 0.87, respectively	• Retrospective data from a single healthcare system, which may limit generalizability • Cohort predominantly white patients • Concerns for selection and survival biases • Reliance on high-quality echo images
Ghorbani et al.[29] 2020	• Convolutional NN model trained to identify intracardiac devices, estimate cardiac function, estimate chamber anatomy and size, LV hypertrophy, LA dilation, and predict systemic risk factors • Images sampled from A4C views on large data set	• Pacemaker lead Identification: AUC: 0.89 • Enlarged LA: AUC: 0.89 • LVH: AUC: 0.75 • LV volumes: $R^2 = 0.74$ (systolic), $R^2 = 0.70$ (diastolic) • LVEF: R^2: 0.50 • Predicted phenotypes age ($R^2 = 0.46$), sex (AUC = 0.88), weight ($R^2 = 0.56$), height ($R^2 = 0.33$)	• Data collected from one ultrasound machine, one patient population at one institution. Concern for lack of generalizability • Used previous imaging study annotations from electronic medical record (EMR) at same institution • Requires rigorous quality control from an institutions' echo laboratory

Contd...

Contd...

Reference	*Aim*	*Results*	*Limitation*
Long et al.[30] 2024	• DL system developed to determine MR severity (none/trace, mild, moderate, and severe) on color Doppler videos from complete 2DTTEs • Reading cardiologist used as reference	• AI showed superiority in MR categorization • Internal test sets: (accuracy: 82%, κappa coefficient = 0.84; AUC: 0.98 for moderate/severe MR) • External test sets: (accuracy: 79%, κ = 0.80; AUC: 0.98 for moderate or more severe MR). Most (63% internal and 66% external) misclassification discrepancies were between none/trace and mild MR	• All studies performed in one city with one vendor, lacks generalizability • Only assessed severity of MR and not the cause or mechanism • Model training and evaluation of model accuracy dependent on cardiologist 2DTTE analyses, subject to technical confines and uncertain reliability
Stowell et al.[31] 2024	• ML LVGLS measurement • NN trained to recognize different LV parts including endocardium in various apical views. End-systolic and diastolic frames identified by 11 experts to create agreement tracings and points • Expert assessment evaluation used for each patient	High AI correlation with expert consensus value of 0.91	• Focused on LVGLS and no other indices of LV function • Did not assess clinical outcomes with LVGLS measurements • Small number of experts • LVGLS calculated from length of complete contour, not from regional tracking of speckles, this may lead to differences
Vrudhula et al.[32] 2024	• DL algorithm for identifying A4C view videos with color Doppler echo and identifying moderate/severe MR from 2DTTE • Comparison with reports of expert echocardiographer	• AI correctly identifying color Doppler information across mitral valve: sensitivity 0.975, specificity 0.999 • MR moderate or greater: AUC: 0.916, severe MR: AUC 0.934	• Poor images resulting in incorrect assessment of MR severity could not be detected by algorithm • Model was trained on clinical evaluation of MR severity which is subjective • Model showed reduced performance when comparing echo assessment of MR severity with CMR
Park et al.[33] 2025	• DL algorithm used to assess AS continuum and automate AS evaluation • TTEs obtained from five tertiary care centers in Korea and evaluated by board-certified cardiologists as reference • System automatically selects necessary views: AS continuum assessed in parasternal long- and short-axis views	• Internal and external validation performed for diagnostic value through different severity of AS and prognosis for: cardiovascular mortality, heart failure, aortic valve (AV) valve replacement • AS severity predicted by a deep learning index for AS continuum; deep learning index increased with worsening AS severity • Discrimination for any AS: AUC 0.92–0.99 • Significant AS: AUC 0.95–0.98 • Severe AS: AUC 0.97–0.99 • Automatic measurements demonstrated correlation with manual measurements with high accuracy for AS staging and similar prognostic usefulness to manually obtained variables	• Retrospectively acquired data from tertiary care centers in Korea, needs further application for generalizability • Observational analysis strategy caused several patients to lose follow up, may lead to selection bias linked to inadequate follow-up period

Contd...

on large datasets, learning to make complex predictions; however, understanding precisely how various factors contribute to a given outcome is often difficult, even for developers. This lack of interpretability poses a substantial challenge in clinical settings, where trust, validation, and transparency are critical for patient care.[34,35]

The issue extends beyond technical transparency to epistemological challenges—questions about the nature and justification of knowledge itself. AI models derive predictions based on patterns in data rather than a human-like rationale, making it hard to ascertain why a specific decision was made. In medicine, where decisions can be life-altering, the inability to clearly explain or justify AI-driven recommendations can erode confidence in these tools.

Philosophically, epistemology explores how we acquire knowledge and what constitutes justified belief. Immanuel Kant, a central figure in this field, posited that our understanding of reality is shaped by innate mental structures rather than purely external truths.[3,36,37] Similarly, AI models, particularly deep learning networks inspired by human cognition, process data through internal mechanisms. These models, like the human mind, filter, interpret, and assign meaning to data in ways that may differ from human reasoning. This analogy underscores the need for critical reflection when entrusting AI with clinical judgments, as its interpretation of reality might not align with that of human clinicians.

Another concern is bias, which is often introduced during the labeling phase of supervised learning. Although labeled data is treated as a reliable standard, it can carry inherent human or systemic biases, potentially skewing AI predictions. As a result, the fairness and accuracy of AI-driven outcomes can be compromised, particularly when models reflect societal or institutional inequities present in their training datasets.[34,38]

AI systems also depend on considerable volumes of high-quality data for effective learning and generalization. In practice, medical images vary widely in quality due to differences in equipment, operator skill, and patient conditions. AI models trained on pristine datasets may struggle with real-word variability, leading to reduced accuracy and reliability.[39-41] This highlights the importance of rigorous data curation and preprocessing to ensure dependable AI performance.

Lastly, there is concern about AI's impact on clinical skills and human connection. If overused, AI might contribute to a decline in the manual and interpretive skills of experienced clinicians, diminishing the art and nuance of echo.[42] Furthermore, AI lacks the capability to comprehend the holistic context of a patient—emotional, social, and environmental factors that influence health outcomes. While AI can offer valuable insights, it cannot replicate the empathy, intuition, and adaptability of a human clinician. Ultimately, AI should be viewed as a complementary tool, enhancing but not replacing the human elements central to compassionate and personalized care.

CONCLUSION

AI continues to reshape the field of cardiology, particularly in echo imaging, with the potential to improve diagnostic accuracy, streamline workflows, and improve patient's outcomes. Its strength lies in early detection, precise classification, and the ability to recognize subtle changes in cardiac function, all of which can contribute to earlier interventions and reduced mortality.

However, ethical, technical, and philosophical challenges persist. The black box nature of AI raises concerns about accountability and trust, while biases in training data and variable data quality can affect accuracy and fairness. These challenges emphasize the need for ongoing research, ethical oversight, and transparency, along with a commitment to preserving human expertise.

It is unlikely that AI will replace clinicians, but it will continue to evolve as a powerful support system, enabling more informed, efficient, and precise decision-making in echo and beyond. The future of AI in medicine lies in a balanced partnership between human intelligence and machine learning.

REFERENCES

1. Mitchell C, Rahko PS, Blauwet LA, Canaday B, Finstuen JA, Foster MC, et al. Guidelines for Performing a Comprehensive Transthoracic Echocardiographic Examination in Adults: Recommendations from the American Society of Echocardiography. J Am Soc Echocardiography. 2018;32(1):1-64.
2. Davis A, Billick K, Horton K, Jankowski M, Knoll P, Marshall JE, et al. Artificial Intelligence and Echocardiography: A primer for cardiac sonographers. J Am Soc Echocardiography. 2020;33(9):1061-6.
3. Karakuş G, Değirmencioğlu A, Nanda NC. Artificial intelligence in echocardiography: Review and limitations including epistemological concerns. Echocardiography. 2022;39(8):1044-53.

4. Seo H, Khuzani MB, Vasudevan V, Huang C, Ren H, Xiao R, et al. Machine learning techniques for biomedical image segmentation: An overview of technical aspects and introduction to state-of-art applications. Med Phys. 2020;47(5):e148-67.
5. Østvik A, Smistad E, Aase SA, Haugen BO, Lovstakken L. Real-Time standard view classification in transthoracic echocardiography using convolutional neural networks. Ultrasound Med Biol. 2018;45(2):374-84.
6. Madani A, Arnaout R, Mofrad M, Arnaout R. Fast and accurate view classification of echocardiograms using deep learning. NPJ Digit Med. 2018;1:6.
7. Narang A, Bae R, Hong H, Thomas Y, Surette S, Cadieu C, et al. Utility of a Deep-Learning algorithm to guide novices to acquire echocardiograms for limited diagnostic use. JAMA Cardiol. 2021;6(6):624.
8. Kusunose K, Haga A, Inoue M, Fukuda D, Yamada H, Sata M. Clinically feasible and accurate view classification of echocardiographic images using deep learning. Biomolecules. 2020;10(5):665.
9. Hasan MK, Zhu H, Yang G, Yap CH. Deep learning image registration for cardiac motion estimation in adult and fetal echocardiography via a focus on anatomic plausibility and texture quality of warped image. Comput Biol Med. 2025;187:109719.
10. Du L, Xue W, Qi Z, Shi Z, Guo G, Yang X, et al. Deep learning framework for interpretable quality control of echocardiography video. Med Phys. 2025;52(6):4039-53.
11. Cheng H, Shi Z, Qi Z, Wang X, Guo G, Fang A, et al. Deep learning-based video-level view classification of two-dimensional transthoracic echocardiography. Biomed Phys Eng Express. 2025;11(2).
12. Asch FM, Poilvert N, Abraham T, Jankowski M, Cleve J, Adams M, et al. Automated echocardiographic quantification of left ventricular ejection fraction without volume measurements using a machine learning algorithm mimicking a human expert. Circ Cardiovas Imag. 2019; 12(9):e009303.
13. Hirata Y, Nomura Y, Saijo Y, Sata M, Kusunose K. Reducing echocardiographic examination time through routine use of fully automated software: a comparative study of measurement and report creation time. J Echocardiography.. 2024;22(3):162-70.
14. Tsang W, Salgo IS, Medvedofsky D, Takeuchi M, Prater D, Weinert L, et al. Transthoracic 3D echocardiographic left heart chamber quantification using an automated adaptive analytics algorithm. JACC Cardiovasc Imaging. 2016;9(7):769-82.
15. He B, Kwan AC, Cho JH, Yuan N, Pollick C, Shiota T, et al. Blinded, randomized trial of sonographer versus AI cardiac function assessment. Nature. 2023;616(7957):520-4.
16. Ali W, Alsabban W, Shahbaz M, Al-Laith A, Almogadwy B. EFNet: estimation of left ventricular ejection fraction from cardiac ultrasound videos using deep learning. PeerJ Comp Sci. 2025;11:e2506.
17. MacKay EJ, Bharat S, Mukaddim RA, Erkamp R, Sutton J, Muhammad AK, et al. Pragmatic evaluation of a Deep-Learning algorithm to automate ejection fraction on Hand-Held, Point-of-Care echocardiography in a cardiac surgical operating room. J Cardiothorac Vasc Anesth. 2024;38(4):895-904.
18. Zhang J, Gajjala S, Agrawal P, Tison GH, Hallock LA, Beussink-Nelson L, et al. Fully automated echocardiogram interpretation in clinical practice. Circulation. 2018; 138(16):1623-35.
19. Knackstedt C, Bekkers SCAM, Schummers G, Schreckenberg M, Muraru D, Badano LP, et al. Fully automated versus standard tracking of left ventricular ejection fraction and longitudinal strain. J Am Coll Cardiol. 2015;66(13):1456-66.
20. Ouyang D, He B, Ghorbani A, Yuan N, Ebinger J, Langlotz CP, et al. Video-based AI for beat-to-beat assessment of cardiac function. Nature [Internet]. 2020;580(7802):252-6.
21. Holste G, Oikonomou EK, Mortazavi BJ, Wang Z, Khera R. Efficient deep learning-based automated diagnosis from echocardiography with contrastive self-supervised learning. Commun Med. 2024;4(1):133.
22. Olaisen S, Smistad E, Espeland T, Hu J, Pasdeloup D, Østvik A, et al. Automatic measurements of left ventricular volumes and ejection fraction by artificial intelligence: clinical validation in real time and large databases. Eur Heart J Cardiovasc Imaging. 2023;25(3):383-95.
23. Salte IM, Østvik A, Olaisen SH, Karlsen S, Dahlslett T, Smistad E, et al. Deep Learning for Improved Precision and Reproducibility of left ventricular strain in Echocardiography: A Test-Retest Study. J Am Soc Echocardiography. 2023;36(7):788-99.
24. Cassianni C, Huntley GD, Castrichini M, Akerman AP, Porumb M, Scott CG, et al. Automated echocardiographic detection of heart failure with preserved ejection fraction using artificial intelligence is associated with cardiac mortality and heart failure hospitalization. J Am Soc Echocardiography.. 2024;37(9):914-6.
25. Liu G, Wang Y, Cheng H, Shi Z, Qi Z, Yao J, et al. Automatic segmentation and evaluation of mitral regurgitation using Doppler echocardiographic images. Bioengineering. 2024;11(11):1131.
26. Sadeghpour A, Jiang Z, Hummel YM, Frost M, Lam CSP, Shah SJ, et al. An Automated Machine Learning–Based quantitative multiparametric approach for mitral regurgitation severity grading. JACC Cardiovasc Imaging. 2025;18(1):1-12.
27. Oikonomou EK, Vaid A, Holste G, Coppi A, McNamara RL, Baloescu C, et al. Artificial intelligence-guided detection of under-recognised cardiomyopathies on point-of-care cardiac ultrasonography: a multicentre study. Lancet Digital Health. 2025;7(2):e113-23.

28. Julakanti RR, Padang R, Scott CG, Dahl J, Al-Shakarchi NJ, Metzger C, et al. Use of artificial intelligence to predict outcomes in mild aortic valve stenosis. Eur Heart J Digital Health. 2024;6(1):63-72.
29. Ghorbani A, Ouyang D, Abid A, He B, Chen JH, Harrington RA, et al. Deep learning interpretation of echocardiograms. NPJ Digital Med. 2020;3(1) 2025;334(4):306-18.
30. Long A, Haggerty CM, Finer J, Hartzel D, Jing L, Keivani A, et al. Deep Learning for Echo Analysis, Tracking, and Evaluation of mitral Regurgitation (DELINEATE-MR). Circulation [Internet]. 2024;150(12):911-22.
31. Stowell CC, Howard JP, Ng T, Cole GD, Bhattacharyya S, Sehmi J, et al. 2-Dimensional echocardiographic global longitudinal strain with artificial intelligence using open data from a UK-Wide collaborative. JACC Cardiovasc Imaging. 2024;17(8):865-76.
32. Vrudhula A, Duffy G, Vukadinovic M, Liang D, Cheng S, Ouyang D. High-ThroughPut Deep Learning detection of mitral regurgitation. Circulation. 2024;150(12):923-33.
33. Park J, Kim J, Jeon J, Yoon YE, Jang Y, Jeong H, et al. Artificial intelligence-enhanced comprehensive assessment of the aortic valve stenosis continuum in echocardiography. EBioMedicine [Internet]. 2025;112:105560.
34. Barry T, Farina JM, Chao CJ, Ayoub C, Jeong J, Patel BN, et al. The role of artificial intelligence in echocardiography. J Imaging. 2023;9(2):50.
35. Dell'Angela L, Nicolosi GL. Artificial intelligence applied to cardiovascular imaging, a critical focus on echocardiography: The point-of-view from "the other side of the coin". J Clin Ultrasound. 2022;50(6):772-80.
36. Swanson LR. The predictive processing paradigm has roots in Kant. Front Syst Neurosci. 2016;79:10.
37. Barlow HB. Possible principles underlying the transformations of sensory messages. Cambridge, MA: The MIT Press eBooks; 2012. pp. 216-34.
38. Yoon YE, Kim S, Chang HJ. Artificial intelligence and echocardiography. J Cardiovasc Imaging. 2021;29(3):193.
39. Akkus Z, Aly YH, Attia IZ, Lopez-Jimenez F, Arruda-Olson AM, Pellikka PA, et al. Artificial Intelligence (AI)-Empowered Echocardiography Interpretation: A State-of-the-Art Review. J Clin Med. 2021;10(7):1391.
40. Krajcer Z. Artificial intelligence in Cardiovascular Medicine: historical overview, current status, and future directions. Texas Heart Inst J. 2022;49(2):e207527.
41. Sengupta PP, Adjeroh DA. Will artificial intelligence replace the human echocardiographer? Circulation. 2018;138(16):1639-42.
42. Wuni G, Wasan V, Nanda NC. Artificial intelligence in echocardiography: Usefulness and limitations. In: Rath PC (Ed). Cardiology Update 2023. New Delhi: Jaypee Brothers Medical Publishers (P) Ltd.; 2024.

Nuclear Imaging and Positron Emission Tomography

CHAPTER 29

Role of Nuclear Perfusion Imaging with SPECT or PET in the Era of Multimodality Imaging

Ciydem Akincioglu, Saurabh Malhotra

INTRODUCTION

Coronary artery disease (CAD) is now the most common cause of mortality and morbidity worldwide.[1] Furthermore, caring for patients with known or suspected CAD poses tremendous economic pressure on healthcare resources, not only due to costs related to testing and treatment but also due to those associated with loss of productivity in afflicted individuals.[1] Therefore, it is expected that more efficient use of resources and focus on improving cardiovascular outcomes in such patients will be prioritized as we continue to move from volume- to value-based care.[2] In addition, there is currently growing emphasis on maximizing the yield of diagnostic testing, such that an imaging modality is not only expected to confirm the presence or absence of a certain diagnosis but also guide post-test decision-making in ways that will improve a patient's prognosis and quality of life.[3]

There are several objectives to be achieved when evaluating patients presenting with chest pain or other angina-equivalent symptoms. Determining the etiology of symptoms and particularly discerning whether they can be attributed to underlying CAD is arguably the principal goal of care in these patients. Once the diagnosis of CAD is confirmed, the next goal would be to stratify those with disease according to their risk of future adverse cardiovascular events based on the anatomic or physiologic extent of the disease. Finally, this information will also be used to guide referrals for more invasive cardiac procedures, such as coronary angiography and revascularization, based on the likelihood that patients will derive more benefit from revascularization compared to medical therapy alone.

Even when obstructive CAD is not identified as the culprit for symptoms, this encounter represents a unique opportunity to assess patients' cardiovascular prognosis and to implement appropriate preventative therapies for those at risk. Detecting markers of "hidden cardiovascular risk", such as incidental subclinical coronary atherosclerosis or coronary microvascular dysfunction, may be used to guide the initiation of therapies, including aspirin and statins, which have been shown to mitigate the risk of cardiac events.

To this end, radionuclide myocardial perfusion imaging (MPI) is a commonly utilized imaging test for evaluation of patients with known or suspected CAD. There is currently a large body of evidence supporting the significant role of MPI in the diagnosis and management of patients with suspected ischemic heart disease, performed using single photon emission computed tomography (SPECT) and positron emission tomography (PET) technologies. This chapter provides an overview of the critical role of nuclear perfusion imaging and highlights its established and growing value despite the availability of other modalities to assess for CAD.

RADIONUCLIDE MYOCARDIAL PERFUSION IMAGING FOR THE DIAGNOSIS OF CORONARY ARTERY DISEASE

Myocardial perfusion imaging forms the backbone for diagnosis of CAD and for the assessment of physiological significance of anatomical stenosis. This reliance on MPI is based on decades of prospective observational data highlighting its ability to provide reliable assessment of the presence and severity of CAD across a wide range of population subgroups. Pooled data from a large number of observational studies suggest the sensitivity and specificity of exercise and pharmacological SPECT-MPI to be 87–89% and 73–75%, respectively.[4] A high normalcy rate of 91% is again indicative of the exceptional diagnostic value of SPECT-MPI to detect normal test results among those with a low likelihood of CAD. The diagnostic performance of SPECT-MPI is further improved using attenuation correction. While most of the evidence has been on the diagnostic performance of MPI with SPECT, recent data from PET suggests a similarly high diagnostic sensitivity and specificity.[5] Addition of myocardial flow reserve (MFR) (normal >2), which is an established advantage of PET, confers a sensitivity and specificity of 96% and 80%, respectively, with an overall accuracy of 92%.

Due to higher spatial resolution and inherent ability to correct for scatter and soft-tissue attenuation, PET MPI provides better image quality, higher interpretive certainty, and superior sensitivity and specificity for the detection of obstructive CAD compared to conventional SPECT.[6,7] Moreover, PET MPI exposes patients to significantly lower radiation dose compared to most conventional SPECT protocols due to the inherent characteristics of PET tracers.[8] Such technical advantages and others have supported growth in PET use in contemporary nuclear laboratories. Despite its diagnostic performance, underestimating the true extent of obstructive epicardial coronary disease (e.g., situations with balanced ischemia) and the inability to determine microvascular dysfunction remain major limitations of stress MPI with conventional SPECT.[9,10] Several perfusion and nonperfusion markers have been proposed to improve the detection of left main or three-vessel coronary disease angiographically when combined with relative perfusion assessment.[11] Additionally, as the use of PET for cardiac applications continues to grow, several PET-derived markers have also been described to improve the diagnostic yield of stress perfusion imaging. A preserved left ventricular ejection fraction (LVEF) reserve with PET—defined as an increase in LVEF between rest and peak hyperemic stress—is associated with a low likelihood of finding angiographically extensive coronary disease.[12] Unlike PET-derived LVEF reserve, however, a negative LVEF reserve with SPECT does carry the same diagnostic utility,[13,14] underscoring the differences in the timing of gated image acquisition between PET and SPECT. Myocardial blood flow (MBF) reserve is another PET-derived marker that improves discrimination between patients with and without left main or three-vessel disease, and finding extensive CAD is unlikely in patients with intact coronary vasomotor function.[15,16] MBF is also a powerful tool that allows for identification of microvessel disease in the absence of significant epicardial CAD **(Fig. 1)**. Dynamic SPECT, with the use of high sensitivity systems, is rapidly evolving and could become a viable alternative for assessment of MBF for laboratories without access to PET.

MYOCARDIAL PERFUSION IMAGING PROTOCOLS FOR THE DIAGNOSIS OF CORONARY ARTERY DISEASE WITH REDUCED RADIATION EXPOSURE

Novel MPI protocols for diagnosing CAD and for evaluating acute chest pain in the emergency department (ED) have been studied that allow for improved laboratory throughput while maintaining the diagnostic and prognostic value of MPI. Since PET MPI tracers have a very short half-life and low radiation exposure, these protocols specifically apply to SPECT-MPI to enhance clinical decision-making with lower radiation while maintaining diagnostic certainty.

Stress-first or Stress-only Myocardial Perfusion Imaging

Numerous studies recently reported the application of stress-first (SF)[17] or stress-only (SO)[19] SPECT-MPI for CAD. Chang et al. reported a retrospective analysis of a large cohort of 16,854 patients who had normal SPECT-MPI by either a SF or stress/rest protocol.[18] Approximately 48% of these patients underwent a SF protocol, and over an average follow-up period of 4.7 years, there were no significant differences in the adjusted annualized mortality rates among those who underwent SF (2.6%) versus those who underwent stress/rest imaging (2.9%), $p = 0.89$. Additionally, there were no differences in outcomes among the two groups by gender, diabetes, known CAD, and Duke treadmill score. Another study by Duvall et al. studied the prognostic value of a normal SO SPECT-MPI protocol among patients with low pretest risk of CAD.[19] Among 1,673 patients with a normal SO SPECT-MPI, the annualized all-cause mortality was <1% over an average follow-up period of 40 months. This was comparable to a cohort of patients with similar low risk who underwent conventional rest/stress protocol ($p = 0.94$). Representative images of a patient with a normal SF SPECT-MPI, despite atherosclerotic disease in the left anterior descending coronary artery (LAD), are shown in **Figures 2A and B**.

Acute Chest Pain Myocardial Perfusion Imaging

Accurate triage of patients presenting to the ED with chest pain is essential for risk assessment and adequate patient management. In majority of the patients presenting to

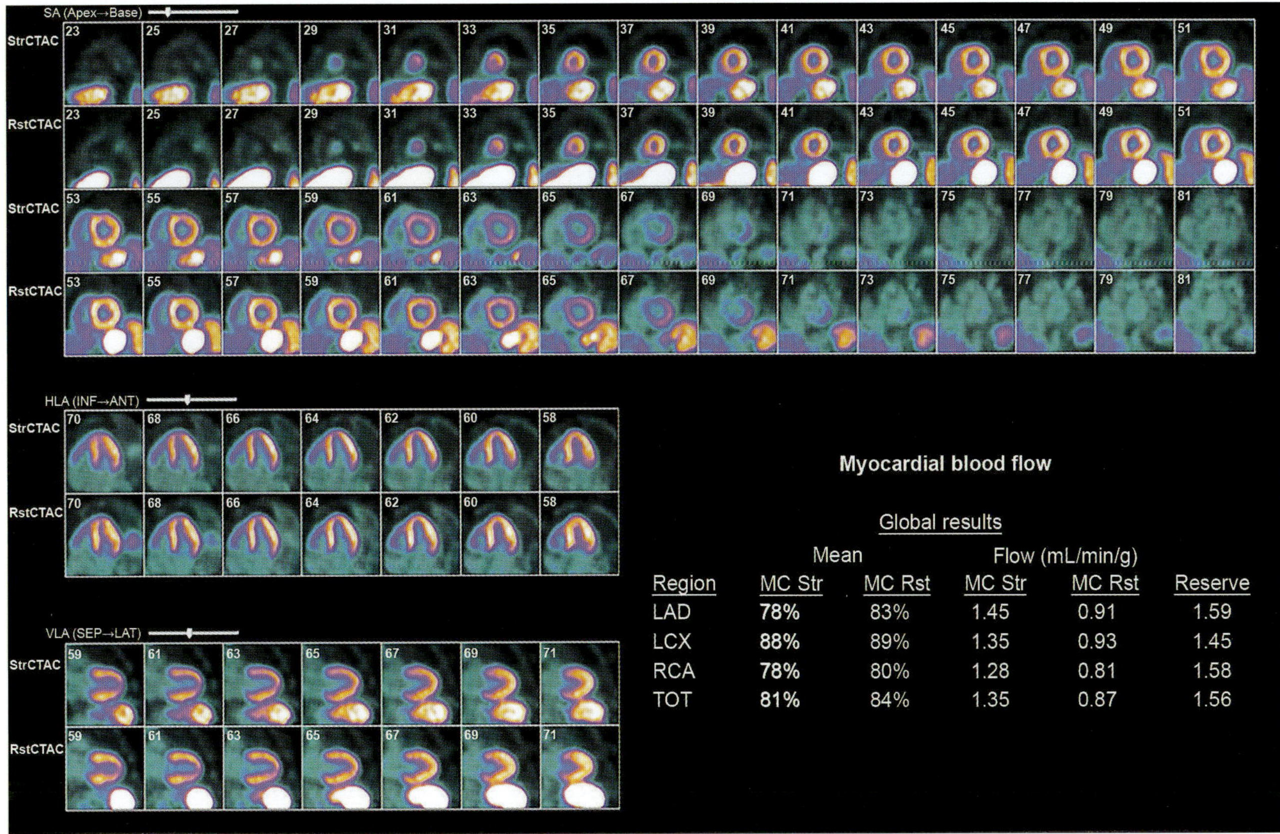

Region	Mean MC Str	Mean MC Rst	Flow (mL/min/g) MC Str	Flow (mL/min/g) MC Rst	Reserve
LAD	78%	83%	1.45	0.91	1.59
LCX	88%	89%	1.35	0.93	1.45
RCA	78%	80%	1.28	0.81	1.58
TOT	81%	84%	1.35	0.87	1.56

Fig. 1: Application of myocardial blood flow for confirmation of microvessel disease. A 70-year-old female with chest pain radiating to the jaw and left arm. She has a history of hypertension, hyperlipidemia, and a remote history of smoking. She underwent coronary angiogram which showed nonobstructive coronary artery disease (CAD) with <30% luminal stenosis in all vessels. She was referred for rubidium-82 rest/vasodilator stress PET MPI, which showed normal relative perfusion and normal left ventricular ejection fraction at 65%. However, myocardial blood flow assessed via dynamic imaging showed significantly reduced global flow reverse, which was compatible with microvessel disease, in the absence of epicardial CAD. (LAD: left anterior descending coronary artery; LCX: left circumflex; MPI: myocardial perfusion imaging; PET: positron emission tomography; RCA: right coronary artery; TOT: total)
Courtesy: Dr Matthieu Pelletier-Galarneau, Institut de cardiologie de Montréal, Montreal, Canada.

the ED, the diagnosis of acute coronary syndrome (ACS) is not always conclusive, and radionuclide imaging can help in triaging of these patients. In patients presenting to the emergency with chest pain, who are suspected of having an ACS, rest imaging during pain can be employed to detect acute myocardial infarction (MI) or ischemia.[20] In this protocol, a standard high dose of technetium-99m (Tc-99m) is injected at rest during chest pain or soon after resolution (within 30 minutes), with gated SPECT imaging performed within 30–60 minutes. A completely normal gated SPECT study virtually excludes the presence of myocardial ischemia. Evaluation of patients with chest pain in the ED with resting SPECT-MPI has shown excellent sensitivity of MPI (92%) for myocardial ischemia, which was significantly greater than that conferred by the first troponin level (39%).[21] A clinical trial of patients with acute chest pain in the ED has highlighted the utility of rest MPI, decreasing the need for hospitalization as well as facilitating early discharge from the ED.[22] SPECT-MPI with Tc-99m is particularly well suited for acute chest pain imaging, due to its 6-hour half-life and no significant redistribution (unlike thallium-201), allowing perfusion to be "fixed" at the time of injection with flexibility in the timing of imaging.

Given the development of ultrafast SPECT systems employing cadmium-zinc-telluride (CZT)[23] technology, these novel protocols have received significant traction for their ability to improve laboratory throughput by eliminating the need for additional imaging, with significant radiation dose reduction.[24] Even with a

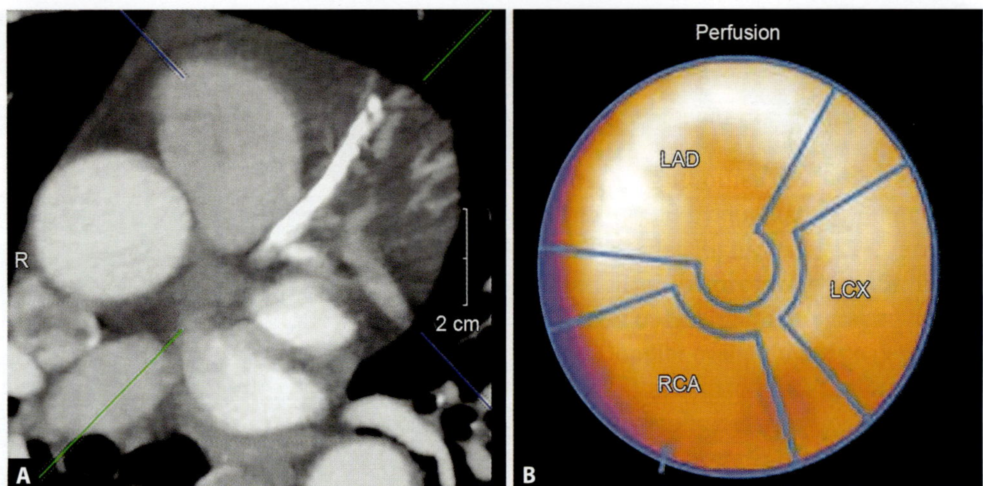

Figs. 2A and B: Normal stress-first SPECT-MPI in a patient with known calcific atherosclerosis. A 57-year-old male with a history of chest pain. He initially underwent a CCTA for the assessment of CAD. CCTA revealed extensive calcific atherosclerosis of the proximal left anterior descending coronary artery (LAD), because of which accurate assessment of underlying luminal stenosis could not be accurately determined. He was referred for a rest/stress SPECT-MPI. Per laboratory protocol, he underwent stress-first imaging that showed normal poststress myocardial perfusion. Rest imaging was thus not performed. (CAD: coronary artery disease; CCTA: cardiac computed tomography angiography; LCX: left circumflex; RCA: right coronary artery; MPI: myocardial perfusion imaging; SPECT: single photon emission computed tomography)

standard Anger camera, a SF/SO protocol or acute chest pain imaging could reduce radiation dose to around 9 mSv considering a total dose of 30 mCi of Tc-99m as a standard high dose for MPI.

RISK STRATIFICATION OF CORONARY ARTERY DISEASE WITH RADIONUCLIDE MYOCARDIAL PERFUSION IMAGING

Several studies have shown the association between the presence and magnitude of myocardial ischemia, risk of cardiac death, and nonfatal MI, with both PET and SPECT.[25,26] An abnormal SPECT-MPI portends a five- to sixfold increase in the rate of cardiac death and nonfatal MI compared to a normal study, whether patients underwent exercise (0.7% vs. 4.3%, respectively) or pharmacologic (1.8% vs. 10%) SPECT-MPI.[27] Similar findings were also shown across the spectrum of cardiovascular risk, including patients with or without CAD, diabetes, and chronic kidney disease. Data from the PET multicenter registry showed a twofold increase in the hazards of cardiac death in patients with a mildly abnormal PET MPI [hazard ratio (HR) 2.3, 95% confidence interval (CI) 1.4–3.8; $p = 0.001$] and almost a fivefold increase in those who had a severely abnormal PET MPI [HR 4.9, 95% CI 2.5–9.6; $p < 0.0001$].[26]

Coronary Flow Reserve: Additive Prognostic Value

The ability to quantify MBF in absolute terms (mL/min/g) has led to increased interest in cardiac applications of PET imaging technology, not only for the diagnostic benefits mentioned earlier but also for the incremental prognostic value provided with the assessment of coronary vasomotor function.[28] Coronary flow reserve (CFR)—defined as the ratio of peak-hyperemic MBF to that at rest—is a physiologic marker of the coronary microcirculatory status, which can now be routinely assessed in clinical practice in addition to relative perfusion assessment.[29] PET-derived CFR measurements are feasible with available PET tracers, including ^{82}Rb, N-13 ammonia, and O-15 water, and flow measurements obtained can be processed across available software packages.[30]

Coronary flow reserve is a stronger predictor of cardiac death compared to peak hyperemic MBF.[31,32] PET-determined CFR has also been shown in several studies to provide incremental risk stratification and to predict adverse cardiovascular events, independent of age, gender, cardiovascular risk factors, and presence and extent of ischemia.[33] Low CFR was associated with a threefold increase in the risk of cardiac death, nonfatal MI, or late revascularization among patients who underwent

N-13 ammonia PET MPI, irrespective of the presence or absence of relative perfusion defects.[34] Similarly, CFR with ^{82}Rb PET MPI was independently predictive of future major adverse cardiac events with comparable estimates of risk.[35-38] The prognostic utility of PET-derived CFR was also demonstrated in other patient cohorts, including women, patients with diabetes, those chronic kidney disease, and those with elevated markers of myocardial injury.[39-44]

RISK STRATIFICATION WITH ISCHEMIC BURDEN ON MYOCARDIAL PERFUSION IMAGING

Observational data has provided therapeutic guidance on an ischemic threshold at which a greater prevalence of adverse outcomes is noted. It is now accepted that patients with greater burden of ischemia [≥10% of the left ventricular (LV) myocardium] have worse prognosis, compared to those with milder degrees of ischemia **(Fig. 3)**. Similar data with PET are available and suggest that the threshold at which patients derive survival benefit with revascularization might be lower. This aspect of prognostication by ischemic burden is underscored by its qualification as a metric of a nuclear laboratory quality, per the recent American Society of Nuclear Cardiology (ASNC) quality standards.[45] While observational data continues to support early revascularization among patients with >10% ischemic myocardium, this was not supported by the results of the ISCHEMIA (International Study of Comparative Health Effectiveness with Medical and Invasive Approaches) study, wherein patients continuing with aggressive medical therapy alone fared similarly when compared to patients with aggressive medical therapy and early revascularization, as long as the significant left main disease was ruled out. An example of the application of findings of the ischemia trial in clinical practice is shown in **Figures 4A and B**.

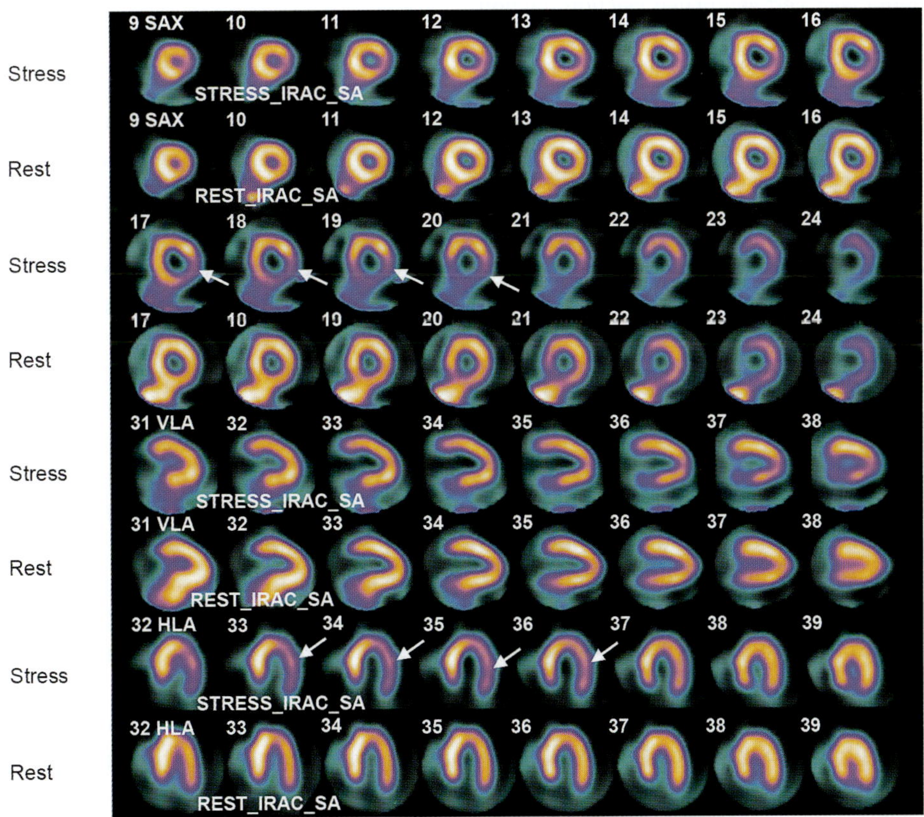

Fig. 3: High burden of myocardial ischemia. A 63-year-old female with known coronary artery disease and prior coronary artery bypass grafting, presenting with 3 months of chest tightness, which is relieved with sublingual nitroglycerine. The patient underwent a rest/dipyridamole SPECT-MPI with attenuation correction on a high-sensitivity cadmium–zinc–telluride system, which showed a large area of moderate-to-severe ischemia in the entire lateral wall, encompassing >10% left ventricular myocardium.

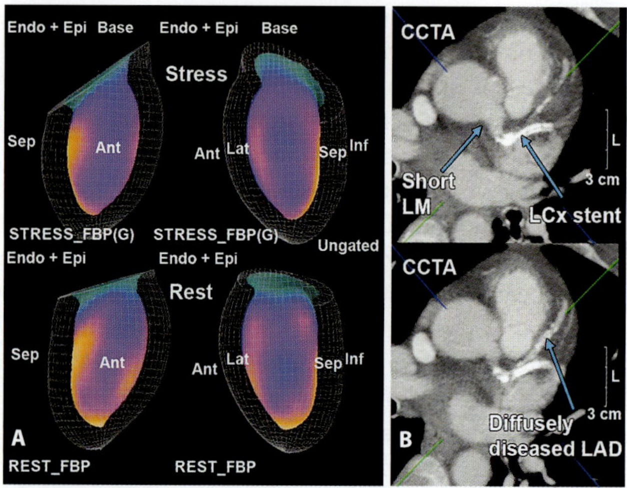

Figs. 4A and B: Complimentary role of functional and anatomical data in the management of a patient with coronary artery disease. A 56-year-old female, with diabetes, severe peripheral arterial disease, and reported history of coronary stent (unknown anatomy) was admitted with critical limb ischemia. The surgical team referred the patient for preoperative risk stratification with a rest/stress SPECT-MPI, which showed a large area of peri-infarct ischemia in the anterior wall. Left ventricular ejection fraction was 45% on gated SPECT-MPI. Given the urgent need for surgery and unknown coronary anatomy, she was referred for cardiac computed tomography angiography (CCTA), which showed no significant left main (LM) stenosis, diffusely diseased left anterior descending coronary artery (LAD), and patent stent in left circumflex (LCX). Given the absence of significant LM disease, a decision was made to continue aggressive medical therapy and proceed with vascular surgery. She tolerated the procedure well and was discharged from the hospital without any perioperative adverse cardiovascular events. (MPI: myocardial perfusion imaging; SPECT: single photon emission computed tomography)

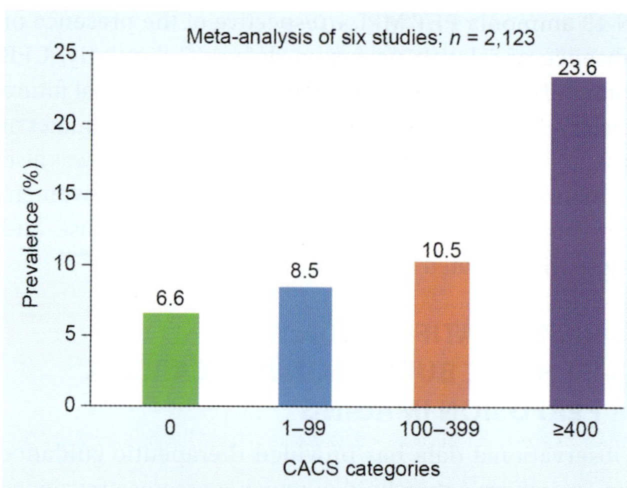

Fig. 5: Prevalence of myocardial ischemia across Coronary Artery Calcium Score (CACS) categories.

INTEGRATION OF RADIONUCLIDE IMAGING WITH CORONARY ARTERY CALCIUM SCORE

While MPI with SPECT is still the most used modality to diagnose CAD, hybrid imaging with the addition of low-dose computed tomography (CT) for attenuation correction and more recently Coronary Artery Calcium Score (CACS) assessment is increasing. This combined approach of using both anatomic and functional information enables improved diagnosis and prognostication of CAD. Several studies have shown increased accuracy of MPI with the addition of low-dose CT by decreasing attenuation artifacts and hence equivocal interpretations.[46,47] Addition of CACS was found particularly helpful in differentiation of ischemic versus nonischemic cardiomyopathy.[48-51] While PET MPI is inherently performed with attenuation correction, the evaluation of coronary atherosclerotic burden using CACS further amplifies the diagnostic and prognostic values of MPI. Integrating MPI with CACS scoring enhances diagnostic accuracy, facilitates early CAD detection before development of ischemia, and optimizes treatment strategies. This hybrid imaging approach improves patient care by providing a more precise and personalized assessment of cardiovascular risk.

Presence of coronary artery calcium (CAC) when perfusion findings are normal has been reported and shown to be related to the intensification of medical therapy and adverse outcomes. Bybee et al.[50] reported a >60% prevalence of CAC among 760 patients with a normal PET MPI. Approximately 30% of these patients had a CACS ≥100. Increasing CACS, despite a normal PET MPI, was related to greater change in medical therapy and institution of statins. Conversely, an increasing burden of CAC is associated with greater likelihood of ischemia on perfusion imaging. This was reported in a meta-analysis of six studies comprising 2,123 patients. Only 6% of the patients had ischemia on perfusion imaging with a CACS of 0, while almost 24% had ischemia when CACS ≥400 **(Fig. 5)**.[52] Furthermore, Chang et al.[51] followed 1,126 asymptomatic or atypical chest pain patients for an average of 6.9 years. In their study, individuals with normal SPECT findings but with a CACS >400 experienced a 3.55-fold relative increase in cardiac events (2.75-fold increase in death/MI) compared to those with minimal CACS (≤10). This incremental prognostic value of CACS has also been reported in conjunction with MBF on PET MPI, wherein increasing CACS allowed for identification of a greater risk for cardiac death and nonfatal MI even when MFR was normal.[53] This risk was the greatest among patients with abnormal MFR across all CACS categories.

For laboratories that may not have access to hybrid technology to allow for calculation of CACS or software to process the data, assessment of visual CACS or visually estimated (VE)-CACS is encouraged. This provides diagnosis of CAD when MPI is normal and has been shown to have good correlation with formally measured CACS using the Agatston method. Furthermore, studies have also shown VE-CACS to predict the likelihood of >70% luminal stenosis and need for coronary revascularization[54] while also providing prognostic value for cardiovascular adverse events.[55] Thus, integrating MPI with CAC scoring enhances diagnostic accuracy, facilitates early CAD detection, and optimizes treatment strategies. This hybrid imaging approach improves patient care by providing a more precise and personalized assessment of cardiovascular risk. CACS adds critical anatomic and prognostic insights to MPI, optimizing CAD management without significant additional radiation or cost. This synergy underscores the need to shift toward hybrid imaging in modern cardiovascular imaging. Adequate training and competency are required to ensure the effective implementation of hybrid imaging in clinical practice.

COMPARATIVE EFFECTIVENESS OF RADIONUCLIDE IMAGING AND OTHER IMAGING MODALITIES

Several studies have compared the performance of MPI for diagnosing CAD with other modalities. Though exercise treadmill stress alone is recommended for individuals at the lowest risk of CAD, its reported sensitivity and specificity of 68% and 77%, respectively, are significantly inferior to those of MPI.[56] Additionally, studies have shown that ischemia on MPI can be present in patients with no evidence of ECG ischemia on treadmill exercise, and this ischemia on MPI is associated with an increased risk of all-cause mortality.[57] When compared to stress perfusion with cardiac magnetic resonance (CMR), nonattenuation-corrected SPECT-MPI has been shown to have similar specificity and positive predictive value for CAD.[58] Additionally, when comparing outcomes, such as invasive angiography rates following stress perfusion imaging, there were no differences in downstream resource utilization and cost with either stress CMR or stress SPECT-MPI. Though a direct comparison between PET and CMR has not been performed, a pooled analysis of 37 CMR studies and 15 PET studies reported a superior area under the curve (AUC) for PET than CMR for CAD.[59] While the diagnostic accuracy of SPECT-MPI and stress echocardiography is generally considered to be comparable, and both have a similarly high negative predictive value, a markedly abnormal SPECT-MPI identifies a significantly higher risk of mortality versus a normal SPECT-MPI.[60] While stress echocardiography provides a similar prognostic stratification,[61] the magnitude of discrimination of risk between a normal and a markedly abnormal stress echocardiogram are substantially lower. Additionally, vasodilator perfusion stress imaging is not routinely performed with echocardiography in contemporary clinical practice, which is a limitation for patients in whom medicines such as beta-blockers cannot be withheld.

Cardiac computed tomography angiography (CCTA), by virtue of anatomical imaging, has excellent sensitivity and comparable specificity for diagnosing CAD; when compared to MPI, it involves administration of iodinated contrast and the need for heart rate control for adequate image quality. The PACIFIC trial reported a superior diagnostic accuracy of PET MPI for detection of hemodynamically significant CAD, when compared to both SPECT and CCTA.[62] In addition, the recently published ReASSESS study reported the diagnostic accuracy of fractional flow reserve derived from computed tomography (FFR-CT) to be comparable to that of conventional SPECT-MPI.[63] Though the sensitivity of FFR-CT was greater, SPECT-MPI had a greater specificity for obstructive CAD, with no difference in overall accuracy. Additionally, the need for CCTA images to be analyzed by a third party to derive the fractional flow reserve (FFR) results makes it costlier with additional time and resources required for diagnosis, when there is no additional diagnostic benefit. The PROMISE (Prospective Multicenter Imaging Study for Evaluation of Chest Pain) trial evaluated the occurrence of major adverse cardiovascular events (MACE) among individuals randomized to either CCTA first or functional testing first strategy.[64] Although MPI was not independently evaluated, two third of the patients in the functional testing arm underwent MPI. Results from the PROMISE trial showed no difference in the occurrence of MACE among those randomized to CCTA versus

TABLE 1: Clinical effectiveness of various imaging modalities for the diagnosis of coronary artery disease.

	Radionuclide perfusion imaging	*Echocardiography*	*Cardiac computed tomography angiography*	*Cardiac magnetic resonance*
Wide availability	+	+	+	–
Type of stress				
• Exercise	+	+	NA	
• Dobutamine	+	+	NA	+
• Vasodilator	+		NA	+
Myocardial blood flow	+			
Imaging with comorbidities				
• Metal implants	+	+	+/–	–
• Renal failure	+	+	–	+/–
• Atrial fibrillation	+	+/–	–	+
• Body habitus/morbid obesity	+		+	+/–
Prognostic value	+	+	+	+

Source: Adapted from Al Baradin and Malhotra.[65]

functional testing, though more patients randomized to CCTA underwent invasive coronary angiography.[11] It should also be noted that only those patients were included in the PROMISE trial whose serum creatinine was <1.5 mg/dL in the last 90 days. This was likely due to the concern for possible contrast-induced nephropathy among those with higher serum creatinine levels, which remains a relative contraindication for CCTA.

CONCLUSION

Radionuclide MPI is a robust technique for the diagnosis of CAD, to guide therapeutic decision-making and to determine the risk of adverse outcomes. Though the field of radionuclide MPI is mature, it continues to evolve, which is evident from the application of new imaging protocols and development of more efficient tracers, along with advances in camera technology, resulting in reduced radiation exposure. Given that radionuclide MPI can be universally employed, without any contraindications, as opposed to other imaging modalities for CAD, its clinical applicability remains unmatched. A comparison of the clinical effectiveness of various imaging modalities is provided in **Table 1**.[65]

REFERENCES

1. Benjamin EJ, Virani SS, Callaway CW, Chamberlain AM, Chang AR, Cheng S, et al; American Heart Association Council on Epidemiology and Prevention Statistics Committee and Stroke Statistics Subcommittee. Heart Disease and Stroke Statistics-2018 Update: A Report From the American Heart Association. Circulation. 2018;137(12):e67-e492.
2. Durand DJ, Lewin JS, Berkowitz SA. Medical-Imaging Stewardship in the Accountable Care Era. N Engl J Med. 2015;373(18):1691-3.
3. Shaw LJ, Blankstein R, Jacobs JE, Leipsic JA, Kwong RY, Taqueti VR, et al; American Heart Association Cardiovascular Imaging and Intervention Subcommittee of the Council on Clinical Cardiology; Council on Cardiovascular Radiology and Intervention; Council on Cardiovascular and Stroke Nursing; Council on Cardiovascular Disease in the Young; and Council on Quality of Care and Outcomes Research. Defining Quality in Cardiovascular Imaging: A Scientific Statement From the American Heart Association. Circ Cardiovasc Imaging. 2017;10(12):e000017.
4. Klocke FJ, Baird MG, Lorell BH, Bateman TM, Messer JV, Berman DS, et al; American College of Cardiology; American Heart Association; American Society for Nuclear Cardiology. ACC/AHA/ASNC guidelines for the clinical use of cardiac radionuclide imaging—executive summary: a report of the American College of Cardiology/American Heart Association Task Force on Practice Guidelines (ACC/AHA/ASNC Committee to Revise the 1995 Guidelines for the Clinical Use of Cardiac Radionuclide Imaging). J Am Coll Cardiol. 2003;42(7):1318-33.
5. Fiechter M, Ghadri JR, Gebhard C, Fuchs TA, Pazhenkottil AP, Nkoulou RN, et al. Diagnostic value of

13N-ammonia myocardial perfusion PET: added value of myocardial flow reserve. J Nucl Med. 2012;53(8):1230-4.
6. Parker MW, Iskandar A, Limone B, Perugini A, Kim H, Jones C, et al. Diagnostic accuracy of cardiac positron emission tomography versus single photon emission computed tomography for coronary artery disease: a bivariate meta-analysis. Circ Cardiovasc Imaging. 2012; 5(6):700-7.
7. Bateman TM, Heller GV, McGhie AI, Friedman JD, Case JA, Bryngelson JR, et al. Diagnostic accuracy of rest/stress ECG-gated Rb-82 myocardial perfusion PET: comparison with ECG-gated Tc-99m sestamibi SPECT. J Nucl Cardiol. 2006;13(1):24-33.
8. Bateman TM. Advantages and disadvantages of PET and SPECT in a busy clinical practice. J Nucl Cardiol. 2012;19 Suppl 1:S3-11.
9. Beller GA. Underestimation of coronary artery disease with SPECT perfusion imaging. J Nucl Cardiol. 2008;15(2):151-3.
10. Berman DS, Kang X, Slomka PJ, Gerlach J, de Yang L, Hayes SW, et al. Underestimation of extent of ischemia by gated SPECT myocardial perfusion imaging in patients with left main coronary artery disease. J Nucl Cardiol. 2007;14(4):521-8.
11. Nakanishi R, Gransar H, Slomka P, Arsanjani R, Shalev A, Otaki Y, et al. Predictors of high-risk coronary artery disease in subjects with normal SPECT myocardial perfusion imaging. J Nucl Cardiol. 2016;23(3):530-41.
12. Dorbala S, Vangala D, Sampson U, Limaye A, Kwong R, Di Carli MF. Value of vasodilator left ventricular ejection fraction reserve in evaluating the magnitude of myocardium at risk and the extent of angiographic coronary artery disease: a 82Rb PET/CT study. J Nucl Med. 2007; 48(3):349-58.
13. Ferro A, Petretta M, Acampa W, Fiumara G, Daniele S, Petretta MP, et al. Post-stress left ventricular ejection fraction drop in patients with diabetes: a gated myocardial perfusion imaging study. BMC Cardiovasc Disord. 2013;13:99.
14. Gomez J, Golzar Y, Fughhi I, Olusanya A, Doukky R. The significance of post-stress decrease in left ventricular ejection fraction in patients undergoing regadenoson stress gated SPECT myocardial perfusion imaging. J Nucl Cardiol. 2018;25(4):1313-23.
15. Naya M, Murthy VL, Taqueti VR, Foster CR, Klein J, Garber M, et al. Preserved coronary flow reserve effectively excludes high-risk coronary artery disease on angiography. J Nucl Med. 2014;55(2):248-55.
16. Ziadi MC, Dekemp RA, Williams K, Guo A, Renaud JM, Chow BJ, et al. Does quantification of myocardial flow reserve using rubidium-82 positron emission tomography facilitate detection of multivessel coronary artery disease? J Nucl Cardiol. 2012;19(4):670-80.
17. Minhas J, Narasimmal SP, M Bull T, Marco T, McConnell JW, Lammi MR, et al. Health-related quality of life and hospitalizations in chronic thromboembolic pulmonary hypertension versus idiopathic pulmonary arterial hypertension: an analysis from the Pulmonary Hypertension Association Registry (PHAR). Pulm Circ. 2021;11(4):20458940211053196.
18. Chang SM, Nabi F, Xu J, Raza U, Mahmarian JJ. Normal stress-only versus standard stress/rest myocardial perfusion imaging: similar patient mortality with reduced radiation exposure. J Am Coll Cardiol. 2010;55(3):221-30.
19. Duvall WL, Wijetunga MN, Klein TM, Razzouk L, Godbold J, Croft LB, et al. The prognosis of a normal stress-only Tc-99m myocardial perfusion imaging study. J Nucl Cardiol. 2010;17(3):370-7.
20. Heller GV, Stowers SA, Hendel RC, Herman SD, Daher E, Ahlberg AW, et al. Clinical value of acute rest technetium-99m tetrofosmin tomographic myocardial perfusion imaging in patients with acute chest pain and nondiagnostic electrocardiograms. J Am Coll Cardiol. 1998;31(5):1011-7.
21. Kontos MC, Jesse RL, Anderson FP, Schmidt KL, Ornato JP, Tatum JL. Comparison of myocardial perfusion imaging and cardiac troponin I in patients admitted to the emergency department with chest pain. Circulation. 1999;99(16):2073-8.
22. Udelson JE, Beshansky JR, Ballin DS, Feldman JA, Griffith JL, Handler J, et al. Myocardial perfusion imaging for evaluation and triage of patients with suspected acute cardiac ischemia: a randomized controlled trial. JAMA. 2002;288(21):2693-700.
23. Imbert L, Poussier S, Franken PR, Songy B, Verger A, Morel O, et al. Compared performance of high-sensitivity cameras dedicated to myocardial perfusion SPECT: a comprehensive analysis of phantom and human images. J Nucl Med. 2012;53(12):1897-903.
24. Depuey EG, Mahmarian JJ, Miller TD, Einstein AJ, Hansen CL, Holly TA, et al. Patient-centered imaging. J Nucl Cardiol. 2012;19(2):185-215.
25. Shaw LJ, Iskandrian AE. Prognostic value of gated myocardial perfusion SPECT. J Nucl Cardiol. 2004;11(2):171-85.
26. Dorbala S, Di Carli MF, Beanlands RS, Merhige ME, Williams BA, Veledar E, et al. Prognostic value of stress myocardial perfusion positron emission tomography: results from a multicenter observational registry. J Am Coll Cardiol. 2013;61(2):176-84.
27. Navare SM, Mather JF, Shaw LJ, Fowler MS, Heller GV. Comparison of risk stratification with pharmacologic and exercise stress myocardial perfusion imaging: a meta-analysis. J Nucl Cardiol. 2004;11(5):551-61.
28. Taqueti VR, Di Carli MF. Clinical significance of noninvasive coronary flow reserve assessment in patients with ischemic heart disease. Curr Opin Cardiol. 2016;31(6):662-9.
29. Murthy VL, Bateman TM, Beanlands RS, Berman DS, Borges-Neto S, Chareonthaitawee P, et al. Clinical Quantification of Myocardial Blood Flow Using PET: Joint Position Paper of the SNMMI Cardiovascular Council and the ASNC. J Nucl Cardiol. 2018;25(1):269-97.

30. Nesterov SV, Deshayes E, Sciagrà R, Settimo L, Declerck JM, Pan XB, et al. Quantification of myocardial blood flow in absolute terms using (82)Rb PET imaging: the RUBY-10 Study. JACC Cardiovasc Imaging. 2014;7(11):1119-27.
31. Gupta A, Taqueti VR, van de Hoef TP, Bajaj NS, Bravo PE, Murthy VL, et al. Integrated Noninvasive Physiological Assessment of Coronary Circulatory Function and Impact on Cardiovascular Mortality in Patients With Stable Coronary Artery Disease. Circulation. 2017;136(24):2325-36.
32. Murthy VL, Lee BC, Sitek A, Naya M, Moody J, Polavarapu V, et al. Comparison and prognostic validation of multiple methods of quantification of myocardial blood flow with 82Rb PET. J Nucl Med. 2014;55(12):1952-8.
33. Al Badarin F, Aljizeeri A, Almasoudi F, Al-Mallah MH. Assessment of myocardial blood flow and coronary flow reserve with positron emission tomography in ischemic heart disease: current state and future directions. Heart Fail Rev. 2017;22(4):441-53.
34. Herzog BA, Husmann L, Valenta I, Gaemperli O, Siegrist PT, Tay FM, et al. Long-term prognostic value of 13N-ammonia myocardial perfusion positron emission tomography added value of coronary flow reserve. J Am Coll Cardiol. 2009;54(2):150-6.
35. Fukushima K, Javadi MS, Higuchi T, Lautamäki R, Merrill J, Nekolla SG, et al. Prediction of short-term cardiovascular events using quantification of global myocardial flow reserve in patients referred for clinical 82Rb PET perfusion imaging. J Nucl Med. 2011;52(5):726-32.
36. Farhad H, Dunet V, Bachelard K, Allenbach G, Kaufmann PA, Prior JO. Added prognostic value of myocardial blood flow quantitation in rubidium-82 positron emission tomography imaging. Eur Heart J Cardiovasc Imaging. 2013;14(12):1203-10.
37. Murthy VL, Naya M, Foster CR, Hainer J, Gaber M, Di Carli G, et al. Improved cardiac risk assessment with non-invasive measures of coronary flow reserve. Circulation. 2011;124(20):2215-24.
38. Ziadi MC, Dekemp RA, Williams KA, Guo A, Chow BJ, Renaud JM, et al. Impaired myocardial flow reserve on rubidium-82 positron emission tomography imaging predicts adverse outcomes in patients assessed for myocardial ischemia. J Am Coll Cardiol. 2011;58(7):740-8.
39. Taqueti VR, Everett BM, Murthy VL, Gaber M, Foster CR, Hainer J, et al. Interaction of impaired coronary flow reserve and cardiomyocyte injury on adverse cardiovascular outcomes in patients without overt coronary artery disease. Circulation. 2015;131(6):528-35.
40. Taqueti VR, Hachamovitch R, Murthy VL, Naya M, Foster CR, Hainer J, et al. Global coronary flow reserve is associated with adverse cardiovascular events independently of luminal angiographic severity and modifies the effect of early revascularization. Circulation. 2015;131(1):19-27.
41. Taqueti VR, Shaw LJ, Cook NR, Murthy VL, Shah NR, Foster CR, et al. Excess Cardiovascular Risk in Women Relative to Men Referred for Coronary Angiography Is Associated With Severely Impaired Coronary Flow Reserve, Not Obstructive Disease. Circulation. 2017;135(6):566-77.
42. Murthy VL, Naya M, Foster CR, Gaber M, Hainer J, Klein J, et al. Association between coronary vascular dysfunction and cardiac mortality in patients with and without diabetes mellitus. Circulation. 2012;126(15):1858-68.
43. Murthy VL, Naya M, Foster CR, Hainer J, Gaber M, Dorbala S, et al. Coronary vascular dysfunction and prognosis in patients with chronic kidney disease. JACC Cardiovasc Imaging. 2012;5(10):1025-34.
44. Shah NR, Charytan DM, Murthy VL, Skali Lami H, Veeranna V, Cheezum MK, et al. Prognostic Value of Coronary Flow Reserve in Patients with Dialysis-Dependent ESRD. J Am Soc Nephrol. 2016;27(6):1823-9.
45. Hage FG, Einstein AJ, Ananthasubramaniam K, Bourque JM, Case J, DePuey EG, et al. Quality metrics for single-photon emission computed tomography myocardial perfusion imaging: an ASNC information statement. J Nucl Cardiol. 2023;30(2):864-907.
46. Malkerneker D, Brenner R, Martin WH, Sampson UK, Feurer ID, Kronenberg MW, et al. CT-based attenuation correction versus prone imaging to decrease equivocal interpretations of rest/stress Tc-99m tetrofosmin SPECT MPI. J Nucl Cardiol. 2007;14(3):314-23.
47. Huang JY, Huang CK, Yen RF, Wu HY, Tu YK, Cheng MF, et al. Diagnostic Performance of Attenuation-Corrected Myocardial Perfusion Imaging for Coronary Artery Disease: A Systematic Review and Meta-Analysis. J Nucl Med. 2016; 57(12):1893-8.
48. Taylor AJ, Bindeman J, Feuerstein I, Cao F, Brazaitis M, O'Malley PG. Coronary calcium independently predicts incident premature coronary heart disease over measured cardiovascular risk factors: mean three-year outcomes in the Prospective Army Coronary Calcium (PACC) project. J Am Coll Cardiol. 2005;46(5):807-14.
49. Berman DS. Complementary roles of coronary calcium scanning and myocardial perfusion SPECT. J Nucl Cardiol. 2004;11(4):379-81.
50. Bybee KA, Lee J, Markiewicz R, Longmore R, McGhie AI, O'Keefe JH, et al. Diagnostic and clinical benefit of combined coronary calcium and perfusion assessment in patients undergoing PET/CT myocardial perfusion stress imaging. J Nucl Cardiol. 2010;17(2):188-96.
51. Chang SM, Nabi F, Xu J, Peterson LE, Achari A, Pratt CM, et al. The coronary artery calcium score and stress myocardial perfusion imaging provide independent and complementary prediction of cardiac risk. J Am Coll Cardiol. 2009;54(20):1872-82.
52. Bavishi C, Argulian E, Chatterjee S, Rozanski A. CACS and the Frequency of Stress-Induced Myocardial Ischemia During MPI: A Meta-Analysis. JACC Cardiovasc Imaging. 2016;9(5):580-9.

53. Aljizeeri A, Ahmed AI, Alfaris MA, Ahmed D, Farea J, Elneama A, et al. Myocardial Flow Reserve and Coronary Calcification in Prognosis of Patients With Suspected Coronary Artery Disease. JACC Cardiovasc Imaging. 2021;14(12):2443-52.
54. Le VT, Knight S, Min DB, McCubrey RO, Horne BD, Jensen KR, et al. Absence of Coronary Artery Calcium During Positron Emission Tomography Stress Testing in Patients Without Known Coronary Artery Disease Identifies Individuals With Very Low Risk of Cardiac Events. Circ Cardiovasc Imaging. 2020;13(1):e009907.
55. Selvaraj S, Khan MS, Vidula MK, Wiener PC, de Feria AE, Rojulpote C, et al. Incremental prognostic value of visually estimated coronary artery calcium in patients undergoing positron emission tomography imaging. Open Heart. 2021;8(1):e001648.
56. Lee TH, Boucher CA. Clinical practice. Noninvasive tests in patients with stable coronary artery disease. N Engl J Med. 2001;344(24):1840-5.
57. Malhotra S, Sharma R, Pasupula DK, Khanna M, Soman P. SPECT imaging provides long-term prognostic value over exercise electrocardiography alone in patients with a normal baseline electrocardiogram. J Am Coll Cardiol. 2015;65:10 Supplement.
58. Greenwood JP, Maredia N, Younger JF, Brown JM, Nixon J, Everett CC, et al. Cardiovascular magnetic resonance and single-photon emission computed tomography for diagnosis of coronary heart disease (CE-MARC): a prospective trial. Lancet. 2012;379(9814):453-60.
59. Jaarsma C, Leiner T, Bekkers SC, Crijns HJ, Wildberger JE, Nagel E, et al. Diagnostic performance of noninvasive myocardial perfusion imaging using single-photon emission computed tomography, cardiac magnetic resonance, and positron emission tomography imaging for the detection of obstructive coronary artery disease: a meta-analysis. J Am Coll Cardiol. 2012;59(19):1719-28.
60. Hachamovitch R, Berman DS, Kiat H, Cohen I, Cabico JA, Friedman J, et al. Exercise myocardial perfusion SPECT in patients without known coronary artery disease: incremental prognostic value and use in risk stratification. Circulation. 1996;93(5):905-14.
61. Marwick TH, Case C, Vasey C, Allen S, Short L, Thomas JD. Prediction of mortality by exercise echocardiography: a strategy for combination with the duke treadmill score. Circulation. 2001;103(21):2566-71.
62. Danad I, Raijmakers PG, Driessen RS, Leipsic J, Raju R, Naoum C, et al. Comparison of Coronary CT Angiography, SPECT, PET, and Hybrid Imaging for Diagnosis of Ischemic Heart Disease Determined by Fractional Flow Reserve. JAMA Cardiol. 2017;2(10):1100-7.
63. Sand NPR, Veien KT, Nielsen SS, Nørgaard BL, Larsen P, Johansen A, et al. Prospective Comparison of FFR Derived From Coronary CT Angiography With SPECT Perfusion Imaging in Stable Coronary Artery Disease: The ReASSESS Study. JACC Cardiovasc Imaging. 2018;11(11):1640-50.
64. Douglas PS, Hoffmann U, Patel MR, Mark DB, Al-Khalidi HR, Cavanaugh B, et al; PROMISE Investigators. Outcomes of anatomical versus functional testing for coronary artery disease. N Engl J Med. 2015;372(14):1291-300.
65. Al Badarin FJ, Malhotra S. Diagnosis and Prognosis of Coronary Artery Disease with SPECT and PET. Curr Cardiol Rep. 2019;21(7):57.

CHAPTER 30

Positron Emission Tomography: The Role of Quantitative Myocardial Perfusion Imaging

Karthik Ananthasubramaniam

INTRODUCTION

Cardiovascular positron emission tomography (PET) with its origins more than 4 decades ago has now entered the mainstream of noninvasive cardiac imaging on a variety of fronts. From ischemia assessment to myocardial viability and extending into infection and inflammation imaging, PET is now widely recognized as a key frontline modality. Beyond visual assessment of myocardial perfusion, PET brings forth unique advantages in its ability to measure myocardial blood flow (MBF) in mL/min/g in stress and rest and hence calculate myocardial flow reserve (MFR), which has been shown to be superior to relative perfusion.[1] As perfusion PET is discussed elsewhere in this book, the main focus of this chapter will be on quantitative PET and case illustrations of value of flow quantification.

FUNDAMENTALS OF FLOW QUANTIFICATION IN POSITRON EMISSION TOMOGRAPHY

Overview of Positron Emission Tomography Radiotracers

The PET radiotracers for evaluation of MBF include well-established tracers, such as ^{15}O-labeled water ($^{15}O\text{-}H_2O$), ^{13}N-labeled ammonia ($^{13}NH_3$),and ^{82}rubidium (^{82}Rb), and newly approved tracers like ^{18}F-Flurpiridaz.[2] $^{15}O\text{-}H_2O$ is generated by a cyclotron (half-life 2 min) and is considered the most ideal perfusion tracer because of its physiological properties. It is freely diffusible and has a high first-pass extraction of 95%. Its uptake is nearly linear with no roll-off in extraction at higher coronary flows, which results in underestimation of MBF. However, because of its short half-life seconds, need for onsite cyclotron, poor tissue accumulation, and challenges with image quality, it is not widely used clinically.[2] $^{13}NH_3$ also requires cyclotron for production (half-life 9.9 min) and is considered the preferred tracer among the available perfusion tracers because of its superior physical properties and pharmacokinetics. $^{13}NH_3$ enters the myocardium either as NH_3 or through Na^+/K^+-ATPase as NH_4^+. The tracer is then converted and trapped intracellularly as ^{13}N-glutamine.

This results in a very high extraction fraction of about 80% at baseline MBF, which decreases nonlinearly with increasing flows due to roll-off.

$^{13}NH_3$ produces high-quality images with excellent resolution because of its long half-life of 9.96 minutes and short mean positron path length. Exercise stress PET is feasible with $^{13}NH_3$.[2] ^{82}Rb is made from strontium-82 (^{82}Sr) using a ^{82}Sr/^{82}Rb generator. Na^+/K^+-ATPase facilitates the uptake of ^{82}Rb into the myocardium. ^{82}Rb has a lower first-pass extraction fraction of 60% at baseline MBF, but at high flows it is affected by greater roll-off. Despite this, studies have shown reliable MBF quantification with ^{82}Rb. ^{82}Rb has longer mean positron range, which explains its lower spatial resolution and degradation in image quality, particularly in larger patients and could pose challenges with flow quantification. One of the very important advantages of ^{82}Rb is it does not require onsite cyclotron as it is eluted from a ^{82}Sr generator, making it the most widely used PET flow tracer in clinical use in the USA. Also, ^{82}Rb's ultrashort half-life of 76 seconds allows for rapid sequential perfusion imaging, although exercise-based testing is not currently practical or feasible.[2] ^{18}F-Flurpiridaz is a long-awaited and just recently approved perfusion radiotracer. It has a longer half-life (110 min), high myocardial extraction fraction independent of flow, excellent spatial resolution, and short mean positron range, which allows for high image resolution. ^{18}F-Flurpiridaz can be acquired and transported from regional cyclotrons and opens the doors of exercise PET imaging given its longer half-life.[2] Importantly, it can be purchased in unit doses which could facilitate centers trying to start a PET program begin offering PET imaging at a smaller scale on a more economically feasible plan rather than a major financial commitment. ^{11}C-Acetate is a PET radiotracer primarily delegated to study oxidative metabolism and is limited to centers with cyclotron capabilities and research applications and is not discussed here. **Table 1** highlights the key clinical characteristics of perfusion radiotracers.

Principles of Positron Emission Tomography Quantitation and Quality Control

The PET flow quantification relies on the fact that proportional to the increase in MBF there is a corresponding increase in uptake of flow radiotracers (^{15}O-H_2O, ^{13}N-NH_3 and ^{18}F-Flurpiridaz). However, a tracer like ^{82}Rb reaches a plateau at high flowrates leading to nonlinear relation **(Figs. 1A and B)** and this along with its intrinsic higher positron energy leads to lower image quality and suboptimal signal to noise ratio due to "roll-off phenomenon". Hence corrections are needed to address these limitations during flow quantification.

In contrast to relative perfusion assessment by visual analysis, PET provides the unique capability of assessing absolute tracer concentrations. A dynamic acquisition is

TABLE 1: Key clinical features of PET perfusion tracers.

Parameter	*$H_2{}^{15}O$*	*$^{13}NH_3$*	*^{82}Rb*	*^{18}F-Flurpiridaz*
Half-life	123 s	9.97 min	76 s	110 min
Production	Cyclotron	Cyclotron	Generator	Cyclotron
Kinetics	Freely diffusible, metabolically inert	Metabolically trapped in myocardium	Metabolically trapped in myocardium	Metabolically trapped in myocardium
Mean positron range in tissue	1.1 mm	0.4 mm	2.8 mm	0.2 mm
Data acquisition	Dynamic	Dynamic, static	Dynamic, static	Dynamic, static
Scan duration	6 min	20 min	6 min	20 min
Gating/LV function	–	+	+	+
Radiation dose	~0.4 mSv	~1 mSv	~3 mSv	~4 mSv
Quantification	Excellent	Good	Moderate	Very good
Image quality	Good (parametric images)	Very good	Good	Excellent

Source: Reproduced from Driessen et al.[2] This is an open access article under creative common license 4.0

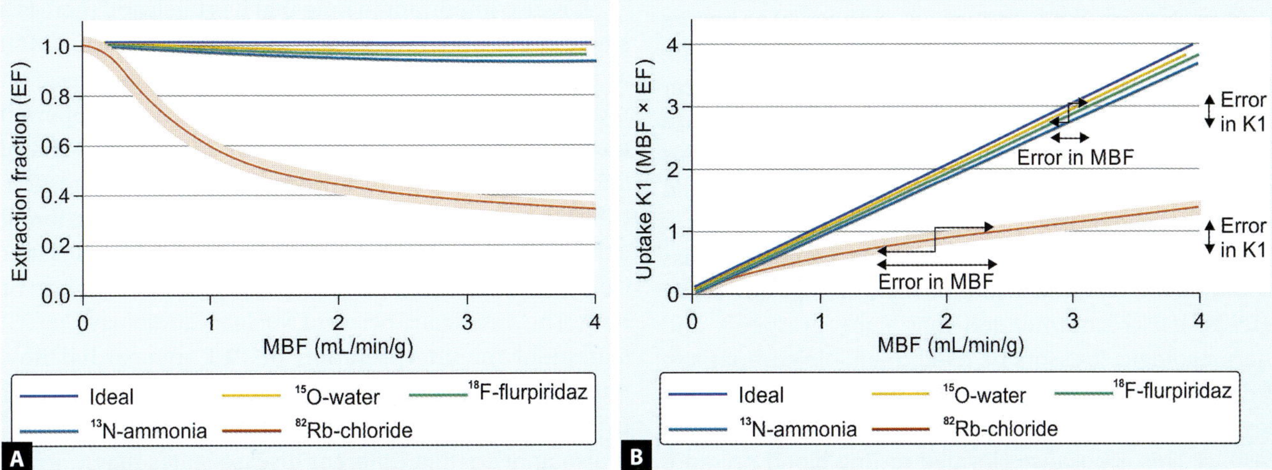

Figs. 1A and B: Extraction characteristics of different positron emission tomography (PET) flow tracers (A) and the impact of slight errors in uptake rate (K_1) between ^{82}Rb and other PET tracers (B).
Source: Reproduced from Dahdal et al.[3] This is an open access article under creative common license 4.0

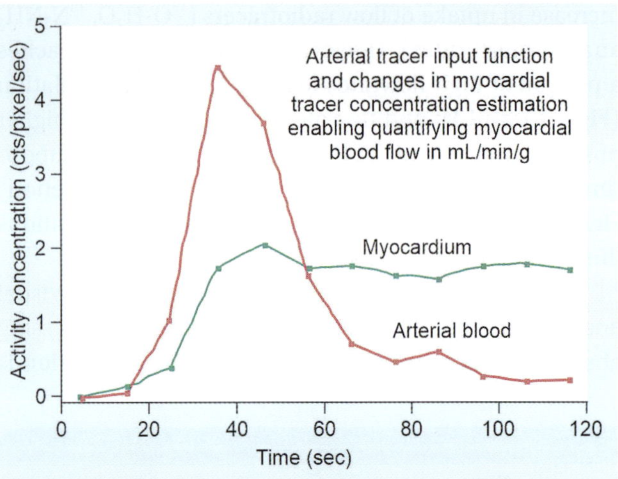

Fig. 2: Positron emission tomography (PET) flow input curves for calculation of myocardial blood flow. The pink curve is the blood pool and the green curve is myocardial uptake of tracer.

typically done (acquiring multiple frames at onset of tracer injection) to generate time activity curves of tracer activity in blood pool and myocardium **(Fig. 2)**. Automated software then uses flow compartmental models depending on tracer (1 or 2 compartmental) to derive MBF (absolute units of mL/min/g) and calculate coronary flow reserve (CFR) otherwise known as myocardial flow reserve. Despite some of the limitations outlined above, each of the flow tracers including the recently approved ^{18}F-Flurpiridaz have been tested against microsphere quantified perfusion which is invasive gold standard. ^{15}O-H_2O and ^{13}N-NH_3 have been well validated and demonstrate low test–retest variability.[4-7]

Important quality control steps are needed to ensure high-quality diagnostic and interpretable data. The PET scanner should begin acquisition before the tracer injection starts to avoid missing key data for "input function" calculation needed to determine MBF. This should be done for rest and stress and the timing should be standardized by using a stopwatch.

A good, free-flowing 18-gauge intravenous access so should be ensured without any kinking. For serial studies, it is recommended that same protocols and pharmacologic stressors be used to enable comparison of data. If patient is anxious and resting vital signs are elevated, allow few minutes of rest to reach baseline if feasible. This is because elevated resting blood pressure and or heart rate can increase rate pressure product and elevated resting blood flow values. This can lead to low MFR calculations skewing interpretation. Adequate working knowledge of the scanner and computational flow models (retention vs. compartmental) is needed by the PET team and physician to understand the nuances of flow analysis. Once flow data is available, the interpretation software QC process should be followed to ensure high-quality data. Specifically, the time activity curves should be evaluated for any errors in acquisition or flow through the tubing (i.e., blunted or double peak curves). Emission and transmission scan registration should be checked and location of blood pool and myocardial region of interest (ROI) should be confirmed. Newer software program have automated motion correction algorithms enabling more robust motion correction; however, the reader should anyhow systematically ensure that the dynamic frames are in the ROI and the spillover maps are in acceptable range. It is paramount that the reading physician never directly interprets flow data without going through systematic QC process specified for the software. When in doubt regarding integrity of flow data parameters, it is best not to report them as otherwise it may lead to inappropriate patient care decision-making.

Normal Values and Diagnostic Yield of Quantitative Positron Emission Tomography

Normal values for resting and hyperemic flow have been published with a wide range for hyperemic flows between 2 and 5 mL/min/g likely due to variations in microvascular resistance and age and sex-dependent inherent variations.[8] Resting blood flow ranges between 0.7 and 1.11 mL/min/g and is affected by resting rate pressure product.

It is also important to note that it is unclear if there is a single cutoff which works best rather than assessing MFR as a continuous variable. Also values may differ based on radiotracer and protocols. Recent studies have supported an hyperemic blood flow cutoff of 2.3 and an MFR of 2.5[9] when compared to invasive fractional flow reserve (FFR) measurements. Cardiac PET MFR is a reflection of epicardial and microvascular disease and hence the latter can be affected by epicardial or microvascular disease or both. The American Society of Nuclear Cardiology (ASNC) statement on interpretation of PET myocardial flow quantification suggests using a cutoff of ≥1.8 mL/min/g for hyperemic stress flow and an MFR of ≥2 as normal values.[10] It also appears that different disease states may warrant different cutoffs. For example, a recent study with ^{15}O-H_2O in CABG (coronary artery bypass graft) patients showed that a hyperemic stress flow of <1.53 mL/min/g best predicted success with percutaneous revascularization and hyperemic stress flow of 1.85 mL/min/g best predicted relief of angina with revascularization.[11]

Cardiac PET perfusion imaging demonstrates higher sensitivity and specificity compared to SPECT (single photon emission computed tomography) perfusion imaging with a reported sensitivity of 84–93% and specificity of 81–88% with invasive angiography as gold standard.[12] The data on quantitative PET accuracy has accumulated over the years showing the value of hyperemic stress flow in diagnostic assessment[13] and MFR in predicting survival benefit with revascularization epicardial coronary artery disease (CAD)[14] **(Figs. 3A and B)**.

Overall, hyperemic blood flow seems to be a better predictor of obstructive CAD than MFR which is affected by epicardial atherosclerosis and microvascular dysfunction.

Key Indications for Quantitative Positron Emission Tomography

Quantitative PET plays a key role in clinical perfusion imaging:

- Accurate assessment of obstructive epicardial CAD or to exclude obstructive CAD beyond relative perfusion
- Identification of multivessel and left main disease in the setting of single territory visual perfusion defect
- In diagnosis of microvascular dysfunction in absence of obstructive CAD or in conjunction with epicardial disease
- Guiding revascularization decisions in patients with obstructive CAD
- Evaluation of coronary allograft vasculopathy (CAV) in heart transplant patients
- Assessing adequacy of vasodilator response to pharmacologic stress

Prognostic Value of Quantitative Positron Emission Tomography Perfusion Imaging

Multiple studies have now shown that incorporating PET quantitative parameters has incremental prognostic value to relative perfusion. In a comprehensive meta-analysis by Smulders et al.,[15] a normal PET scan was associated with a low event rate comparable to many other imaging modalities **(Fig. 4)**. Gupta et al. in a large study of over 4,000 patients undergoing quantitative PET demonstrated the superior prognostic valve of MFR over hyperemic stress flow and defined unique patients subsets based on MFR and hyperemic stress flow.[16] A positive correlation

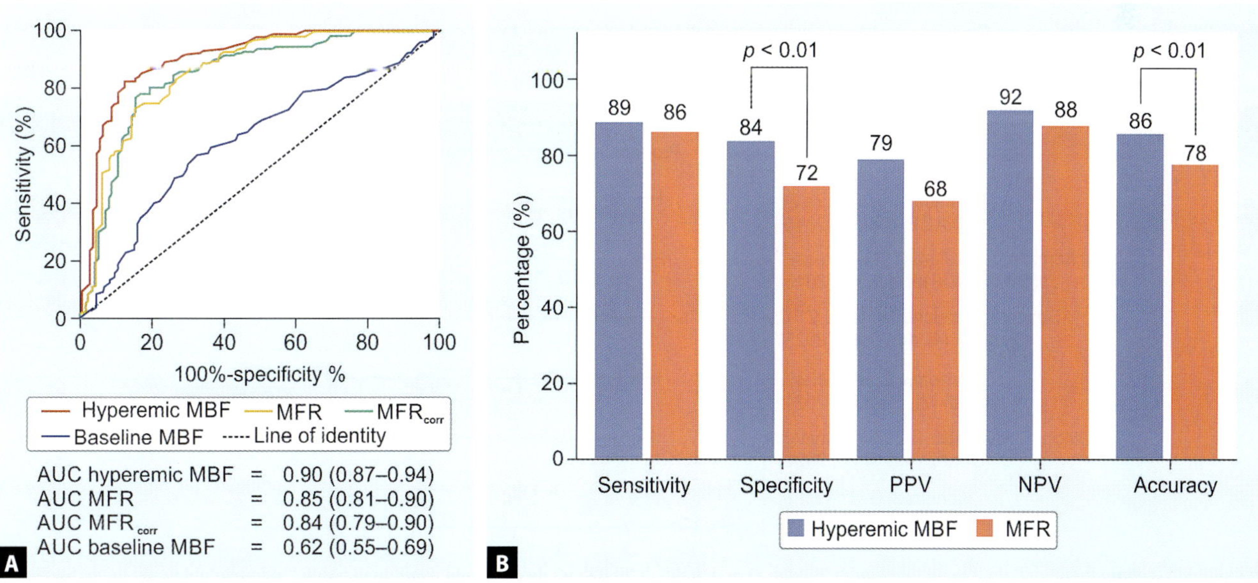

Figs. 3A and B: Value of PET quantitative parameters by ROC analysis (A); and sensitivity and specificity, positive and negative predictive values, and overall accuracy (B).

Source: reproduced from Dahdal et al.[3] This is an open access article under creative common license 4.0

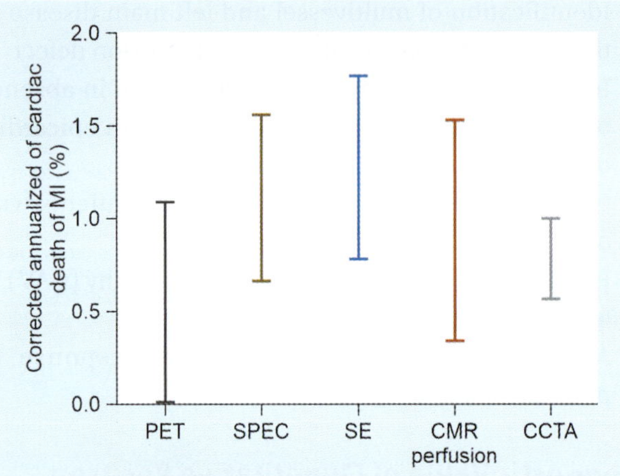

Fig. 4: Prognostic value of negative stress imaging modalities. Annualized event rates for death and myocardial infarction adjusted for population event risk and prevalence of coronary artery disease (CAD).

Source: Reproduced from Dahdal et al.[3] This is an open access article under creative common license 4.0

to adverse outcomes has also been demonstrated also associated with extent and severity of perfusion defects (ischemic burden) similar to SPECT data.[17]

A recent meta-analysis of 13 studies encompassing 11,864 participants with known or suspected CAD followed for 7.1 years showed a hazard ratio of 1.93 (CI 1.64–2.27) for major adverse events [death, myocardial infarction (MI), heart failure, and late revascularization] in the group with the lowest MFR.[18] Most prognostic studies have utilized ^{82}Rb as the perfusion agent with varying MFR cutoff values of <1.6 to <2.

Figures 5A and B below demonstrate the independent prognostic value of quantitative PET parameters even after adjustment of clinical risk, CAD extent of angiography, coronary calcium score, and extent and severity of perfusion defect.

To further enhance the prognostic value of hybrid PET CT data further provide atherosclerosis-related

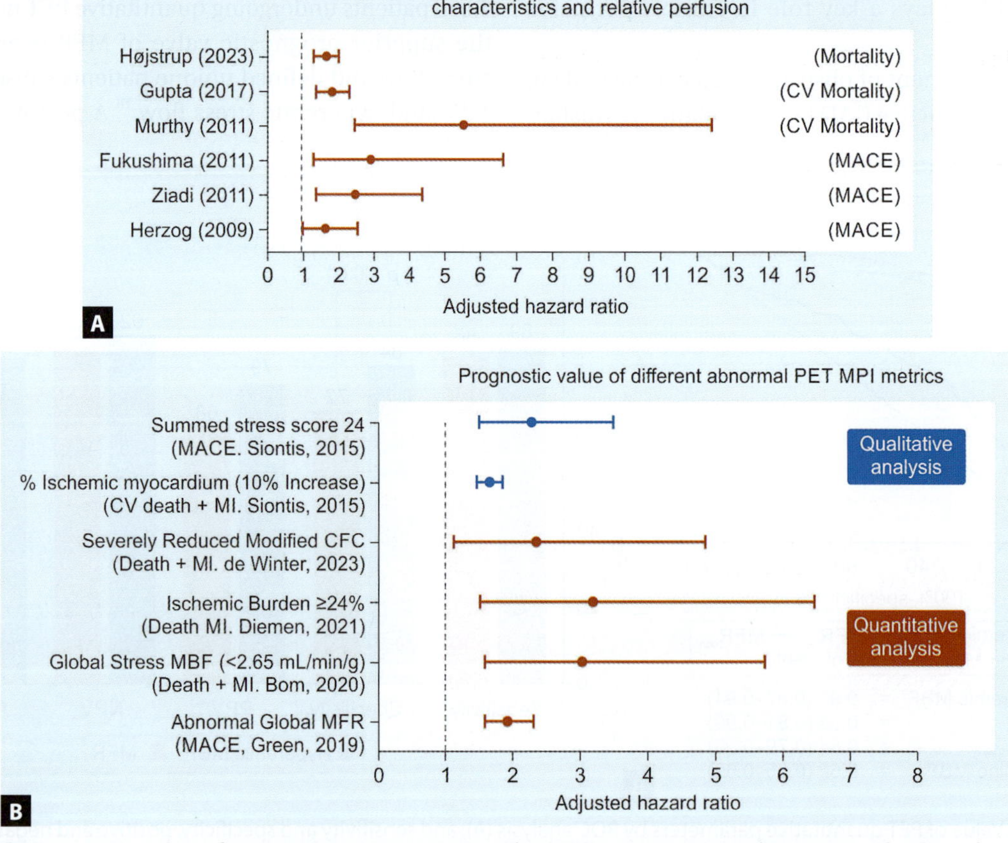

Figs. 5A and B: Prognostic value of positron emission tomography (PET) parameters and incremental value of quantitative PET incorporating hyperemic flow and myocardial flow reserve (MFR). Annualized event rates for death and myocardial infarction adjusted for population event risk and prevalence of coronary artery disease (CAD).

Source: Reproduced from Dahdal et al.[3] This is an open access article under creative common license 4.0

information with calcium burden (visual and quantitative) and had incremental prognostic value over PET.[19] It appears that ischemic burden on PET provides short-term prognostic information while atherosclerosis burden on CT provides long-term prognostic value. Hence the combination provides a comprehensive prognostic assessment in patients.

More recently artificial intelligence-based diagnostic and prognostic data have emerged for PET with an integrated assessment of PET and cardiac computed tomography angiography (CCTA). In this study after integrating clinical CCTA and PET data, PET was able to enhance prediction of adverse events up to 4 years based on machine learning analysis.[20]

Limitations of Quantitative Positron Emission Tomography

As per ASNC guiding document diagnostic interpretation quantitative PET parameters,[10] conditions such as prior CABG, large prior MI, severe cardiomyopathy, and end-stage renal disease are highlighted as scenarios where MFR and flow data has not been well studied and may provide conflicting information. Hence it is recommended not to routinely use flow data for decision-making in such scenarios. However, this author feels that if hyperemic stress flow are normal in patients with CABG and chronic renal disease that may help to exclude obstructive CAD despite MFR being abnormal as latter can be affected by epicardial or microvascular dysfunction.

CASE ILLUSTRATIONS OF VALUE OF QUANTITATIVE POSITRON EMISSION TOMOGRAPHY PERFUSION IMAGING

Normal Relative Perfusion and Normal Quantitative PET

A 73-year-old female, BMI 47, with bilateral knee replacement presented with dyspnea and intermittent chest discomfort at rest lasting few minutes. Regadenoson ^{82}Rb PET was performed for assessment of CAD.

Rest and stress EKG was normal, resting EF 54%, stress EF 62%, and there was no transient ischemic dilation (TID) **(Figs. 6A and B)**.

Single-vessel Disease by Relative Perfusion and Quantitative Positron Emission Tomography

A 72-year-old male diabetic, smoker with new chest discomfort, with prior nondiagnostic treadmill test was referred for Regadenoson ^{82}Rb PET.

Resting EKG was normal; stress EKG 1 mm inferolateral ST depression; TID present; with rest EF 49% and stress EF 50% **(Figs. 7A and B)**.

Multivessel Disease by Relative Perfusion and Quantitative Positron Emission Tomography

An 80-year-old male presented with new intermittent dyspnea. Risk factors included hypertension, hyperlipidemia, prediabetes, and stage 2 chronic kidney disease. Regadenoson ^{82}Rb PET was performed.

Rest and stress EKG was normal, with rest EF 52%, stress EF 51%, and EF reserve <0 **(Figs. 8A and B)**.

Single-vessel Disease by Relative Perfusion but Multivessel Disease by Quantitative Positron Emission Tomography

A 76-year-old male for major vascular surgery presented with new right bundle branch block and poor exercise capacity. Regadenoson ^{82}Rb PET was performed.

Resting EKG showed normal sinus rhythm and right bundle branch block. Stress EKG showed no definitive ischemia; rest EF 54%; stress EF 52% **(Figs. 9A and B)**.

Normal Relative Perfusion and Abnormal Myocardial Flow Reserve: Likely Microvascular Disease

A 66-year-old woman with obesity, hypertensive, and polycystic ovarian disease presented with intermittent chest discomfort. Coronary CT was performed showing no obstructive disease. She remained symptomatic and was sent for a regadenoson ^{82}Rb PET for evaluation of microvascular function. Resting EKG was normal. Stress EKG showed diffuse 1 mm ST depression consistent with ischemia. PET perfusion was normal, with rest EF 60% and stress EF 64% **(Figs. 10A and B)**.

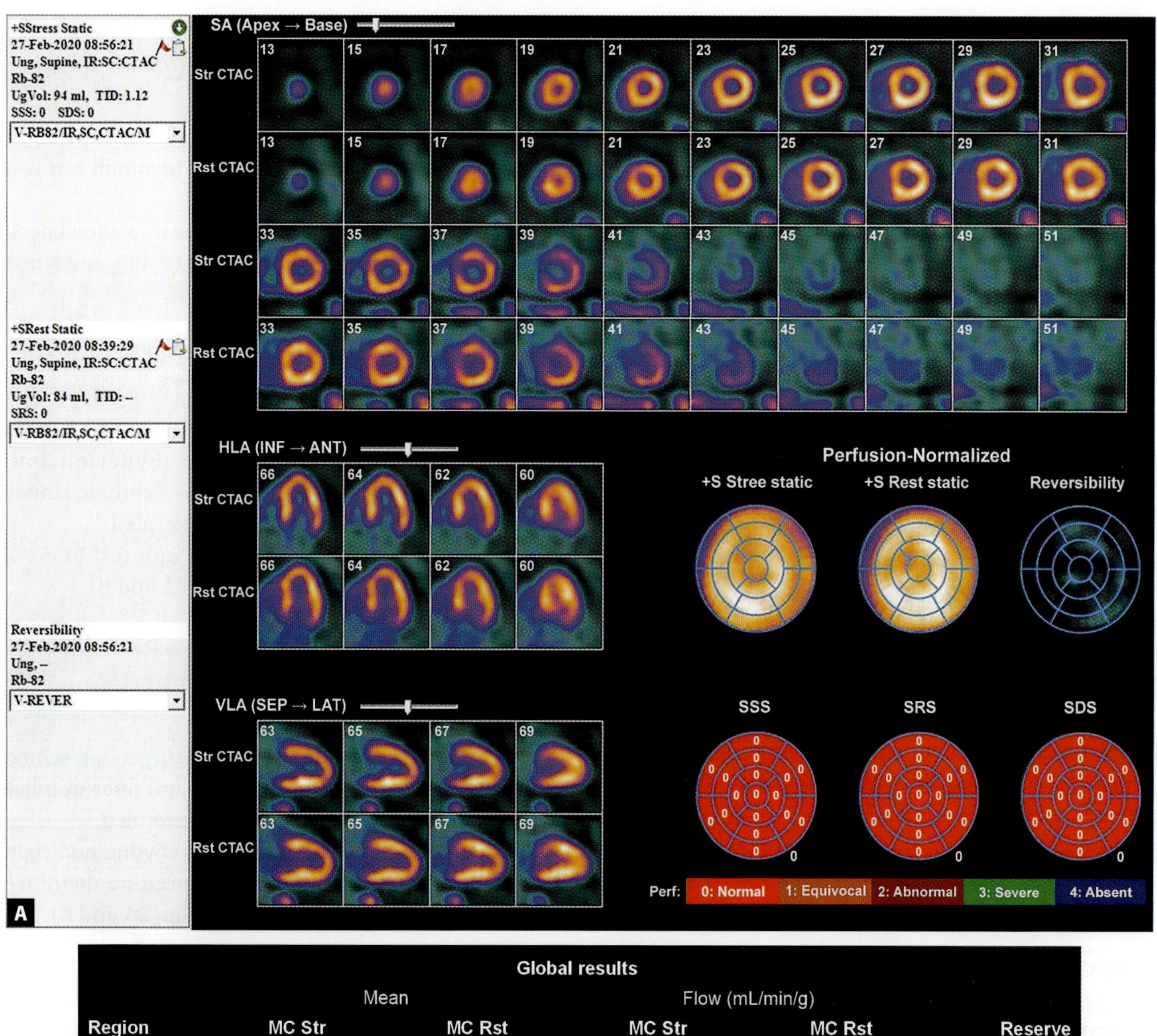

Global results

Region	Mean MC Str	Mean MC Rst	Flow (mL/min/g) MC Str	Flow (mL/min/g) MC Rst	Reserve
LAD	83%	82%	2.58	1.04	2.48
LCX	80%	81%	2.42	0.85	2.56
RCA	87%	85%	2.72	0.95	2.86
TOT	83%	83%	2.55	0.98	2.60

B

Figs. 6A and B: Normal perfusion. PET flow analysis shows normal resting and peak hyperemic flows and normal MFR confirming normal study with added value of low risk of future cardiac events. (LAD: left anterior descending; LCX: left circumflex; RCA: right coronary artery)

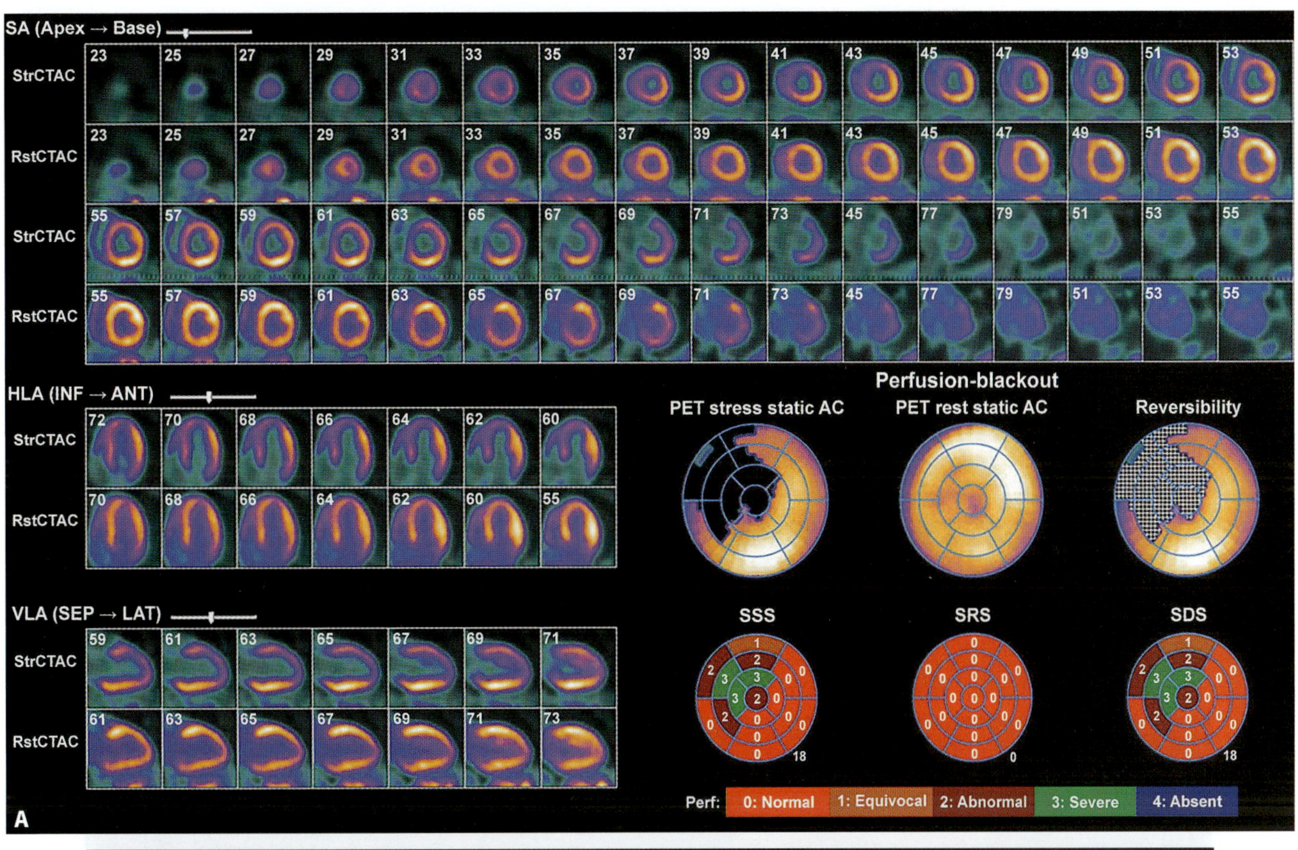

Global results					
	Mean		Flow (mL/min/g)		
Region	MC Str	MC Rst	MC Str	MC Rst	Reserve
LAD	64%	79%	1.44	0.92	1.57
LCX	82%	82%	2.37	1.04	2.29
RCA	82%	78%	2.16	0.88	2.45
TOT	73%	79%	1.90	0.94	2.02

B

Figs. 7A and B: Perfusion images show large area of anteroseptal and apical ischemia. Quantitative PET confirms blunted hyperemic stress flow and MFR in left anterior descending distribution and normal stress flow in left circumflex and right coronary territory confirming single-vessel disease as shown by perfusion images. Global MFR is in low normal range.

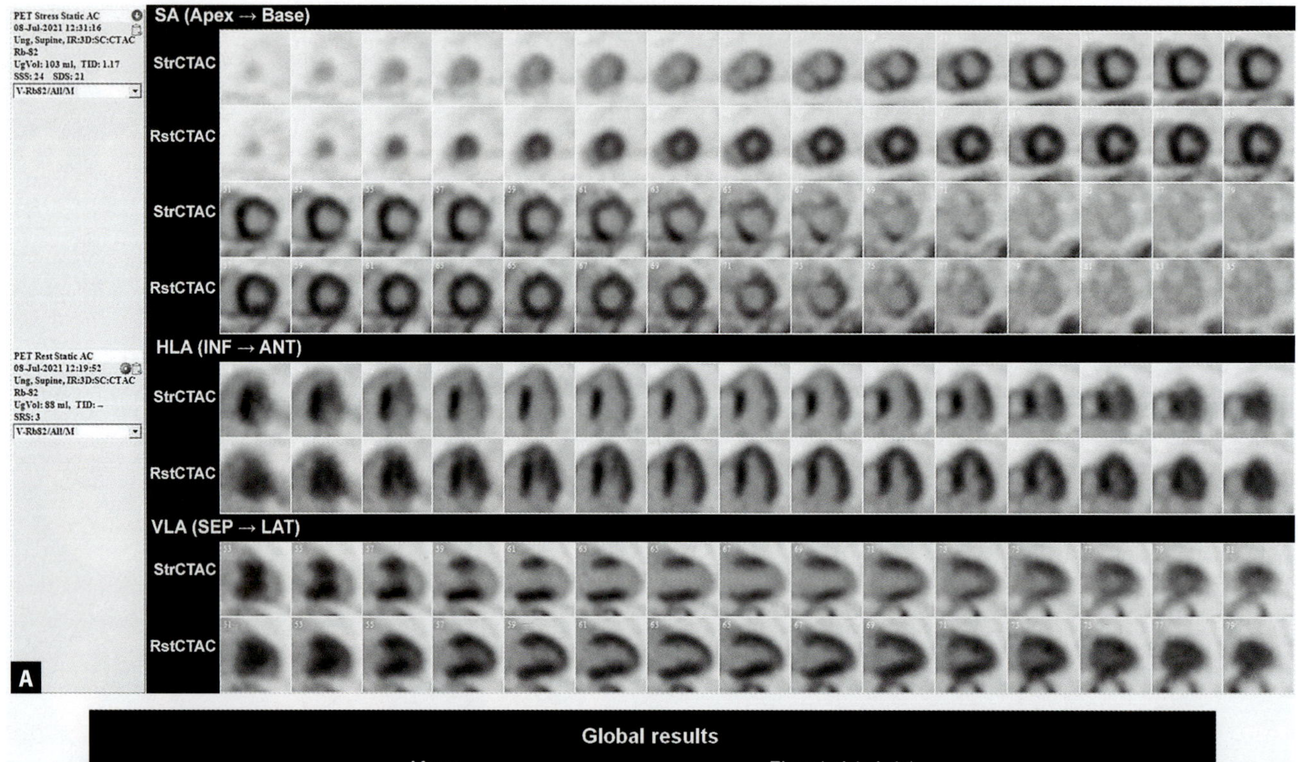

Global results

Region	Mean MC Str	Mean MC Rst	Flow (mL/min/g) MC Str	Flow (mL/min/g) MC Rst	Reserve
LAD	76%	79%	1.50	1.12	1.34
LCX	72%	77%	1.36	0.94	1.45
RCA	86%	81%	1.73	0.90	1.91
TOT	78%	79%	1.52	0.99	1.53

B

Figs. 8A and B: Perfusion images show anteroseptal, apical, and inferolateral ischemia concerning for multivessel disease. TID present. Quantitative PET shows global reduction in peak hyperemic flow with reduced MFR confirming multivessel disease. Coronary angiography showed severe LAD and LCX stenosis.

Hybrid Imaging with Computed Tomography Atherosclerosis and Value of Quantitative Positron Emission Tomography

A 60-year-old male with strong family history (FMH) of premature coronary disease, hypertension, hyperlipidemia, and BMI 34 presented with multivessel coronary calcification on chest CT with dyspnea on daily activities. Regdenoson ^{82}Rb PET showed normal perfusion. Rest and Stress EKG were normal; rest EF 60% and stress EF 62% **(Figs. 11A and B)**.

Evaluation of Coronary Allograft Vasculopathy

A 60-year-old female with history of heart transplant 5 years ago now presented with progressive dyspnea. Echocardiogram showed minimal pericardial effusion, mild biventricular hypertrophy, EF 57%, and reduction in global longitudinal strain at –15%. Regadenoson ^{82}Rb PET was done for evaluation of coronary disease and assessment for CAV **(Figs. 12A and B)**.

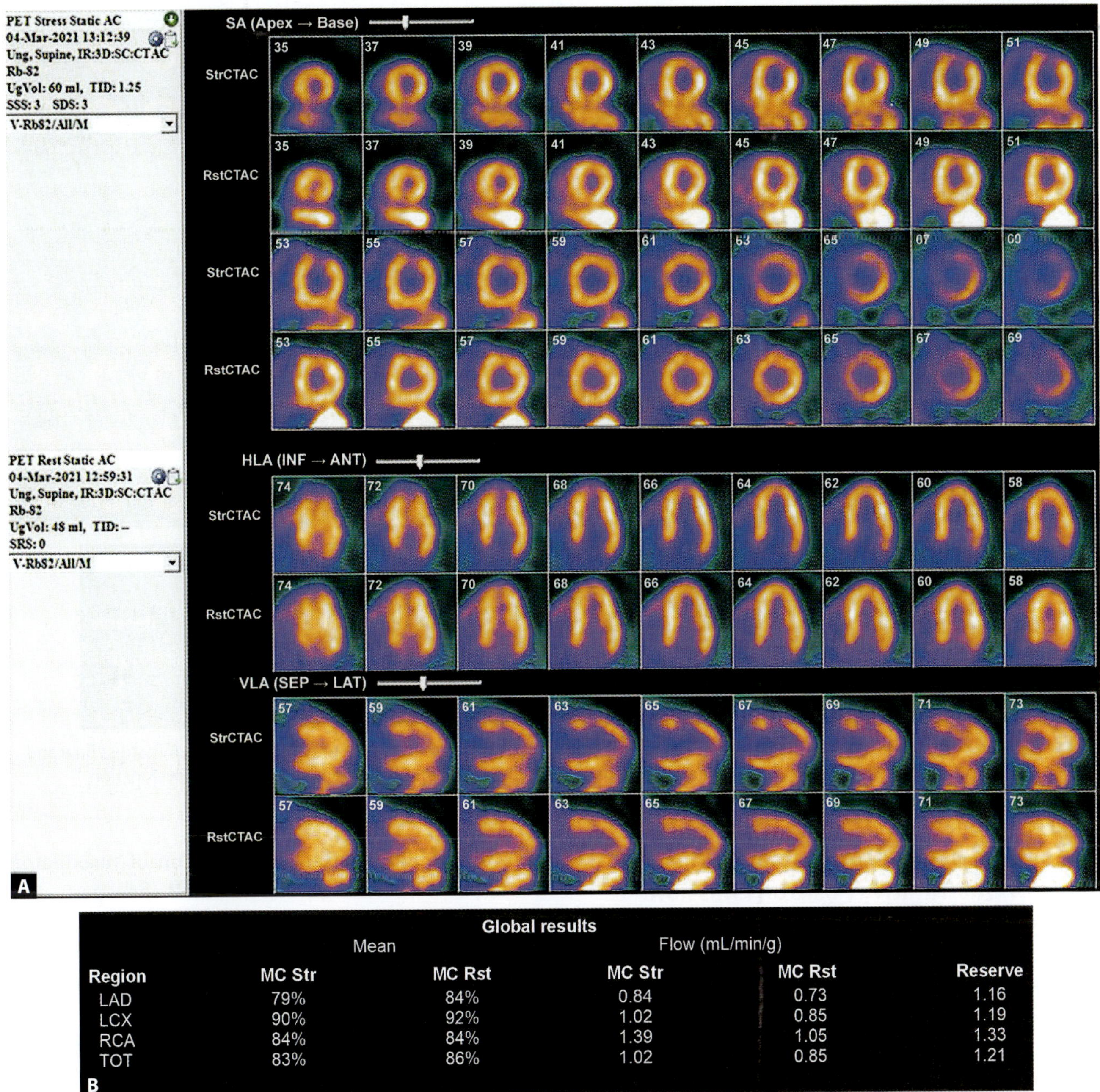

Global results

Region	Mean MC Str	Mean MC Rst	Flow (mL/min/g) MC Str	Flow (mL/min/g) MC Rst	Reserve
LAD	79%	84%	0.84	0.73	1.16
LCX	90%	92%	1.02	0.85	1.19
RCA	84%	84%	1.39	1.05	1.33
TOT	83%	86%	1.02	0.85	1.21

Figs. 9A and B: Relative perfusion images although suboptimal quality show focal small anterior wall reversible defect. TID was present. However, PET flow analysis shows diffuse multivessel flow reduction and abnormal MFR raising concern for multivessel disease. Coronary angiography confirmed multivessel obstructive disease requiring CABG (coronary artery bypass graft).

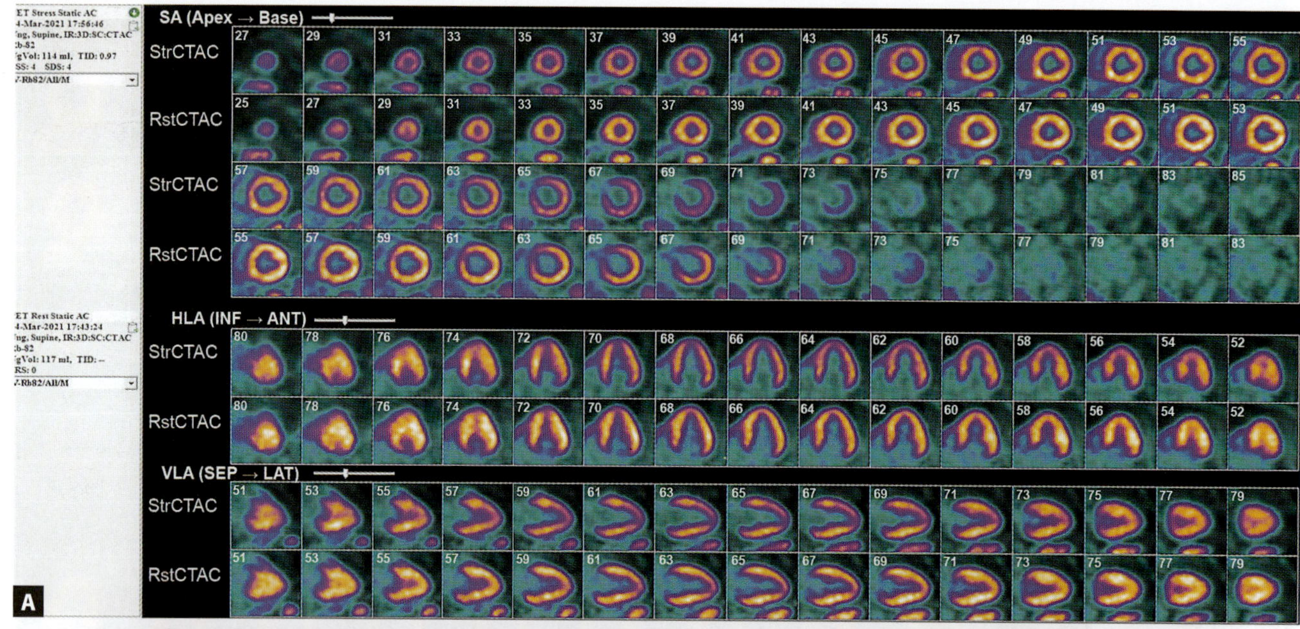

Global results

	Mean		Flow (mL/min/g)		
Region	**MC Str**	**MC Rst**	**MC Str**	**MC Rst**	**Reserve**
LAD	77%	79%	1.44	1.10	1.32
LCX	87%	90%	1.60	1.25	1.28
RCA	89%	88%	1.95	1.17	1.67
TOT	83%	84%	1.63	1.16	1.41

B

Figs. 10A and B: Perfusion images were normal. No TID. PET flow analysis shows mild diffuse reduction in hyperemic stress flow and abnormal MFR. With the absence of epicardial disease, this constellation of findings favors microvascular dysfunction.

Evaluation of Vasodilator Nonresponsiveness: Value of Quantitative Positron Emission Tomography

A 64-year-old male with history of known nonobstructive coronary disease by coronary CTA 1 year ago, hypertension, and hyperlipidemia presented for a regadenoson ^{82}Rb PET for ischemic evaluation given recent exertional chest pain. Initial outpatient PET showed normal perfusion with known LV dysfunction, without appreciable changes in heart rate, blood pressure, or rest versus stress EF (52% and 51%, respectively). Rest and stress EKG were normal. Further analysis of PET MBF showed no increase in stress MBF across all coronary territories (global stress flow of 1.14 versus rest flow of 1.18) and severely reduced MFR of 0.97. This raised the suspicion of vasodilator nonresponsiveness. **Figures 13A and B** show perfusion images and flow analysis.

Patient was brought back another day after strict instructions on avoiding caffeine for 12 hours and scan repeated. Perfusion images remained normal. Rest EF was 52% and stress EF was 58%. As given in **Figure 13C**, flow analysis showed increased in peak stress flow albeit blunted (1.51) along with reduced MFR at 1.49. This suggested better response to vasodilator with overall conclusion of likely nonobstructive atherosclerosis ± microvascular dysfunction-related reduction in peak flow and MFR. Thus PET flow analysis was able to identify nonresponsiveness to vasodilator challenge in the first scan in this case.

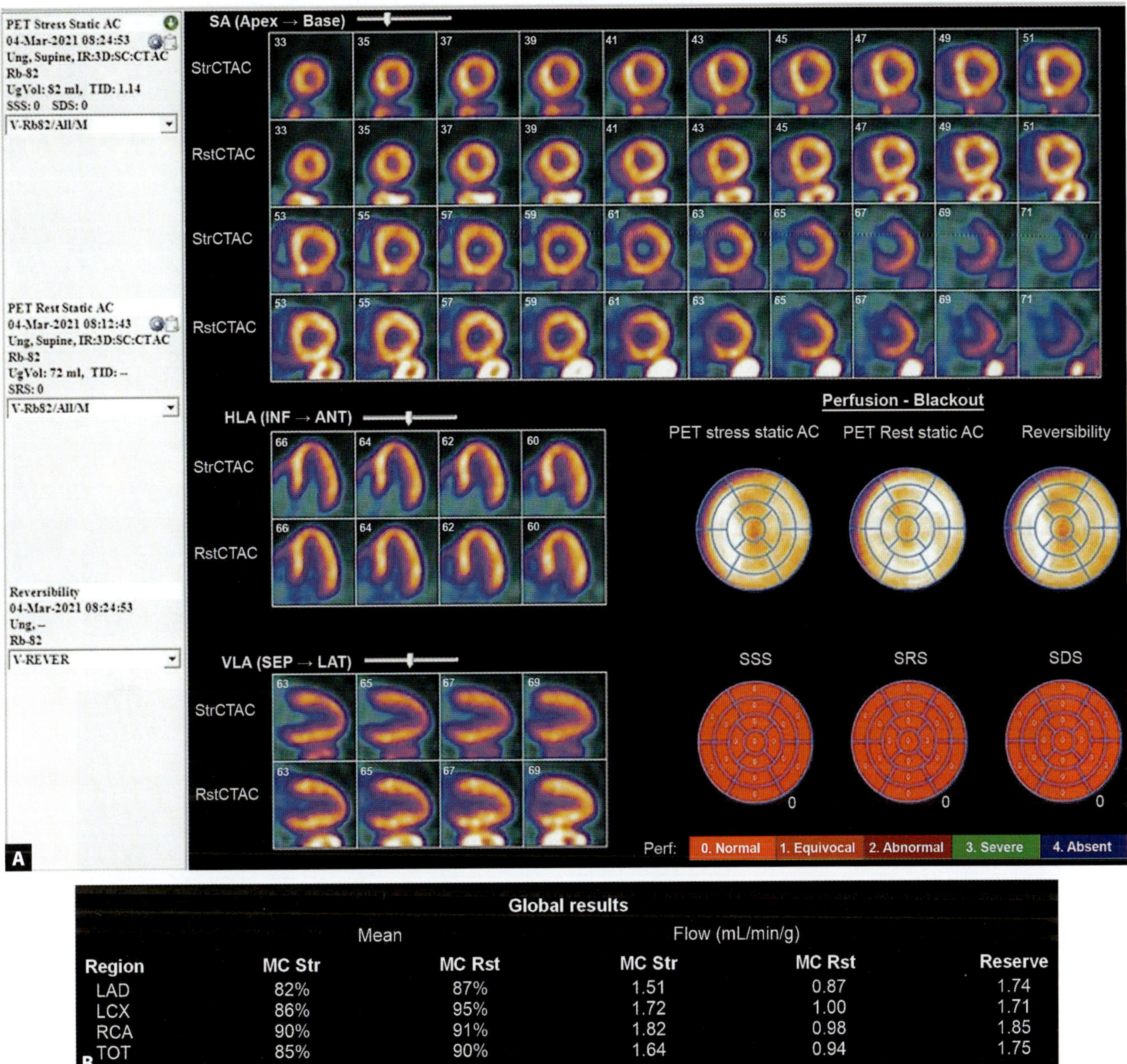

Global results

Region	Mean MC Str	Mean MC Rst	Flow (mL/min/g) MC Str	Flow (mL/min/g) MC Rst	Reserve
LAD	82%	87%	1.51	0.87	1.74
LCX	86%	95%	1.72	1.00	1.71
RCA	90%	91%	1.82	0.98	1.85
TOT	85%	90%	1.64	0.94	1.75

Figs. 11A and B: Perfusion images were normal. Quantitative PET showed mild diffuse reduction in peak hyperemic flow with no flow gradient and reduced MFR. Coronary angiography showed diffuse nonobstructive atherosclerosis. In this case abnormal peak flow and MFR was likely a reflection of diffuse atherosclerosis ± coexistent microvascular disease.

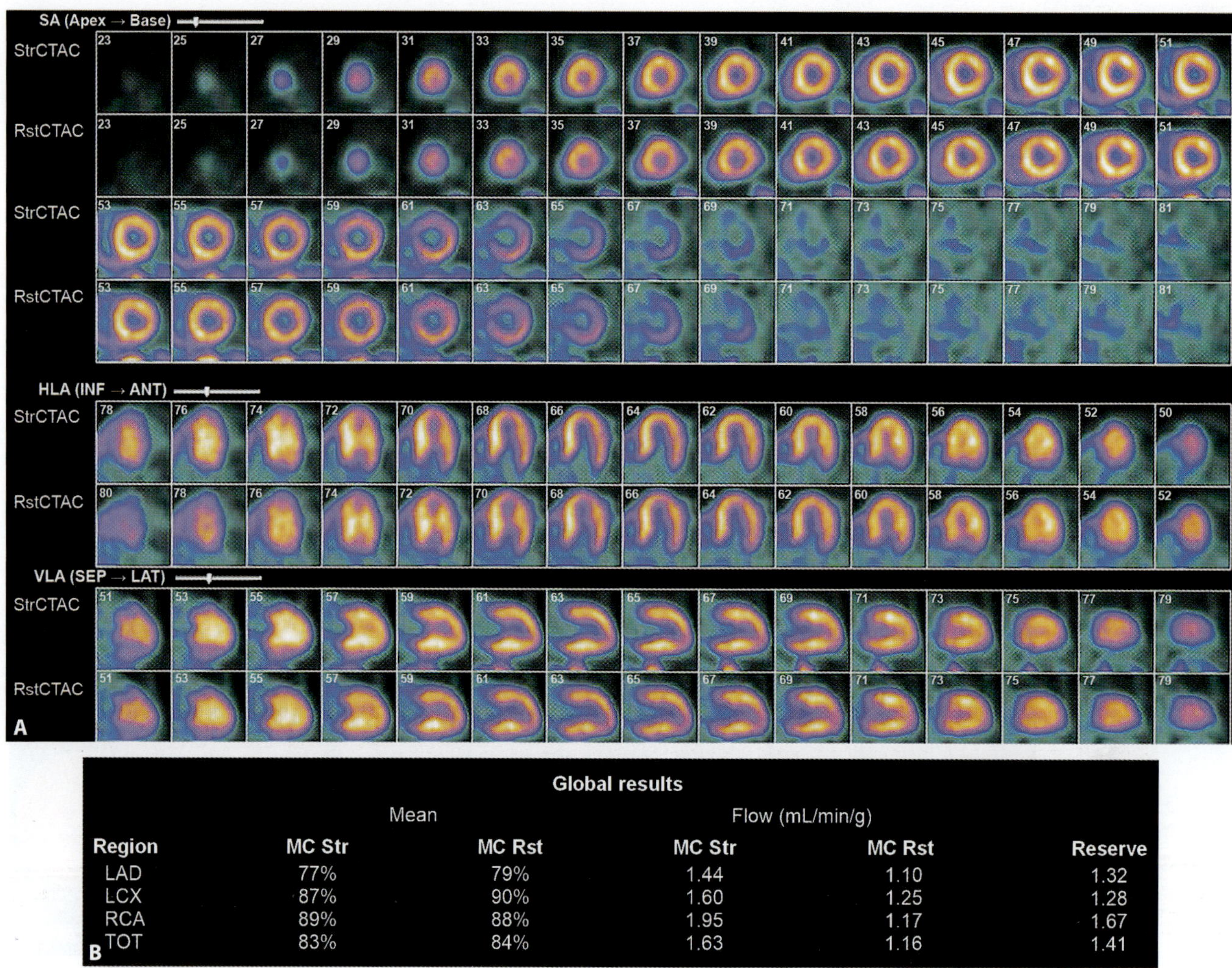

Global results

Region	Mean		Flow (mL/min/g)		
	MC Str	MC Rst	MC Str	MC Rst	Reserve
LAD	77%	79%	1.44	1.10	1.32
LCX	87%	90%	1.60	1.25	1.28
RCA	89%	88%	1.95	1.17	1.67
TOT	83%	84%	1.63	1.16	1.41

Figs. 12A and B: Perfusion images show normal perfusion. Rest and stress EKG were normal, with rest EF 60% and stress EF 68%. PET flow analysis shows blunting of global hyperemic stress flow (1.63), rate pressure product corrected MFR was abnormal at 1.4 and coronary vascular resistance (mean arterial pressure/peak stress flow) was >55. Based on published evidence on value of PET in CAV these parameters indicate CAV is likely. Patient underwent coronary angiography with intravascular ultrasound confirming ISHLT Grade 2 CAV.

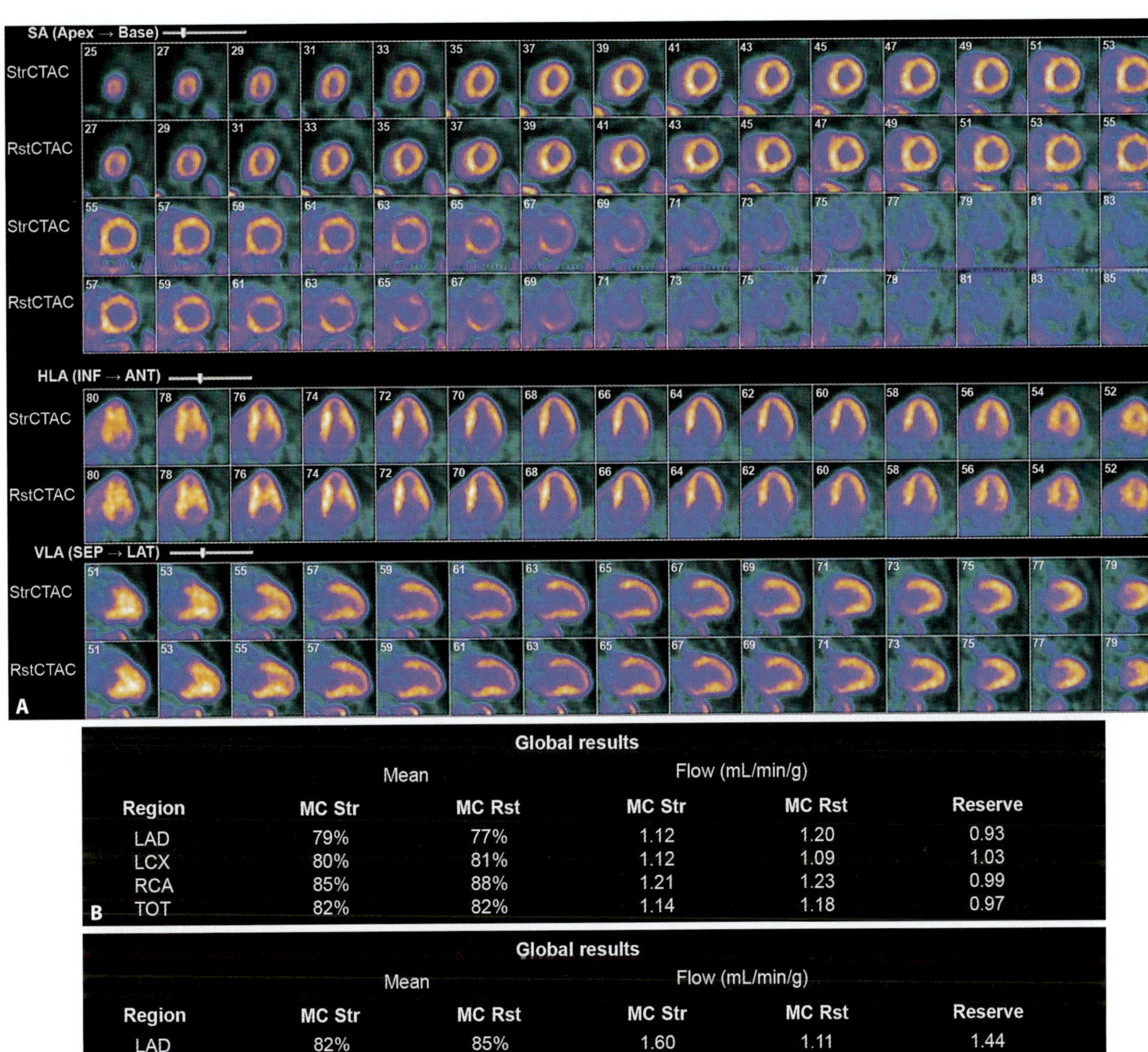

B

Global results

Region	Mean MC Str	Mean MC Rst	Flow (mL/min/g) MC Str	Flow (mL/min/g) MC Rst	Reserve
LAD	79%	77%	1.12	1.20	0.93
LCX	80%	81%	1.12	1.09	1.03
RCA	85%	88%	1.21	1.23	0.99
TOT	82%	82%	1.14	1.18	0.97

C

Global results

Region	Mean MC Str	Mean MC Rst	Flow (mL/min/g) MC Str	Flow (mL/min/g) MC Rst	Reserve
LAD	82%	85%	1.60	1.11	1.44
LCX	81%	83%	1.42	1.00	1.42
RCA	85%	87%	1.47	0.90	1.63
TOT	83%	85%	1.51	1.01	1.49

Figs. 13A to C: (A) First and second perfusion PET scans show normal perfusion; (B) No increases in stress flow or flow reserve in setting of normal perfusion suggesting vasodilator non-responsiveness in first scan; (C) Second scan data and shows blunted but increased stress flow and flow reserve after caffeine abstinence suggesting vasodilator response but likely in setting of microvascular dysfunction and diffuse atherosclerosis without ischemia.

CONCLUSION

This chapter and its illustrative cases highlight the incremental value provided by quantitative PET over relative perfusion and superiority to SPECT. Cardiac PET with flow quantitation is now a Class 2A indication for evaluation of chest pain when pharmacologic testing is considered in the 2021 American College of Cardiology Chest Pain guidelines. Cardiac PET is poised to become even more widely adopted with the recent approval of ^{18}F-Flurpiridaz which could enable exercise PET to become a reality given longer half-life of tracer along with better flow characteristics due to tracer uptake properties and easier adoption of PET due to unit dosing capability.

REFERENCES

1. Gould KL, Johnson NP, Bateman TM, Beanlands RS, Bengel FM, Bober R, et al. Anatomic versus physiologic assessment of coronary artery disease. Role of coronary flow reserve, fractional flow reserve, and positron emission tomography imaging in revascularization decision-making. J Am Coll Cardiol. 2013;62:1639-53.
2. Driessen SR, Raijmakers PG, Stuijfzand FJ, Knaapen P. Myocardial perfusion imaging with PET. Int J Cardiovasc Imaging. 2017;33:1021-31.
3. Dahdal J, Jukema RA, Harms HJ, Cramer MJ, Raijmakers PG, Knaapen P, et al. PET myocardial perfusion imaging: Trends, challenges, and opportunities. J Nucl Cardiol. 2024; 40:102011.
4. Kauffman PA, Gnecci-Ruscone T, Yap JT, Rimoldi O, Camici PG. Assessment of the reproducibility of baseline and hyperemic myocardial blood flow measurements with 15O-labeled water and PET. J Nucl Med. 1999;40:1848-56.
5. Slomka PJ, Alexanderson E, Jácome R, Jiménez M, Romero E, Meave A, et al. Comparison of clinical tools for measurements of regional stress and rest myocardial blood flow assessed with 13N-ammonia PET/CT J Nucl Med. 2012;53:171-81.
6. Dekemp RA, Declerck J, Klein R, Pan XB, Nakazato R, Tonge C, et al. Multisoftware reproducibility study of stress and rest myocardial blood flow assessed with 3D dynamic PET/CT and 1-tissue-compartment model of 82Rb kinetics. J Nucl Med. 2013;54:571-7.
7. Packard RR, Huang SC, Dahlbom M, Czernin J, Maddahi J. Absolute quantitation of myocardial blood flow in human subjects with or without myocardial ischemia using dynamic flurpiridaz F18 PET. J Nucl Med. 2014;55:1438-44.
8. Chareonthaitawee P, Kaufmann PA, Rimoldi O, P G Camici PG. Heterogeneity of resting and hyperemic myocardial blood flow in healthy humans. Cardiovasc Res. 2001; 50;151-61.
9. Danad I, Uusitalo V, Kero T, Saraste A, Raijmakers PG, Lammertsma AA, et al. Quantitative assessment of myocardial perfusion in the detection of significant coronary artery disease: cutoff values and diagnostic accuracy for quantitative [(15)O]H2O PET imaging. J Am Coll Cardiol. 2014;64:1464-75.
10. Bateman TM, Heller GV, Beanlands R, Calnon DA, Case J, deKemp R, et al. Practical guide for interpreting and reporting Cardiac PET measurements of myocardial blood flow: An information statement from the American Society of Nuclear Cardiology, and the Society of Nuclear Medicine and Molecular Imaging. J Nuc Cardiol. 2021;28(2):768-87.
11. Vester M, Madsen S, Kjærulff MLG, Tolbod LP, Nielsen BRR, Kristensen SD, et al. Myocardial perfusion imaging with $^{15}O\text{-}H_2O$ positron emission tomography predicts clinical revascularization procedures in symptomatic patients with previous coronary artery bypass graft. Eur Heart J Open. 2023;3(3):oead044.
12. Mc Ardle BA, Dowsley TF, deKemp RA, Wells GA, Beanlands RS. Does rubidium-82 PET have superior accuracy to SPECT perfusion imaging for the diagnosis of obstructive coronary disease?: A systematic review and meta-analysis. J Am Coll Cardiol. 2012;60:1828-37.
13. Cho SG, Lee SJ, Ma MH, Choi YY, Bom HH. Comparison of diagnostic accuracy of PET-derived myocardial blood flow parameters: A meta-analysis. J Nucl Cardiol. 2020;27(6):1955-566.
14. Patel KK, Spertus JA, Chan PS, Sperry BW, Al Badarin F, Kennedy KF, et al. Myocardial blood flow reserve assessed by positron emission tomography myocardial perfusion imaging identifies patients with a survival benefit from early revascularization. Eur Heart J. 2020;41(6):759-68.
15. Smulders MW, Jaarsma, C, Nelemans, PJ, Bekkers SCAM, Bucerius J, Leiner T, et al. Comparison of the prognostic value of negative non-invasive cardiac investigations in patients with suspected or known coronary artery disease—a meta-analysis. Eur Heart J Cardiovasc Imaging. 2017;18(9):980-7.
16. Gupta A, Taqueti VR, van de Hoef TP, Bajaj NS, Bravo PE, Murthy VL, et al. Integrated noninvasive physiological assessment of coronary circulatory function and impact on cardiovascular mortality in patients with stable coronary artery disease. Circulation. 2017;136(24):2325-36.
17. Dorbala S, Hachamovitch R, Curillova Z, Thomas D, Vangala D, Kwong RY, et al. Incremental prognostic value of gated Rb-82 positron emission tomography myocardial perfusion imaging over clinical variables and rest LVEF. JACC Cardiovasc Imaging. 2009;2(7);846-54.
18. Green R, Cantoni V, Acampa W, Assante R, Zampella E, Nappi C, et al. Prognostic value of coronary flow reserve in patients with suspected or known coronary artery disease referred for PET myocardial perfusion imaging: A meta-analysis. J Nucl Cardiol. 2021;28(3):904-18.
19. Dobrolinska MM, Jukema RA, van Velzen SGM, van Diemen PA, Greuter MJW, Prakken NHJ, et al. The prognostic value of visual and automatic coronary calcium scoring from low-dose computed tomography [15O]-water positron emission tomography. Eur Heart J Cardiovasc Imaging. 2024;25(9):1186-96.
20. Lehtonen E, Kujala I, Tamminen J, Maaniitty T, Saraste A, Teuho J, et al. Incremental prognostic value of downstream positron emission tomography perfusion imaging after coronary computed tomography angiography: a study using machine learning. Eur Heart J Cardiovasc Imaging. 2024;24(2):285-92.

Global Supply Chain of Radiotracers and Challenges in the Security of Supplies

Aruna Korde, Meera Venkatesh, N Ramamoorthy

INTRODUCTION

Cardiac imaging using radiopharmaceuticals (RPh) is an important element in the management of numerous patients of cardiac disorders. Myocardial perfusion imaging has been the most widely used procedure in nuclear cardiology, while there are also many other procedures used to varying extent. The short half-life ($t_{½}$) of the radionuclide (RN) component of the RPh (e.g., ^{18}F—110 min; ^{99m}Tc—6 h; ^{201}Tl—74 h) requires reliable periodic supplies to—availability at—nuclear medicine (NM) centers. The major RPh/RN used in nuclear cardiology and associated advances have been covered in previous chapters in the books on cardiac imaging.[1,2] The current chapter aims to project the features of RPh/RN supply chain involved and inevitable challenges faced at times to avail the RPh/RN as and when required for (cardiac) patient studies. Most of these aspects are applicable for all other RPh (and not limited to cardiac RPh), e.g., of ^{131}I, ^{177}Lu (lutetium-177), ^{68}Ge-^{68}Ga, and hence the scope of the current chapter is designed to cover important RN in NM.

Nuclear medicine centers serving patients are the end users of RPh/RN and the entities requiring to address and manage the supply chain challenges (faced to varying extent) can be of the following types: (1) Individual radiopharmacy (dedicated) unit in NM centers; (2) Central/commercial radiopharmacy units serving several NM centers; (3) National laboratories/centers in many countries dealing with supplies of RPh/RN; (4) Entrepreneurs driven initiatives engaged in supplies in many countries; and (5) Global industrial (corporate) entities. Medical cyclotron (MC) facilities in operation serving NM centers will be mostly under (3), (4), (5) and some of the MC facilities may be also handling the roles of (2) above.

Out of these, the first entity is invariably an integral part of NM center and gets its supplies from the entities (2) to (5). Supply chain issues pose greater challenges to entities listed as (2), (3), and (4). The corporate entities under (5) are also subject to supply chain issues, but invariably they are more resilient and better equipped to cope with challenges.

BACKGROUND TO SUPPLY CHAIN MANAGEMENT

The practice of NM procedures is solely dependent on the use of RPh, mostly administered intravenously. The physical half-life of the RN/radioisotope (RI) component of the RPh is usually short (minutes to hours to a few days) and in turn, the shelf-life of RPh is limited (cf. conventional pharma products). This fact underpins the challenges in the availability and accessibility to RN and RPh and in turn, the NM procedures to deliver timely benefits. Consequently, the supply chain management of RPh/RN is of crucial importance to sustainably offer the benefit of NM procedures to the patients requiring diagnostic imaging or therapy procedure. While this has been known all along, the growth of the field and wider use of NM procedures in numerous countries have increased the pressure on the supply chain. Insurance claims-related matters as well as patients' rights to sue medical centers, if they fail to honor treatment appointments, add to the list of issues/challenges.

Reactor-based RNs such as ^{131}I, ^{99}Mo-^{99m}Tc, ^{177}Lu are of importance at all times.[3,4] The continual growth of (medical) cyclotron-based RN—especially ^{18}F, ^{68}Ga for use with positron emission tomography (PET)/CT—has slightly reduced the demand for ^{99m}Tc in some cases. Reactor facility is invariably under national nuclear centers (functioning mostly on government support), while MC have wider ownership beyond national laboratories, e.g., medical centers/hospitals, industry, entrepreneurs, academic institutes.

Among the various advantages of the use of ^{99m}Tc in NM, its availability from a RN generator (^{99}Mo-^{99m}Tc), eluted as and when needed at NM center, has been an important feature (though availability of the generator itself at regular intervals of 10–12 days is to be also ensured). Thus, when ^{201}Tl (74 h) entered the clinical scene in late 1970s for myocardial perfusion imaging,[1,2] periodic procurement of the same was needed. While it is necessary to serve patients for cardiac imaging as and when they are referred for the same, holding stock of ^{201}Tl was not practical for multiple reasons. This was also one of the reasons in the search for alternatives to ^{201}Tl and especially based on ^{99m}Tc. Development and launch of ^{99m}Tc-sestamibi and ^{99m}Tc-tetrofosmin followed in the 1980s, though ^{201}Tl held its place for a long time, due to its more favorable biological features.[1,2] Other RPh obtained from MC-produced RN came into regular use much later, e.g., $^{13}NH_3$, ^{18}FDG, especially after 2001 with increasing availability of PET/CT in most NM centers (and also recently ^{18}F-flurpiridaz).[2]

Matters concerning the global availability of important RN—^{99}Mo and ^{131}I in particular—were shaken up in the fall of 2008, when a sudden, prolonged shutdown of the Canadian reactor (NRU), providing a huge share of the global supply of ^{99}Mo, occurred. This became a wake-up call for the NM community and other stakeholders in almost all parts of the world.[3,5,6] The crisis lasted for over 2 years, and several initiatives and measures followed to address the supply chain issues and evolve robust means of ensuring cooperation, collaboration among major entities supporting production of RN. Both the IAEA (International Atomic Energy Agency) and Nuclear Energy Agency, a wing of the Organisation for Economic Co-operation and Development (NEA-OECD) anchored several of the above efforts and helped interested member states to enhance access to RN/RPh and avoid disruptions in NM services.[5-7] Subsequently, the COVID-19 global pandemic led to near total disruption of transportation options of RPh/RN and posed another round of challenges to the practice of NM (Medical Radioisotopes still Produced but Facing Distribution Challenges Globally, Data Collected by IAEA Shows | IAEA). Sustainable operation of the irradiation facilities as well as of post-irradiation processing facilities (including pre-established back-up facilities for both irradiation and processing), facile access to (enriched) targets cum fair stock inventory and means of transportation of finished products (and also of irradiated targets, where necessary) are all of vital importance toward ensuring effective management of supply chain. The salient features of the efforts and measures taken in this context are outlined in this chapter, mainly covering the most widely used RN in diagnostic imaging,* viz., ^{99}Mo-^{99m}Tc, ^{68}Ga, ^{89}Zr, and ^{64}Cu and therapy products, viz., ^{131}I, ^{177}Lu, ^{90}Y, ^{161}Tb, and ^{225}Ac.

SUSTAINABILITY OF SUPPLIES OF ^{99}Mo AND ^{99M}Tc STRENGTHENED

As alluded earlier, the convenience of availing ^{99m}Tc from a ^{99}Mo-^{99m}Tc RN generator and the possibility of imaging almost every organ/metabolic system in the body (thanks to the versatile chemistry of technetium and the enormous efforts worldwide through the 1980s to develop suitable RPh) rendered ^{99m}Tc the most widely used diagnostic RN and rightfully named the "Workhorse of NM". Advances in imaging instrumentation, especially arrival of SPECT (single photon emission computed tomography) and hybrid SPECT/CT, expanded further the benefits of using ^{99m}Tc. By the end of last century, almost 90% of the diagnostic scans were performed using ^{99m}Tc-based RPh.

In this backdrop, the supply shortage witnessed due to the unplanned shutdown of the NRU reactor in Canada (which was the major producer of medical RNs, especially ^{99}Mo), followed by outages in other aged ^{99}Mo-producing research reactors, during the 2008–2009 period, shook the entire system of production of RNs and practice of NM. While the NM fraternity tried to manage the situation through different strategies including austerity in use, enhanced use through the sharing of generators with nearby NM centers, and shifting to non-^{99m}Tc RPs (mainly ^{18}F based RPs) wherever possible, the suppliers' community put in enormous efforts to strengthen the entire supply chain to achieve robust sustainable supply of medical RNs, particularly ^{99}Mo. The efforts, which began immediately after the crisis in 2009, continued rigorously till 2018,[5-7] under the umbrella of NEA-OECD at the behest

*Large-scale production of ^{18}F and its RPh, on a virtually daily basis, in numerous centers across the world has been well established, thanks to continual advances in water target technology, recovery of ^{18}F, ^{18}F-RPh synthesis modules, possible reuse of enriched water target, etc. Except for the inevitable logistics constraints, due to the 110-min half-life of ^{18}F, there are no major issues in the supply chain. Accessing enriched water target from more than one source, ensuring availability of water target-related components/ systems, and regularly availing vendors' support are some of the measures in practice.

of its member countries. The following are the actions put in place for fostering reliable and sustained supply of ^{99}Mo and ^{99m}Tc.

Based on Canada-led remediation efforts, NEA brought all the stakeholders from around the world involved in global supply of medical RNs, to analyze the situation threadbare and evolve mechanisms and strategies to strengthen the supply of ^{99}Mo and other RNs. The NEA set-up a high-level group on the Security of Supply of Medical Radioisotopes (HLG-MR) in April 2009, comprising representatives from the major member countries, all major stakeholder entities such as the irradiators who produce ^{99}Mo in reactors, processors who process the irradiated targets and supply ^{99}Mo, generator manufacturers who avail ^{99}Mo and produce and supply ^{99}Mo/^{99m}Tc generators, representatives from healthcare sectors (NM professionals, international societies, and insurance companies), and the IAEA—the relevant international organization of larger global representation to complement NEA member countries. The HLG-MR examined the causes of supply disruptions and developed a policy approach, including principles and supporting recommendations to address these causes.

The "Association of Imaging Producers and Equipment Suppliers (AIPES)", a professional body of relevant stakeholders expanded its roles to coordinate at the international level, the scheduling of reactors' operation that produce ^{99}Mo to help plan adequate, uninterrupted target irradiation capacity and in turn minimize supply risks. This group assembles multiple times each year and maintains ongoing, continuous communications outside of formal meetings to harmonize reactor scheduling. The major ^{99}Mo producers around the world participate in this initiative to ensure reactor availability for planned irradiations, mobilize support for replacement of closed/aging reactors, and have coordinated actions to increase capacity toward securing the reliable supply of ^{99}Mo.

A major positive outcome of all the above has been the coordinated (and congenial) working of the entire supply chain market players who are often competitors, which has led to a robust system being followed to date for ensuring sustained supply.

Independent of the above, other production options for ^{99}Mo involving irradiation of molybdenum trioxide including in power reactors, use of accelerators, and enriched ^{100}Mo targets by (gamma, n) reaction were also developed by research groups in association with potential users toward diversifying options to avail ^{99}Mo and ^{99m}Tc.[8] Scope for direct production of ^{99m}Tc in large quantities was also demonstrated using accelerators/cyclotrons and very highly enriched ^{100}Mo targets by (p,2n) reaction.[9] Some of these R&D initiatives were also funded and supported by the Governments of US and Canada, with some degree of success. These approaches are, however, limited in capacity and the extent of possible utilization, while they can help reduce the burden of sole dependency on large-scale ^{99}Mo and generator producers. IAEA's Coordinated Research Project (CRP) mechanism was also well leveraged to support these needs-based developments, especially cyclotron production of ^{99m}Tc and accelerator production of ^{99}Mo and their evaluation for possible adoption.[9]

Although several alternate routes to avail ^{99}Mo and ^{99m}Tc were successfully demonstrated, reactor produced fission-based ^{99}Mo continues to be the most viable economic model for large-scale supply of ^{99}Mo-^{99m}Tc generators worldwide. And, despite the shifts in the use of ^{99m}Tc-based RPs worldwide, it continues to be a widely used RN in diagnostic imaging, accounting for about 80% of scans globally. The cooperative functioning of the irradiating reactor facilities, processors, and generator manufacturers has been successful in avoiding major supply shortages and managing planned outages, although unplanned outages caused occasional short-term supply issues in the past decade. A plan to combat such unexpected shortages was built through "*outage reserve capacity*" wherein the production is augmented to have a reserve to take care of unexpected shortages—which would of course increase the cost; yet is acceptable to the NM community in general as the patients would not suffer. It is noteworthy that the severe crisis experienced during 2009–10 period, brought many governments to take note of the vital role of NM and ^{99m}Tc in the health sector, and extend their bit to support to make the system to become more robust and sustainable. However, due to unfavorable economics of operations, there will be less interest in developing new facilities for ^{99}Mo (compared to investments on production of other RN). This likelihood, taken along with the issue of aging of reactors serving RN industry, may cause more concerns in future.

FOSTERING ENHANCED UTILIZATION OF ^{68}Ge-^{68}Ga GENERATOR AND DIRECT PRODUCTION OF $^{68}GaCl_3$

Gallium-68 ($t_{½}$ 68 min) is now the second most widely used RI for PET imaging (after ^{18}F). ^{68}Ga is a suitable tracer of

M(III) element for chelation with desired targeting ligands, as well as for pairing with therapeutic radio(metal)nuclide ^{177}Lu. The same chelator-binder moiety and RPh design can be used thus with both these RNs.[3,4]

Currently, the most common method for obtaining ^{68}Ga is from ^{68}Ge-^{68}Ga generator. Generators are convenient to use at hospital radiopharmacy for preparation of short-lived ^{68}Ga RPh for many applications. The long half-life of the parent nuclide ^{68}Ge ($t_{½}$ 270.93 days) allows long shelf life for generator and the 4-hour equilibrium time between ^{68}Ge and ^{68}Ga permits repeated elution of ^{68}Ga and need-based RPh preparations multiple times every day. Early technologies of ^{68}Ge-^{68}Ga generator used eluents which were not directly suitable for further compounding—formulation of ^{68}Ga-RPh. Subsequent advances have addressed this concern, and more synthesis-friendly eluents have been developed. However, the activity of ^{68}Ga available is limited (1–4 GBq) based on the loaded expensive parent RN ^{68}Ge activity. Further, there is always a potential risk for breakthrough of long-lived parent ^{68}Ge in the eluate, especially over the long shelf-life of the generator. This requires effective quality control (QC) measures with periodic testing at the user end. Also, ^{68}Ge supply is limited to a few producers (who also seem to be constrained to limit supplies only to specific purchase contract holders—that is, not freely commercially available); and the cost of pharmaceutical grade generators is continually showing upward trend in the past several years.

Central radiopharmacies can use generators more efficiently and economically to cater to the needs of NM centers nearby (cf. captive generator for each NM center). Concept of "shared use of generator" has also emerged in some cities/regions among interested NM centers. What would be more useful, and worthy of promotion, is to consider "licensed portable generator", which can be taken to NM centers within certain distances to deliver in-situ eluted ^{68}Ga. This would be more efficient, by making use of the secular equilibrium time duration (about 4 h) for transport of the generator, than transporting the eluted ^{68}Ga or its RPh itself due to inevitable decay loss.

Exploring other options to avail ^{68}Ga by a different route has led to developing direct production of ^{68}Ga via ^{68}Zn (p,n) ^{68}Ga reaction using small-to-medium energy MC.[10,11] Thanks to the established liquid target technology with MC for ^{18}F production from water target, good progress was achieved using Zinc-68 (^{68}Zn) salt solution as a target for production of ^{68}Ga in fairly sufficient quantities.[10,11] This really became a turning point as an alternate option to the use of ^{68}Ge-^{68}Ga generator. It is feasible to adapt both liquid target and solid target systems of ^{68}Zn depending on MC features and overall requirements of envisaged production. Commercial liquid target systems are available; e.g., when target solution comprising 1.0 M $^{68}Zn(NO_3)_2$ in 0.3 M HNO_3 is irradiated at 30–35 μA of beam current, with 14.3 MeV protons for 60 minutes, one can produce 4.6 ± 0.4 GBq of ^{68}Ga at end of bombardment in a typical run. The high density of ^{68}Zn solid target material allows high-yield of ^{68}Ga.

Direct production of ^{68}Ga has, however, certain technical challenges associated with it. Reliable, rapid radiochemical processing is needed along with availability of automated modules for ease and (radiation) safety of all post-irradiation operations. It is heartening to report that adequate progress has been accomplished thanks to development of radiochemical separation methods (mostly involving ion exchange chromatography and acidic eluents) and industrial support for access to "easy-to-reliably-operate" modules. These are primarily meant to ensuring complete removal of target (metallic) material and other trace impurities as well as achieve the requisite purity standards applicable for medical use of ^{68}Ga (matching pharmacopeial standards). While the use of generator is based on manufacturer's roles and responsibilities for product quality, direct production of ^{68}Ga shifts the same on MC operators. Dealing with the 68-minute half-life RN post end of irradiation is demanding due to inevitable decay losses. Furthermore, recovery and reuse of the expensive enriched target ^{68}Zn would be necessary for better techno-economics of operations. Technology and regulatory aspects in this context have to be satisfactorily addressed for regular adoption.

The column chromatography-based chemical separation methods are amenable to automation. Different options of synthesizer are now available commercially, that ease out target dissolution and further processing processes[†]. Removal of bulk of target material and associated metallic impurities is necessary to achieve efficient radiolabeling of different ligands. For easy adaption to established synthesis procedures particularly adaptable with synthesis module, it is necessary to have matching

[†]IBA launches CASSY®, a new compact radiochemistry module to enhance efficiency in radiopharmaceuticals production | IBA-Radio Pharma Solutions
Synthera® Extension | IBA - Radio Pharma Solutions
MultiSyn | iPHASE technologies
ALCEO - Solid Target Processing System

parameters such as concentrations and pH with that of generator produced ^{68}Ga. Despite all these challenges, it is still a feasible alternative for wider availability of ^{68}Ga considering large number of MC facilities that are available globally. The IAEA has supported collaboration among interested MS through its CRP and fostered developments in this context (Production of cyclotron-based Gallium-68 radioisotope and related radiopharmaceuticals | IAEA).

ADDRESSING ACCESS TO EMERGING DIAGNOSTIC RADIONUCLIDES

The recognition of the vital roles of PET/CT imaging for patient management and their wider deployment in many countries drove the search for additional PET tracers of preferably longer half-life, of several hours to a few days. Accordingly, during the last decade radiometal RNs such as $^{64/61}$Cu, ^{89}Zr, ^{43}Sc, ^{155}Tb, etc. are gaining increasing attention due to different potential applications.[10-13] ^{64}Cu ($t_{½}$ 12.3 h) and ^{89}Zr ($t_{½}$ 3.2 days) have been already fairly deployed in clinical studies and are likely to see further growing use. It would be ideal to have consensus-based selection of one or two such RNs for regular use from the point of view of effective management of supply chain, although the list of potential candidate RN is expectedly large. Key considerations will include ease of access to target and high-yield production in MCs. ^{89}Zr is thus a highly favorable candidate RN likely to be promoted for regular clinical use.[10-13] The most common production route is the ^{89}Y(p,n) ^{89}Zr reaction on mononuclidic yttrium-89 target. Use of widely available natural target material is advantageous for RPh/RN, compared to other RNs such as ^{64}Cu that require expensive, isotopically highly enriched ^{64}Ni target material. Invariably, very highly enriched target is necessary for accelerator/cyclotron irradiations. This is due to the potential for trace RN impurities that can come from concomitant reaction(s) on other nuclides present in target (however, small their content may be in target). This adds to the cost as well as need to explore recycling of such precious target.

Both liquid and solid target systems are used for production of ^{89}Zr. Even though production methods appear straight forward, it is critical to remove metallic trace contaminants, stemming from cooling water, cooling helium, collimators, degraders, and backing material. Metal contamination even if present at ppm levels can affect subsequent radiolabeling and may decrease effective specific activity. PET imaging using ^{89}Zr has opened possibilities of visualization of in-vivo processes with slow pharmacokinetics of emerging bio-vectors such as monoclonal antibodies, cell tracking agents, nucleotides, and nanoparticle systems. Recent IAEA CRPs focused on standardization of production of important radiometals, including ^{68}Ga, ^{89}Zr and ^{64}Cu, are helping toward ease of availability of these RI and allied RPh (Production of Zirconium-89 and the Development of Zr-89 Radiopharmaceuticals | IAEA).

ENSURING AVAILABILITY OF RADIONUCLIDES FOR THERAPY

Targeted therapy using RPh/RN is an attractive option as even the deep-seated lesions can be treated with radiation and particulate emitters with high LET (linear energy transfer) are the choice for such internal therapy. With the availability of a wide variety of RNs suitable for therapy as well as targeting molecules (peptides, antibodies, etc.), targeted therapy has grown well beyond Na^{131}I treatment of well-differentiated metastatic thyroid cancer.[3,4,10,11,13,14] While several particle emitter RNs with therapeutic potential have been explored to various extent,[13,14] not all have reached clinics for routine use. Some of these with very attractive features which were approved for use in clinics did not witness growth as expected and in fact declined due to varied reasons—e.g., Xevalin-^{90}Y, Xofigo ^{223}Ra, ^{188}Re-lipiodol, and Bexxar-^{131}I. Yet, the interest in these RI lingers on. Interest in hard beta emitter ^{90}Y seems to have reemerged in the recent times (Eckert & Ziegler Signs Contract Manufacturing Agreement for Yttrium-90-based PentixaTher with Pentixapharm).

Therapies using in-house produced ^{177}Lu RPh using target binder (vector) conjugate have become commonplace in many NM centers and India has played a leading role in this context.

For credible, assured treatment planning, availability of the RPh/RN at the desired time is a non-compromisable prerequisite. In the case of thyroid cancer patients to be treated, they would have been prepared by being taken off medication (thyroxine) to enhance absorption of ^{131}I for treatment efficacy. Hence any sudden inability to administer radioiodine at the planned time will cause (avoidable) inconvenience and trauma/discomfort to the patients. In the case of emerging and promising modes of targeted therapy, a delay or uncertainty in offering the treatment procedure will discourage future referrals by the physicians. It is hence of utmost importance to have reliable effective supply chain for such RPh.

Iodine-131

Reliability of supplies of ^{131}I is by and large quite high, thanks to its 8-day half-life and two major methods of production in vogue—viz., neutron irradiation of tellurium targets in reactor and recovery of ^{131}I; fission-produced ^{131}I separated from irradiated LEU target (by facilities producing fission-produced ^{99}Mo in bulk quantity). Commercial vendors in many countries also ensure exports to interested NM centers in most parts of the world, though occasionally certain logistics issues have been known. Yet, the supply chain issues in the case of ^{131}I is relatively low, except where the source of supply is linked to a single reactor operation, as in the case of India. The ease of imports by private vendors has been a boon in this context to complement the indigenous production and supply of ^{131}I by the national centers, BARC and BRIT.

There are two important lessons learnt during the 2008–2010 crisis referred to earlier. The first is the scope for ^{131}I recovery to be encouraged to be explored by all manufacturers handling fission-based production of ^{99}Mo in bulk (as it is otherwise being left in the radioactive waste stream for management—disposal). The second is the need for establishing/ensuring regulatory approval for clinical use of ^{131}I obtained by both the above production routes (even when only a single source of ^{131}I may be normally in use). A major country faced a regulatory exigency during the initial part of the crisis period to accommodate need-based sourcing of nonfission-based ^{131}I for use in its NM centers, as it did not have this addressed prior to the crisis.

Lutetium-177

Lutetium-177 is currently one of the most widely used therapeutic RN beyond ^{131}I, although it entered the market only at the beginning of this century, understandably due to its excellent decay characteristics and scope for ease of availability.[4,10,11,13,14] In brief, emission of β^- particles with E_{max} of 497 keV (78.6%), 384 keV (9.1%), and 176 keV (12.2%), which have a relatively short range in soft tissue, make it suitable for several applications, especially small-size lesions (<3 mm diameter), while sparing deep tissue penetration and the associated undesired crossfire effects. Emission of gamma photons of adequate energy and low abundance (113 keV, 6.4%, 208 keV, 11%), enables *in vivo* quantification by SPECT imaging, including vital dosimetry calculations. Being a lanthanide, its chemistry is amenable and well-studied, for coupling with a variety of biomolecules. Its physical half-life of 6.7 days is another advantage from multiple angles, such as long-term dose delivery, compatible with RPh having slower pharmacokinetics, and logistics convenience for production and distribution over large distances.

The production logistics for availing ^{177}Lu are also very attractive. ^{177}Lu can be produced via ^{176}Lu (n, gamma) reaction in large quantities as the reaction cross-section is extremely high (2100 barn). Research reactors with moderate neutron flux ($\geq 1 \times 10^{14}$ n cm^{-2} s^{-1}) can be used for ^{177}Lu production and several such facilities (around 30) are available around the world.[3,13,14]

However, soon after the use of ^{177}Lu started to rise, the issue of radionuclidic impurity of ^{177m}Lu (half-life of 160.4 days) in ^{177}Lu was debated from waste disposal angle, especially as some countries have highly restrictive limits for discharge. Use of highly enriched ^{176}Lu targets and shorter durations of high-flux irradiations (7–10 days in place of 3–4 weeks) help minimize the ^{177m}Lu burden. High specific activity ^{177}Lu, or better "no carrier added" ^{177}Lu (nca), is more suited for targeted therapies such as peptide receptor radionuclide therapy (PRRT) to enable using very low quantities of binder-vector ligand (to avoid saturation of binding sites in lesion). This has led to the wider use of production of ^{177}Lu by either irradiating enriched ^{176}Lu target (up to 97% enriched ^{176}Lu targets being used cf. natural abundance of ^{176}Lu 2.6%), or by irradiating highly enriched ^{176}Yb target—(^{176}Yb(n,γ)^{177}Yb $\rightarrow$ ^{177}Lu)—to get nca grade ^{177}Lu. It is important to note that enriched targets are necessary in both these cases. ^{176}Yb enriched to 97% is irradiated in high flux research reactors as the reaction cross section is just only 2.85 b. Availability of enriched targets, development of efficient target processing and recovery methods for ^{176}Yb-enriched target for reuse that are adaptable for large-scale production, and management of radioactive waste are some of the challenges for production of nca ^{177}Lu. 6.7 days half-life of ^{177}Lu provides favorable logistics for international supply, and currently GMP grade $^{177}LuCl_3$ is widely available from a few commercial suppliers. Bruce Power, Isogen, and ITM in partnership are supplying nca ^{177}Lu in recent years as innovative technology for irradiation system was developed for CANDU reactors for irradiating ^{176}Yb targets.[‡] This development following the earlier efforts in

‡Canadian Candu produces cancer therapy isotope - World Nuclear News
Cernavoda reactor to produce Lutetium-177 - Nuclear Engineering International

crisis period (from 2009) to produce (n, gamma) ^{99}Mo in power reactors is significant, as ^{177}Lu production in large quantities has been commercially accomplished. Another approach of using linear accelerators is also being tried for large-scale production of RI including ^{177}Lu by US-based commercial company currently. Such ventures can help to meet envisaged growth in demand for ^{177}Lu in future.

Terbium-161

Terbium is a M(III) element with unique advantage in terms of having a quadruplet of RNs—$^{149/152/155/161}$Tb—with potential for diagnostics and therapy in NM. Among these, ^{161}Tb ($t_{½}$ 6.95 days) is attractive as a potential superior alternative to ^{177}Lu. ^{161}Tb emits low-energy beta particles of average energy 0.154 MeV and also emits Auger and conversion electrons (both well suited for therapy) apart from gamma radiation suitable for SPECT imaging. Due to similarity of decay characteristics with ^{177}Lu and with additional Auger/conversion electron emissions, ^{161}Tb is called "beta plus therapeutic RN". ^{161}Tb is produced by neutron irradiation of highly enriched $^{160}Gd_2O_3$ target material. The recovery and purification of ^{161}Tb from target are based on the use of combination of chromatography methods. Multiple ongoing clinical trials are investigating the safety and efficacy of RPh of ^{161}Tb. One such study is the VIOLET study, which is a phase I/II trial that evaluates (^{161}Tb)-Tb-PSMA-I&T radioligand treatment in men with metastatic castration-resistant prostate cancer. First results demonstrated that radiation-absorbed doses from this RPh are within a safe and expected range for normal organs with physiological uptake.[15,16] There is much interest to explore further, while current availability of ^{161}Tb is limited; Dutch companies TerThera and Isotopia Isreal are the main commercial sources of ^{161}Tb. Requirement of enriched target material is a constraint for production of ^{161}Tb, similar to the case of ^{177}Lu, and efforts are ongoing to meet the demands.[§]

ALPHA EMITTER RADIONUCLIDES

Radium-223 (^{223}Ra) dichloride, Xofigo from Bayer, is the only approved alpha emitter-based RPh, approved in 2013. The interest in ^{223}Ra as calcium analog, and of very high LET highly suited for metastatic bone pain palliation, led to initially finding significant benefits for management of patients with prostate cancer (P-Ca). However, subsequent findings have not been satisfactory. It is the launch of ^{225}Ac ($t_{½}$ 10 days) in 2014, in place of beta emitter ^{177}Lu, with PSMA binder ligand (PSMA-617)—first patient of P-Ca treated with ^{225}Ac-PSMA-617 at Heidelberg, Germany—that triggered high clinical interest in targeted alpha therapy (TAT) and growing demand to using ^{225}Ac.[10,11,14,17] Also, interest in other alpha emitters (including ones under exploration since many years) emerged.[10,11,14,17-20] Currently, there is a handful of such alpha emitters in limited clinical studies, e.g., ^{213}Bi (obtained from precursor RN chain coming from ^{225}Ac), ^{212}Pb-^{212}Bi [beta emitter ^{212}Pb ($t_{½}$ 10.64 h)] obtained from precursor RN chain coming from ^{224}Ra ($t_{½}$ 3.66 d) decays in vivo to alpha emitter ^{212}Bi ($t_{½}$ 60.6 min), ^{211}At, and ^{227}Th.[19,20] Lack of ready availability of the required alpha emitter RNs is a bottleneck for larger number of clinical studies required to better understand in vivo fate, efficacy, and toxic effects of different TAT agents.

Actinium-225 is the main alpha emitter of clinical importance currently for TAT and the expected demand for ^{225}Ac is very large going by the prevalence of P-Ca. However, current availability is hardly 60 GBq/year, mainly coming from limited legacy stocks of ^{229}Th and radiochemical separation. Large capital/commercial investments in high-energy proton accelerators, rhodotrons, electron accelerators are notable to support producing large quantities of ^{225}Ac, via spallation on Th targets, and photonuclear reaction or (p,2n) reaction on ^{226}Ra targets. The latter methods have led to coordinated efforts to retrieve the safely disposed ^{226}Ra from radioactive waste storage facilities and developing suitable safe target system for using in accelerators. IAEA support is also evident for such measures to avail radium-226.[||] In the case of ^{225}Ac, it is the limited supplies currently available that pose challenges to supply chain management. In the long-term, availability may become better, while its relatively high cost will still be a challenge in its supply chain.

CONCLUSION

It is evident that supply chain issues of RPh/RN have been receiving attention, especially over the past about 15 years. Some of the basic concepts in addressing nuclear and radiation safety, namely defense in depth, redundancy, diversity, etc., are very much relevant and valid when trying to strengthen supply chain management of RPh/

§https://nusano.com/nusano-stable-isotope-program-enriches-gadolinium-160-to-99-2-purity/

||IAEA Enables Safe Management of Radium-226 Legacy Sources | IAEA

RN and of enriched targets. They have been well adopted as demonstrated in the case of enhancing access to ^{99}Mo, ^{99m}Tc, and ^{68}Ga. Diverse options for production of the important RNs have emerged to advantage, though their capacity may be limited in many cases. Further the techno-economics of the alternative option may not be necessarily favorable in most cases than that of the main (established) method. Also, cost and availability of the enriched targets pose concerns.

Lessons learnt in the past need to be judiciously taken into account when requiring to deal with new products of promise for clinical use. Ease of wider production feasibility (both RN and RPh) matching the envisaged demands should be a key driving factor. Similarly, choice of enriched target vis-à-vis natural target for RN production would be another key factor for consideration.

There are responsibilities for every stakeholder involved in the supply chain of RPh/RN. Complexity of certain facilities like reactor and high-energy accelerator, techno-economics of overall operations, not-so-easily available key materials, vendors commercial competition, etc. are inescapable facts. Remaining engaged with the management of major facilities, e.g., reactors, is an imperative need. Also, scope for exploring public–private–partnership (PPP) model is known and worthy of adoption wherever possible.

The fact that all radioactive material cargo is branded under "dangerous goods" classification (Class 7) has been a well-known point of concern and debate in many a forum. Efforts to get RPh and allied products under a different new classification have been unfortunately unsuccessful. Considering the global growth of NM centers and procedures, it is necessary to revisit this matter, as RPh and allied RN are transported invariably as Type-A package only.[¶] The concerned UN bodies like IAEA, World Health Organization (WHO) remaining engaged with International Civil Aviation Organization (ICAO) is much needed (IAEA and ICAO to enhance cooperation on transport of vital radioactive materials | IAEA). Furthermore, greater harmonization and simplification of practical requirements for road transport of such goods, especially over short distances within cities, and/or nearby areas (mostly for products like, ^{18}F, ^{68}Ga, ^{99m}Tc—distributed from a central/commercial radiopharmacy unit, MC facility), merit early attention, support, and suitable facilitation.

As the overarching goal is to enable patient benefits in a timely manner, all efforts to facilitate sustainable functioning of supply chain of RPh/RN should be ensured, as well as supported by all stakeholders. NM practice cannot go on without using RPh, and there are vital roles of NM as unique support for patient care (e.g., cancer mets imaging with PET/CT; RPh therapy of P-Ca) or as significant value addition to patient care (e.g., imaging myocardial perfusion, imaging infection). Consequently, strong commitment to effective management of supply chain by vendor-like service providers, national laboratories, central radiopharmacies, and individual NM centers is imperative to sustainably deliver the benefits of NM to the innumerable patients requiring the same.

REFERENCES

1. Ramamoorthy N, Venkatesh M Myocardial imaging products' evolution: Change for the better. In: Mahapatra G, Manoria PC, Jain D (Eds). Cardiac Imaging Update 2017. New Delhi: Jaypee Brothers Medical Publishers; 2017.
2. Ramamoorthy N, Venkatesh M. Myocardial imaging—Status update. In: Mahapatra G, Manoria PC, Jain D (Eds). Cardiac Imaging Update 2023. New Delhi: Evangel Publishing; 2023.
3. Das T, Ramamoorthy N, Radiopharmaceuticals: Evolution and accomplishments at DAE. In: Tyagi AK, Rao V (Eds). Atomic Energy in India: Accomplishments since Independence; Mumbai: HBNI; 2023. pp. 163-79.
4. Ramamoorthy N. Role of radiopharmaceuticals: Perspectives, future trends and requirements. In: Das T, Bhardwaj YK, Mohapatra PK (Eds). Applications of Radioisotopes and Radiation Technology. Mumbai: BARC; 2024. pp. 131-44.
5. Perkins A, Hilson A, Hall J. Global shortage of medical isotopes threatens nuclear medicine services. BMJ. 2008; 337:a1577.
6. OECD; NEA. (2021). The Supply of Medical Radioisotopes: Final Report of the Fourth Mandate of the High-level Group on the Security of Supply of Medical Radioisotopes (HLG-MR). [online] Available from https://www.oecd-nea.org/jcms/pl_55496/the-supply-of-medical-radioisotopes-final-report-of-the-fourth-mandate-of-the-high-level-group-on-the-security-of-supply-of-medical-radioisotopes-hlg-mr?details=true [Last accessed September, 2025].

[¶]In future, package containing certain RN, particularly alpha emitters, may have to go under Type-B when containing above a certain quantity of alpha emitter activity. This is due to ongoing revisions of certain safety documents based on considerations of potential for exposure due to any damage of such a package (not covered here further, being beyond the scope of the current chapter).

7. OECD; NEA. (2023). The Security of Supply of Medical Radioisotopes. Nuclear Technology Development and Economics NEA/NDC/R(2023)1. [online] Available from https://www.oecd-nea.org/upload/docs/application/pdf/2023-10/nea_ndc_r_2023_1.pdf [Last accessed September, 2025].
8. International Atomic Energy Agency. Photonuclear Production of Radioisotopes, IAEA-TECDOC-2051, Vienna: IAEA; 2024.
9. International Atomic Energy Agency. Cyclotron Based Production of Technetium-99m, IAEA Radioisotopes and Radiopharmaceuticals Reports No. 2. Vienna: IAEA; 2017.
10. International Atomic Energy Agency. Trends in Radiopharmaceuticals (ISTR-2019), IAEA/STI/PUB/1913. Vienna: IAEA; 2020.
11. Jalilian AR, Decristoforo C, Denecke M, Elsinga PH, Hoehr C, Korde A, et al. Proceedings of international symposium of trends in radiopharmaceuticals 2023 (ISTR-2023). EJNMMI Radiopharm Chem. 2023;8:39.
12. International Atomic Energy Agency. Copper-64 Radiopharmaceuticals: Production, Quality Control and Clinical Applications, IAEA Radioisotopes and Radiopharmaceuticals Series No. 7. Vienna: IAEA; 2022.
13. Venkatesh M, Kang KW. Medicine: Radionuclides used in nuclear medicine. Medical, Industrial and Agricultural Applications of Nuclear Technology. In: Greenspan E (Ed). Encyclopedia of Nuclear Energy, 1st edition. Amsterdam: Elsevier Publication; 2021.
14. Vogel WV, van der Marck SC, Versleijen MWJ. Challenges and future options for the production of lutetium-177. Eur J Nucl Med Mol Imaging. 2021;48:2329-35.
15. Buteau JP, Kostos L, Alipour R, Jackson P, McInstosh L, Emmerson B, et al. Clinical Trial Protocol for VIOLET: A Single-Center, Phase I/II Trial Evaluation of Radioligand Treatment in Patients with Metastatic Castration-Resistant Prostate Cancer with [^{161}Tb]Tb-PSMA-I&T. J Nucl Med. 2024;65(8):1231 8.
16. Gracheva N, Müller C, Talip Z, Heinitz S, Köster U, Zeevaart JR, et al. Production and characterization of no-carrier-added ^{161}Tb as an alternative to the clinically-applied ^{177}Lu for radionuclide therapy. EJNMMI Radiopharm Chem. 2019;4:12.
17. Apostolidis C, Molinet R, Rasmussen G, Morgenstern A. Production of Ac-225 from Th-229 for targeted alpha therapy. Anal Chem. 2005;77:6288-91.
18. Al-Ibraheem A, Zimmermann R, Abdlkadir AS, Herrmann K. Radiotheranostics Global Market and Future Developments. Semin Nucl Med. 2024;54:622-33.
19. Radchenko V, Cutler CS, Burgoyne A, Jalilian AR. Practical aspects, status, and future perspectives of application of alpha-emitting radionuclides for Targeted Alpha Therapy (TAT). Nucl Med Biol. 2025.
20. Jalilian AR, Kleynhans J, Bouziotis P, Bruchertseifer F, Chakraborty S, De Blois E, et al. IAEA activities to support the member states in the production of targeted alpha therapy radiopharmaceuticals. 2025;144-145:109008.

Appropriate Use Criteria in Nuclear Cardiology: Where do We Stand Today?

Prajwal Chauhan, Siddharth Sharma, Manish Ora, Sanjay Gambhir

INTRODUCTION

Cardiovascular diseases (CVDs) are the leading cause of morbidity and mortality. It necessitates early diagnosis and management. Apart from coronary artery disease (CAD), inflammatory diseases such as aortoarteritis, cardiac infiltrative diseases, and valvular infections are becoming significant concerns. Assessment includes detailed clinical history, risk factor assessment, biochemical markers, exercise testing, and invasive and noninvasive imaging. Noninvasive imaging remains integral to CVD and CAD management for management and prognostication. It helps to decide the optimal treatment and avoid unnecessary interventions.

Commonly used imaging modalities are echocardiography (echo), computed tomography (CT), cardiac magnetic resonance (CMR), single photon emission computed tomography (SPECT), and positron emission tomography (PET). Intravascular ultrasound, computed tomography coronary angiography (CTCA), and hybrid imaging (SPECT-CT and PET/CT) have an evolving role. SPECT and PET utilize various radiopharmaceuticals for myocardial perfusion imaging (MPI). Unlike anatomical imaging like CT and CMR, nuclear cardiology emphasizes functional assessment of myocardial perfusion, receptor imaging, or inflammatory cell uptake. These offer critical insight into myocardial perfusion, cellular viability, receptor expressions, and metabolic activity. Although beneficial, most cardiology imaging techniques are inherently associated with variable radiation exposures (CT, PET, and SPECT) and noteworthy healthcare expenses. There is a difference in regional availability and expertise of these modalities. Implementing Appropriate Use Criteria (AUC) is essential for the optimal utilization of available resources cost-effectively and for curtailing avoidable radiation exposure.[1]

This chapter will analyze nuclear cardiology AUC's evolving role in CVD. It aims to help clinicians, researchers, and policymakers benefit from nuclear cardiology, minimizing low-yield studies and reducing interprovider variability in imaging requisitions.

HISTORICAL CONTEXT AND CURRENT STATE OF APPROPRIATE USE CRITERIA IN NUCLEAR CARDIOLOGY

Fast progress in cardiac imaging, especially CTCA, coronary calcium scoring, fractional flow rate (FFR), and intravascular ultrasound, has increased diagnostic choices for cardiac imaging. Each modality has its benefits and limitations, making test selection for a particular indication multifaceted and complicated. Guidelines are periodically accessed to integrate these modalities, depending on availability, expertise, and cost-effectiveness.[2] AUC offer a systematized approach to prioritize the imaging modality with substantial clinical evidence. The essence of AUC is to sustain diagnostic accuracy by circumventing redundant diagnostic delay, cost, radiation exposure, and patient discomfort.[3] Professional societies, including the American College of Cardiology (ACC), European Society of Cardiology (ESC), American Society of Nuclear Cardiology (ASNC), and American Heart Association (AHA), have made efforts to optimize these guidelines.[4-6] These cover several relevant clinical indications, including chest pain, suspected CAD, patients with known CAD, risk stratification after myocardial infarction (MI), and assessment of myocardial viability. Recent guidelines also include cardiovascular, inflammatory, and infectious diseases.

RISK FACTORS FOR CARDIOVASCULAR DISEASE

Risk Stratification divides patients into low-, intermediate-, or high-risk categories. It helps patient management by

TABLE 1: Risk factors for CVD.

Risk-enhancing factors	*Criteria/details*
Family history of premature atherosclerotic CVD	*Men:* Age < 55 years, *Women:* Age <65 years
Primary hypercholesterolemia	*LDL:* 160–189 mg/dL
Metabolic syndrome	Waist circumference
	Elevated triglycerides (>175 mg/dL), Low HDL-C (<40 mg/dL in men; <50 mg/dL in women)
	Elevated blood pressure or glucose
Chronic kidney disease	eGFR: 15–59 mL/min/1.73 m^2
Chronic inflammatory conditions	
History of premature menopause	< 40 years
Noncoronary vascular disease	
Elevated high-sensitivity C-reactive protein, lipoprotein A protein, and apolipoprotein B	
Coronary calcifications	
Prior chest radiation or vasotoxicity chemotherapy	

(CVD: cardiovascular disease; eGFR: estimated glomerular filtration rate; HDL-C: high-density lipoprotein-cholesterol; LDL: low-density lipoprotein)
Source: Adapted from Winchester DE, et al.[4]

ensuring that imaging is necessary, safe, and cost-effective while minimizing potential radiation and contrast-related side effects and avoidable procedures. Incidental findings in low-risk individuals with low impact on clinical outcomes may lead to anxiety, follow-up investigations, and interventions **(Table 1)**.

CLINICAL INDICATION AND APPROPRIATE USE CRITERIA IN NUCLEAR CARDIOLOGY

Suspected Coronary Artery Disease

Early detection of CVD is paramount. Screening individuals without a documented CAD history helps identify patients "at risk".

Symptomatic Patients with no Known Cardiac Catheterization and no Prior Testing

The first step is to identify the familial and modifiable risk factors. Based on the Framingham model, patients are stratified into low, moderate, or high risk.[7] Based on precipitating factors, location, and response to nitroglycerin or physical activity, chest discomfort is subdivided into nonanginal, atypical, or typical angina types. The patients are stratified into very low risk (10-year absolute risk of CAD 5%), low (~10%), intermediate (~10–90%), and high risk.[2] Stress MPI is appropriate for symptomatic patients without cardiac catheterization or testing. It benefits younger individuals (<50 years) with zero or one cardiovascular risk factor. It is also indicated in older patients (>50 years) with two or more risk factors.[4] The ESC recommended CCTA in patients with a low to intermediate clinical likelihood. Alternatively, functional testing using stress imaging modalities is recommended for accessing myocardial ischemia.[5] Functional imaging is recommended in cases with a high (>50–85%) likelihood of obstructive CAD.[5] The 2025 ACC/AHA updates prioritize CCTA's role due to technological improvements in plaque characterization and fractional flow reserve estimation via CT.

Symptomatic Patients Without Known Coronary Artery Disease and with Prior Testing

Stress MPI is indicated if exercise stress testing is inconclusive or abnormal. It also includes patients with moderate stenosis (50–69%) on CCTA. Stress MPI is also considered appropriate in individuals with high coronary artery calcium scores (100–299, or above 300), and invasive coronary angiography reveals intermediate stenosis severity.[4]

Other Cardiovascular Conditions Without Symptoms of Ischemia

Stress MPI is also indicated in certain nonischemic cardiovascular conditions. It assesses ischemia as a contributing factor in newly diagnosed heart failure with reduced or preserved ejection fraction. It is helpful in certain arrhythmias, such as exercise-induced ventricular tachycardia (VT), sustained VT, ventricular fibrillation, and syncope, when initial evaluation suggests a potential cardiovascular cause. Stress MPI is vital in evaluating symptomatic and asymptomatic patients and providing critical information on myocardial perfusion, ischemia, and viability.[4]

Preoperative Evaluation

Cardiovascular disease remains the leading cause of morbidity and death in the perioperative conditions. Perioperative cardiovascular risk stratification is based on history and physical examination. Stress MPI is recommended in patients undergoing high-risk noncardiac elective surgery having poor functional capacity and a high likelihood of CAD. Stress MPI is also recommended in asymptomatic high-risk patients with a history of revascularization. It may be considered for intermediate-risk patients with suspected ischemia.[8]

Patients with Known Coronary Artery Disease

Symptomatic Patients with Prior Myocardial Infarction or Revascularization

The presence of inducible ischemia is paramount in evaluating incomplete revascularization in patients with prior percutaneous coronary intervention (PCI) and coronary artery bypass grafting (CABG) who present with chest pain. Stress MPI plays a critical role in guiding further management in these patients. Patients with a history of MI who were not revascularized and remain symptomatic should undergo stress MPI to assess for ischemia and viability assessment.[4]

Asymptomatic Patients with Prior Revascularization or Myocardial Infarction

Stress MPI may be indicated in asymptomatic patients who have undergone prior PCI or CABG. This is important for individuals at high risk of future events or silent ischemia in this subset of patients.

Asymptomatic Patients Undergoing Assessment for an Exercise Program or Cardiac Rehabilitation

Stress MPI helps identify underlying ischemia in patients preparing for an unsupervised exercise program or cardiac rehabilitation. Stress imaging can help stratify risk and guide exercise recommendations.

Following Revascularization

Patients with PCI are at risk for recurrent cardiovascular events, such as thrombosis, restenosis, and disease progression.[9,10] Residual untreated disease and partial revascularization may be present. The AHA/ACC guidelines for cardiac radionuclide imaging mark myocardial perfusion scintigraphy (MPS) unsuitable for asymptomatic individuals within 2 years following PCI. The "uncertain" category requires clinical judgment and risk factors. Among these asymptomatic individuals, high-risk individuals with ventricular dysfunction, multivessel disease or proximal left anterior descending disease, and diabetes mellitus may require follow-up testing. Follow-up and risk categorization after CABG remains challenging, particularly in asymptomatic patients. The AHA/ACC recommends testing to be reasonable for asymptomatic patients >5 years after CABG.[11]

Chronic Coronary Artery Disease and Fluorodeoxyglucose-positron Emission Tomography Viability Study in Guiding Revascularization

Fluorodeoxyglucose (FDG)-positron emission tomography is commonly used for assessing myocardial viability and is particularly helpful in differentiating infarcted and hibernating viable myocardium. A meta-analysis by Allman et al. demonstrated a significant reduction in mortality with revascularization in patients with viable myocardium (3.2% vs. 16% annual mortality, $p < 0.0001$).[12] The PARR-2 (Positron emission tomography And Recovery following Revascularization-2) study reinforced this by showing better outcomes in those with more significant PET mismatch.[13] A large area of ischemia (>10%) detected by the functional testing is a criterion for revascularization.[14] Thus, imaging is crucial in guiding revascularization by identifying hibernating myocardium that may benefit from intervention.

At the same time, the STICH (Surgical Treatment for Ischemic Heart Failure) trial questioned the survival benefit of viability testing.[15] However, it faced criticism accounting for the various limitations of using less accurate imaging modalities (SPECT/dobutamine echo instead of PET) and incomplete viability testing.[16-18] FDG-PET is a valuable tool for predicting left ventricular functional recovery. Noninvasive stress imaging, including CMR, stress echo, SPECT, or PET, can help evaluate myocardial ischemia and viability in patients with heart failure and CAD who are being considered for revascularization.[14]

CARDIOMYOPATHIES

Cardiac Sarcoidosis

Cardiac sarcoidosis (CS) is caused by granulomatous inflammation, leading to conduction disturbances, arrhythmias, and ventricular dysfunction. Its prevalence is increasing, but a definitive diagnosis is often challenging. Instead of a simple, obvious diagnosis, it is considered a disease spectrum ranging from definite to unlikely. Treatment usually involves immunosuppression, mostly corticosteroids in symptomatic patients, and active inflammation.[19] CMR and FDG-PET are essential in diagnosing myocardial fibrosis (CMR) and inflammation (FDG-PET). Combining resting MPS with FDG-PET helps to identify fibrosis, excluding CAD, and identifying CS-compatible patterns. The location, extent, and distribution of late gadolinium enhancement (LGE) and FDG uptake contribute to accurate diagnosis and prognosis. Right ventricular involvement is related to morbidity and mortality.[19-21]

Clinical Cardiology guidelines such as the Heart Rhythm Society, Japanese Cardiology Society, World Association of Sarcoidosis and Other Granulomatous Disorders, and AHA include the FDG uptake on FDG-PET in a pattern compatible with CS as a major criteria for CS.[19-22] Diagnostic criteria include FDG avidity, uptake location (right ventricle involvement), intensity of FDG avidity [maximum standardized uptake value (SUVmax)], and perfusion defects.[19,22] The recent guidelines also include positive gallium-68 (68Ga) in a pattern compatible with CS.[19,22]

Cardiac Amyloidosis

Cardiac amyloidosis is a cardiac infiltrative disease and a significant cause of heart failure, with preserved ejection fraction. It is associated with high morbidity and mortality. Imaging helps in early diagnosis and improves prognostication and management.[21] Nuclear cardiology plays a unique role in the noninvasive diagnosis with bone-seeking tracers like technetium-99m (99mTc)-labeled diphosphonate and pyrophosphate to diagnose transthyretin amyloidosis (ATTR) cardiac amyloidosis.[23] A multicenter study (1,498 patients) including patients with an echocardiogram or CMR consistent with or suggestive of cardiac amyloidosis in the absence of monoclonal protein using urine and serum with immunofixation electrophoresis showed a positive predictive value of 100% for ATTR cardiac amyloidosis. However, it was not very specific.[23] The ratio of heart-to-contralateral lung uptake, heart-to-whole-body retention, and heart-to-bone ratio are being used to aid in diagnosis. Combined ASNC/AHA/American Society of Echocardiography (ASE)/European Association of Nuclear Medicine (EANM)/Heart Failure Society of America (HFSA)/International Society of Amyloidosis (ISA)/Society for Cardiovascular Magnetic Resonance (SCMR)/Society of Nuclear Medicine and Molecular Imaging (SNMMI) Expert Consensus guideline recommends (AUC > 8) 99mTc-labeled diphosphonate and pyrophosphate cardiac imaging in identifying cardiac involvement in asymptomatic *ATTR* gene carriers. It is helpful for screening in new symptomatic heart failure patients (African-Americans of age > 60 years, increased LV wall thickness, familial amyloidosis, and neuropathy).[24] PET tracers such as 11C-PIB, 18F-florbetapir, and 18F-florbetaben targeting amyloid receptors are highly specific for amyloid deposits by binding to both light-chain amyloidosis (AL) and ATTR.[25]

Large-vessel Vasculitis

Takayasu arteritis (TAK) is an uncommon variant of large-vessel vasculitis characterized by granulomatous inflammation of the aorta and its major branches.[26] Assessment of disease activity is intrinsic to managing autoimmune inflammatory diseases. Active disease leads to initiation or intensification of immunosuppression. In TAK, pathology sites are problematic for biopsy. Clinical assessment of disease activity relies on a multifactorial evaluation of clinical features, inflammatory markers, and imaging.[27,28] 18-FDG-PET-CT denotes metabolic activity in the blood vessels and the positron emission tomography vascular activity score (PETVAS), summing the uptake grades in different arteries. PET-CT is superior to erythrocyte sedimentation rate (ESR) and C-reactive protein (CRP) in identifying active TAK. Follow-up scans after treatment demonstrated the resolution of PET-CT activity. PET-CT can show uptake in clinically inactive patients with elevated acute phase reactants or even when ESR and CRP are normal.[29,30] American College of Rheumatology/Vasculitis Foundation recommends using noninvasive imaging [CT, magnetic resonance (MR) angiography, or FDG-PET] to access vascular wall inflammation over catheter-based dye angiography (accesses lumen) as a disease activity assessment. It is also recommended in remission but with signs of inflammation in new vascular territories.[31,32]

Prosthesis Valve Endocarditis

A substantial and life-threatening complication of implanted cardiac devices is infection. Anatomical changes of prosthesis valve endocarditis (PVE), such as wall thickening, fluid collection, abscess, or fistulae formation, are detected by echo and CT. However, these changes can be nonspecific, leading to an equivocal diagnosis. FDG-PET/CT can provide confirmatory evidence under these circumstances.[21,33] FDG-PET/CT findings are a major criterion to the modified Duke Criteria, increasing the diagnostic sensitivity from 52–70% to 91–97% without compromising specificity. It reclassifies most "possible" cases to "definite" diagnoses. Similar diagnostic performance is seen in cardiac implantable electronic devices, intracardiac lead-related infection, and endocarditis.[21,33] 18-FDG-PET/CT is recommended in all cases of "possible" PVE and in some patients of "definitive" PVE to detect septic emboli or primary source of infection.[21,33] It helps identify primary infection sources, differentiate infection from inflammation, and monitor response to antimicrobial treatment.[21]

IMPACT OF APPROPRIATE USE CRITERIA IN NUCLEAR CARDIOLOGY

The quality, effectiveness, and clinical relevance of imaging have significantly increased since AUC was introduced in nuclear cardiology.[2] AUC improves patient outcomes by preventing inappropriate testing and guiding clinicians toward more effective imaging modalities.[34] The role of nuclear cardiology has expanded to PVE and inflammatory heart diseases.[35]

CHALLENGES, OPPORTUNITIES, AND FUTURE DIRECTIONS IN APPROPRIATE USE CRITERIA FOR NUCLEAR CARDIOLOGY

Challenges that impede AUC's implementation include physician resistance, lack of awareness, clinical workflow integration, and rapid evolution of imaging technology.[2] Variability in clinician interpretation further complicates its use.[36] Successful implementation requires collaboration. Implementing standardized "one-size-fits-all" criteria in patients with multiple comorbidities and complex clinical presentations is difficult. AUC are still evolving as novel tracers for cardiac PET imaging.[25] Advanced data analytics and machine learning techniques might have a possible role in integrating vast datasets to generate personalized risk assessments. Artificial intelligence algorithms may help identify complex patterns and improve AUC accuracy.[37] The continuous refinement of AUC is needed to enhance patient care and optimize resource utilization.

CONCLUSION

The evolving role of CTCA and magnetic resonance imaging (MRI) challenges the role of nuclear cardiology. However, nuclear cardiology still plays a dominant role in noninvasive functional imaging, especially in accessing ischemia in intermediate anatomy lesions, atypical chest pain, viability assessment, and cardiac inflammatory pathology. It is vital to note the availability, expertise, and cost-effectiveness of the suggested imaging modality (CTCA, CT-FFR, and CMR) in the Indian scenario before directly adapting the other guidelines. This chapter describes AUC in nuclear cardiology and attempts to provide insight into the advantages, disadvantages, and quickly changing nature of diagnostic criteria. By decreasing redundant, nonspecific studies, AUC improves the appropriate application of nuclear cardiology. It may reduce medical expenses and radiation exposure while raising the standard of care and patient outcomes.

REFERENCES

1. Hong AS, Levin D, Parker L, Rao VM, Ross-Degnan D, Wharam JF. Trends in Diagnostic Imaging Utilization among Medicare and Commercially Insured Adults from 2003 through 2016. Radiology. 2020;294(2):342-50.
2. Hendel RC, Berman DS, Di Carli MF, Heidenreich PA, Henkin RE, Pellikka PA, et al. ACCF/ASNC/ACR/AHA/ASE/SCCT/SCMR/SNM 2009 appropriate use criteria for cardiac radionuclide imaging: a report of the American College of Cardiology Foundation Appropriate Use Criteria Task Force, the American Society of Nuclear Cardiology, the American College of Radiology, the American Heart Association, the American Society of Echocardiography, the Society of Cardiovascular Computed Tomography, the Society for Cardiovascular Magnetic Resonance, and the Society of Nuclear Medicine. Circulation. 2009;119(22):e561-87.

3. Mettler FA, Thomadsen BR, Bhargavan M, Gilley DB, Gray JE, Lipoti JA, et al. Medical radiation exposure in the U.S. in 2006: preliminary results. Health Phys. 2008;95(5):502-7.
4. Winchester DE, Maron DJ, Blankstein R, Chang IC, Kirtane AJ, Kwong RY, et al.; Multimodality Writing Group for Chronic Coronary Disease. ACC/AHA/ASE/ASNC/ASPC/HFSA/HRS/SCAI/SCCT/SCMR/STS 2023 Multimodality Appropriate Use Criteria for the Detection and Risk Assessment of Chronic Coronary Disease. J Am Coll Cardiol. 2023;81(25):2445-67.
5. Vrints C, Andreotti F, Koskinas KC, Rossello X, Adamo M, Ainslie J, et al. 2024 ESC Guidelines for the management of chronic coronary syndromes: Developed by the task force for the management of chronic coronary syndromes of the European Society of Cardiology (ESC) Endorsed by the European Association for Cardio-Thoracic Surgery (EACTS). Eur Heart J. 2024;45(36):3415-537.
6. American Society of Nuclear Cardiology. Clinical Guidelines - ASNC. [online] Available from https://www.asnc.org/clinical-guidelines-tools/clinical-guidelines/ [Last accessed September, 2025].
7. D'Agostino RB Sr, Grundy S, Sullivan LM, Wilson P; CHD Risk Prediction Group. Validation of the Framingham coronary heart disease prediction scores: results of a multiple ethnic groups investigation. JAMA. 2001;286(2):180-7.
8. Halvorsen S, Mehilli J, Cassese S, Hall TS, Abdelhamid M, Barbato E, et al.; ESC Scientific Document Group. 2022 ESC Guidelines on cardiovascular assessment and management of patients undergoing non-cardiac surgery: Developed by the task force for cardiovascular assessment and management of patients undergoing non-cardiac surgery of the European Society of Cardiology (ESC) Endorsed by the European Society of Anaesthesiology and Intensive Care (ESAIC). Eur Heart J. 2022;43(39):3826-924.
9. Cottin Y, Rezaizadeh K, Touzery C, Barillot I, Zeller M, Prevot S, et al. Long-term prognostic value of 201Tl single-photon emission computed tomographic myocardial perfusion imaging after coronary stenting. Am Heart J. 2001;141(6):999-1006.
10. Zellweger MJ, Weinbacher M, Zutter AW, Jeger RV, Mueller-Brand J, Kaiser C, et al. Long-term outcome of patients with silent versus symptomatic ischemia six months after percutaneous coronary intervention and stenting. J Am Coll Cardiol. 2003;42(1):33-40.
11. Hendel RC, Abbott BG, Bateman TM, Blankstein R, Calnon DA, Leppo JA, et al. The role of radionuclide myocardial perfusion imaging for asymptomatic individuals. J Nucl Cardiol. 2011;18(1):3-15.
12. Allman KC, Shaw LJ, Hachamovitch R, Udelson JE. Myocardial viability testing and impact of revascularization on prognosis in patients with coronary artery disease and left ventricular dysfunction: a meta-analysis. J Am Coll Cardiol. 2002;39(7):1151-8.
13. D'Egidio G, Nichol G, Williams KA, Guo A, Garrard L, deKemp R, et al. Increasing benefit from revascularization is associated with increasing amounts of myocardial hibernation: a substudy of the PARR-2 trial. JACC Cardiovasc Imaging. 2009;2(9):1060-8.
14. Neumann FJ, Sousa-Uva M, Ahlsson A, Alfonso F, Banning AP, Benedetto U, et al. 2018 ESC/EACTS Guidelines on myocardial revascularization. Eur Heart J. 2019;40(2).87-165.
15. Bonow RO, Maurer G, Lee KL, Holly TA, Binkley PF, Desvigne-Nickens P, et al. Myocardial Viability and Survival in Ischemic Left Ventricular Dysfunction. N Engl J Med. 2011;364(17):1617-25.
16. Daggubati R, Arumugham P, Ferguson TB. The world post STICH: is this a "Game Changer?" A surgeon's perspective--revascularization is still the treatment of choice. Prog Cardiovasc Dis. 2013;55(5):470-5.
17. Gramze NL, Shah DJ. Is there a need to assess myocardial viability in patients presenting with heart failure? Curr Opin Cardiol. 2016;31(5):501-9.
18. Athanasuleas C, Buckberg G, Conte J. The STICH trial data: Keep it simple. J Thorac Cardiovasc Surg. 2015;149(6):1682-3.
19. Cheng RK, Kittleson MM, Beavers CJ, Birnie DH, Blankstein R, Bravo PE, et al. Diagnosis and Management of Cardiac Sarcoidosis: A Scientific Statement From the American Heart Association. Circulation. 2024;149(21):e1197-216.
20. Birnie DH, Sauer WH, Bogun F, Cooper JM, Culver DA, Duvernoy CS, et al. HRS Expert Consensus Statement on the Diagnosis and Management of Arrhythmias Associated With Cardiac Sarcoidosis. Heart Rhythm. 2014;11(7):1304-23.
21. Arbelo E, Protonotarios A, Gimeno JR, Arbustini E, Barriales-Villa R, Basso C, et al; ESC Scientific Document Group. 2023 ESC Guidelines for the management of cardiomyopathies: Developed by the task force on the management of cardiomyopathies of the European Society of Cardiology (ESC). Eur Heart J. 2023;44(37):3503-626.
22. Terasaki F, Azuma A, Anzai T, Ishizaka N, Ishida Y, Isobe M, et al.; apanese Circulation Society Joint Working Group. JCS 2016 Guideline on Diagnosis and Treatment of Cardiac Sarcoidosis—Digest Version. Circ J. 2019;83(11):2329-88.
23. Gillmore JD, Maurer MS, Falk RH, Merlini G, Damy T, Dispenzieri A, et al. Nonbiopsy Diagnosis of Cardiac Transthyretin Amyloidosis. Circulation. 2016;133(24):2404-12.
24. Witteles RM, Bokhari S, Damy T, Elliott PM, Falk RH, Fine NM, et al. Screening for Transthyretin Amyloid Cardiomyopathy in Everyday Practice. JACC Heart Fail. 2019;7(8):709-16.
25. Dorbala S, Vangala D, Semer J, Strader C, Bruyere JR, Di Carli MF, et al. Imaging cardiac amyloidosis: a pilot study using 18F-florbetapir positron emission tomography. Eur J Nucl Med Mol Imaging. 2014;41(9):1652-62.

26. Pugh D, Karabayas M, Basu N, Cid MC, Goel R, Goodyear CS, et al. Large-vessel vasculitis. Nat Rev Dis Primers. 2022;7(1):1-23.
27. Misra DP, Jain N, Ora M, Singh K, Agarwal V, Sharma A. Outcome Measures and Biomarkers for Disease Assessment in Takayasu Arteritis. Diagnostics. 2022;12(10):2565.
28. Aghayev A, Steigner ML, Azene EM, Burns J, Chareonthaitawee P, Desjardins B, et al. ACR Appropriateness Criteria® Noncerebral Vasculitis. J Am Coll Radiol. 2021;18(11):S380-93.
29. Santhosh S, Mittal BR, Gayana S, Bhattacharya A, Sharma A, Jain S. F-18 FDG PET/CT in the evaluation of Takayasu arteritis: An experience from the tropics. J Nucl Cardiol. 2014;21(5):993-1000.
30. Nassarmadji K, Vanjak A, Bourdin V, Champion K, Burlacu R, Mouly S, et al. 18-Fluorodeoxyglucose positron emission tomography/computed tomography for large vessel vasculitis in clinical practice. Front Med (Lausanne). 2023;10:1103752.
31. Maz M, Chung SA, Abril A, Langford CA, Gorelik M, Guyatt G, et al. 2021 American College of Rheumatology/Vasculitis Foundation Guideline for the Management of Giant Cell Arteritis and Takayasu Arteritis. Arthritis Rheumatol. 2021;73(8):1349-65.
32. Grayson PC, Alehashemi S, Bagheri AA, Civelek AC, Cupps TR, Kaplan MJ, et al. Positron Emission Tomography as an Imaging Biomarker in a Prospective, Longitudinal Cohort of Patients with Large Vessel Vasculitis. Arthritis Rheumatol. 2018;70(3):439-49.
33. Tanis W, Scholtens A, Habets J, van den Brink RBA, van Herwerden LA, Chamuleau SAJ, et al. CT Angiography and 18F-FDG-PET Fusion Imaging for Prosthetic Heart Valve Endocarditis. JACC Cardiovasc Imaging. 2013;6(9):1008-13.
34. Patel MR, Bailey SR, Bonow RO, Chambers CE, Chan PS, Dehmer GJ, et al. ACCF/SCAI/AATS/AHA/ASE/ASNC/HFSA/HRS/SCCM/SCCT/SCMR/STS 2012 appropriate use criteria for diagnostic catheterization: a report of the American College of Cardiology Foundation Appropriate Use Criteria Task Force, Society for Cardiovascular Angiography and Interventions, American Association for Thoracic Surgery, American Heart Association, American Society of Echocardiography, American Society of Nuclear Cardiology, Heart Failure Society of America, Heart Rhythm Society, Society of Critical Care Medicine, Society of Cardiovascular Computed Tomography, Society for Cardiovascular Magnetic Resonance, and Society of Thoracic Surgeons. J Am Coll Cardiol. 2012;59(22):1995-2027.
35. Doherty JU, Kort S, Mehran R, Schoenhagen P, Soman P. ACC/AATS/AHA/ASE/ASNC/HRS/SCAI/SCCT/SCMR/STS 2017 Appropriate Use Criteria for Multimodality Imaging in Valvular Heart Disease: A Report of the American College of Cardiology Appropriate Use Criteria Task Force, American Association for Thoracic Surgery, American Heart Association, American Society of Echocardiography, American Society of Nuclear Cardiology, Heart Rhythm Society, Society for Cardiovascular Angiography and Interventions, Society of Cardiovascular Computed Tomography, Society for Cardiovascular Magnetic Resonance, and Society of Thoracic Surgeons. J Am Coll Cardiol. 2017;70(13):1647-72.
36. Wolk MJ, Bailey SR, Doherty JU, Douglas PS, Hendel RC, Kramer CM, et al. ACCF/AHA/ASE/ASNC/HFSA/HRS/SCAI/SCCT/SCMR/STS 2013 Multimodality Appropriate Use Criteria for the Detection and Risk Assessment of Stable Ischemic Heart Disease: A Report of the American College of Cardiology Foundation Appropriate Use Criteria Task Force, American Heart Association, American Society of Echocardiography, American Society of Nuclear Cardiology, Heart Failure Society of America, Heart Rhythm Society, Society for Cardiovascular Angiography and Interventions, Society of Cardiovascular Computed Tomography, Society for Cardiovascular Magnetic Resonance, and Society of Thoracic Surgeons. J Am Coll Cardiol. 2014;63(4):380-406.
37. Betancur J, Commandeur F, Motlagh M, Sharir T, Einstein AJ, Bokhari S, et al. Deep Learning for Prediction of Obstructive Disease from Fast Myocardial Perfusion SPECT: A Multicenter Study. JACC Cardiovasc Imaging. 2018;11(11):1654-63.

Imaging with Fibroblast Activation Imaging Inhibitors: Potential Role in Cardiovascular Imaging

Diwakar Jain, Perry Gerard

INTRODUCTION

A unique strength of nuclear imaging is its ability to allow us to image molecular and cellular receptors, transporters, and other cell membrane proteins; matrix composition; and biochemical and metabolic processes and pathways in the animal models as well as in humans.[1-3] This involves an identification of a molecular target inside the body, which is highly specific for a particular disease process, is abundantly expressed, and is amenable to an exogenously administered molecular probe. The next step requires the development of new ligand(s) specific for that particular target and its radiolabeling with a suitable radiotracer to image the target. This has helped us to understand various complex biological phenomena in various pathological conditions. This has also helped us to identify several targets for diagnostic imaging and for therapeutic interventions.[1-3] Fibroblast activation protein (FAP) and radiolabeled FAP inhibitors (FAPI) are highly promising modalities for imaging as well as treating several cancers. These modalities are also highly promising for imaging various complex cardiovascular disease. This article provides a brief background of these agents in oncology and an overview of the underlying principles and potential applications in cardiovascular medicine.

FIBROBLAST ACTIVATION PROTEIN

Fibroblast activation protein is a cell surface serine protease that has emerged as an important diagnostic and therapeutic target in oncology, particularly for targeted radiotherapy.[4] FAP is a type II transmembrane glycoprotein, with 760 amino acids in humans. This protein is a member of dipeptidyl peptidase family (DPP family) with a molecular weight of ~97 kDa. This protein is a serine protease, with DPP activity, which cleaves proteins after proline residues. This protein has both exopeptidase and endopeptidase activities. This protein also has collagenase activity and can degrade type I collagen.

Normal Physiological Functions of Fibroblast Activation Protein

- *Wound healing and tissue repair:* FAP is expressed by activated fibroblasts during wound healing and repair.[5] FAP breaks down and reorganizes collagen. FAP also helps in angiogenesis. Normally, its expression is transient. It turns off when healing is complete.
- *Embryonic development:* FAP plays critical role during embryogenesis in tissue morphogenesis; organogenesis and shaping; and cell migration guidance. It gets silenced in healthy adult tissues.
- *Inflammatory responses:* This gets activated during inflammation in various tissues and during tissue remodeling after injury.[6] This facilitates immune cell migration. This also helps in the resolution of inflammatory responses.

FAP expression in most healthy adult tissues is very low or absent. Under normal conditions, in adults, it is only transiently expressed during wound healing, inflammation, and tissue repair processes.

FIBROBLAST ACTIVATION PROTEIN IN CANCER

Fibroblast activation protein is highly expressed in cancer stroma, playing a significant role in the propagation of cancer.[7-9] Cancer-associated fibroblasts (CAFs) show a very high expression of FAP in most solid tumors. FAP serves as a stromal activation marker and indicates "turned on" fibroblasts in the tumors. FAP plays tumor-promoting functions rather than tumor-suppression. FAP expression in tumors is persistent unlike transient expression during normal wound healing. FAP results in tumor stromal remodeling and matrix degradation, which create paths for cancer spread, invasion and metastasis. FAP degrades basement membrane, which allows cancer cell to escape into the adjacent and remote tissues. It also promotes tumor angiogenesis, by releasing proangiogenic factors. FAP also facilitates the activation of tumor growth factors, and facilitates an immunosuppressive environment by T-cell exclusion from tumors and immune checkpoint activation, which suppresses antitumor immunity. Several cancers such as pancreatic adenocarcinoma, colorectal cancers and triple-negative and invasive type breast cancers, and lung cancers have high FAP expression. Tumor FAP expression is a prognostic marker. High FAP expression often correlates with poor prognosis, increased metastasis, and treatment resistance.

A tumor-selective expression makes FAP a very attractive imaging as well as therapeutic target in oncology. Since this is a cell surface protein, this is readily accessible for antibody/small molecule targeting. FAP-targeted CAR-T cells and bispecific antibodies targeting FAP and immune effector cells and FAP-directed immunoconjugates (FAP antibodies with cytotoxic payloads) are also under development. Since FAP is overexpressed in a wide range of tumors, these therapeutic modalities will have a very wide therapeutic spectrum antitumor activity. FAP represents a promising therapeutic target.

FIBROBLAST ACTIVATION PROTEIN INHIBITORS

Fibroblast activation protein inhibitors are molecules designed to bind to and target FAP for both diagnostic imaging and therapeutic applications in oncology.[10] These are quinoline-based small molecules that bind specifically to FAP with high affinity and selectivity, and inhibit FAP. These molecules can be radiolabeled for imaging and/or for therapy of cancer. In early 2010s, first FAP inhibitor was developed for cancer therapy. Subsequently, these agents were radiolabeled for tumor imaging.[11] Several FAPI agents have been developed. Gallium-68 radiolabeled FAPI (^{68}Ga-FAPI-04) is the most widely used agent for clinical imaging.[12,13] ^{68}Ga is a PET emitter with a half-life of 68 minutes, and is eluted from a Germanium-68/Gallium-68 generator. ^{68}Ga-FAPI-04 has high FAP affinity and selectivity with rapid clearance from the blood pool and from normal tissues. Several other FAPI agents, such as FAPI-46 and FAPI-74, have improved tumor retention compared to FAPI-04, with better pharmacokinetics for imaging and therapy. However, FAPI-4 remains the most studied agent in clinical studies.

^{68}Ga-FAPI-04 PET imaging is used for cancer staging, treatment planning and for monitoring treatment response. ^{68}Ga-FAPI imaging has several advantages over FDG-PET: superior contrast in many cancer types, low background activity, and no dietary restrictions. Several cancers such as pancreatic adenocarcinoma, colorectal cancers, lung cancer, ovarian cancer, head and neck cancers have excellent FAPI uptake, sometimes better than FDG uptake. FAPI can also be radiolabeled with β-emitter or even α-emitting radiotracers for their use to treat FAP overexpressing tumors. Several radiolabeled FAPI agents such as ^{177}Lu-FAPI, ^{90}Y-FAPI, ^{225}Ac-FAPI are in various stages of clinical or preclinical therapy studies. In pancreatic cancer, radiolabeled FAPI imaging is dramatically superior to FDG-PET imaging with nearly 100% detection of primary tumors, with excellent metastasis detection. This modality has changed management of pancreatic cancer. FAPI represents a major breakthrough in nuclear oncology and is a major milestone in theranostics and targeted cancer therapy in oncology, where the same target is used for imaging and therapy. FAPI's use is still investigational in most countries.

Fibroblast Activation Protein Inhibitors Imaging in Cardiovascular Disease

This is an emerging and promising application that leverages FAP expression by activated cardiac fibroblasts.[14,15] This represents a significant expansion beyond FAPI's primary oncological uses. In the normal hearts, there is only minimal FAP expression in the healthy myocardium, which is undetectable by FAPI imaging. However, under several pathological conditions, activated cardiac fibroblasts express high levels of FAP. Inflammatory and fibrotic responses and myocardial tissue remodeling are associated with an increase of FAP expression, which can be imaged by radiolabeled FAPI.

Potential Clinical Applications in Cardiovascular Medicine

- *Myocardial infarction:* Following an acute myocardial infarction, inflammatory response during the healing process leads to FAP expression, with peak radiotracer uptake typically seen 3–7 days post-MI.[16-18] Infarct zone can be delineated clearly by FAPI imaging. The extent of abnormal radiotracer uptake correlates with the extent of myocardial injury and predicts outcomes. In the chronic phase, scar formation may be associated with residual faint FAPI uptake. However, persistent, high intensity FAPI uptake postmyocardial infarction is indicative of remodeling assessment and indicates poor prognosis. FAPI imaging may find a useful place in monitoring response to cardioprotective therapies in these patients.

- *Dilated cardiomyopathy:* Diffuse FAPI uptake can be seen throughout the myocardium.[19] This correlates with the extent and degree of fibrosis. This can predict the progression to advanced heart failure. Changes in FAPI uptake can be used to monitors treatment response.
- *Ischemic cardiomyopathy:* Regional FAPI uptake corresponds to prior infarcts. However, diffuse or remote uptake can be used to detect myocardial remodeling. FAPI imaging may also find some application in the differentiation of viable myocardium from scar.[20]
- *Hypertrophic cardiomyopathy:* Focal FAP uptake may be observed in areas of fibrosis and may correlated with sudden death risk.[21]
- *Myocarditis:* In inflammatory cardiomyopathies, intense FAPI uptake may be observed during active inflammation. This may be observed before conventional imaging techniques can detect inflammation. Serial monitoring can be used to detect the resolution of inflammatory process. Viral myocarditis is associated with patchy uptake patterns characteristic of inflammation. Treatment response can also be monitored by serial FAPI imaging.
- *Cardiac sarcoidosis:* Sarcoidosis is a chronic granulomatous inflammation of the lungs, lymphatic system, skin, and several other organ systems in the body, with a long-drawn smoldering course with periods of exacerbations and remissions. Cardiac involvement is seen in a relatively small proportion of patients with sarcoidosis of other organ systems. The clinical presentation and symptoms of cardiac involvement are highly variable and relatively nonspecific and can be very challenging to diagnose. Rarely, heart may be the only organ system involved by sarcoidosis. Nevertheless, cardiac involvement by sarcoidosis is associated with a poor prognosis and risk of sudden death. Therefore, it is very important to detect cardiac sarcoidosis as early as possible. Clinical examination, electrocardiography, echocardiography, and coronary angiography are often not helpful in confirming the diagnosis of cardiac sarcoidosis. Cardiac magnetic resonance imaging, FDG PET-CT imaging, and endomyocardial biopsy are often useful in confirming the diagnosis of cardiac sarcoidosis. However, each modality has important limitations. It is not uncommon that several of these diagnostic modalities are needed to confirm the diagnosis of cardiac sarcoidosis. Cardiac FDG PET-CT allows us to image the extent and severity of myocardium with active inflammation. Inflammatory cells are highly FDG avid. This requires a very rigorous patient preparation: high fat and low carbohydrate diet for 2–3 days and a prolonged fasting (12–16 hours) prior to cardiac FDG PET-CT imaging. This preparation results in a suppression of FDG uptake by the normal myocardium, whereas myocardium with active inflammation continues to show significantly higher FDG uptake compared to the normal myocardium as well as the background activity. Adequate patient preparation can be a major challenge in some patients particularly in those with diabetes mellitus.

  Since myocardial inflammation is associated with high FAP expression in the active sarcoid lesions, FAPI imaging can be very helpful in the detection of cardiac sarcoidosis.[22] In fact, this offers some theoretical advantages over FDG PET-CT imaging: such as lower background uptake and no need for a rigorous dietary preparation. Similar to FDG PET-CT imaging, serial FAPI imaging may also be highly useful for evaluating the response to therapy.
- *Cardiac amyloidosis:* Systemic amyloidosis is associated with an abnormal deposition of degraded and polymerized fibrillar proteins in the interstitium and extracellular matrix of various organs in the body, with a resultant dysfunction of these organs.[23] Several proteins have a predilection for dissociating into its component polypeptide chains in the circulation and misfold while trying to reconstitute and reassemble, and these misfolded proteins degrade into fibrillar structures which deposit in various organ systems. Transthyretin (TTR), a tetrameric protein is produced in the liver and released into the circulation, where it transports thyroxine and retinol-binding protein. The TTR tetramers can dissociate in the circulation and degrade into amyloidogenic fibrils. These fibrils have a predilection for depositing into the intercellular space of the myocardium, peripheral nerves, and tendons and ligaments. Similarly, the light chains (LC) of immunoglobulins can also degrade into fibrillar

structures, if overproduced in the body due to an abnormal clonal proliferation of LC producing B cells. The LC fibrils deposit in several organs including the kidneys, liver, and myocardium resulting in LC amyloidosis. TTR and LC are responsible for over 95% of cases with cardiac amyloidosis. Cardiac amyloidosis is suspected in patients with persistent diastolic dysfunction and an abnormal thickening of the myocardium on echocardiography and confirmed by ^{99m}Tc-pyrophosphate imaging (for TTR amyloidosis), elevated levels of LC (LC amyloidosis) and by endomyocardial biopsy. A potential role of FAPI imaging in diagnosing cardiac amyloidosis; differentiating TTR from LC amyloidosis and in evaluating the response to therapy and disease progression warrants clinical evaluation.[24,25]

CONCLUSION

FAPI imaging in cardiovascular disease represents a paradigm shift toward molecular cardiac imaging, where molecular-level information about cardiac fibroblast activation can be obtained by imaging. Currently, there is no simple way to obtain this kind of information by any diagnostic modality. FAPI imaging represents an exciting potential development in nuclear cardiology, offering insights into cardiac pathophysiology that were not previously possible with conventional imaging. So far, cardiovascular FAPI imaging has only been evaluated in case series and small cohort studies, mostly for demonstrating proof-of-concept. The results of these small studies have been highly encouraging and large scale are warranted.

REFERENCES

1. Jain D, He ZX. Direct myocardial ischemia imaging with exercise (18)FDG. J Nucl Cardiol. 2015;22:111-4.
2. Jain D, He ZX, Lele V. Cardiac Hot Spot Imaging With (18) FDG. Semin Nucl Med. 2014;44:375-85.
3. Panjrath GS, Jain D. Apoptosis for Nuclear Physicians. Indian J Nucl Med. 2004;19:68-74.
4. Park JE, Lenter MC, Zimmermann RN, Garin-Chesa P, Old LJ, Rettig WJ. Fibroblast activation protein, a dual specificity serine protease expressed in reactive human tumor stromal fibroblasts. J Biol Chem. 1999;274:36505-12.
5. Prabhu S, Frangogiannis NG. The biological basis for cardiac repair after myocardial infarction—From inflammation to fibrosis. Circ Res. 2016;119:91-112.
6. Humeres C, Frangogiannis NG. Fibroblasts in the infarcted, remodeling, and failing heart. J Am Coll Cardiol Basic Trans Sci. 2019;4:449-67.
7. Teichgräber V, Monasterio C, Chaitanya K, Boger R, Gordon K, Dieterle T, et al. Specific inhibition of fibroblast activation protein (FAP)-alpha prevents tumor progression in vitro. Adv Med Sci. 2015;60:264-72.
8. Loktev A, Lindner T, Mier W, Debus J, Altmann A, Jäger D, et al. A tumor-imaging method targeting cancer-associated fibroblasts. J Nucl Med. 2018;59:1423-9.
9. van den Hoven AF, Keijsers RGM, Lam MGEH, Glaudemans AWJM, Verburg FA, Vogel WV, et al. Current research topics in FAPI theranostics: a bibliometric analysis. Eur J Nucl Med Mol Imaging. 2023;50:1014-27.
10. Lindner T, Loktev A, Altmann A, Giesel F, Kratochwil C, Debus J, et al. Development of quinoline-based theranostic ligands for the targeting fibroblast activation protein. J Nucl Med. 2018;59:1415-22.
11. Privé BM, Boussihmad MA, Timmermans B, van Gemert WA, Peters SMB, Derks YHW, et al. Fibroblast activation protein-targeted radionuclide therapy: background, opportunities, and challenges of first (pre)clinical studies. Eur J Nucl Med Mol Imaging. 2023;50:1906-18.
12. Kiani M, Jokar S, Hassanzadeh L, Behnammanesh H, Bavi O, Beiki D, et al. Recent Clinical Implications of FAPI: Imaging and Therapy. Clin Nucl Med. 2024;49:e538-56.
13. Bailly M, Dupont AC, Domain G, Darsin-Bettinger D, Courtehoux M, Metrard G, et al. Gallium-Labeled PET Radiopharmaceuticals in Cardiovascular Disease. Pharmaceuticals (Basel). 2025;18:387.
14. Higuchi T, Serfling SE, Leistner DM, Speer T, Werner RA. FAPI-PET in Cardiovascular Disease. Semin Nucl Med. 2024;54:747-52.
15. Jain D. Molecular Imaging of Tumor Specific Markers and their Expression in Other Organs (Editorial). J Nucl Cardiol. 2021;28:822-4.
16. Nagaraju CK, Dries E, Popovic N, Singh AA, Haemers P, Roderick HL, et al. Global fibroblast activation throughout the left ventricle but localized fibrosis after myocardial infarction. Sci Rep. 2017;9:10801.
17. Christia P, Bujak M, Gonzalez-Quesada C, Chen W, Dobaczewski M, Reddy A, et al. Systematic characterization of myocardial inflammation, repair, and remodeling in a mouse model of reperfused myocardial infarction. J Histochem Cytochem. 2013;61:555-70.
18. Varasteh Z, Mohanta S, Robu S, Braeuer M, Li Y, Omidvari N, et al. Molecular imaging of fibroblast activity after myocardial infarction using a 68Ga-labelled fibroblast activation protein inhibitor FAPI-04. J Nucl Med. 2019;60:1743-9.
19. Siebermair J, Köhler M, Kupusovic J, Nekolla S, Kessler L, Ferdinandus J, et al. Cardiac fibroblast activation detected by Ga-68 FAPI PET imaging as a potential novel biomarker of cardiac injury/remodeling. J Nucl Cardiol. 2021;28:812-21.

20. Frangogiannis NG, Shimoni S, Chang SM, Ren G, Dewald O, Gersch C, et al. Active interstitial remodeling: an important process in the hibernating human myocardium. J Am Coll Cardiol. 2002;39:1468-74.
21. Ding J, Zhang H, Chen X, Wang H, Wang W, You Z, et al. Enhanced detection of damaged myocardium and risk stratification in hypertrophic cardiomyopathy using integrated [(68)Ga]Ga-FAPI-04 PET/CMR imaging. Eur J Nucl Med Mol Imaging. 2024;52:98-108.
22. Lartey DA, Schilder LA, Zwezerijnen GJC, D'Haens GRAM, Grootjans J, Löwenberg M. FAPi PET/CT Imaging to Identify Fibrosis in Immune-Mediated Inflammatory Diseases. Biomedicines. 2025;13:775.
23. Wang A, Mahmood U, Feldman J, Pan S, Aronow WS, Jain D. Amyloidosis of the heart: pathophysiology, diagnosis, and treatment. Expert Opin Pharmacother. 2025;26:731-41.
24. Zheng Y, Wang Y, Zhang X. ^{68}Ga-FAPI-04 PET/CT for the Assessment of Light-Chain Cardiac Amyloidosis: A Promising Risk- Stratification Imaging Modality. Curr Cardiol Rep. 2025;27:83.
25. Jafari E, Juweid ME, Bahtouee M, Pourbehi M, Esmaeilinejad K, Jokar N, et al. Beyond Cancer: The Role of Radiolabeled Fibroblast Activation Protein Inhibitors (FAPI) in Non-Oncological Molecular Imaging. Acad Radiol. 2025:S1076-6332(25)00704-4.

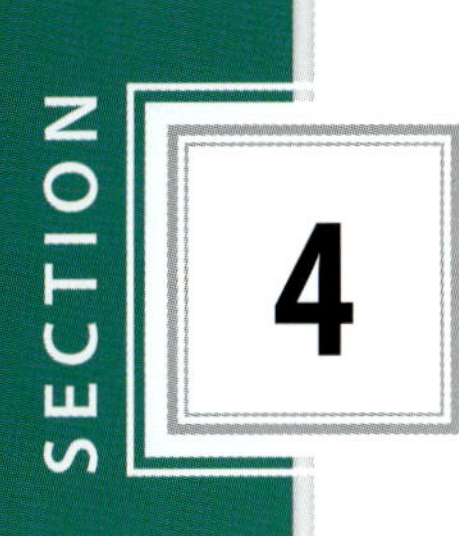

Cardiodiabetology

Heart Failure in Diabetes: Pathophysiology and Management

S Arulrhaj, Aarathy Kannan, Dhinesh Kumar

INTRODUCTION

About 422 million people worldwide have diabetes, the majority living in low- and middle-income countries. In India, there are estimated 77 million people above the age of 18 years who are suffering from diabetes (type 2) and nearly 25 million are prediabetics; 1.5 million deaths are directly attributed to diabetes each year.

HEART FAILURE: PREVALENCE

- Heart failure is a major public health problem.
- Overall prevalence of HF is 1–12%.
- Indian populations will range from 3% at younger age group to 10–24% at the age of 65 years.
- Lifetime risk of HF at the age of 55 years—23% for men, 19% women
- High mortality—more than 40% die
- Around 29% readmitted within 1 year of first hospitalization

OCCURRENCE OF HEART FAILURE IN DIABETES

The prevalence of HF in people with diabetes is between 9 and 22%, while in the general population, it is 2.3% **(Fig. 1)**.

This research paper examines all possible mechanisms of HF in diabetes and the sustainable, practical, and scalable approaches to treat HF in DM, highlighting the evidence base, and serves as an interim update for practitioners looking to fill the practical knowledge gap on this topic in conventional heart failure guidelines.

Global mortality variations observed in the International Congestive Heart Failure (INTER-CHF) study in patients with heart failure is shown in **(Figures 2 and 3)**.

People with diabetes are at increased risk of heart failure

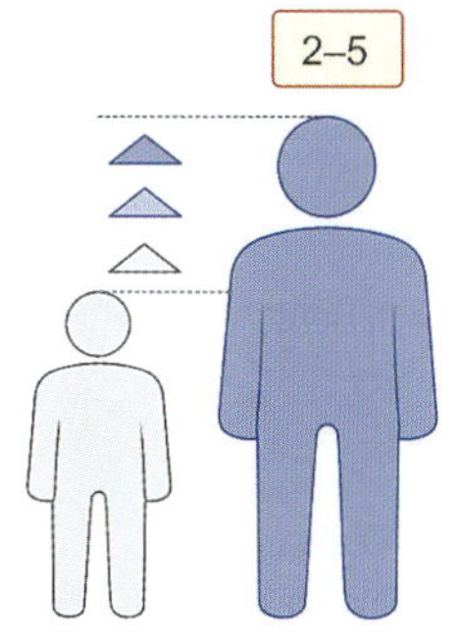

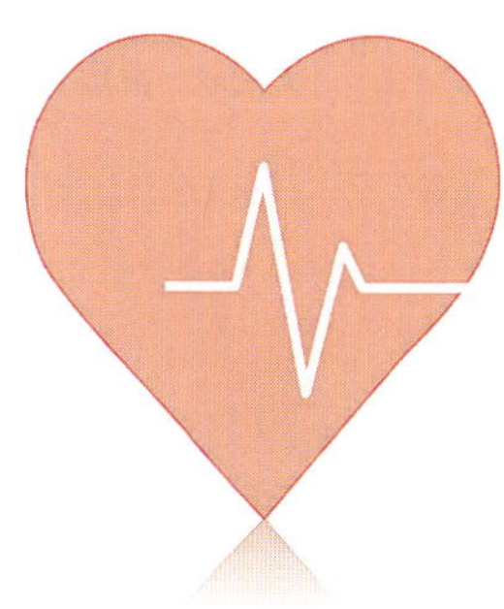

Fig. 1: Prevalence of HF in people with diabetes. (HF: heart failure)

DEFINITIONS

- *Heart failure:* Heart failure is a condition in which the heart muscle cannot pump enough blood to meet the body's needs for blood and oxygen.
- *Systolic heart failure:* Characterized by reduced ejection fraction and enlarged ventricle size.
- *Diastolic heart failure:* Characterized by increased resistance to filling due to increased filling pressures.
- *Acute heart failure:* Develops rapidly may result from cardiopulmonary bypass surgery, acute infection, acute myocardial infarction, and valve dysfunction
- *Chronic heart failure:* Long-term condition that is associated with the heart undergoing adaptive responses (e.g., dilation, hypertrophy) to a precipitating cause.

ETIOLOGY

Coronary artery disease (CAD)—70%, valve disease, and cardiomyopathies each account for 10%. Other causes

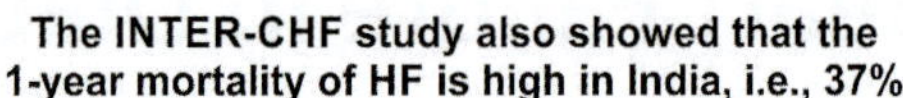

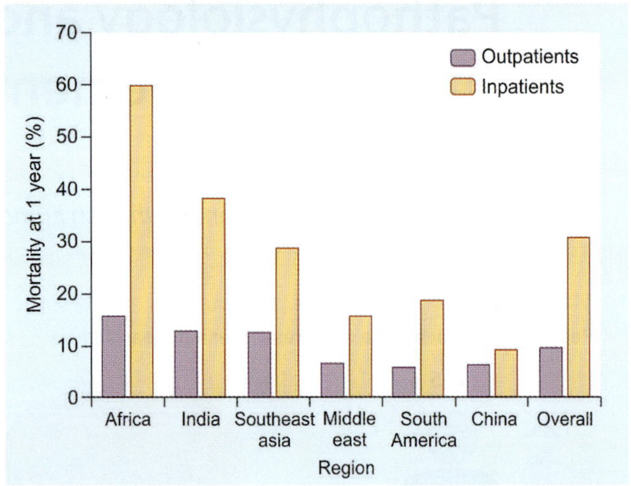

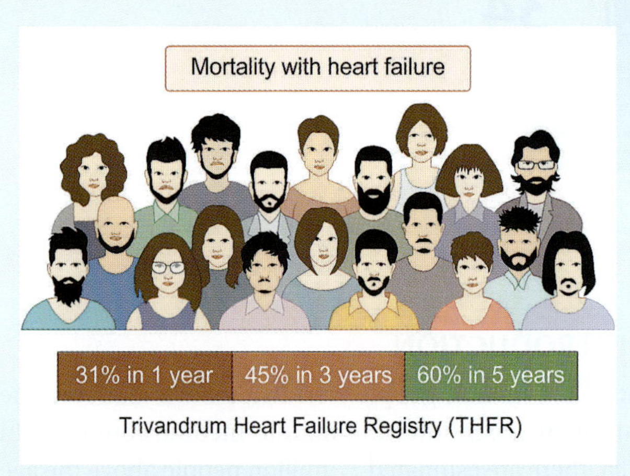

Fig. 2: Mortality variations in patients with HF. (HF: heart failure)

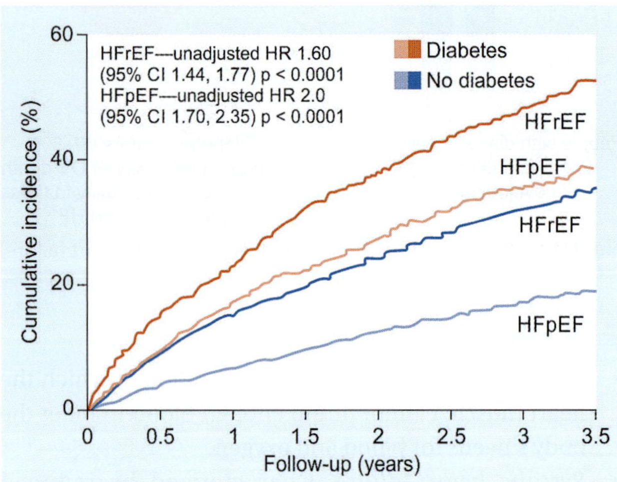

Fig. 3: Illustrates the presence of diabetes worsens HF prognosis. (HF: heart failure)

include hypertension, drugs, toxins, endocrine disorders, and infiltrative disorders.

Risk Factors for Developing Heart Failure in Patients with Diabetes

- *Cardiac risk factors:* Ischemic heart disease, myocardial infarction, hypertension, valvular heart disease, arrythmias
- *Noncardiac risk factors:* Age, chronic kidney disease, increased BMI, longer duration of illness, smoking, alcohol excess

CLASSIFICATION OF HEART FAILURE (FLOWCHARTS 1 AND 2)

2022 AHA classification of heart failure.

PATHOPHYSIOLOGY

Pathophysiology of diabetes contributing to heart failure is shown in **Figures 4 to 7**.

TREATMENT OF HEART FAILURE (TABLE 1)

Treatment of HFrEF (LVEF ≤40%) as per the 2022 AHA/ACC/HFSA HF guidelines is given below.[2]

Quadruple therapy:

- Guideline-directed medical therapy mainly targeting the sympathetic nervous system and renin-angiotensin-aldosterone system (RAAS) has led to improved survival and a reduction in HF hospitalization.
- Heart failure practice guidelines strongly recommend the use of four classes of medications to **(Fig. 8)**:
  1. Renin-angiotensin-aldosterone system inhibitors, particularly angiotensin receptor neprilysin inhibitor (ARNI)
  2. Beta-blockers
  3. Mineralocorticoid receptor antagonist (MRA)
  4. Sodium glucose co-transporter 2 inhibitors (SGLT2i)
- The STRONG-HF (Safety, Tolerability and Efficacy of Up-Titration of Guideline Directed Medical Therapies for Acute Heart Failure) trial demonstrated that rapid

Flowchart 1: 2022 AHA classification of heart failure.

HFrEF
HF with reduced ejection fraction
LVEF < 40%
HFimpEF
HF with improved ejection fraction
Previous LVEF < 40 and on follow-up LVEF > 40%
2021 ESC guidelines do not distinguish this category
HFmrEF
HF with mildly reduced ejection fraction
LVEF 41–49%
Evidence of spontaneous or provokable increased LV filling pressures (elevated BNP, non invasive/invasive hemodynamic measurements)
HFpEF
HF with preserved ejection fraction
LVEF > 50%
Evidence of spontaneous or provokable increased LV filling pressures (elevated BNP, non invasive/invasive hemodynamic measurements)

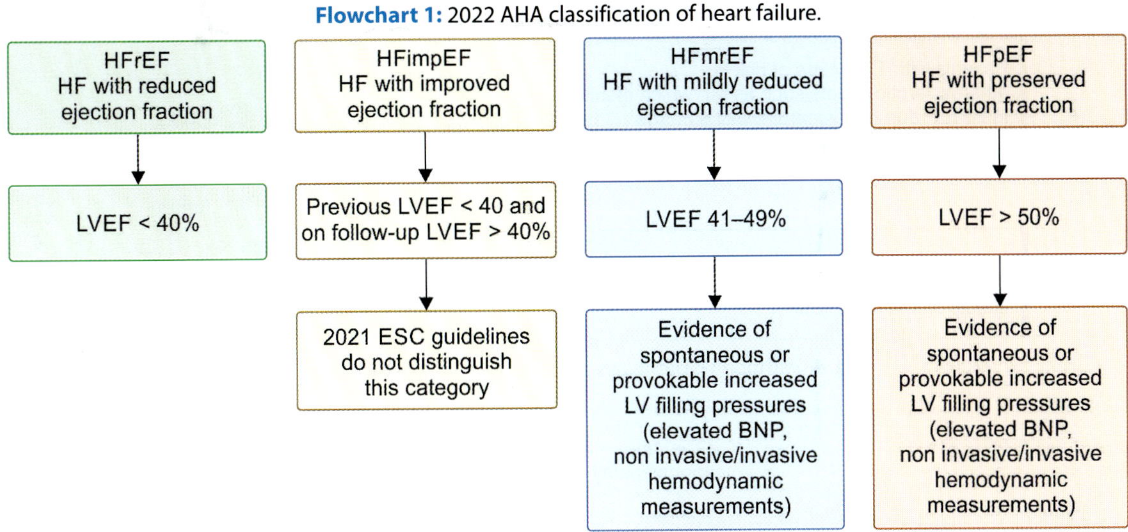

(LVEF: left ventricular ejection fraction)

Source: Heidenreich PA, Bozkurt B, et al. 2022 AHA/ACC/HFSA guideline for the management of heart failure: a report of the American College of Cardiology/American Heart Association Joint Committee on Clinical Practice Guidelines. Journal of the American College of Cardiology. 2022;79(17):e263-421.

Flowchart 2: Classification of heart failure.

Heart failure
Inability of the heart to pump out blood to meet the physiological demands of the body
Low cardiac output heart failure
Cardiac output is low and fails to increase normally with exertion
High cardiac output heart failure
Output is normal/increased in the face of increased needs
Right-sided heart failure
Edema, ascites, hepatomegaly, nausea, anorexia
Left-sided heart failure
Dyspnea, poor exercise tolerance, orthopnea, PND, wheeze, nocturnal cough (+/- pink frothy sputum)
Systolic failure (HFrEF)
Inability of ventricle to contract normally and fail to pump enough blood into circulation. EF <40%
Diastolic failure (HFpEF)
Inability of ventricle to relax and fill normally. EF >50%
Common causes:
• Left ventricular failure
• Pulmonary stenosis
• Lung disease (cor pulmonale)
• Ischemic heart disease
• Dilated cardiomyopathy
• Valvular disease
• Hypertension
• Hypertension
• Restricted cardiomyopathy
• Constrictive pericarditis
• Pericardial tamponade
• Anemia
• Pregnancy
• Hyperthyroidism
• Arteriovenous malformation

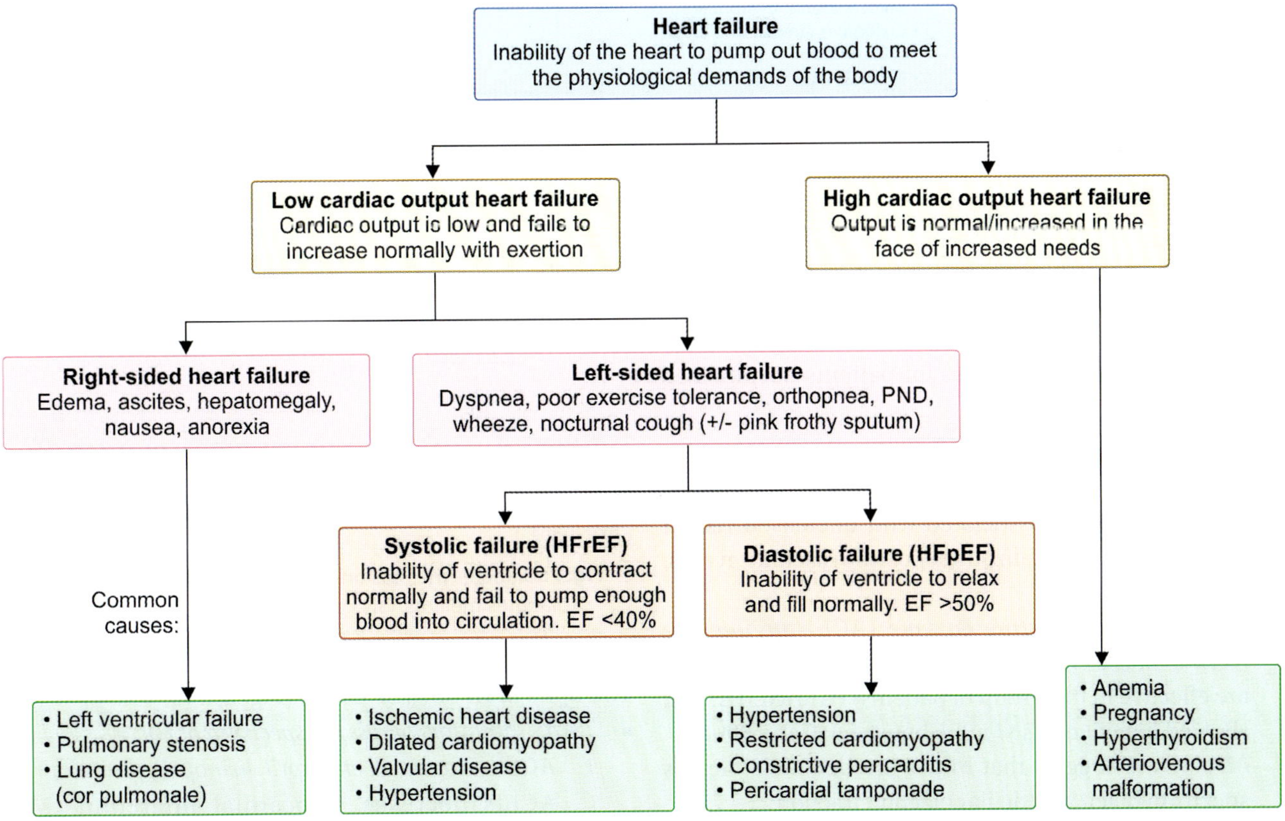

(HFpEF: heart failure with preserved ejection fraction; HFrEF: heart failure with reduced ejection fraction)

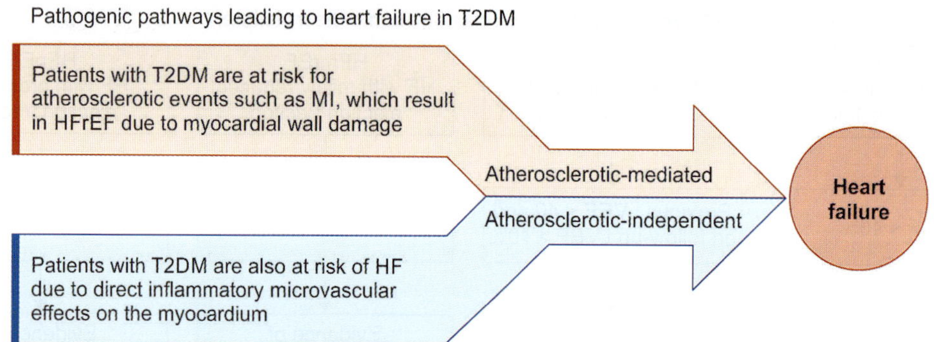

Fig. 4: Pathogenic pathways. (T2DM: type 2 diabetes mellitus)

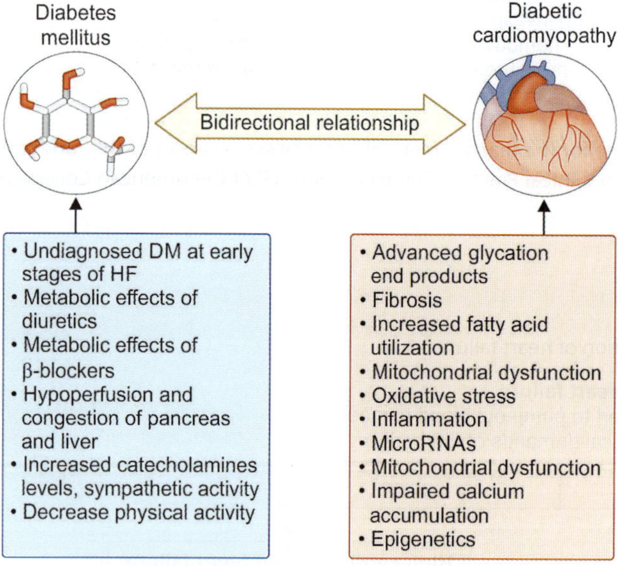

Fig. 5: Link between diabetes and heart failure.

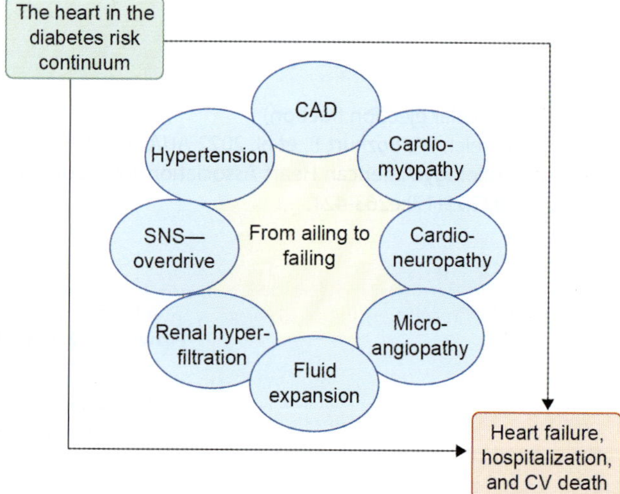

Fig. 6: Heart failure in diabetes—"Ominous Octet". (CAD: coronary artery disease; CV: cardiovascular; SNS: sympathetic nervous system)

in hospital initiation and post discharge up-titration of GDMT with close follow-up safely and substantially improves clinical outcomes for patients hospitalized for HF.

Guideline recommendations in HFmrEF:

- *Diuretics:* As needed for volume control and symptoms
- *SGLT2 inhibitors:* associated with decreased risk of heart failure hospitalizations, cardiovascular events, and mortality
- *Angiotensin-converting enzyme (ACE)/angiotensin receptor blocker (ARB)/ARNI:* data suggest that all three are effective in this group of patients; PARAGLIDE trial showed benefit of ARNI in EF between 40 and 60%
- *MRA:* Data suggest that MRAs are beneficial across spectrum of left ventricular ejection fraction
- *Beta blocker:* Benefit for LVEF 41–50% in sinus rhythm

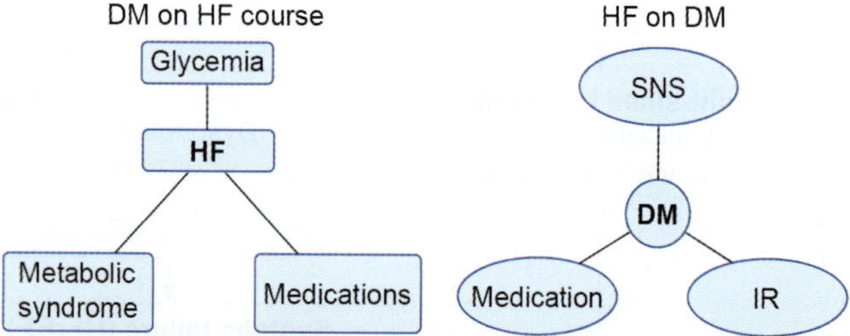

Fig. 7: Diabetes mellitus on heart failure and heart failure on diabetes mellitus. (SNS: sympathetic nervous system)

Therapies in HFpEF (EF ≥50%) ***(Fig. 9)****:*

- *RAAS inhibitors across the spectrum of HF:*
  - *ACEIs—ramipril, enalapril, lisinopril, perindopril:* ACEIs decrease myocardial infarction (MI), mortality, and HF significantly within 30 days of

TABLE 1: Guideline-directed medical therapy (GDMT) for heart failure (HF).

GDMT across HF stages				
Stage A ***At Risk for HF***	***Stage B*** ***Pre-HF***	***HFrEF: LVEF ≤ 40%***	***Stage C and D*** ***Stage C: Symptomatic HF and*** ***Stage D: Advanced HF*** ***HFmrEF: LVEF 41–49%***	***HFpEF: LVEF ≥ 50%***
SGLT2i in patients with DM Class 1	SGLT2i in patients with DM Class 1	ARNI in NYHA II-III; ACEI or ARB in NYHA II-IV Class 1	Diuretics as needed Class 1	Diuretics as needed Class 1
Management of risk factors for HF	ACEI Class 1	β-blocker Class 1	SGLT2i Class 2a	SGLT2i Class 2a
	ARB if ACEI intolerant: Class 1	MRA Class 1	ACEI, ARB, ARNI Class 2b	ARNI Class 2b
	β-blocker: Class 1	SGLT2i Class 1	MRA Class 2b	MRA Class 2b
		Diuretics as needed: Class 1	β-blocker Class 2b	ARB Class 2b
		Hydral-nitrates for NYHA III-IV in Black patients: Class 1		

(HFpEF: heart failure with preserved ejection fraction; HFrEF: heart failure with reduced ejection fraction)

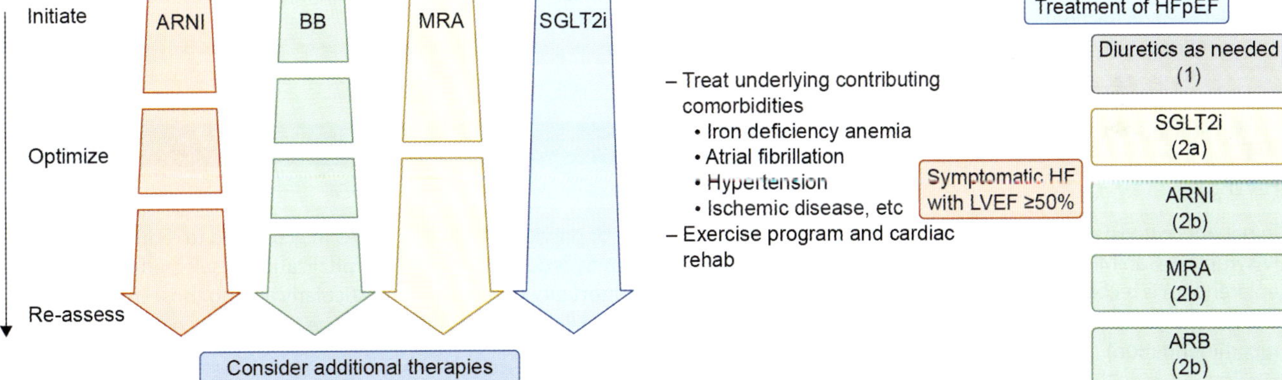

Fig. 8: Quadruple therapy. (ARNI: angiotensin receptor-neprilysin inhibitor; BB: β-blocker; MRA: mineralocorticoid receptor antagonist; SGLT2i: sodium-glucose cotransporter-2 inhibitor)

Fig. 9: Treatment therapy for HFpEF (EF≥50%). (ARNI: angiotensin receptor-neprilysin inhibitor; HFpEF: heart failure with preserved ejection fraction; LVEF: left ventricular ejection fraction; MRA: mineralocorticoid receptor antagonist; SGLT2i: sodium-glucose cotransporter-2 inhibitor)

initiation. ACEI should be started at low doses and slowly increased over 1–2 weeks to the target level, which has been shown in trials to reduce the risk of cardiovascular (CV) events.

- *ARBs—telmisartan and losartan:*
  Although not superior to ACEIs in reducing mortality or morbidity, they were certainly better tolerated. ARBs can be considered as an alternative therapy for those who are intolerant to ACEi or ARNI to reduce CV death and HF hospitalization.
- *ARNI:* ARNI significantly reduced the composite endpoint of CV death or HF hospitalization by 20% compared to enalapril. Patients with HFrEF,

sacubitril/valsartan combination is recommended as a replacement for an ACEis to reduce the risk of HF hospitalization and CV death (Class IB recommendation).

- *Beta-blockers across the spectrum of HF* **(Table 2)**: Carvedilol, bisoprolol, and metoprolol are safe. BBs upregulate the β-receptors in the heart, suppress the cardiotoxic effects of catecholamines, and prolong the diastolic phase, thus increasing coronary blood flow. BBs also reduce the blood pressure and burden of arrhythmias.
- *Mineralocorticoid receptor antagonists across the spectrum of HF* **(Table 3)**: The commonly used MRAs are spironolactone (nonselective aldosterone antagonist) and eplerenone (selective to the aldosterone receptor). Trials have shown morbidity and mortality benefits with spironolactone and eplerenone respectively in patients with HFrEF. Finerenone is a nonsteroidal MRA, and its use in diabetic patients with chronic kidney disease (CKD) has been shown to reduce urinary protein or albumin excretion.
- *SGLT2 inhibitors across the spectrum of HF* **(Table 4; Fig. 10)**.
- *Diuretics across the spectrum of HF* **(Flowchart 3)**: Loop diuretics are the preferred in HF patients.

In patients with diuretic resistance, metolazone or chlorothiazide can be added for sequential nephron blockade and further diuresis **(Flowchart 4)**.

TABLE 2: Beta-blockers across the spectrum of HF.

HFrEF	*HFmrEF*	*HFpEF*
Patients with current or prior HF symptoms evidence-based BBs are recommended to reduce morbidity and mortality. (Class I recommendation)	Evidence-based BBs may be used to reduced HF hospitalization in selected patients, particularly among those in the lower EF spectrum. (Class IIb recommendation)	BBs may be used in patients with symptomatic CAD, for treatment of hypertension (history of MI), or atrial fibrillation (AF).

(HFmrEF: heart failure with mildly reduced ejection fraction; HFpEF: heart failure with preserved ejection fraction; HFrEF: heart failure with reduced ejection fraction)

TABLE 3: Mineralocorticoid receptor antagonists across the spectrum of HF.

HFrEF	*HFmrEF*	*HFpEF*
In patients with HFrEF and NYHA class II to IV symptoms, an MRA (spironolactone or eplerenone) is recommended to reduce CV morbidity and mortality. (Class I recommendation)	In patients with current or previous symptoms of HF, MRAs may reduce HF hospitalisation and CV mortality particularly among those in the lower EF range. (Class IIb recommendation)	MRAs may be used to reduce HF hospitalization in selected patients, particularly among those in the lower EF range (Class IIb recommendation)

(HFmrEF: heart failure with mildly reduced ejection fraction; HFpEF: heart failure with preserved ejection fraction; HFrEF: heart failure with reduced ejection fraction)

TABLE 4: SGLT2 inhibitors across the spectrum of HF.

SGLT2i (to reduce HF hospitalization and CV mortality)	*HFrEF*	*HFmrEF*	*HFpEF*
2023 ESC guidelines recommendation	Class I A	Class I A	Class I A
2022 ACC/AHA/HFSA guidelines recommendation	Class I A	Class II A	Class II A

(HFmrEF: heart failure with mildly reduced ejection fraction; HFpEF: heart failure with preserved ejection fraction; HFrEF: heart failure with reduced ejection fraction; SGLT2i: sodium-glucose cotransporter-2 inhibitor)

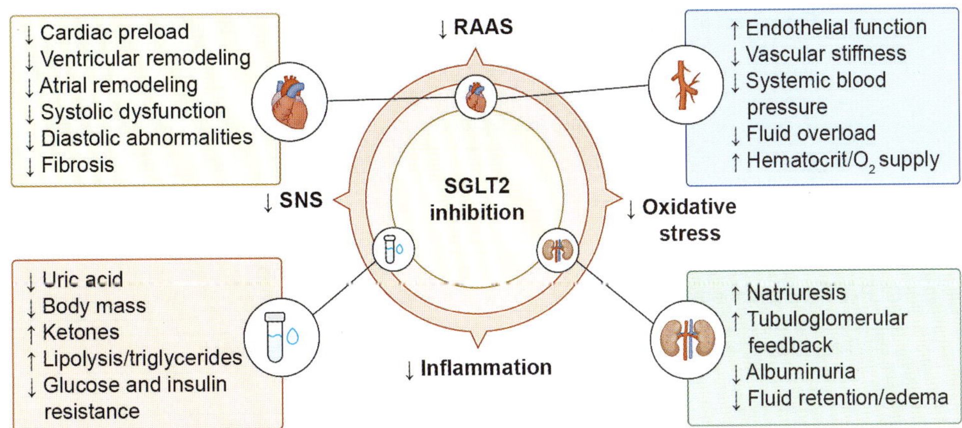

Fig. 10: DAPA-HF and EMPEROR-Reduced: Adding SGLT2i to ARNI. (ARNI: angiotensin receptor-neprilysin inhibitor; RAAS: renin-angiotensin-aldosterone system; SGLT2i: sodium-glucose cotransporter-2 inhibitor)

Flowchart 3: Diuretics for decongestion and to reduce HF hospitalization.

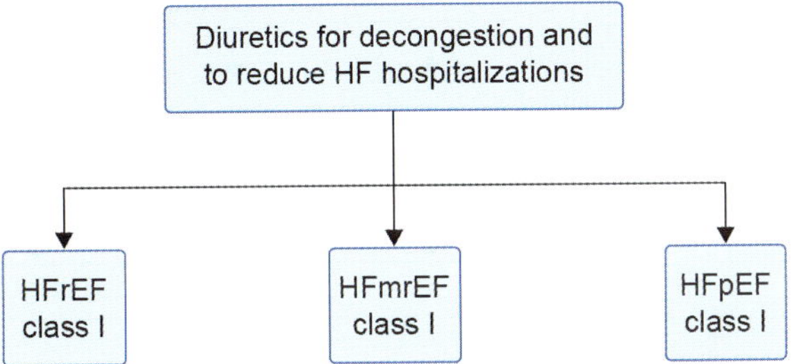

(HFmrEF: heart failure with mildly reduced ejection fraction; HFpEF: heart failure with preserved ejection fraction; HFrEF: heart failure with reduced ejection fraction)

Flowchart 4: Sequential blocking using loop diuretics in heart failure patients.

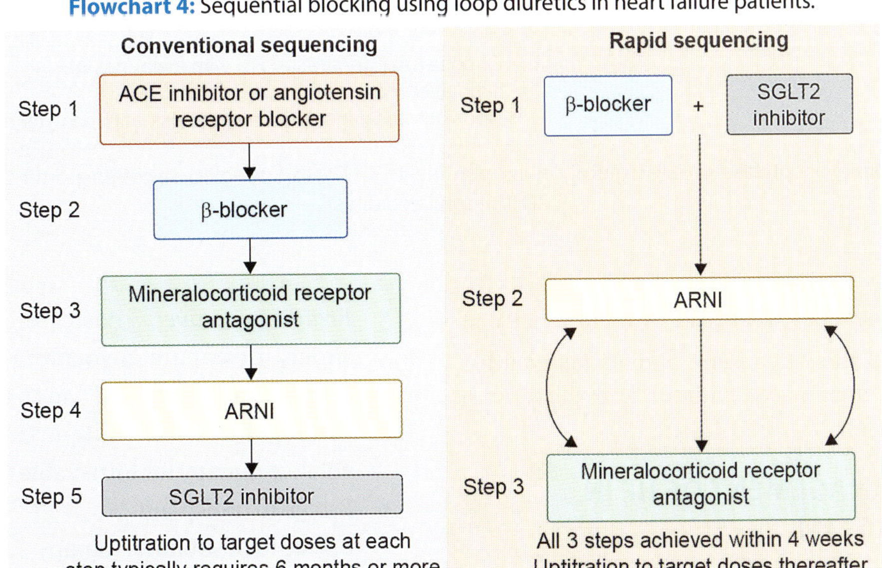

(ACE: angiotensin-converting enzyme; ARNI: angiotensin receptor-neprilysin inhibitor; SGLT2: sodium-glucose cotransporter-2)

Flowchart 5: Treatment for type 2 DM in HF with drug naïve patients.

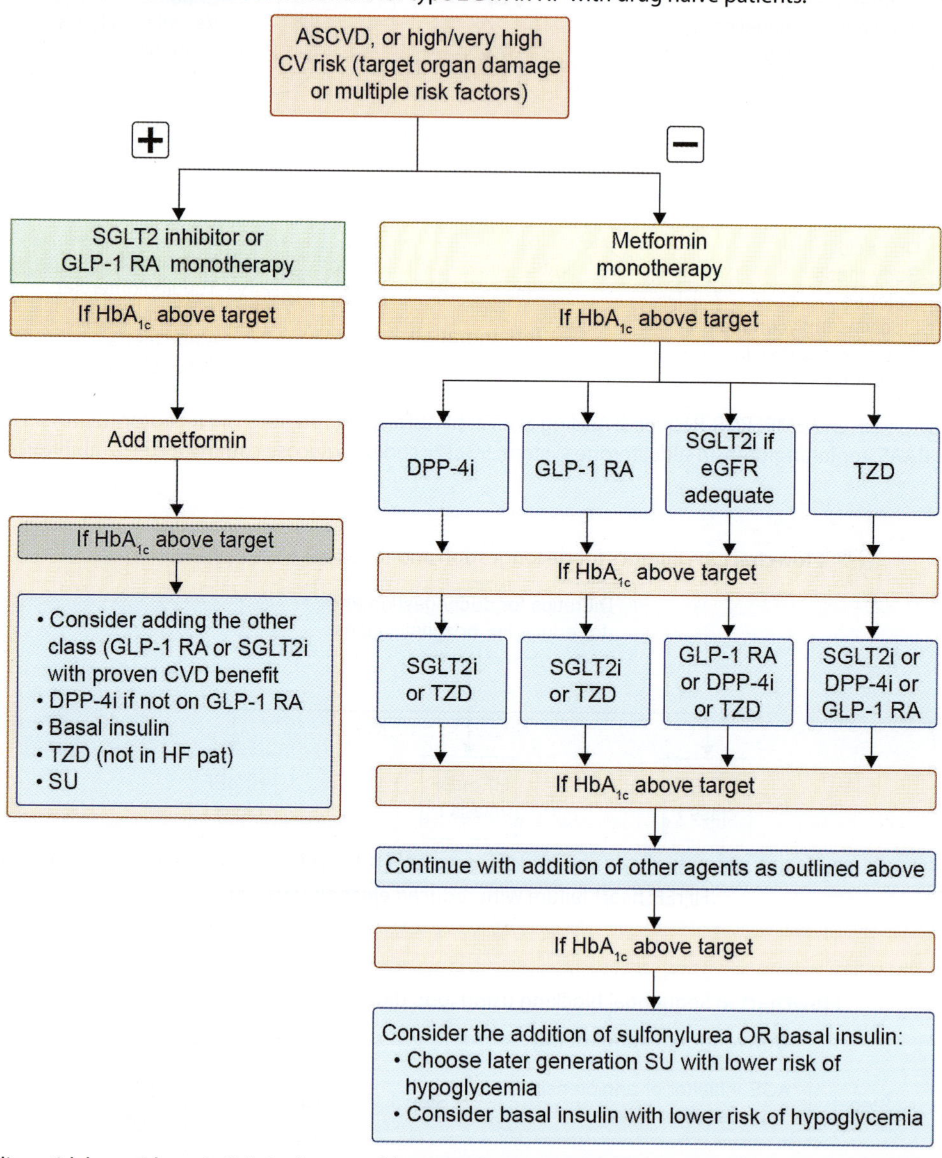

(DPP: dipeptidyl peptidase-4; GLP-1: glucagon-like peptide-1; SGLT2i: sodium-glucose cotransporter-2 inhibitor; TZD: thiazolidinediones)

Treatment of Diabetes Mellitus in Heart Failure

Flowcharts 5 and 6 show treatment of diabetes mellitus in heart failure in drug naive patients and those with metformin respectively.[3]

CURRENT MANAGEMENT OF HF IN DIABETES (FIG. 11)

Nonpharmacological Therapy

- *Left ventricular assist device (LVAD)*
    - *Bridge to recovery:* Postcardiotomy cardiogenic shock, postacute myocardial infarction (MI), cardiogenic shock, myocarditis-induced cardiogenic shock, support during medical or ablative therapy for intractable dysrhythmias
    - Bridge to transplant
    - Bridge to destination therapy
- Extracorporeal membrane oxygenation (ECMO)
- Cardiac transplant

Flowchart 6: Treatment for type 2 DM in HF with patient on metformin.

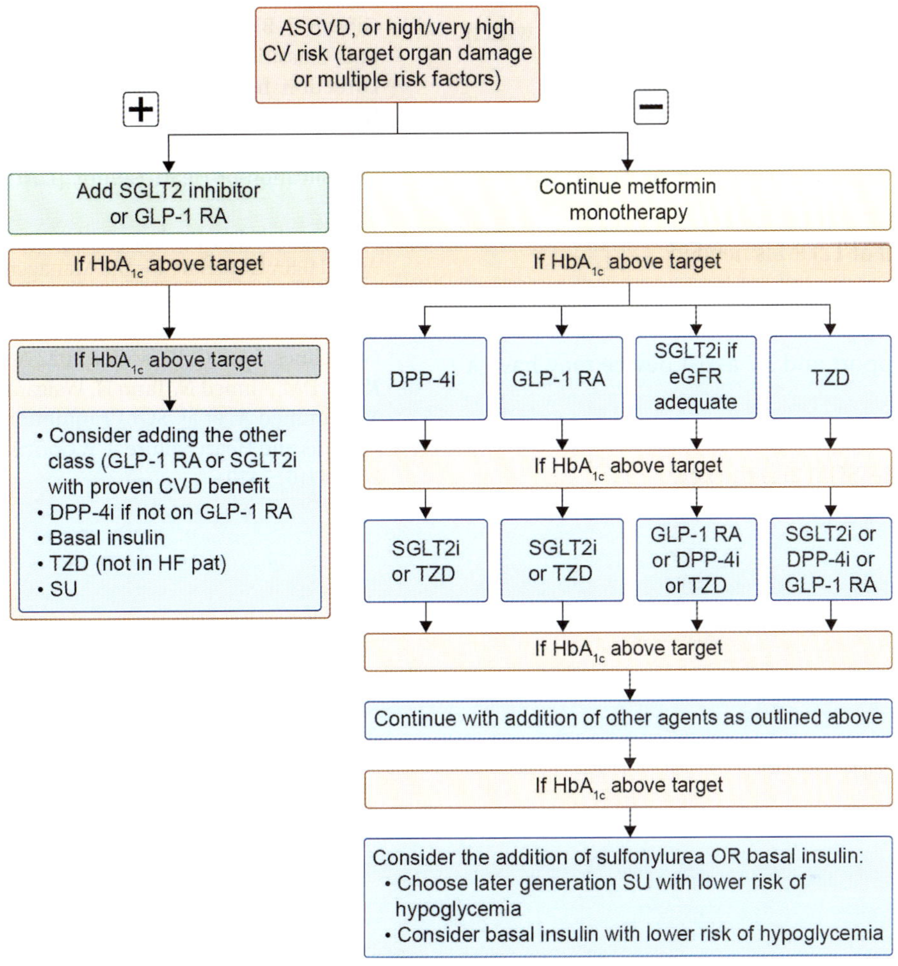

Note: Hypoglycemia dangerous in heart failure—avoid

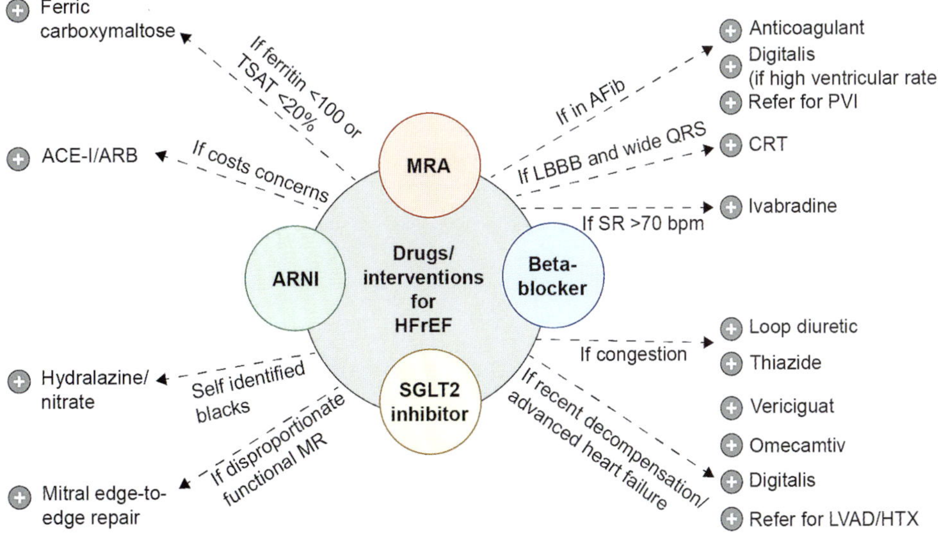

Fig. 11: Current management of HF in diabetes.

CONCLUSION

- GDMT for HFrEF requires four medications which include SGLT2i, ARNI, MRA, β-blockers.
- SGLT2i has role in HFmrEF.
- HFpEF requires SGLT2i, MRA, and ARNI.
- Care of iron deficiency anemia, HTN, T2DM, AF, and CAD has good outcome.
- Effective control of T2DM is needed.
- *Revascularization:* Mechanical or surgery may have a role.
- Mechanical support and LV assist device may have a standby role.
- Heart transplant is final.

Heart failure in DM—SGLT2i is the key.

REFERENCES

1. Gibson G, Blumer V, Mentz RJ. (2021). Universal Definition and Classification of Heart Failure: A Step in the Right Direction from Failure to Function. [online] Available from https://www.acc.org/Latest-in-Cardiology/Articles/2021/07/12/12/31/Universal-Definition-and-Classification-of-Heart-Failure. [Last accessed September, 2025]
2. Heidenreich PA, Bozkurt B, Aguilar D, et al. 2022 AHA/ACC/HFSA Guideline for the Management of Heart Failure: A Report of the American College of Cardiology / American Heart Association Joint Committee on Clinical Practice Guidelines. J Am Coll Cardiol. 2022 Apr 1.
3. Keller DM, Ahmed N, Tariq H, Walgamage M, Walgamage T, Mohammed A, et al. SGLT2 Inhibitors in Type 2 Diabetes Mellitus and Heart Failure — A Concise Review. J Clin Med. 2022;11(6):1470.

CHAPTER 35

Diabetes Management in 2025

Vijay Panikar

INTRODUCTION AND CHALLENGES

With the advancements in medical technology and treatment options, managing diabetes has evolved significantly over the years. Yet, in 2025, healthcare providers continue to face numerous challenges in delivering optimal care to diabetes patients.

The global prevalence of diabetes has been rising at an alarming rate, with India and Southeast Asia experiencing particularly high growth.[1] This surge necessitates a robust healthcare system to manage the increasing patient load and ensure timely interventions.[2]

"Technological Integration and Access" is still issue even in developed countries. While continuous glucose monitoring (CGM) systems, artificial pancreas systems, and smart insulin pens have transformed diabetes management, equitable access remains a significant issue.[3] Patients in low-resource settings often struggle to afford or access these advanced technologies, creating a disparity in care quality. With the integration of artificial intelligence (AI) and digital health tools in diabetes management, there is an increased risk of data breaches and privacy concerns. Healthcare providers need robust data protection measures to safeguard patient information. Furthermore, interoperability between different health management systems remains a challenge, requiring a unified digital platform for seamless data integration.

The shift toward personalized treatment plans poses both opportunities and challenges. While personalized care can significantly improve outcomes, it requires sophisticated infrastructure, skilled healthcare professionals, and substantial investment in training and resources. Keeping up with the latest pharmaceutical developments and tailoring treatment to individual needs demand continuous education and adaptation.

Managing coexisting conditions such as obesity, hypertension, and chronic kidney disease (CKD) becomes more complex when paired with diabetes. Managing diabetes involves not only physical but also psychological and social challenges. Patients often face stigma, mental health issues, and social isolation. Healthcare providers should adopt a holistic approach, offering support groups, mental health services, and patient's education programs to address these barriers effectively.

INNOVATIONS IN DIABETES MANAGEMENT–GOING MAINSTREAM IN 2025

Technological Innovations

Advancements in technology have transformed diabetes care, with innovations like continuous glucose monitoring, insulin pumps, and telemedicine playing pivotal roles. Though access remains a challenge particularly in India, still acceptance has increased tremendously in India. The social media and peer-to-peer exchange of information has fueled the acceptance of technology among diabetes patients:

- *Continuous glucose monitoring (CGM) systems:* These systems have become more sophisticated, offering real-time insights into blood glucose levels. The latest CGM devices are smaller, more accurate, and user-friendly, featuring advanced algorithms that predict glucose trends and integration with smartphones and wearable devices has also improved, enabling seamless data sharing with healthcare providers and caregivers. The acceptance in India has increased by app-based weight loss and diabetes reversal programs and these programs are primarily lifestyle modification programs with help of CGMS, diet tracking, and personalized coaches to keep patients motivated.
- *Artificial pancreas systems:* Combining CGM and insulin pump technology, these systems automatically adjust insulin delivery based on glucose readings. The Medtronic MiniMed™ 780G insulin pump with

guardian CGMS sensors is hybrid closed loop system which automatically adjusts and corrects insulin delivery every 5 minutes to help to maintain stable glucose levels. This system is part of an automated insulin delivery setup, integrating with a guardian CGM to provide real-time glucose data and reduce the need for manual interventions, closely mimicking the body's natural insulin response.

- *Smart insulin pens:* Enhanced connectivity allows users to track insulin doses, monitor injection sites, and receive reminders for missed doses. AI integration provides personalized dosing recommendations based on individual glucose patterns, lifestyle, and dietary habits.

Pharmaceutical Developments

- *Novel insulin formulations:* New insulin formulations offer more predictable pharmacokinetics and pharmacodynamics. Ultra-rapid-acting insulins provide faster onset and shorter duration of action, while once-weekly basal insulin formulations reduce injection frequency. Insulin icodec, a once weekly injectable basal insulin, is about to launch in India in 2025[4] and it will definitely increase acceptance in Indian patients who are not willing for multiple injections.
- *Noninsulin therapies:* The landscape of noninsulin therapies has expanded with glucagon-like peptide-1 (GLP-1) receptor agonists, sodium-glucose cotransporter 2 (SGLT-2) inhibitors, and dual agonists showing promise in controlling blood glucose levels and addressing comorbidities such as obesity and cardiovascular disease. The most significant development in GLP-1 therapy is the emergence of "dual incretin" drugs, like tirzepatide, which simultaneously activate both the GLP-1 and gastric inhibitory polypeptide (GIP) receptors, leading to significantly improved blood sugar control and greater weight loss compared to traditional GLP-1 receptor agonists alone;[5] this advancement offers a more potent treatment option for type 2 diabetes mellitus and obesity management by leveraging the combined effects of both incretin hormones. India already has oral version of semaglutide (GLP-1 agonist) available, and injectable formulation is about to launch in this year only. Similarly, widely popular tirzepatide (GLP-1 and GIP dual coagonists) will also be launched simultaneously this year in India. Though these two are unofficially getting imported to India and sold via gray market. These two launches in India will definitely revolutionize diabesity care in India in 2025.

  Building on the success of dual GIP/GLP-1 receptor coagonists, the first triple GLP-1/GIP/glucagon receptor triagonist—retatrutide was started under development.[6] This approach aimed to enhance efficacy through the synergistic action of three gastrointestinal hormones, surpassing the dual hormone method. Research demonstrated that the GLP-1/GIP/glucagon-receptor triagonist outperformed earlier dual coagonists, showing greater effectiveness in reducing body weight, improving lipid profiles, and lowering insulin secretion.

  Acceptance of SGLT2 inhibitors (SGLT2i) in India has skyrocketed after availability of generic dapagliflozin, and this will be further boosted as empagliflozin patent has expired on 11th March 2025. Empagliflozin is another SGLT2i with robust cardiovascular benefits. And not only physicians and diabetologists, but also cardiologists have been writing empagliflozin left and right. With availability of generic empagliflozin flooding the Indian market in 2025, use will be going high simultaneously. The major concern will be avoiding genitourinary side effects, when using these molecules in more and more patients due to reduced cost. Hydration, hygiene, and patient's education will be key to reduce these side effects.
- *Personalized medicine:* Advancements in genomics and biomarker research enable personalized treatment plans based on genetic profiling, maximizing therapeutic benefits and minimizing adverse effects. Though it seems to be more of a future initiative, individualized treatment depending upon patients' individual characteristics such as weight, cardiovascular disease (CVD) risk, atherosclerotic cardiovascular disease (ASCVD), chronic kidney disease (CKD), affordability, hypoglycemia risk, etc. has been the main focus for all major national and international guidelines.

Lifestyle Interventions

- *Digital health platforms:* These platforms offer personalized coaching, dietary planning, and exercise programs tailored to individual needs. AI-driven applications provide real-time feedback and motivation, while gamification elements increase patient's engagement. With the popularity of social media and mobile devices, actually addiction to mobile devices getting.

- *Exercise and physical activity:* Tailored exercise programs, integrated with virtual reality (VR) and augmented reality (AR) technologies, provide immersive and engaging experiences, making exercise more accessible and enjoyable.

REFINING TYPE 2 DIABETES MELLITUS: CLUSTER-BASED CLASSIFICATION

Current treatment options have not succeeded in halting disease progression or preventing chronic complications. A key issue lies in diagnosing diabetes based on a single metabolite, glucose, despite the disease's heterogeneous nature in clinical presentation and progression. Classification primarily distinguishes type 1 diabetes mellitus from type 2 diabetes mellitus based on autoantibodies targeting pancreatic islet β-cells and age at onset, with 75–85% of cases falling under type 2 diabetes mellitus. A third category, latent autoimmune diabetes in adults (LADA), defined by the presence of glutamic acid decarboxylase antibodies (GADA), initially resembles type 2 diabetes mellitus but increasingly exhibits characteristics of type 1 diabetes mellitus over time. Gene sequencing has further identified rare monogenic forms like maturity-onset diabetes of the young and neonatal diabetes.

An enhanced classification system could significantly improve the identification of individuals at diagnosis who are at higher risk of complications, thereby facilitating personalized treatment plans. Similar to how genetic diagnoses guide optimal care for monogenic diabetes, Emma Ahlqvist and colleagues introduced a new diabetes classification.[7] This novel approach utilizes unsupervised, data-driven cluster analysis of six routinely measured variables and compares the results metabolically, genetically, and clinically to existing classifications across four distinct populations in Sweden and Finland. This classification framework divides diabetes into five distinct subgroups or clusters, based on six easily measurable clinical factors:[8] age at diagnosis, body-mass index (BMI) at diagnosis, glycated hemoglobin (HbA1c) levels, presence of glutamic acid decarboxylase antibodies (GADA), β-cell function (determined using the Homeostasis Model Assessment 2-beta, HOMA2-β), and insulin resistance (assessed by HOMA2-IR, using fasting glucose and C-peptide levels). The identified subgroups include:

- Severe autoimmune diabetes (SAID)
- Severe insulin-deficient diabetes (SIDD)
- Severe insulin-resistant diabetes (SIRD)
- Mild obesity-related diabetes (MOD)
- Mild age-related diabetes (MARD)

Following their identification within the Scandinavian population, efforts have been undertaken to evaluate the applicability of these clusters in more diverse populations globally.

MANAGING HUGE BURDEN OF NEWLY DIAGNOSED YOUNG TYPE 2 DIABETES MELLITUS PATIENTS

Durable Control

As we discussed earlier, there is exponential rise in type 2 diabetes mellitus in recent times getting diagnosed at young age. Looking back at the pathophysiology of type 2 diabetes mellitus, these young individuals have more years to live with diabetes and thus will have more complications and at an earlier age and this will have tremendous impact on families, both socially and economically. Simultaneously, it will be difficult to keep them just on oral drugs as most patients require insulin injections in second decade after diagnosis.

To give these young individuals a longer, complications free life and without insulin at earlier stage, we need treatment with durable control. Pioglitazone, being a true insulin sensitizer, along with metformin can give young patients great durable control without undue weight gain or any undesirable side effects. Along with that we need to start with at least dual drugs to keep patients on good control for longer duration as per VERIFY Trial.[9]

Using Newer Generation Antiobesity Drugs and Remission of Diabetes

With blockbuster success of GLP1-receptor agonists and upcoming dual and triple incretin agonists, for weight loss in range of 15–25 % of bodyweight which was unheard before. We have learnt from DIRECT TRIAL[10] that a 15% weight loss can give majority of patients a pharmacological remission. With new antiobesity drugs with rapid and sustainable weight loss exceeding 15%, we can now aim to achieve diabetes remission in newly diagnosed obese individuals and explore the possibilities of diabetes drug free life with lifestyle modifications only and maintenance of weight loss.

Prevention and Early Detection

The rise in type 2 diabetes mellitus cases in 2025, particularly among younger populations, highlights the need for proactive prevention and early detection strategies. Community initiatives promoting healthy lifestyles, regular screenings, and education are crucial to mitigate the onset of diabetes. However, these initiatives require sustained funding and community engagement to be effective. But, this will be our only way to make our society healthy and free of grave complications of diabetes in society where diabetes is getting in each and every household.

CONCLUSION

Diabetes management in 2025 reflects a decisive shift toward precision, durability, and holistic care. Breakthrough technologies, once-weekly insulin, and potent dual/triple incretin therapies have transformed treatment, while SGLT2 inhibitors have strengthened cardiometabolic protection. However, unequal access, rising diabetes in the young, and the need for durable control remain major challenges. Future success will depend on integrating personalized therapy, prevention, sustained lifestyle intervention, and equitable delivery systems to achieve not just glycemic control, but long-term remission and complication-free survival.

REFERENCES

1. Gupta R, Upadhyay A, Kohli S, Khadgwat R. Evolving Landscape of Diabetes Epidemic in Southeast Asia: Insights from National Family Health Survey. Indian J Endocrinol Metab. 2023;27(6):492-500.
2. Schwarz P. Diabetes care in India and Southeast Asia: the way forward. Int J Diabetes Dev Ctries. 2025:45(1):1-2.
3. Agarwal S, Simmonds I, Myers AK. The Use of Diabetes Technology to Address Inequity in Health Outcomes: Limitations and Opportunities. Curr Diab Rep. 2022;22(7): 275-81.
4. MoneyControl.com. Efforts on to Launch Once-a Week- Insulin in India by Mid-2025: Novo Nordisk MD (no date). [online] Available from https://www.moneycontrol.com/news/trends/health/efforts-on-to-launch-once-a-week-insulin-in-india-by-mid-2025-novo-nordisk-md-10290811.html. [Last accessed Sept., 2025].
5. Mathiesen DS, Bagger JI, Bergmann NC, Lund A, Christensen MB, Vilsbøll T, et al. The Effects of Dual GLP-1/GIP Receptor Agonism on Glucagon Secretion-A Review. Int J Mol Sci. 2019;20(17):4092.
6. Jakubowska A, Roux CWL, Viljoen A. The Road towards Triple Agonists: Glucagon-Like Peptide 1, Glucose-Dependent Insulinotropic Polypeptide and Glucagon Receptor—An Update. Endocrinol Metab (Seoul). 2024;39(1):12-22.
7. Ahlqvist E, Storm P, Käräjämäki A, Martinell M, Dorkhan M, Carlsson A, et al. Novel subgroups of adult-onset diabetes and their association with outcomes: a data-driven cluster analysis of six variables. Lancet Diabetes Endocrinol. 2018;6(5):361-9.
8. Abdel-Sater KA. New Paradigms of Diabetes Classification: Implications for Complication. Am J Pharmacol. 2024; 7(1):1039.
9. Matthews DR, Paldánius PM, Proot P, Chiang Y, Stumvoll M, Del Prato S; VERIFY study group. Glycaemic durability of an early combination therapy with vildagliptin and metformin versus sequential metformin monotherapy in newly diagnosed type 2 diabetes (VERIFY): a 5-year, multicentre, randomised, double-blind trial. Lancet. 2019;394(10208):1519-29.
10. Leslie WS, Ford I, Sattar N, Hollingsworth KG, Adamson A, Sniehotta FF, et al. The Diabetes Remission Clinical Trial (DiRECT): protocol for a cluster randomised trial. BMC Fam Pract. 2016;17:20.

Early Diagnosis and Management of Gestational Diabetes Mellitus

Banshi Saboo, Subhajyoti Ghosh

INTRODUCTION

Gestational diabetes mellitus (GDM) is defined as glucose intolerance first detected in pregnancy, often in the second trimester, posing risks such as hypertensive disorders, macrosomia, neonatal hypoglycemia, and future type 2 diabetes in mothers. Rising global prevalence is linker to increasing obesity and diabetes rates. Early detection and careful management are crucial to reducing complications.

DEFINITIONS

Gestational diabetes mellitus is defined as any degree of glucose intolerance with onset or first recognition during pregnancy.

Gestational Diabetes Mellitus

Gestational diabetes mellitus refers to hyperglycemia diagnosed between 24 and 28 weeks of pregnancy by the standard criteria [conventionally International Association of Diabetes and Pregnancy Study Groups (IADPSG) or two-step oral glucose tolerance test (OGTT)] but falling short of the levels for overt diabetes.[1,2]

Overt Diabetes or Diabetes in Pregnancy

This refers to hyperglycemia diagnosed during pregnancy, satisfying the standard criteria [American Diabetes Association (ADA) or WHO] for diabetes mellitus (DM) in nonpregnant individuals.[3]

Early Gestational Diabetes Mellitus

Early gestational diabetes mellitus (eGDM) refers to intermediate degrees of hyperglycemia detected before 24 weeks of pregnancy that fulfill the criteria for conventional gestational diabetes mellitus (cGDM) but fall short of the threshold for overt diabetes.[4,5]

RATIONALE FOR EARLY DIAGNOSIS

Risks of Untreated Gestational Diabetes Mellitus

- Maternal complications include gestational hypertension, preeclampsia, cesarean section, and the future development of type 2 diabetes.[6,7]
- Neonatal risks include macrosomia, shoulder dystocia, birth injuries, respiratory distress, and neonatal hypoglycemia.[8]

Early-onset Gestational Diabetes Mellitus

Screening in the first trimester can identify preexisting diabetes or early-onset GDM, enabling prompt glycemic control and reducing adverse outcomes.

Epidemiologic Trends

Globally and in India, GDM prevalence is rising, making early identification an urgent public health priority.[9]

Screening Timing Across Global Guidelines

- *American Diabetes Association (2025 Standards):*
  - Routine screening at *24–28 weeks* in individuals without prior diabetes.
  - Those not screened pre-pregnancy should be tested *before 15 weeks;* early screening may be universal in high-risk groups.
- *American College of Obstetricians and Gynecologists (ACOG)/US Preventive Services Task Force (USPSTF) (United States):*
  - *Endorse a two-step approach:* Begin with a 50 g glucose challenge at 24–28 weeks; if positive, followed by a diagnostic 100 g OGTT using Carpenter–Coustan criteria.
  - No recommendation for routine screening before 24 weeks, citing insufficient evidence.

- *Postpartum Screening (ADA and ACOG):*
  - Recommend 75 g OGTT *4–12 weeks postpartum* to detect persistent dysglycemia; *immediate postpartum testing before discharge* is reasonable to improve adherence.
  - Lifelong glucose screening every *1–3 years* for women with a history of GDM.
- *Screening of GDM:* The screening methodologies for diagnosing hyperglycemia early in pregnancy as recommended by various organizations:
  - *American Diabetes Association:*
    - *Tests:* Fasting plasma glucose (FPG), 2-hour OGTT (75 g), HbA1c, or random plasma glucose (RPG).
    - *Criteria:* Overt diabetes if FPG ≥126 mg/dL (7.0 mmol/L), 2-hour PG ≥200 mg/dL (11.1 mmol/L), HbA1c ≥6.5%, or RPG ≥200 mg/dL with symptoms. GDM criteria are not clearly defined.
    - *Timing:* First prenatal visit.
    - *Target population:* Women with risk factors.
    - *Comments:* Recognizes limitations of applying IADPSG or 2-step criteria in early pregnancy.
  - *American College of Obstetricians and Gynecologists:*
    - *Tests:* ADA diagnostic criteria for nonpregnant individuals
    - *Criteria:* Standard ADA criteria
    - *Timing:* Preferably at initiation of prenatal care
    - *Target Population:* Women with risk factors
    - *Comments:* HbA1c may be used but is less sensitive than OGTT.
  - *International Association of Diabetes and Pregnancy Study Groups:*
    - *Tests:* FPG, HbA1c, or RPG.
    - *Criteria:* Overt diabetes if FPG ≥126 mg/dL (7.0 mmol/L), HbA1c ≥6.5%, or RPG ≥200 mg/dL with confirmation. GDM if FPG ≥92 mg/dL (5.1 mmol/L) but <126 mg/dL (7.0 mmol/L).
    - *Timing:* First prenatal visit.
    - *Target population:* Decision to test all pregnant women or only high-risk groups depends on population prevalence and local circumstances.
  - *National Institute for Health and Care Excellence (NICE):*
    - *Tests:* 75 g OGTT (FPG and 2-hour PG).
    - *Criteria:* GDM if FPG ≥100 mg/dL (5.6 mmol/L) or 2-hour PG ≥140 mg/dL (7.8 mmol/L).
    - *Timing:* After booking (first or second trimester).
    - *Target population:* Risk-based assessment at booking.
    - *Comments:* Advises against using FPG, RPG, HbA1c, GCT, or urinalysis for glucose to determine GDM risk.

DIAGNOSIS OF GESTATIONAL DIABETES MELLITUS

- *American Diabetes Association (ADA), Endocrine Society, WHO, FIGO, and ADIPS:*
  - *Criteria:* IADPSG (International Association of the Diabetes and Pregnancy Study Group).
  - *Method:* One-step 75 g OGTT
  - *Tests:* Fasting plasma glucose (FPG), 1-hour plasma glucose (PG), and 2-hour PG.
  - *Interpretation:* GDM is diagnosed if any of the following thresholds are met:
    - FPG ≥92 mg/dL (5.1 mmol/L)
    - 1-hour PG ≥180 mg/dL (10.0 mmol/L)
    - 2-hour PG ≥153 mg/dL (8.5 mmol/L)
- *American College of Obstetricians and Gynecologists (ACOG):*
  - *Criteria:* Carpenter–Coustan or National Diabetes Data Group (NDDG).
  - *Method: Two-step approach:*
    - *Step 1:* Non-fasting 50 g glucose challenge test (GCT)
    - *Step 2:* 3-hour 100 g OGTT if GCT exceeds thresholds
  - *Tests:* FPG, 1-hour PG, 2-hour PG, 3-hour PG
  - *Interpretation:* GDM is diagnosed if two or more thresholds are met:
    - *Carpenter–Coustan:* FPG ≥95 mg/dL (5.3 mmol/L), 1-hour PG ≥180 mg/dL (10.0 mmol/L), 2-hour PG ≥155 mg/dL (8.6 mmol/L), 3-hour PG ≥140 mg/dL (7.8 mmol/L)
    - *National Diabetes Data Group:* FPG ≥105 mg/dL (5.8 mmol/L), 1-hour PG ≥190 mg/dL (10.6 mmol/L), 2-hour PG ≥165 mg/dL (9.2 mmol/L), 3-hour PG ≥145 mg/dL (8.0 mmol/L)
- *National Institute for Health and Care Excellence (NICE):*
  - *Criteria:* One-step 75 g OGTT
  - *Tests:* FPG and 2-hour PG
  - *Interpretation:* GDM is diagnosed if:
    - FPG ≥100 mg/dL (5.6 mmol/L)
    - 2-hour PG ≥140 mg/dL (7.8 mmol/L)

- *Management of GDM—lifestyle, pharmacology, and technology:*
- *Glycemic targets (2025 ADA guidance)—Updated glucose goals across pregnancy types:*
  - *Fasting/pre-prandial:* 70–95 mg/dL
  - *1-hour postprandial:* 110–140 mg/dL
  - *2-hour postprandial:* 100–120 mg/dL
- *Lifestyle and nutrition:*
  - Lifestyle changes, including diet and exercise, are essential and may suffice for many individuals with GDM.
  - Insulin is the preferred medication for managing hyperglycemia in GDM, while metformin and glyburide are not recommended as first-line treatments.
  - Telehealth visits combined with in-person care can improve outcomes for pregnant individuals with GDM.
- *Medical nutrition therapy for GDM:* Individualized nutrition plans are crucial for managing gestational diabetes effectively.
  - A nutrition plan should provide adequate calories, focusing on a minimum of 175 g of carbohydrates and 71 g of protein daily.
  - Emphasis should be placed on nutrient-dense foods, including healthy fats and high-quality carbohydrates, to control glucose levels.
  - *Emphasize plant-based diets*: Fruits, vegetables, whole grains, lean proteins, and healthy fats
  - Monitoring carbohydrate intake is essential to avoid excessive postprandial glucose spikes.
- *Physical activity recommendations:* Regular physical activity is beneficial for managing glucose levels in individuals with gestational diabetes.
  - Exercise interventions have shown improvements in glucose outcomes and reduced insulin requirements.
  - Recommended exercise includes moderate-intensity activities for 20–50 minutes, 2–7 days a week.
- *Pharmacologic therapy:*
  - *Pharmacologic therapy for GDM:* Pharmacological treatment may be necessary for managing gestational diabetes when lifestyle changes are insufficient.
    - Insulin is the first-line treatment for GDM, while metformin and glyburide are not recommended due to safety concerns for the fetus.
    - Sulfonylureas, such as glyburide, can cross the placenta and are associated with increased neonatal hypoglycemia.
  - *Glyburide in gestational diabetes management:* Glyburide is associated with higher neonatal risks compared to insulin or metformin.
    - Glyburide linked to increased neonatal hypoglycemia, macrosomia, and abdominal circumference.
    - It was not found non-inferior to insulin based on composite outcomes.
    - Long-term safety data for offspring exposed to glyburide is lacking.
  - *Metformin's role in pregnancy:* Metformin shows benefits in reducing neonatal hypoglycemia and maternal weight gain but raises concerns about long-term effects on offspring.
    - Associated with lower risk of neonatal hypoglycemia and less maternal weight gain than insulin.
    - Crosses the placenta, leading to umbilical cord blood levels comparable to maternal levels.
    - Studies show heavier offspring and increased obesity risk at ages 4 and 9 years.
    - Not recommended for those with hypertension or preeclampsia due to potential risks.
  - *Insulin management in diabetes during pregnancy:* Insulin is the preferred treatment for managing type 1 and type 2 diabetes in pregnancy.
    - Multiple daily injections or insulin pumps are both effective delivery methods.
    - Frequent blood glucose monitoring is essential due to changing insulin requirements.
    - No human insulin preparations have been shown to cross the placenta.
  - *Type 1 diabetes considerations in pregnancy:* Pregnant individuals with type 1 diabetes face unique risks and management challenges.
    - Increased risk of hypoglycemia in the first trimester and altered hypoglycemia awareness.
    - Diabetic ketoacidosis (DKA) risk is higher at lower blood glucose levels.
    - Rapid implementation of euglycemia is crucial, especially in the context of retinopathy.
  - *Type 2 diabetes management during pregnancy:* Type 2 diabetes management during pregnancy requires careful monitoring and weight management.

        - Recommended weight gain is 15–25 lb for those with overweight and 10–20 lb for those with obesity.
        - Insulin is the preferred treatment, with higher doses often needed.
        - Associated risks include hypertension and increased pregnancy loss in the third trimester.
    - *Preeclampsia prevention with aspirin:* Low-dose aspirin is recommended to lower the risk of preeclampsia in pregnant individuals with diabetes.
        - Recommended dosage is 100–150 mg/day starting at 12–16 weeks of gestation.
        - Low-dose aspirin <100 mg is ineffective in reducing preeclampsia risk.
        - Individuals with GDM may also benefit from aspirin if they have high-risk factors.
- *Technology in management:*
    - *Automated insulin delivery (AID) systems and insulin pumps* with pregnancy-specific glucose targets are now endorsed for type 1 diabetic pregnancies.
    - *Continuous glucose monitoring (CGM)* increasingly integrated—allowing better glycemic control and reduced neonatal complications.
- *Fetal surveillance and timing of delivery:*
    - For well-controlled diet-managed (A1GDM), induction/delivery may be deferred to *39–40+ weeks.*
    - Medication-treated (A2GDM) or poorly controlled cases may warrant earlier surveillance and individualized delivery planning, possibly *37–38 weeks* depending on control and fetal size.
- *Postpartum care, prevention, and equity:*
    - *Postpartum follow-up and risk reduction:* Postpartum care is crucial for managing diabetes and preventing future complications.
        - Insulin requirements decrease dramatically postpartum, often to about half of prepregnancy levels.
        - Screening for diabetes should occur 4–12 weeks postpartum using a 75-g oral glucose tolerance test.
        - Breastfeeding is encouraged for its health benefits for both mother and child.
    - *Preconception counseling:* Preconception counseling is vital for individuals with diabetes to ensure optimal health before conception.
        - Counseling should start at puberty for those with diabetes and childbearing potential.
        - Effective contraception should be used until A1C levels are optimized for pregnancy.
        - Achieving near-normal glucose levels before conception reduces risks of congenital anomalies and other complications.
        - Preconception care should involve an interprofessional team, including endocrinologists and dietitians.
    - *Long-term diabetes risk after GDM:* Individuals with a history of gestational diabetes have a significantly increased risk of developing type 2 diabetes.
        - Estimated lifetime risk of diabetes is 50–60% for those with a history of GDM.
        - Risk increases linearly over time, with approximately 20% at 10 years and 60% at 50 years.
        - Healthy eating patterns can lower subsequent diabetes risk.
    - *Long-term offspring risks:*
        - In-utero hyperglycemia exposure heightens risk of childhood obesity, hypertension, and future type 2 diabetes.
        - Preventive strategies and early lifestyle interventions could mitigate intergenerational transmission of metabolic disease—but require further study.
    - *Contraception and family planning:* Effective contraception is essential for individuals with diabetes to prevent unplanned pregnancies.
        - Family planning options should be reviewed regularly for those of childbearing potential.
        - Long-acting reversible contraception is recommended to minimize the risk of unplanned pregnancies.
- *Emerging research insights:*
    - *Early detection benefits:* A March 2025 study assessed outcomes of early detection and treatment of GDM—evaluating cesarean rates, preterm birth, and neonatal macrosomia.[10] While details are pending full publication, this study underlines the growing focus on early intervention's potential benefits.
    - *The ADA 2025 Standards Emphasis:* The ADA's *2025 standards of care* reinforce integration of advanced pharmacotherapies (e.g., GLP-1 receptor agonists), technological tools (CGM, AID systems), and personalized patient-centered care strategies.

CONCLUSION

Early, risk-based screening and individualized management of GDM via lifestyle interventions, timely pharmacotherapy, technology integration and structured postpartum follow-up can aid in reduction of maternal and neonatal risks while improving long-term health for both mother and child.

REFERENCES

1. Carpenter MW and Coustan DR. Criteria for screening tests for gestational diabetes. Am J Obstet Gynecol. 1982;144(7):768-73.
2. ACOG Practice Bulletin No. 190: Gestational Diabetes Mellitus. Obstet Gynecol. 2018;131(2):e49-e64.
3. World Health Organization. (2006). International Diabetes Federation. Definition and Diagnosis of Diabetes Mellitus and Intermediate Hyperglycaemia: Report of a WHO/IDF Consultation. [online] Available from: http://www.who.int/diabetes/publications/diagnosis_diabetes2006/en/ (Lats accessed 16 September 2025).
4. International Association of Diabetes and Pregnancy Study Groups Consensus Panel; Metzger BE, Gabbe SG, Persson B, Buchanan TA, Catalano PA, et al. International Association of Diabetes and pregnancy study groups recommendations on the diagnosis and classification of hyperglycemia in pregnancy. Diabetes Care. 2010;33(3):676-82.
5. Expert Committee on the Diagnosis and Classification of Diabetes Mellitus. Report of the expert committee on the diagnosis and classification of diabetes mellitus. Diabetes Care. 2003;26 (Suppl 1):S5-20.
6. Will JS, Crellin H. Gestational Diabetes Mellitus: Update on Screening, Diagnosis, and Management. Am Fam Physician. 2023;108(3):249-258.
7. American Diabetes Association Professional Practice Committee; 15. Management of Diabetes in Pregnancy: Standards of Care in Diabetes—2025. Diabetes Care. 2025;48 (Supplement_1): S306-20.
8. Davitt C, Flynn KE, Harrison RK, Pan A, Palatnik A. Current practices in gestational diabetes mellitus diagnosis and management in the United States: survey of maternal-fetal medicine specialists. Am J Obstet Gynecol. 2021;225(2):203-4.
9. Bastian B, Smithers LG, Pape A, Davis W, Fu K, Francois M. Early screening and diagnosis of gestational diabetes mellitus (GDM) and its impact on perinatal outcomes. Diabetes Res Clin Pract. 2024;217:111890.
10. García-Patterson A, Balsells M, Solà I and Corcoy R. Detection and treatment of early gestational diabetes mellitus: a systematic review and meta-analysis of randomized controlled trials. Am J Obstet Gynecol. 2025:S0002-9378(25)00290-X.

CHAPTER 37

Diabetes Distress Syndrome

Vijay Negalur

INTRODUCTION

Diabetes distress syndrome (DDS) refers to the emotional and psychological burden that individuals face while managing diabetes. This condition encompasses feelings of stress, guilt, frustration, and anxiety specifically tied to the daily demands of diabetes self-management and the potential long-term complications associated with the disease. Unlike clinical depression or general stress, diabetes distress is a distinct emotional response that arises from the unique challenges of living with diabetes.

Differentiation from Clinical Depression and General Stress

Diabetes distress is often confused with clinical depression; however, it is essential to recognize that DDS does not imply a psychological disorder. While both conditions may share overlapping symptoms, diabetes distress is a reaction to the specific challenges posed by diabetes management rather than a general mood disorder. For instance, individuals experiencing diabetes distress may feel overwhelmed by their treatment regimen but do not necessarily exhibit the pervasive sadness or anhedonia characteristic of major depressive disorder.[1,2]

Prevalence of Diabetes Distress Globally and in India

Globally, diabetes distress is prevalent among individuals with diabetes, affecting nearly 18% to 35% of this population.[3] A recent study in type 1 diabetes found that diabetes distress and depressive symptoms were prevalent in 27.8% and 38.3% of individuals, respectively, with 19.6% experiencing both conditions.[4] In India, studies show varying prevalence rates, with the latest meta-analysis indicating that diabetes distress among individuals with type 2 diabetes ranges from 8.45% to 61.48%, with a pooled estimate of 33% (95% CI: 21%–45%), as measured by the diabetes distress scale-17 (DDS-17).[5]

Overall, DDS appears to be more common than clinical depression among diabetes patients but remains underrecognized in clinical settings.

Underrecognition of Diabetes Distress Syndrome

Despite its higher prevalence, DDS often remains underdiagnosed and undertreated compared to clinical depression. This underrecognition can be attributed to several factors:

Overlap with Clinical Depression

Many individuals may experience symptoms of both conditions, leading to confusion in diagnosis. However, DDS specifically relates to the emotional strain of managing diabetes rather than a broader depressive disorder.[4,6]

Lack of Screening

Routine screening for DDS is less common in clinical practice compared to screening for depression. This oversight means that many patients may not receive the support they need to manage their emotional well-being effectively.[7,8]

Stigma and Awareness

There may be a lack of awareness among healthcare providers regarding the significance of DDS, which can contribute to stigma and further delay appropriate interventions.[9]

KEY TRIGGERS AND RISK FACTORS

Diabetes distress is a significant emotional burden experienced by individuals managing diabetes,

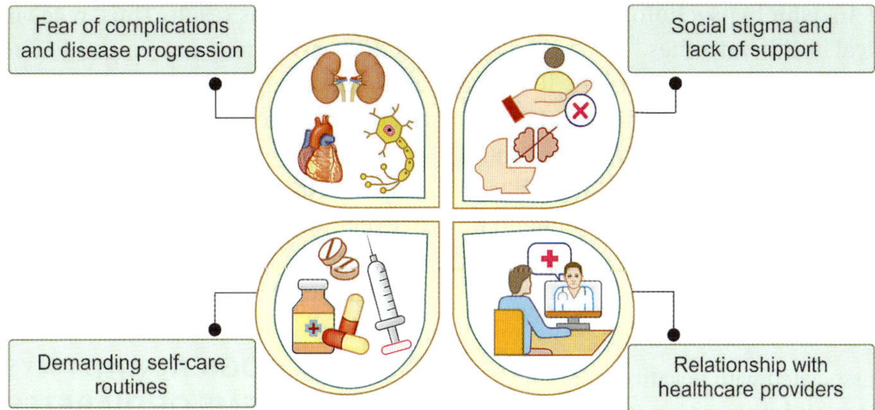

Fig. 1: Key triggers of diabetes distress.

characterized by feelings of anxiety, frustration, and overwhelm related to their condition. Understanding the key triggers and risk factors associated with diabetes distress is crucial for effective management and support **(Fig. 1)**.

Key Triggers of Diabetes Distress

- *Demanding self-care routines:* Managing diabetes involves routine blood glucose monitoring, adherence to prescribed medications, and lifestyle modifications. Although crucial for maintaining health, these responsibilities can become overwhelming and contribute to emotional stress. Patients often find it challenging to balance these demands, impacting their overall well-being. Moreover, the emotional burden of diabetes, including feelings of fear and being overwhelmed by its long-term management, adds to the strain of living with the condition.[10,11]
- *Fear of complications and disease progression:* The anticipation of complications such as neuropathy, retinopathy, and cardiovascular conditions often generates significant fear among patients. This ongoing concern can heighten anxiety and sometimes lead to avoidance behaviors, which may negatively affect diabetes management and overall health. Additionally, many patients experience interpersonal distress, feeling unsupported by family and friends in their efforts to manage diabetes, further compounding emotional and psychological challenges.[9]
- *Social stigma and lack of support:* Social stigma associated with diabetes frequently contributes to feelings of isolation among patients. This sense of isolation may be exacerbated by inadequate support from family and friends, further challenging patients' ability to effectively manage their condition and maintain emotional well-being.[9,12]
- *Relationship with healthcare providers:* Ineffective communication with healthcare providers can result in misunderstandings regarding treatment plans and expectations, contributing to feelings of frustration and dissatisfaction among patients. When patients perceive a lack of support or understanding from their healthcare team, they are more prone to experiencing diabetes-related distress. A significant component of this is physician-related distress, characterized by concerns about the quality of care, access to adequate expertise, and the level of support provided by their healthcare providers.[9,13]

Risk Factors

- *Demographics:* Higher levels of diabetes distress are associated with feminine gender, younger age, and poorer educational achievement. Due to the lack of direct support networks, those who live alone are also more vulnerable.[9,14]
- *Clinical factors:* Distress levels are significantly elevated in patients with a history of diabetes-related complications. Moreover, the perceived challenges in managing these risks contribute to heightened distress, particularly among those on insulin therapy or experiencing frequent episodes of hypoglycemia.[12,15]
- *Psychosocial factors:* Increased distress is associated with poor diets, less social support, and lower perceived self-efficacy in treating diabetes. Chronic illness management's emotional toll frequently creates

a vicious cycle in which psychological variables exacerbate physical health outcomes.[12,14]

- *Health status:* Diabetes distress is more likely to develop in people who have concomitant diseases (such as depression) or who have poor glycemic control (high HbA1c levels). Understanding how physical and mental health interact is essential to comprehending the entire effects on individuals.[9,15]

IMPACT ON DIABETES OUTCOME

Diabetes mellitus is associated with negative emotions such as anxiety, depression, and distress, and these emotions have been associated with poor clinical consequences including medication nonadherence and glycemic outcomes.[16-18] Diabetes distress is the emotional reaction to the challenges, anxieties, and worries connected to the wider demands of diabetes and represents negative sentiments surrounding the condition.[19] The discomfort stems from the inconveniences and demands of managing the condition on a daily basis, concerns about inadequate glucose control, anxieties about complications related to diabetes, inadequate support from significant others, stigma, and financial challenges.[10,20-22]

Long-term diabetes distress that is not recognized and treated leads to burnout in patients, which exacerbates feelings of powerlessness, despair, and dissatisfaction with diabetes care in general. Sometimes, an acute hyperglycemic crisis might cause physiological burnout.[16,23]

Individuals who experience significant discomfort linked to their diabetes are more prone to exhibit inadequate self-management.[23] All these negative emotions can eventually cause patients to fail to follow health advice, medications, medical follow-ups, which can lead to a worsening of their personal perceptions about of self-care and that leads to excessive smoking, uncontrolled eating, and arguments with their significant others. One of the reasons that may link to depression which results in adverse health outcomes in diabetics is poor glycemic control. All of this reason can results in the recurrence of diabetes symptoms and related complications even with increased medication.[24] It is now well understood that people with type 1 and type 2 diabetes have a doubled risk for comorbid depression, compared with healthy people. Fact is that depression among diabetics is linked to decreased quality of life, increase microvascular problems, cardiovascular disease, and death which are the highlights of this result. Thus, receiving effective therapy for depression may have a good effect on both physical and emotional well-being. Diabetes-specific emotional distress has been found to be substantially connected with both depression and poor glycemic control, and it has been proposed that diabetes-distress mediates the relationship between depression and glycemic control. Moreover, to date, psychological depression treatment has shown small but significant positive effects on glycemic outcomes.[18,25,26]

PSYCHOLOGICAL AND PHYSIOLOGICAL MECHANISMS OF DIABETES DISTRESS SYNDROME

The hypothalamic-pituitary-adrenal (HPA) axis plays a critical role in regulating the body's response to stress. Chronic stress leads to prolonged activation of the HPA axis, causing excessive cortisol release (hypercortisolemia) and disrupting its negative feedback mechanism. In diabetes, this dysfunction exacerbates hyperglycemia, insulin resistance, and flattened cortisol rhythms, with higher nighttime cortisol levels associated with depression and anxiety. Persistent activation also triggers systemic inflammation, immunosuppression, and metabolic disturbances, contributing to conditions such as central obesity and metabolic syndrome, creating a vicious cycle of stress and metabolic dysregulation. The connection between diabetes and mental health disorders further amplifies this problem. Diabetic patients have a higher risk of depression and anxiety than non-diabetics, and these comorbidities can impair self-care and blood glucose management, increasing the likelihood of complications and reducing the quality of life. This also adds to the financial and social burden of diabetes. Simultaneously, prolonged physiological stress activates both the HPA axis and the sympathetic nervous system. Elevated glucocorticoids and catecholamines enhance glucose intolerance and contribute to insulin resistance. While acute hyperglycemia during stress may benefit the body by providing glucose to insulin-independent tissues, chronic stress shifts this response toward harmful effects. Prolonged stress also intensifies inflammation, with inflammatory cytokines further promoting the development or worsening of diabetes. This interplay between stress, mental health, and physiological mechanisms underscores the complex and self-perpetuating nature of diabetic distress syndrome, emphasizing the need for integrated management approaches.[27,28]

MEASUREMENT AND SCREENING

Diabetic patients who participate in behavioral intervention programs have shown improvements in glycemic control and self-management behaviors over time, which further supports diabetic distress as a crucial intervention point. In order to assist people, start to anticipate and identify the distress that they may experience as a result of having a chronic illness, as well as address its impact on their disease management. It can be extremely beneficial to address distress through diabetes education or during normal clinical visits. One important factor influencing medication adherence behavior is diabetes distress. Therefore, integrating regular distress screening into the health system's standard diabetic care and encouraging medical professionals to manage diabetes using a biopsychosocial approach will be crucial context-specific interventions to enhance the health of those living with diabetes.[29]

Routine Screening for Diabetes Distress is Increasingly Recognized as Part of Diabetes Care

The PAID scale (Problem Areas in Diabetes scale) and the DDS scale (Diabetes Distress scale) are tools used to assess diabetes distress, a psychological condition that affects many individuals with diabetes.[30]

Problem Areas in Diabetes Scale

The problem areas in diabetes (PAID) scale is a 20-item questionnaire designed to measure emotional distress related to living with diabetes. It assesses areas such as feelings of guilt, frustration, fear, and lack of support. It is widely used in clinical and research settings to monitor psychological well-being and provide insight into the emotional burden of diabetes.[30]

Diabetes Distress Scale

The DDS is a 17-item questionnaire that evaluates the psychological distress specifically related to diabetes management. It focuses on four domains—emotional burden, physician-related distress, regimen-related distress, and interpersonal distress. The DDS is used to identify diabetes distress in patients and guide appropriate interventions.[30]

Both scales help clinicians identify patients who may be struggling with emotional aspects of managing diabetes, facilitating tailored support and treatment.

MANAGEMENT STRATEGIES FOR DIABETIC DISTRESS

When dealing with the difficulties of treating diabetes, diabetic distress is a typical psychological reaction. Diabetes patients' quality of life can be considerably enhanced by effective management techniques, which include behavioral support, psychological therapies, and healthcare participation (**Fig. 2**).

Psychological Interventions

- *Cognitive-behavioral therapy (CBT):* It has been demonstrated that CBT is useful in treating the emotional components of managing diabetes. It lessens the distress and anxiety that come with managing diabetes by assisting people in recognizing and changing harmful thought patterns linked with their illness.[31,32]
- *Mindfulness:* By encouraging patients to concentrate on the here and now, mindfulness techniques can reduce stress and enhance emotional control. Better self-management practices and general psychological well-being in diabetics have been associated with this strategy.[33,34]
- *Problem-solving therapy:* This therapeutic approach gives patients the tools they need to address certain diabetes management difficulties. People can feel more powerful and less overwhelmed by their situation by improving their problem-solving skills.[32,35]

Behavioral Support

- *Diabetes education:* It is essential to provide thorough instruction regarding diabetes control. This entails being aware of dietary decisions, physical exercise, and medication compliance. Patients who are well-informed are more likely to practice good self-management.[33,36]
- *Peer support groups:* By interacting with others who have gone through similar things, one might lessen feelings of loneliness and promote a sense of community. Peer support can significantly enhance

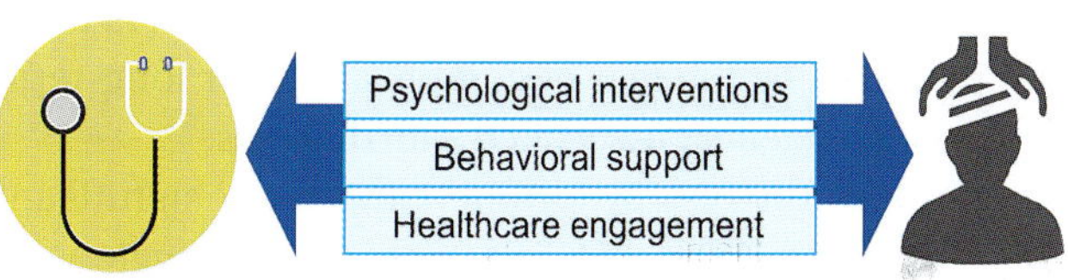

Fig. 2: Management strategies for diabetes distress.

glucose management and general health outcomes, according to studies.[34,35]

- *Family involvement:* Support networks can be strengthened by involving family members in diabetes treatment. Effective self-care requires both practical and emotional assistance, which family members can offer. Family support has been linked in studies to enhanced psychological well-being and better self-management practices.[35,36]

Healthcare Engagement

- *Empathy-driven care:* Healthcare providers who demonstrate empathy can significantly impact patient outcomes. Empathetic care fosters trust and encourages open communication, allowing patients to express their concerns about managing diabetes without fear of judgment.[33,34]
- *Shared decision-making:* Involving patients in their care decisions promotes a sense of ownership over their health. Shared decision-making encourages collaboration between healthcare providers and patients, leading to tailored treatment plans that align with the patient's preferences and lifestyle.[32,35,36]

For management of diabetes distress there is significance of multifaceted approach that incorporates psychological interventions, behavioral support, and empathetic healthcare engagement. These strategies not only improve clinical outcomes but also enhance the overall quality of life for individuals living with diabetes.

CHALLENGES FACED IN REAL WORLD

Psychological Aspects and Marital Aspects

Psychologically, DDS can lead to feelings of frustration, burnout, and helplessness due to the constant management required for diabetes care. The chronic nature of the disease, coupled with the need for frequent monitoring of blood sugar levels, medication adherence, and lifestyle changes, often leads to anxiety and depression. The emotional toll of managing a condition that requires daily attention can cause individuals to experience a loss of control over their lives, heightening feelings of distress and affecting self-esteem. This emotional strain is often compounded by the fear of complications or long-term health consequences associated with diabetes.[37]

Diabetes distress syndrome can create significant stress within relationships. Partners may struggle with understanding the complexities of the condition, leading to communication breakdowns. The caregiving aspect, where one partner may assume a more active role in managing the condition, can create imbalances in the relationship, leading to feelings of resentment or role strain.[38] Additionally, the chronic nature of the condition means that the partner's distress is ongoing, which may overshadow the emotional needs of the other partner, leading to frustration and conflict. Marital satisfaction may decline as one or both partners feel overwhelmed by the constant demands of managing the disease, impacting intimacy and emotional connection.[39]

Effective management of DDS requires a holistic approach, including psychological support and relationship counseling. Couples are encouraged to engage in open communication, share responsibilities, and seek therapy when needed to address both the emotional and relational challenges that diabetes distress presents. Recognizing the interconnectedness of psychological and marital aspects in managing DDS can promote better overall health outcomes and relationship stability.[7,40]

Physician–Patient Conversation

Effective communication between healthcare providers and patients is crucial in addressing diabetes distress. Research indicates that many patients with diabetes are unaware of the concept of diabetes distress and have never been asked about their emotional well-being. This gap in communication can hinder the identification of distress and the implementation of supportive interventions.[2]

Physicians should adopt a more proactive approach by:

- *Inquiring about emotional well-being:* Regularly asking patients about their feelings related to diabetes management can help identify those experiencing distress.
- *Using standardized screening tools:* Implementing tools such as the DDS can facilitate the assessment of emotional burdens and guide appropriate interventions.[4]
- *Encouraging open dialogue:* Creating a safe environment for patients to express their concerns can foster trust and improve patient engagement in their care.

Counseling

Counseling plays a vital role in managing diabetes distress. Evidence suggests that tailored psychological interventions can significantly alleviate symptoms of diabetes distress. For instance, studies have shown that emotion-focused interventions yield the most consistent benefits in reducing diabetes distress compared to traditional education-based approaches.[12]

Key strategies for effective counseling include:

- *Emotion-focused interventions:* Programs that specifically target emotional aspects of living with diabetes, such as the "TunedIn" program, have demonstrated substantial reductions in distress levels.[2]
- *Peer support:* Incorporating peer support elements into counseling can help normalize feelings of distress and provide coping strategies through shared experiences.[1]
- *Cognitive behavioral techniques:* Utilizing CBT techniques can help patients reframe negative thoughts associated with diabetes management and enhance coping skills.[4]

Building Trust and Addressing Emotional Challenges

Building a trusting relationship between healthcare providers and patients is essential for addressing the emotional challenges associated with diabetes. Trust facilitates open communication, making it easier for patients to discuss their struggles with diabetes distress.[41,42]

Strategies to build trust include:

- *Consistent follow-up:* Regular follow-ups can demonstrate commitment to patient care and encourage ongoing dialogue about emotional well-being.[42]
- *Holistic care approaches:* Integrating mental health support into routine diabetes care acknowledges the interconnectedness of physical and emotional health, leading to more comprehensive patient management.[41]
- *Training for healthcare professionals:* Providing training for healthcare providers on recognizing and addressing psychological aspects of diabetes can enhance their ability to support patients effectively.[1,41]

CONCLUSION

Overcoming diabetes distress requires a concerted effort from healthcare providers to enhance communication, provide effective counseling, and build trusting relationships with patients. By prioritizing emotional well-being alongside medical management, healthcare professionals can significantly improve the quality of life for individuals living with diabetes.

REFERENCES

1. Kreider KE. Diabetes Distress or Major Depressive Disorder? A Practical Approach to Diagnosing and Treating Psychological Comorbidities of Diabetes. Diabetes Ther. 2017;8(1):1-7.
2. Sekhri S, Verma A. Study of Depression and Its Associated Factors Among Patients of Diabetes Mellitus (DM) and Hypertension (HTN) Attending a Primary Health Center (PHC) in a Rural Area of New Delhi, India. Cureus. 2023; 15(1):e33826.
3. Fisher L, Skaff MM, Mullan JT, Arean P, Mohr D, Masharani U, et al. Clinical depression versus distress among patients with type 2 diabetes: not just a question of semantics. Diabetes Care. 2007;30(3):542-8.
4. AlOzairi A, Irshad M, AlKandari J, AlSaraf H, Al-Ozairi E. Prevalence and predictors of diabetes distress and depression in people with type 1 diabetes. Front Psychiatry. 2024;15:1367876.
5. Sinha R, Priya A, Sinha A, Hifz Ur Rahman M. Prevalence of diabetes distress among type 2 diabetes mellitus patients in India: a systematic review and meta-analysis. Health Psychol Behav Med. 2024;12(1):2324091.
6. Nanayakkara N, Pease A, Ranasinha S, Wischer N, Andrikopoulos S, Speight J, et al. Depression and diabetes distress in adults with type 2 diabetes: results from the Australian National Diabetes Audit (ANDA) 2016. Sci Rep. 2018;8(1):7846.
7. Wojujutari AK, Idemudia ES, Ugwu LE. Psychological resilience mediates the relationship between diabetes distress and depression among persons with diabetes in a multi-group analysis. Sci Rep. 2024;14:6510.
8. Farooqi A, Gillies C, Sathanapally H, Abner S, Seidu S, Davies MJ, et al. A systematic review and meta-analysis to compare the prevalence of depression between people with and without Type 1 and Type 2 diabetes. Prim Care Diabetes. 2022;16(1):1-10.
9. Wardian JL, Kanzler KE, True MW, Glotfelter MA, Sauerwein TJ. Is It Distress, Depression, or Both? Exploring Differences in the Diabetes Distress Scale and the Patient Health Questionnaire in a Diabetes Specialty Clinic. Clin Diabetes. 2019;37(2):124-30.
10. Diabetes Canada Clinical Practice Guidelines Expert Committee, Robinson DJ, Coons M, Haensel H, Vallis M, Yale JF. Diabetes and Mental Health. Can J Diabetes. 2018;42 Suppl 1:S130-41.
11. Bhaskara G, Budhiarta AAG, Gotera W, Saraswati MR, Dwipayana IMP, Semadi IMS, et al. Factors Associated with Diabetes-Related Distress in Type 2 Diabetes Mellitus Patients. Diabetes Metab Syndr Obes Targets Ther. 2022;15:2077-85.
12. Kirk BO, Khan R, Davidov D, Sambamoorthi U, Misra R. Exploring facilitators and barriers to patient-provider communication regarding diabetes self-management. PEC Innov. 2023;3:100188.

13. Geleta BA, Dingata ST, Emanu MD, Eba LB, Abera KB, Tsegaye D. Prevalence of Diabetes Related Distress and Associated Factors Among Type 2 Diabetes Patients Attending Hospitals, Southwest Ethiopia, 2020: A Cross-Sectional Study. Patient Relat Outcome Meas. 2021;12:13-22.
14. German J, Kobe EA, Lewinski AA, Jeffreys AS, Coffman C, Edelman D, et al. Factors Associated with Diabetes Distress Among Patients with Poorly Controlled Type 2 Diabetes. J Endocr Soc. 2023;7(5):bvad031.
15. Kretchy IA, Koduah A, Ohene-Agyei T, Boima V, Appiah B. The Association between Diabetes-Related Distress and Medication Adherence in Adult Patients with Type 2 Diabetes Mellitus: A Cross-Sectional Study. J Diabetes Res. 2020;2020:4760624.
16. Hessler DM, Fisher L, Polonsky WH, Masharani U, Strycker LA, Peters AL, et al. Diabetes distress is linked with worsening diabetes management over time in adults with Type 1 diabetes. Diabet Med J Br Diabet Assoc. 2017;34(9):1228-34.
17. Van Bastelaar KMP, Pouwer F, Geelhoed-Duijvestijn PHLM, Tack CJ, Bazelmans E, Beekman AT, et al. Diabetes-specific emotional distress mediates the association between depressive symptoms and glycaemic control in Type 1 and Type 2 diabetes. Diabet Med. 2010;27(7):798-803.
18. Fisher L, Mullan JT, Arean P, Glasgow RE, Hessler D, Masharani U. Diabetes Distress but Not Clinical Depression or Depressive Symptoms Is Associated with Glycemic Control in Both Cross-Sectional and Longitudinal Analyses. Diabetes Care. 2010;33(1):23-8.
19. Fisher L, Polonsky WH, Hessler DM, Masharani U, Blumer I, Peters AL, et al. UNDERSTANDING THE SOURCES OF DIABETES DISTRESS IN ADULTS WITH TYPE 1 DIABETES. J Diabetes Complications. 2015;29(4):572-7.
20. Delahanty LM, Grant RW, Wittenberg E, Bosch JL, Wexler DJ, Cagliero E, et al. Association of diabetes-related emotional distress with diabetes treatment in primary care patients with Type 2 diabetes. Diabet Med. 2007;24(1):48-54.
21. Schabert J, Browne JL, Mosely K, Speight J. Social Stigma in Diabetes. Patient - Patient-Centered Outcomes Res. 2013;6(1):1-10.
22. Levitt NS. Diabetes in Africa: epidemiology, management and healthcare challenges. Heart. 2008;94(11):1376-82.
23. Fritschi C, Quinn L. Fatigue in Patients with Diabetes: A Review. J Psychosom Res. 2010;69(1):33-41.
24. Chew BH, Mohd-Sidik S, Shariff-Ghazali S. Negative effects of diabetes–related distress on health-related quality of life: an evaluation among the adult patients with type 2 diabetes mellitus in three primary healthcare clinics in Malaysia. Health Qual Life Outcomes. 2015;13:187.
25. Schram MT, Baan CA, Pouwer F. Depression and Quality of Life in Patients with Diabetes: A Systematic Review from the European Depression in Diabetes (EDID) Research Consortium. Curr Diabetes Rev. 2009;5(2):112-9.
26. Fisher L, Skaff MM, Mullan JT, Arean P, Glasgow R, Masharani U. A longitudinal study of affective and anxiety disorders, depressive affect and diabetes distress in adults with Type 2 diabetes. Diabet Med J Br Diabet Assoc. 2008; 25(9):1096-101.
27. Tareen RS, Tareen K. Psychosocial aspects of diabetes management: dilemma of diabetes distress. Transl Pediatr. 2017;6(4):383-96.
28. Mangoulia P, Milionis C, Vlachou E, Ilias I. The Interrelationship between Diabetes Mellitus and Emotional Well-Being: Current Concepts and Future Prospects. Healthcare. 2024;12(14):1457.
29. Albright D, Wardell J, Harrison A, Mizokami-Stout K, Hirschfeld E, Garrity A, et al. Screening for diabetes distress and depression in routine clinical care for youth with type 1 diabetes. J Pediatr Psychol. 2024;49(5):356-64.
30. Welch GW, Jacobson AM, Polonsky WH. The Problem Areas in Diabetes Scale: An evaluation of its clinical utility. Diabetes Care. 1997;20(5):760-6.
31. Pendley JS, Kasmen LJ, Miller DL, Donze J, Swenson C, Reeves G. Peer and Family Support in Children and Adolescents with Type 1 Diabetes. J Pediatr Psychol. 2002; 27(5):429-38.
32. Pamungkas RA, Chamroonsawasdi K, Vatanasomboon P. A Systematic Review: Family Support Integrated with Diabetes Self-Management among Uncontrolled Type II Diabetes Mellitus Patients. Behav Sci. 2017;7(3):62.
33. Diriba DC, Leung DYP, Suen LKP. Effects of family-based diabetes self-management education and support programme on support behaviour amongst adults with type 2 diabetes in Western Ethiopia. Sci Rep. 2023;13:20867.
34. Werner JJ, Ufholz K, Yamajala P. Recent Findings on the Effectiveness of Peer Support for Patients with Type 2 Diabetes. Curr Cardiovasc Risk Rep. 2024;18(5):65-79.
35. Baig AA, Benitez A, Quinn MT, Burnet DL. Family interventions to improve diabetes outcomes for adults. Ann N Y Acad Sci. 2015;1353(1):89-112.
36. Mphasha MH, Mothiba TM, Skaal L. Family support in the management of diabetes patients' perspectives from Limpopo province in South Africa. BMC Public Health. 2022;22:2421.
37. Chew BH, Vos RC, Metzendorf M, Scholten RJ, Rutten GE. Psychological interventions for diabetes-related distress in adults with type 2 diabetes mellitus. Cochrane Database Syst Rev. 2017;2017(9):CD011469.
38. Helgeson VS, Allen NA, Tracy EL, Butner J, Berg CA. Diabetes stress contagion among romantic partners: a daily diary investigation. J Behav Med. 2022;45(5):716-27.
39. Poole L, Hackett RA. Diabetes distress: the psychological burden of living with diabetes. Lancet Diabetes Endocrinol. 2024;12(7):439-41.
40. Hernar I, Cooper JG, Nilsen RM, Skinner TC, Strandberg RB, Iversen MM, et al. Diabetes Distress and Associations with Demographic and Clinical Variables: A Nationwide

Population-Based Registry Study of 10,186 Adults with Type 1 Diabetes in Norway. Diabetes Care. 2024;47(1):126-31.

41. Stenov V, Cleal B, Willaing I, Christensen JN, Jensen CG, Mouritsen JD, et al. An Evidence-Based Nurse-Led Intervention to Reduce Diabetes Distress Among Adults with Type 1 Diabetes and Diabetes Distress (REDUCE): Development of a Complex Intervention Using Qualitative Methods Informed by the Medical Research Council Framework. JMIR Form Res. 2024;8(1):e58658.
42. Misra R, Shawley-Brzoska S, Khan R, Kirk BO, Wen S, Sambamoorthi U. Addressing Diabetes Distress in Self-Management Programs. J Appalach Health. 2021;3(3):68-85.

CHAPTER 38

Diabetes and Infection

Jayanta K Panda, Manoranjan Behera

INTRODUCTION

Diabetes mellitus (DM) is considered as a secondary immune deficiency disorder by the World Health Organization (WHO) as the disease is characterized by frequent, severe, prolonged, and recurrent infections due to alteration of at least one of the immune response mechanisms, and elimination of the underlying cause leads to resolution.[1] This immunocompromised state predisposes the patient to an increased risk of infection and sepsis which are contributing factors for increasing the rate of morbidity and mortality in diabetic subjects.[2] The incidence of infection is higher in patients with diabetes and also difficult to treat than nondiabetic counterparts. This hampers the glycemic control and worsens the prognosis in diabetics. So, there is a bidirectional relationship between diabetes and infection. Infection may be the first presenting clinical feature of undiagnosed DM in many people. The focus of infection, when remains unrecognized and untreated, becomes systemic with bacteremia and toxemia, leading to "sepsis".

DIABETES MELLITUS AND RISK OF INFECTION

Certain infections are common, and few infections are most commonly associated with DM **(Box 1)**.[3]

In comparison to general population, people with diabetes (PWD) have a 1.5-fold increased risk of infection presenting in an outpatient setting and a two- to fourfold increased risk of infection-related hospitalization by infection-type foot infection (6.0- to 14.7-fold), osteomyelitis (4.4- to 15.7-fold), kidney infection (3.0- to 4.9-fold), and also increased risk for influenza, pneumonia, skin infection, tuberculosis (TB), general sepsis, and surgical site infection. Diabetes confers a twofold higher rate of death from COVID-19.[4]

BOX 1: Specific infections in diabetes mellitus.[3]

Infections associated with increased incidence:
- *Genitourinary tract infections:*
  - Cystitis
  - Pyelonephritis
  - Renal and perinephric abscess
  - Balanoposthitis and vulvovaginitis
- *Respiratory tract infections:*
  - *Staphylococcus aureus* pneumonia
  - Gram-negative pneumonia
  - Tuberculosis
  - Lung abscess
- *Skin and soft-tissue infections:*
  - Surgical wound infection
  - Pyomyositis
  - Foot infection
- *Abdominal infections:*
  - *Salmonella enteritidis*
  - *Campylobacter jejuni*

Infections predominantly associated with diabetes:
- Malignant otitis externa
- Rhinocerebral mucormycosis
- Emphysematous cholecystitis
- Emphysematous pyelonephritis
- Emphysematous cystitis
- Necrotizing fasciitis
- Fournier's gangrene

Though studies revealed infection rates in type 1 DM and type 2 DM separately, the risk ratios were generally higher for type 1 DM than type 2 DM.

Mechanisms by which Infection may Worsen Glycemia (Flowchart 1):[4]

Infection and its treatment often affect glucose homeostasis through effects on insulin resistance and insulin secretion and increase the risk of hyperglycemia.[4]

Many viruses, in particular enteroviruses (especially coxsackie B1, B4), cytomegalovirus (CMV), rubella, and mumps, infect β cells, resulting in diminished insulin secretion and have been associated with type 1 DM, though the link has not been conclusively proven in humans. Severe acute respiratory syndrome coronavirus (SARS-CoV)-2 can infect and replicate in human β cells by gaining entry via angiotensin-converting enzyme (ACE)-2 receptors. Though a few early studies suggested an increased incidence of type 1 DM, not all longer-term studies have confirmed.[4]

Infection induces a stress reaction, leading to the production of counter-regulatory hormones (glucocorticoids, catecholamines, growth hormone, and glucagon) and cytokines like tumor necrosis factor α (TNF-α) and interleukin (IL)-1. This combination accelerates insulin resistance, leading to failure to suppress hepatic neoglucogenesis and glucose uptake by skeletal muscle. Hepatitis C virus (HCV) and human immunodeficiency virus (HIV) have been associated with type 2 DM.[4]

Flowchart 1: Mechanisms by which infection may worsen glycemia.[4]

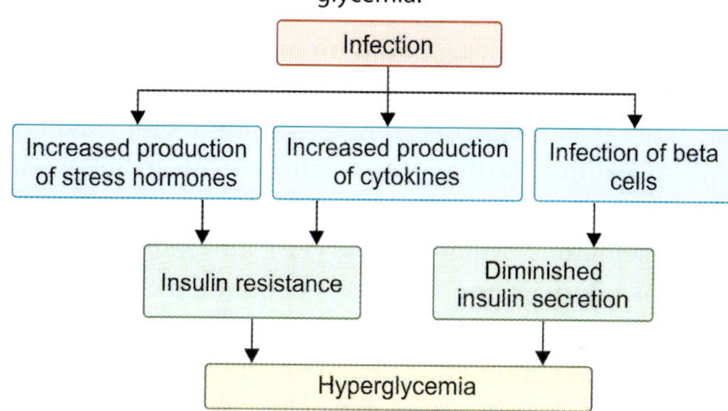

Mechanisms that Increase the Risk of Infection in Diabetes ***(Fig. 1)***:[4]

Several factors contribute to increased propensity for infection in patients with diabetes, which includes, importantly, an altered immunity. The innate immunity is predominantly affected, manifesting as dysfunction of polymorphonuclear cells (PMNs), which includes dysfunction in adhesion, impaired migration, altered chemotaxis, reduced phagocytosis, oxidative burst, and capacity of microbial killing.[5] Abnormalities in monocyte/macrophage chemotaxis and phagocytic function have also been found.[6] Pro-inflammatory cytokines such as TNF-α, IL-1, IL-6, and IL-8 are increased in diabetic patients in basal state.[7,8] Advanced glycation end-products lead to low-grade persistent activation and ultimately exhaustion of PMNs.[7] There is an impaired sequential pattern of cytokine production and an increase in the duration of cytokine response (e.g., TNF-α) in diabetic individuals, leading to more persistent inflammation and tissue damage.[9] There is impaired local cytokine production (e.g., diabetic women with bacteriuria present with lower urinary levels of IL-6 and IL-8).[10] This cytokine dysregulation associated with hyperglycemia could be one of the factors responsible for more severe infection noted

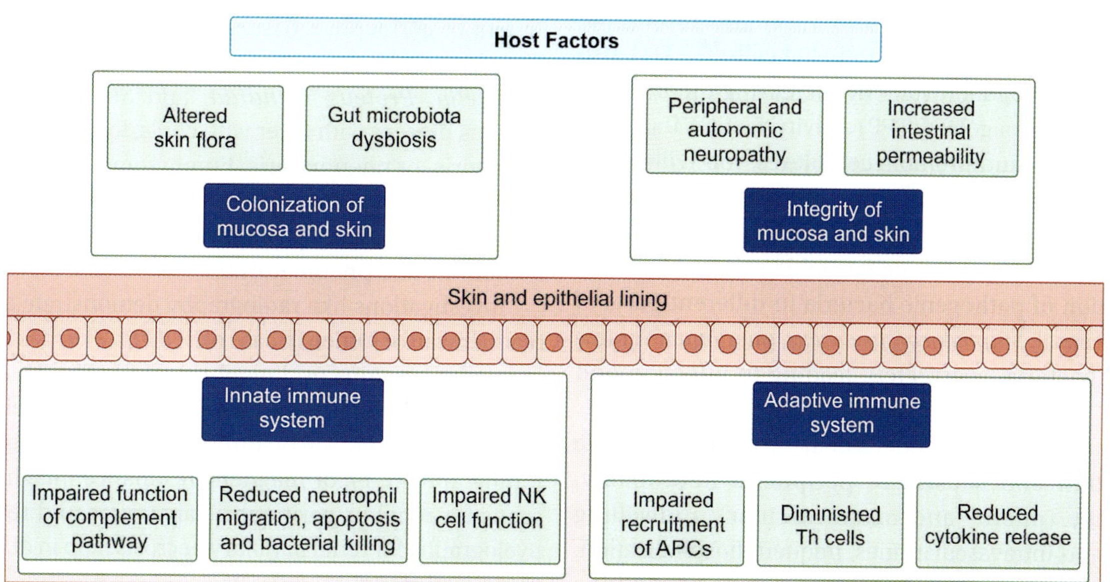

Fig. 1: Mechanisms that increase the risk of infection in people with diabetes.[4]
(APCs: antigen-presenting cells; NK: natural killer; Th: T helper)

in diabetics than their nondiabetic counterparts. The complements are affected in diabetic patients by which they are less able to opsonize pathogenic bacteria. Glucose attacks the thioester bond of complement C3 (opsonic binding site) and prevents it from binding to the bacterial surface. This also increases the susceptibility to *Candida* infection.[11]

Diabetes has direct inhibitory effect on the adaptive immune system as well. There is an impaired proliferative response against different antigens and delayed hypersensitivity reaction of T-cell function in diabetic patients, which is attributed to dysregulation between pro-inflammatory and anti-inflammatory cytokines as well as defects at the level of antigen-presenting cells.[12]

Diabetic patients with poor long-term glucose control [elevated glycated hemoglobin (HbA1c) levels] were found to have not only quantitative defects, i.e., decrease in the amounts of global and specific circulating antibodies, but also qualitative defects, i.e., lower functionality of immunoglobulin G (IgG) antibodies and impairment of antigen binding due to nonenzymatic glycosylation of antibodies.[13,14] Despite all these antibody alterations, a good antibody response to vaccine challenge is found in diabetic patients.[7]

Diabetes mellitus induces endothelial dysfunction. Hyperglycemia and oxidative bursts directly activate cell adhesion molecules [e.g., vascular cell adhesion molecule-1 (VCAM-1), intercellular adhesion molecule-1 (ICAM-1), and E-selectin], and vascular endothelial growth factor signaling in endothelial cells.[5,8,15] DM also induces a procoagulant state by increasing the levels of tissue factor procoagulant (TFP) activity, factor VIIa, factor VIII, thrombin—antithrombin complexes, von Willebrand factor, tissue factor procoagulant inhibitor (TFPI) activity, and a decrease plasminogen activator inhibitor-1 (PAI-1) activity.[16] DM also provides a favorable soil for increased colonization of pathogenic bacteria in different parts of the body (nasal: *Staphylococcus aureus*, pharyngeal: gram-negative bacteria, yeast, etc.), leading to infection and sepsis.

Other factors which render a diabetic more susceptible to infection and sepsis are peripheral neuropathy, angiopathy (micro- and macrovascular), indwelling catheter and intravascular lines, frequent hospitalization, diabetic ketoacidosis (DKA), chronic renal failure requiring dialysis and blood transfusion, gastroparesis, and frequent minor and major surgery.

COMMON INFECTIONS IN DIABETES MELLITUS

Urinary Tract Infections

Urinary tract infection (UTI) is the most common infection seen in diabetes, and it is a common cause of hospitalization as well. Symptomatic as well as asymptomatic UTI is commonly encountered in diabetic patients with a higher incidence of bacteriuria seen as compared to controls. The main risk factors for UTI in DM are long duration of diabetes, impaired glycemic control, diabetic autonomic neuropathy, impaired bladder distension, increased residual urine volume, vesicoureteral reflux, decreased urinary cytokine excretion, increased *Escherichia coli* adhesion, diabetic microangiopathy, neutrophil dysfunction, and recurrent vaginitis.[17] Other concomitant causes such as cystocele, rectocele, and indwelling catheterization also contribute to a higher incidence.[7] Common organisms responsible for UTI are *E. coli, Klebsiella, Proteus,* and *Candida.*

Acute pyelonephritis is more common with classical clinical features like that in nondiabetics with an increased risk of complications such as perinephric or renal abscess, emphysematous pyelonephritis (EP), and renal papillary necrosis.[7] Perinephric abscess is common in DM due to enteric gram-negative bacilli with palpable mass in loin and perirenal suppuration due to inflammatory reaction.

Emphysematous pyelonephritis is a necrotizing infection of the renal parenchyma with gas in collecting system or perinephric tissues. It is most commonly found in women and is caused by *E. coli, Enterobacter aerogenes, Klebsiella, Proteus, Candida,* and *Streptococcus*. The patients present with fever with chills, loin pain, vomiting, hematuria, or pneumaturia. Emphysematous cystitis (EC) is also common in diabetics with presence of gas in urinary bladder. The patients present with lower abdominal pain, hematuria, and pneumaturia.

Investigations like radiography demonstrate air in the bladder wall or lumen in case of EC **(Fig. 2)** or gas in kidney in emphysematous pyelonephritis (EP) **(Fig. 3)**. At times, it can involve two intra-abdominal organs, namely kidney and gallbladder. Ultrasonography (USG), computed tomography (CT), or magnetic resonance imaging (MRI) scans for renal or perinephric abscesses and retrograde pyelography for renal papillary necrosis help in diagnosing complications.[7]

Treatment consists of good glycemic control by insulin, appropriate antibiotics (6–8 weeks), and surgical

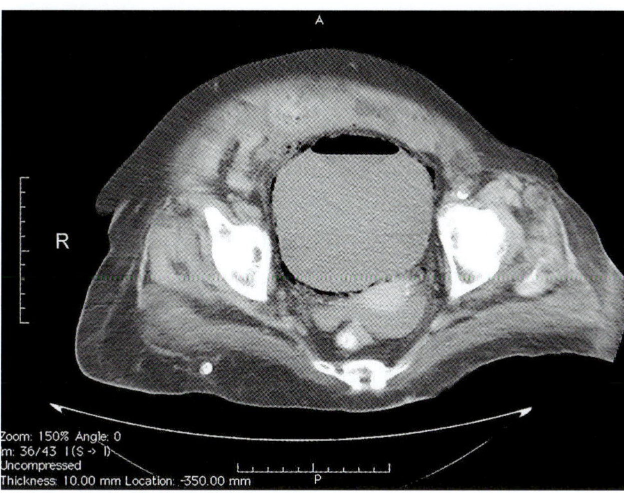

Fig. 2: Computed tomography (CT) scan showing emphysematous cystitis.

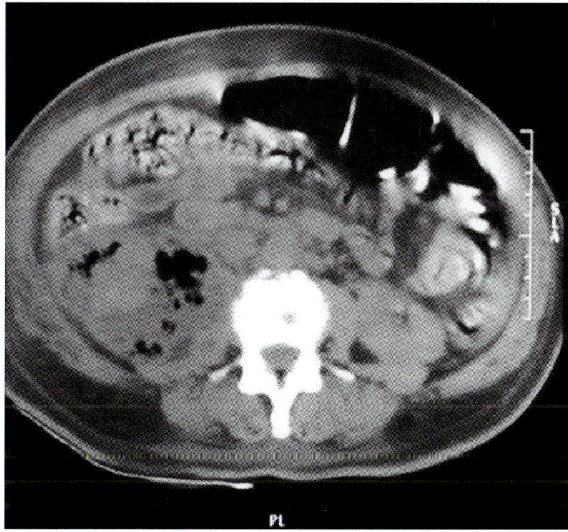

Fig. 3: Computed tomography (CT) scan showing emphysematous pyelonephritis.

intervention including nephrectomy according to the disease severity. Mortality in these emphysematous disorders is 60–80% with medical therapy alone. With the use of newer agents [sodium-glucose cotransporter-2 (SGLT2) inhibitors], counseling regarding genital hygiene is mandatory to reduce the risk of urogenital infections.

Respiratory Tracts Infections

The overall incidence of community-acquired pneumonia (CAP) is not higher in patients with diabetes.[18] However, diabetic patients with pneumonia when hospitalized have a higher mortality than nondiabetics.[19] The incidence of bacteremia, delayed resolution of pneumonia, and recurrence of infection may also be higher in these patients. There is prolonged viral shedding following influenza virus infection in diabetics.[20]

Certain organisms such as *S. aureus*, gram-negative bacteria, and *Mycobacterium tuberculosis* infect diabetics more often, while some microorganisms such as *Streptococcus pneumoniae*, *Legionella*, and influenza virus are responsible for increase in morbidity and mortality in patients with diabetes.[21] Influenza and bacterial pneumonia also increase the risk of acute coronary events.

There is increased colonization of upper airway by *S. aureus* and gram-negative bacteria in diabetics, which may be responsible for an increased incidence of bacterial pneumonias.[7] Colonization by *S. aureus* makes patients susceptible to lower respiratory tract infection following an infection by influenza virus, which affects mucociliary activity.[7] Fungal infections like aspergillosis and *Cryptococcus neoformans* can also cause primary pneumonia.

It is recommended that diabetics should receive influenza vaccine annually and pneumococcal vaccine.[22]

Gastrointestinal and Liver Infections

Diabetic patients are susceptible to certain enteric pathogens because of gastrointestinal dysmotility syndrome. *Salmonella enteritidis* and *Campylobacter* infections are reported with increased frequency. DM is also a risk factor for infection with *Listeria monocytogens* with higher than nondiabetic counterparts.

Oropharyngeal and esophageal candidiasis are commonly found in patients with diabetes due to *Candida albicans* with increased production of proteinase and phospholipase along with increased virulence. The association of DM and *Helicobacter pylori* is controversial. The efficiency of *H. pylori* eradication is lower, and reinfection rates are higher in persons with DM.[23]

Patients suffering from HCV infection are three times more likely to develop DM than those who are HCV-negative. It has been found that 13–33% of HCV-infected patients had type 2 DM compared to 4–10% in HCV-negative cohort. HCV-positive diabetics have more severe liver disease and increased fibrosis compared to nondiabetic HCV patients. Type 2 DM is considered as an extrahepatic manifestation of HCV infection.[24]

Emphysematous cholecystitis is a rare complication of acute cholecystitis found in diabetics due to gas-producing microorganisms such as *Clostridium perfringens, E. coli, and Bacillus fragilis,* leading to ischemia of gallbladder wall and collection of air in lumen and wall of gallbladder. This affects males more commonly (75%), and gallstones are present in 50% of patients. Perforation (30 times) and gangrene (5–10 times) are many-fold higher compared to nonemphysematous cholecystitis. Clinical features are as those of acute cholecystitis with marked toxicity and jaundice. Crepitus on abdominal palpation is an ominous sign. The common complications are pericholecystic abscess, gallbladder necrosis, and generalized or biliary peritonitis. Surprisingly, mortality is higher in younger population. It can be diagnosed with plain abdominal X-ray or ultrasound abdomen in 95% cases, but CT scan of the abdomen is the most sensitive diagnostic modality which shows gas in the gallbladder **(Fig. 4)**. Air, if found in hypochondrium, suggests perforation. It needs broad-spectrum antibiotics and at times emergency cholecystectomy.

Genital Infections

Vulvovaginitis in women and balanoposthitis in men are common with *C. albicans*. Treatment of choice is with oral or topical azoles.

Skin and Soft-tissue Infections

Intertrigo due to fungal infections and tinea infections are common in diabetics. Infections involving the skin, nails, and subcutaneous tissues are very common in DM **(Fig. 5)**. Peripheral neuropathy, micro- and macroangiopathy, and poor glycemic control are predisposing factors. Infection is polymicrobial, caused by Streptococci, anaerobes, *C. albicans*, and gram-negative bacilli.

Necrotizing Fasciitis

About 75% of patients with necrotizing fasciitis have DM.[25] It is a life-threatening, rapidly spreading infection of deep-seated subcutaneous tissue with progressive destruction of fascia, fat, and muscles. The infection is usually polymicrobial and categorized as type 1 (If caused by an anaerobe in combination with facultative anaerobes like Streptococci or enterobacteriaceae) and type 2 (if caused by group A beta-hemolytic Streptococci alone or in combination with Staphylococci).[26] Common sites affected include lower limbs, abdominal wall, nape of neck, back, and perineum. It usually follows trauma, insect bites, and abrasions. Clinically characterized by fever, local pain, violaceous discoloration of the skin, ulceration and gangrene occur following necrosis of superficial fascia **(Fig. 6)**. It needs aggressive surgical debridement along with broad-spectrum antibiotics. Despite appropriate therapy, mortality is nearly 60%.

Fournier's Gangrene

Fournier's gangrene is a specific form of necrotizing fasciitis involving the perineum, scrotum, and penis. An estimated 40–60% of the patients with this condition are associated with DM. Predisposing genitourinary pathologies responsible for this condition are urethral trauma, instruments like chronic indwelling catheter, scrotal abscess, injury, and perianal abscess.

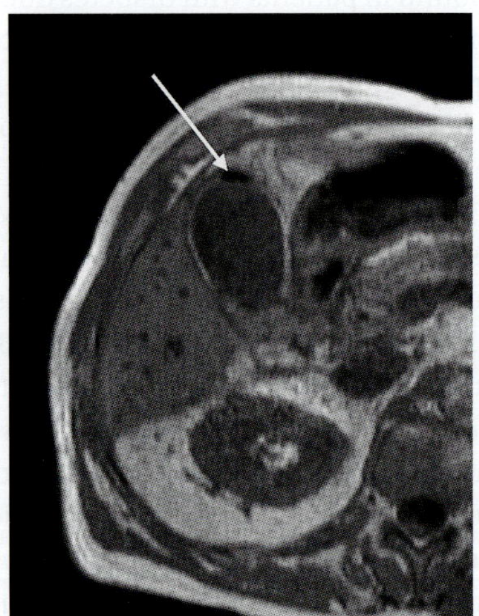

Fig. 4: Computed tomography (CT) scan showing emphysematous cholecystitis.

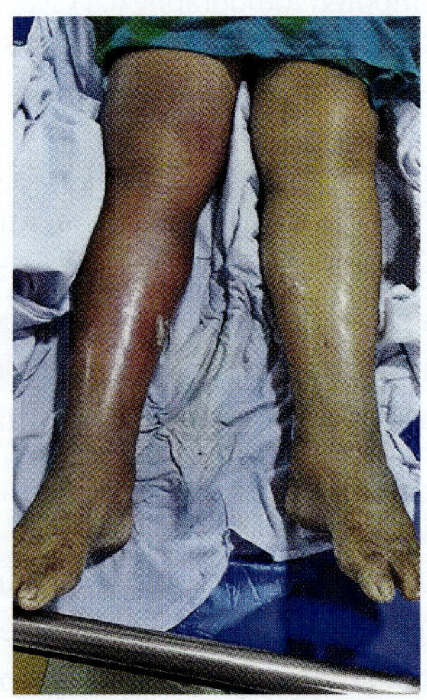

Fig. 5: Cellulitis on right lower limb.

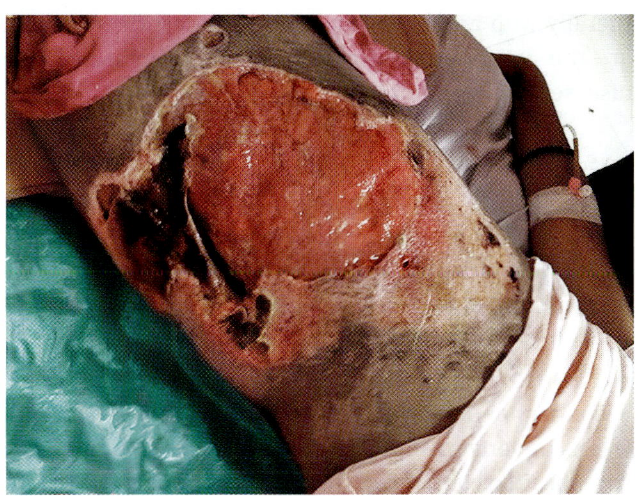

Fig. 6: Necrotizing fasciitis.

There is extensive tissue destruction and thrombosis of blood vessels, with rapid spread to abdominal wall, buttocks, or thighs through facial planes **(Fig. 7)**. Crepitus may be present and testicles are usually spared.[27]

Infection is polymicrobial which includes *Clostridium*, gram-negative bacilli, *Bacteroides*, and anaerobic Streptococci. Despite best of treatment, mortality ranges between 20 and 35%.

Foot Infection

Foot infections are extremely common in diabetics and the leading cause of lower limb amputations. Clinically manifest neuropathy is present in 25% of cases, and up to 40% of patients with a foot ulcer will require amputation within 3 years. The factors that contribute to increased susceptibility to foot infections are presence of peripheral neuropathy, peripheral vascular disease (PVD), minor trauma, and paronychia, which result in entrance of pathogens, leading to life-threatening infection.

Foot infections are classified into non-limb-threatening and limb-threatening infections. The non-limb-threatening infections are mild and superficial with minimum cellulitis of <2 cm and no evidence of systemic toxicity and vascular (ischemic) or bone involvement. The serious limb-threatening infections are severe and deep with >2 cm cellulitis with vascular, systemic, bone, and joint involvement **(Fig. 8)**.[28] Infections are mono- or polymicrobial.

Assessment of ischemic and neuropathic foot should be done. Samples for culture and sensitivity test from wounds should be sent, and deep-tissue biopsy is to be done if needed. Good glycemic control, broad-spectrum antibiotics (active against *S. aureus, Pseudomonas, and* enterococci), surgical debridement, and treatment of ischemia and neuropathy along with footwear advice are essential in all cases.

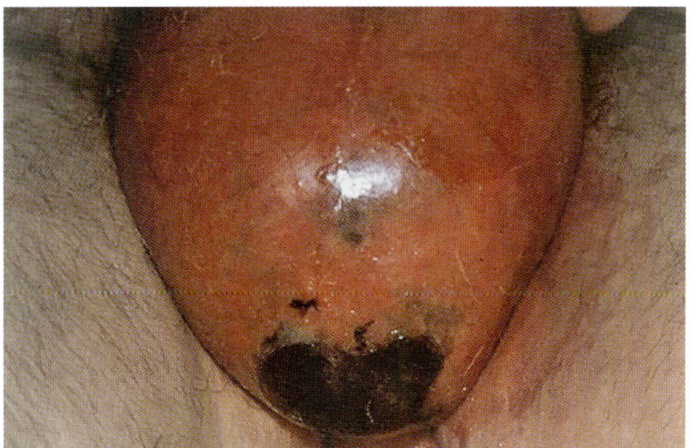

Fig. 7: Fournier's gangrene.

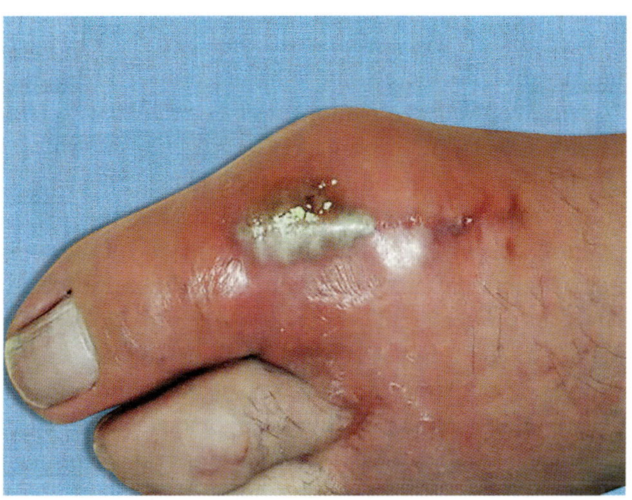

Fig. 8: Diabetic foot.

Malignant External Otitis

Malignant external otitis is an invasive infection of the external auditory canal and skull base, which typically occurs in elderly patients with DM. Majority of the cases are caused by *Pseudomonas*, sometimes secondary to colonization by *Aspergillus* of the external auditory canal, rarely by *S. aureus, Proteus mirabilis,* and *Klebsiella oxytoca*. Patients present with severe otalgia, otorrhea, and headache. The important predisposing factors are increased pH in diabetic cerumen, microangiopathy of ear canal, poor glycemic control, use of hearing aids, swimming in contaminated swimming pools, and use of nonsterile water for ear irrigation.

Management includes surgical debridement of necrotic tissue and appropriate antipseudomonal therapy (ciprofloxacin for 6–8 weeks and cefepime/ceftazidime if osteomyelitis is suspected).[29,30]

Rhino-orbital Cerebral Mucormycosis

Rhino-orbital cerebral mucormycosis (ROCM) is a rare, rapidly progressive and often fatal opportunistic fungal infection that usually occurs in immunocompromised patients. DM is the most common predisposing factor. It is caused by a fungus of the order Mucorales. *Mucor* is a ferrophilic, acidophilic, and angioinvasive fungus. Angioinvasion with thrombosis and tissue necrosis is the key pathological feature. Altered iron metabolism is a critical factor in the pathogenesis of patients with DM, particularly DKA.[31] The presenting features are nasal congestion, dark blood-tinged rhinorrhea or epistaxis, sinus tenderness, retro-orbital headache, fever, and malaise. Rapid extension into cranial cavity leads to neurological deficits like proptosis, ophthalmoplegia, visual loss, and cranial nerve palsies **(Fig. 9)**. Biopsy with histopathological examination of tissue collected from sinuses demonstrating wide, thick-walled, and ribbon-like aseptate hyphae branching at right angles establishes the diagnosis. CT and MRI scan of sinuses and brain can further aid in delineating the extension of lesion. Early diagnosis, rapid correction of glycemic status, medical therapy with amphotericin B, and surgical debridement are the cornerstone of management. If untreated, the disease is universally fatal.

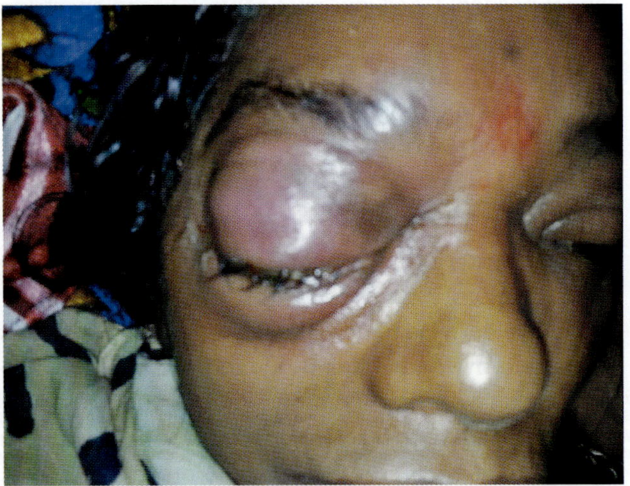

Fig. 9: Diabetic with ROCM showing proptosis and drooping of right eyelid. (ROCM: rhino-orbital cerebral mucormycosis)

Periodontal Infections

The increased susceptibility of periodontal disease in patients of DM is multifactorial. Periodontitis and gingivitis are associated with systemic and local inflammatory responses, thus adversely affecting glycemic status.[32]

Endophthalmitis

Secondary endophthalmitis by *E. coli* and *Klebsiella* with UTI as underlying sources of infection or as postoperative complications of cataract surgery is common in DM.[33]

Tuberculosis

Diabetes mellitus almost triples the risk of developing TB.[34] Although the definite pathophysiological mechanism of the effect of DM as a predisposing risk factor for TB is unknown, some hypotheses are suggested: Depressed cellular immunity, dysfunction of alveolar macrophages, low level of interferon-γ, pulmonary microangiopathy, and micronutrient deficiency.[35] In DM, TB has the following characteristics: Relative paucity of physical signs and diagnosis made at a far advanced stage, multilobar disease or presence of multiple cavities, limited pleural involvement, greater tendency of hemoptysis, less chance of extrapulmonary involvement and endobronchial TB, more cases of sputum-positive disease, more multidrug-resistant TB, treatment failures, or deaths. Treatment regimens are the same as those of nondiabetic patients. Rifampicin may affect glycemic control by increasing the metabolism of oral antidiabetic drugs.

Coronavirus

Studies during the COVID-19 pandemic have revealed that diabetes was associated with a higher mortality rate and adverse outcome. Between 13% and 58% of people with COVID-19 required ICU admission and between 17% and 35% of people who succumbed had preexisting diabetes. Globally, diabetes was responsible for 10% of severe forms and 17% of COVID-19-related death. Glycemic level appears to affect the outcome of COVID-19.[4]

CONCLUSION

Many specific infections and some exclusive ones are commonly seen in patients with diabetes. This predilection is due to various host factors and immune mechanisms. Some unique infections are associated with increased morbidity and mortality which need early recognition. Defective innate immunity contributes to increased susceptibility to infection, and mostly immune deficiencies are linked to glycemic control. Early recognition, judicious antimicrobial therapy, surgical intervention when necessary, and immunization schedule along with glycemic control are the cornerstones of management to reduce morbidity and mortality.

REFERENCES

1. World Health Organization. Immunodeficiency: Report of a scientific group. Technical report series 630. World Health Organ Tech Rep Ser. 1978;(630):3-80.
2. Muller LMAJ, Gorter KJ, Hak E, Goudzwaard WL, Schellevis FG, Hoepelman AI, et al. Increased risk of common infections in patients with Type 1 and Type 2 diabetes mellitus. Clin Infect Dis. 2005;41(3):281-8.
3. Bhadada SK. Acute infections in diabetes mellitus. In: Chandalia HB (Ed). RSSDI Textbook of Diabetes Mellitus, 3rd edition. New Delhi: Jaypee Brothers Medical Publishers; 2014. pp. 819-27.
4. Holt RIG, Cockram CS, Ma RCW, Luk AOY. Diabetes and infection: review of the epidemiology, mechanisms and principles of treatment. Diabetologia. 2024;67(7):1168-80.
5. Delamaire M, Maugendre D, Moreno M, Le Goff MC, Allannic H, Genetet B. Impaired leucocyte functions in diabetic patients. Diabet Med. 1997;14(1):29-34.
6. Geerlings SE, Hoepelman A. Immune dysfunction in patients with diabetes mellitus (DM). FEMS Immunol Med Microbiol. 1999;26(3-4):259-65.
7. Calvet HM, Yoshikawa TT. Infections in diabetes. Infect Dis Clin North Am. 2001;15 (2):407-21.
8. Stegenga ME, van der Crabben SN, Dessing MC, Pater JM, van den Pangaart PS, de Vos AF, et al. Effect of acute hyperglycemia and/or hyperinsulinemia on proinflammatory gene expression, cytokine production and neutrophil function in humans. Diabet Med. 2008; 25(2):157-64.
9. Graves DT, Naguib G, Lu H, Leone C, Hsue H, Krall E. Inflammation is more persistent in Type1 Diabetic mice. J Dent Res. 2005;84(4):324-8.
10. Geerlings SE, Brouwer EC, Van Kessel KC, Gaastra W, Stolk RP, Hoepelman AI. Cytokine secretion is impaired in women with diabetes mellitus. Eur J Clin Invest. 2000; 30(11):995-1001.
11. Hostetter MK. Handicaps to host defence. Effects of hyperglycemia on C3 and candida albicans. Diabetes. 1990;39:271-5.
12. Spatz M, Eibl N, Hink S, Wolf HM, Fischer GF, Mayr WR, et al. Impaired primary immune response in Type 1 Diabetes. Functional impairment at the level of APCs and T-cells. Cell Immunol. 2003;221(1):15-26.
13. Liberatore RR Jr, Barbosa SF, Alkimin Md, Bellinati-Pires R, Florido MP, Isaac L, et al. Is immunity in diabetic patients influencing the susceptibility to infections? Immunoglobulins, complement and phagocytic function in children and adolescents with Type1 Diabetes mellitus. Pediatr Diabetes. 2005;6(4):206-12.
14. Lapolla A, Tonani R, Fedela D, et al. Non-enzymatic glycation of IgG : an in -vivo study. Horm Metab Res. 2002; 34:260-4.
15. Matsumoto K, Sera Y, Miyake S, Ueki Y. Serum levels of adhesion molecules correlate with insulin resistance. Atherosclerosis. 2002;161:243-4.
16. Stegenga ME, van der Crabben SN, Blümer RM, Levi M, Meijers JC, Serlie MJ, et al. Hyperglycemia enhances coagulation and reduces neutrophil degranulation, whereas hyperinsulinemia inhibits fibrinolysis during human endotoxemia. Blood. 2008;112(1):82-9.
17. Geerlings SE. Urinary tract infections in patients with diabetes mellitus: Epidemiology, pathogenesis and treatment. Int Antimicrob Agents. 2008;31S:S54-7.
18. Woohead MA, Macfarlane JT, Mc Cracken JS, Rose DH, Finch RG. Prospective study of aetiology and outcome of pneumonia in the community. Lancet. 1987;1(8534):671-74
19. Fine MJ, Smith MA, Carson CA, Mutha SS, Sankey SS, Weissfeld LA, et al. Prognosis and outcome of patients with community-acquired pneumonia. A meta-analysis. JAMA. 1996;275(2):134-41.
20. Lee N, Chan PK, Hui DS, Rainer TH, Wong E, Choi KW, et al. Viral loads and duration of viral shedding in adult patients hospitalized with influenza. J Infect Dis. 2009; 200(4):492-500
21. Kozicl II, Kozicl MJ. Pulmonary complications of diabetes mellitus. Pneumonia. Infect Dis Clin North Am. 1995;9:65-96.
22. American Diabetes Association (ADA). Standards of medical care in diabetes. Diabetes Care. 2011;33:S11-61.
23. Ojetti V, Pellicano R, Fagoonee S, Migneco A, Berrutti M, Gasbarrini A. Helicobacter pylori infection and diabetes. Minerva Med. 2010;101(2):115-9.
24. Elhawary EI, Mahmoud GF, EI-Daly MA, Mekky FA, Esmat GG, Abdel-Hamid M. Association of HCV with diabetes mellitus: An Egyptian case control study. Virol J. 2011;8:367.
25. Wheat LJ. Infection and diabetes mellitus. Diabetes Care. 1980;3:187-97.
26. Giuliano A, Lewis F Jr, Hadley K, Blaisdell FW. Bacteriology of necrotizing fasciitis. Am J Surg. 1977;134(1):52-7.
27. Montoya CR, Izquierda ME, Nicolae PB, et al. Fournier's gangrene. Descriptive analysis of 20 cases and literature review. Actas Urol ESP. 2009;33:873-80.
28. Joseph WS, Lipsky BA. Medical therapy of diabetic foot infections. J Vasc Surg. 2010;52(3):S67-71.

29. Sapico F, Bessman A. Infections in the diabetic patient. Infect Dis Clin Pract. 1995;1:339.
30. Carfrae MJ, Kesser BW. Malignant otitis externa. Otolaryngol Clin North Am. 2008;41:537-49.
31. Gamaletsou MN, Sipsas NV, Roilides E, Walsh TJ. Rhino-Orbital-Cerebral-Mucormycosis. Curr Infect Dis Rep. 2012;14:423-34.
32. Nagasawa T, Noda M, Katagiri S, Takaichi M, Takahashi Y, Wara-Aswapati N, et al. Relationship between periodontitis and diabetes -importance of clinical study to prove the vicious cycle. Intern Med. 2010;49(10):881-5.
33. Karaclal H, Kymes SM, Apte RS. Retrospective analysis of etiopathogenesis of all cases of endophthalmitis at a large tertiary referral center. Int Ophthalmol. 2007;27:251-9.
34. Stevenson CR, Forouhi NG, Roglic G, Williams BG, Lauer JA, Dye C, et al. Diabetes and tuberculosis: the impact of the diabetic epidemic on tuberculosis incidence. BMC Public Health. 2007;7:234.
35. Ottmani SC, Murray MB, Jeon CY, Baker MA, Kapur A, Lönnroth K, et al. Consultation meeting on tuberculosis and diabetes mellitus: meeting summary and recommendations. Int J Tuber Lung Dis. 2010;14(12):1513-7.

Computed Tomography and Magnetic Resonance Imaging

CHAPTER 39

Cardiac Magnetic Resonance Imaging in Myocardial Viability

Priya Jagia, Akshit Kumar

INTRODUCTION

The rationale of myocardial viability assessment in individuals presenting with left ventricular (LV) systolic dysfunction secondary to ischemic cardiomyopathy stems from the advent of coronary revascularization. Revascularization of regions with dysfunctional yet viable myocardium holds the potential to augment LV function. The imaging techniques used for this purpose include stress echocardiography, perfusion scintigraphy, positron emission tomography (PET), and cardiac magnetic resonance imaging (CMR). This chapter will review the role of CMR in assessing myocardial viability and its significance in the currently established management protocols for ischemic heart disease.

NEED FOR VIABILITY IMAGING: THE CURRENT EVIDENCE

Ischemic cardiomyopathy has a high overall mortality of 62.5% in 10 years, even with guideline-directed medical therapy.[1] Coronary artery bypass grafting (CABG) is preferred in patients with profound LV dysfunction and multivessel coronary artery disease (CAD).[2]

A range of studies based on perfusion scintigraphy, PET, and a few CMR-based studies have shown improved function after revascularization. In a meta-analysis with more than 3,000 patients and a mean left ventricular ejection fraction (LVEF) of 32%, myocardial viability was assessed using thallium perfusion imaging, PET, or dobutamine echocardiography (but not CMR). It was found that in patients with viable myocardium who undergo revascularization, a reduction of 79.6% in annual mortality rate was observed as opposed to patients with viable myocardium who were treated medically.[3]

Recently, Gerber et al. concluded that survival rates were significantly lower in patients who were medically managed than revascularization in the presence of myocardial viability assessed by delayed enhancement (DE)-CMR. Patients were classified as having viable myocardium if at least four segments showing dysfunction had ≤50% transmural late gadolinium enhancement (LGE).[4]

However, the STICH (Surgical Treatment for Ischemic Heart Failure) trial study contradicted the results of previous retrospective studies and reported no impact of viability imaging on all-cause mortality in patients with ischemic severe heart failure (HF). Single-photon emission computed tomography (SPECT) or dobutamine echocardiography was used in the STICH trial for preoperative viability assessment, and surgical revascularization was compared to medical management in patients with an ejection fraction of <35%. The trial had several methodologic problems: The original study design, patient selection, and poor standardization of nuclear protocol. Also, there has been debate over whether employing imaging modalities like PET or CMR, which offer superior sensitivity and specificity, might have changed the study outcomes.

It is plausible that an actual interaction occurs between myocardial viability and the efficacy of revascularization; however, the therapeutic benefits of revascularization may not be comprehensively elucidated by a single myocardial viability assessment. This is particularly true when such assessments do not account for the spectrum of viability (rather than the mere presence or absence of viability) or the nuanced interplay between ischemic zones, collateral circulation, and the metabolic state of the myocardium. These factors collectively influence the potential for functional recovery post revascularization, thus requiring a more multidimensional approach to interpret the full therapeutic landscape.

Although the benefits of viability assessment on functional improvement after revascularization are not fully elucidated, the European Society of Cardiology (ESC)/

TABLE 1: European Society of Cardiology (ESC)/European Association for Cardio-Thoracic Surgery (EACTS) 2018 recommendations.

Recommendations	*Class of recommendation*	*Level of evidence*
Noninvasive stress imaging (CMR, stress echocardiography, SPECT, or PET) may be considered for the assessment of myocardial ischemia and viability in patients with HF and CAD (considered suitable for coronary revascularization) before the decision on revascularization	IIb	B

(CAD: coronary artery disease; CMR: cardiac magnetic resonance imaging; HF: heart failure; PET: positron emission tomography; SPECT: single-photon emission computed tomography)

European Association for Cardio-Thoracic Surgery (EACTS) 2018 Guidelines **(Table 1)** on myocardial revascularization recommend the use of noninvasive stress imaging in patients with HF and CAD before deciding on revascularization (class IIb level B recommendation).[5]

MYOCARDIAL VIABILITY

The term "viable myocardium" is used for severely ischemic myocardium, which is dysfunctional at baseline, but its function recovers with time either spontaneously (myocardial stunning) or following revascularization (hibernating myocardium).

Myocardial stunning is a viable myocardium in a state of perfusion-contraction mismatch, where transient myocardial dysfunction occurs after severe ischemia or a brief coronary artery occlusion, followed by a restoration of normal myocardial perfusion. No significant ultrastructural alterations exist in the stunned myocardium, and functional recovery is usually spontaneous after several hours or days. Stunned myocardium has a good contractile reserve that can be elicited by catecholamines (dobutamine or epinephrine).[6]

Hibernating myocardium is also a viable myocardium in a state of persistent dysfunction due to chronic reduction of myocardial perfusion, or flow reserve. Herein, the myocyte metabolism is impaired, and the myocardium utilizes glucose rather than free fatty acids, termed a flow-metabolic mismatch.

Myocardial hibernation was first thought to be an adaptive mechanism for chronic reduction in resting myocardial flow. However, studies have shown that chronic dysfunction can also develop after repeated episodes of transient ischemia due to impaired coronary vasodilator reserve. So, reduced flow reserve and not necessarily reduced perfusion at rest can result in chronic myocardial dysfunction.[7] Ultrastructural changes like reduced number and function of mitochondria, intracellular glycogen accumulation, or intercellular fibrosis may be present. The contractile reserve is usually present but depends on the extent of fibrosis, beta-receptor density, and flow reserve.[8] After dobutamine, hibernating myocardium shows a biphasic response—transient increase in myocardial thickening, followed by reduced contraction due to increased oxygen demand in the presence of low flow reserve.

CARDIAC MAGNETIC RESONANCE IMAGING TOOLS FOR MYOCARDIAL VIABILITY IMAGING

Thickness and Transmurality of Scar

The concept of the "wave front phenomenon of myocardial death" explains how the size of an infarct grows from the endocardium and progresses outward to the epicardium as the duration of coronary blockage increases.[9] Thinning of the LV wall is a characteristic feature of chronic, transmural myocardial infarction (MI) that develops after 3–6 months of remodeling.[10]

Healed nontransmural infarcts usually do not develop severe thinning, and some layers of epicardial myocardium are preserved. Therefore, preserved myocardial rim on late gadolinium images in a patient with a known chronic infarct represents nontransmural infarction.

Nonetheless, in some instances, patients with minor subendocardial infarctions might exhibit regional wall thinning even with significant (>50% of wall thickness) viable myocardium remaining, as reported by Kim et al. In their study, the diastolic LV wall thickness measured on LGE-CMR was only 5 mm, with the subendocardial scar extending just 1.5 mm into the myocardium, suggesting considerable viable tissue. This viable myocardium showed functional recovery postrevascularization.[11]

Shah et al., in their study, found that if the transmural extent of the infarct is ≤50% of total myocardium, complete recovery of function with an increase in end-diastolic wall thickness may occur following revascularization.[12] However, in a study where CMR was done in patients after

3 months of revascularization, out of 125 segments with an end-diastolic wall thickness of <5.5 mm, only 12 segments recovered. The end-diastolic wall thickness ≥5.5 mm has a negative predictive accuracy of 90% but a positive predictive accuracy of only 62% for predicting recovery after revascularization.[13]

This is because measuring myocardial wall thickness via standard CMR imaging does not delineate the extent of viable myocardium since it includes both viable and nonviable tissue within the measurement. Gadolinium-enhanced CMR is essential to identify the remaining viable myocardial rim's thickness. This contrast between enhanced (scarred) and nonenhanced (viable) myocardium allows for precise differentiation of the viable rim **(Figs. 1 and 2)**.

Contractile Reserve of Myocardium

Viable myocardium responds to sympathomimetics with increased contractility; scarred tissue does not; the commonly used sympathomimetic agent is low-dose

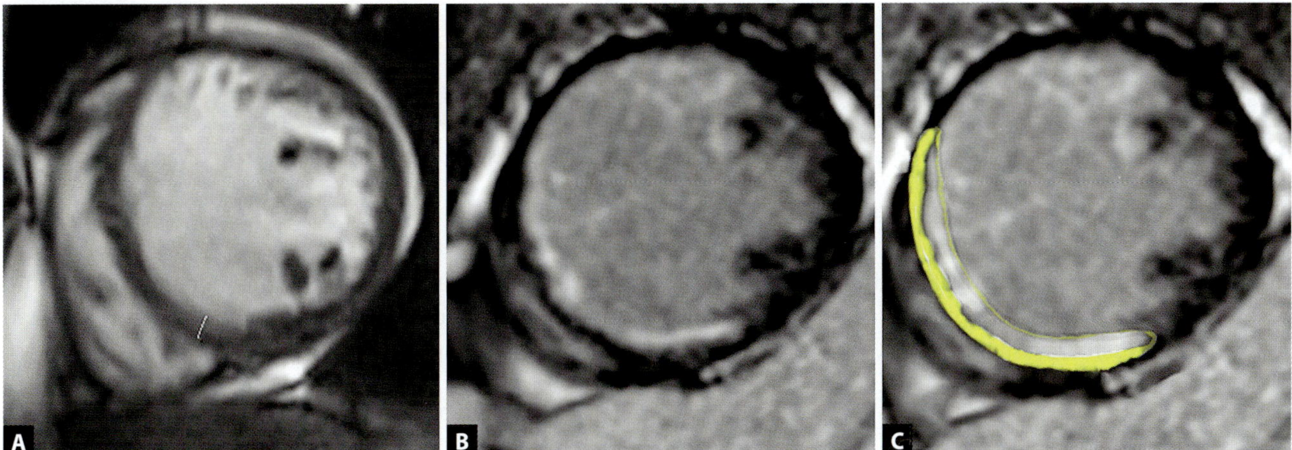

Figs. 1A to C: (A) Short-axis end-diastolic cine image showing thinned-out (measures 5.4 mm) basal septal segments; (B) and (C) Short-axis LGE images show >50% thick subendocardial scar with a preserved thin rim of the myocardium. (LGE: late gadolinium enhancement)
Note: Even a thinned-out septum can preserve the myocardium. Thus, the extent of transmurality of the scar is a more reliable predictor of viability than the absolute thickness of the myocardium.

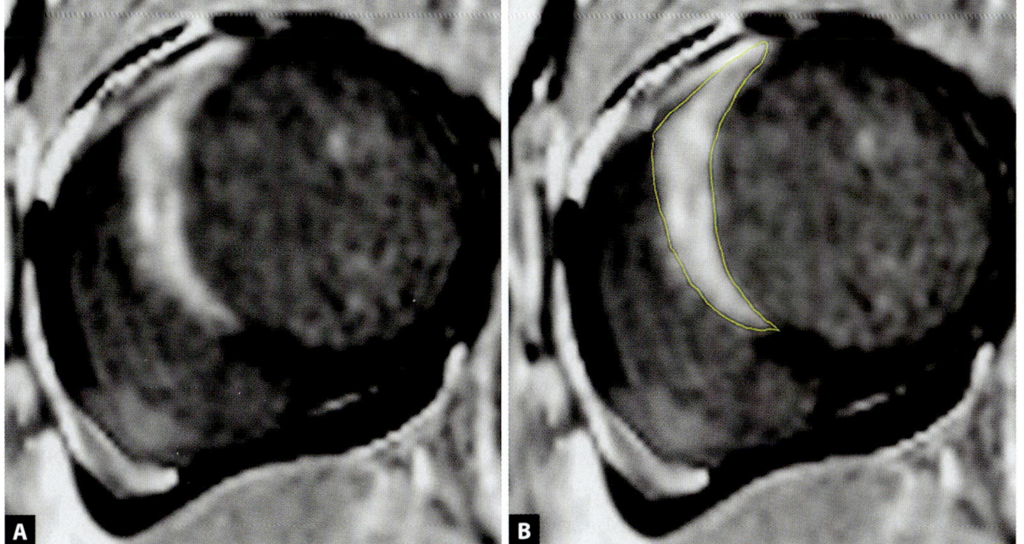

Figs. 2A and B: Short-axis LGE images show a transmural scar with no preserved rim of the myocardium. (LGE: late gadolinium enhancement)
Note: Scar thickness >75% is a poor predictor of viability.

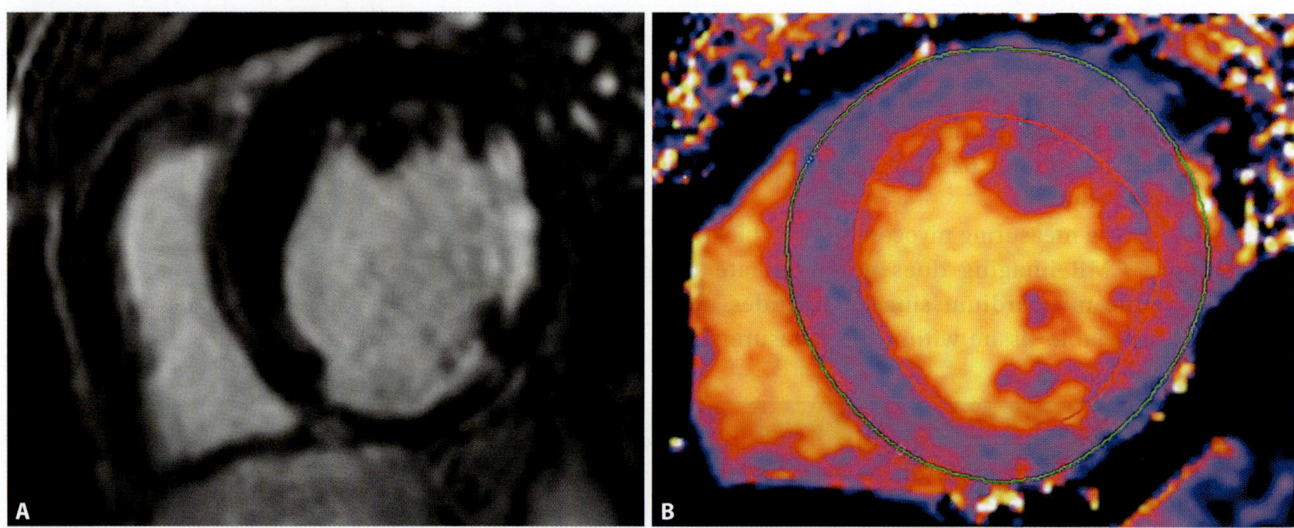

Figs. 3A and B: (A) Short-axis LGE images show subendocardial scar; (B) The corresponding T1 map shows raised values, depicted by orange shade with normal myocardium as violet.
Note: Parametric mapping can help predict the extent of infarct.

dobutamine (5–10 μg/kg/min). If there is contractile reserve, the heart muscle typically regains its function following successful revascularization.

Myocardial Edema

Early signs of ischemia include intracellular edema and sarcolemmal rupture, visible within 30–120 minutes via electron microscopy. T2-weighted (T2W) CMR sequences can detect this edema, differentiating acute from chronic myocardial infarcts.

Late Gadolinium Enhancement in Infarcted Tissue

Gadolinium chelates are extracellular magnetic resonance imaging (MRI) contrast agents that shorten both T1 and T2 relaxation times. During the acute phase of myocardial injury, the rupture of myocyte membranes increases the volume where gadolinium can distribute, leading to a more significant shortening of these relaxation times. Chronic myocardial scars are primarily composed of fibroblasts and collagen, with significant intercellular spaces, which retain gadolinium than the normal myocardium, where tightly packed myocytes restrict its penetration.

In normal myocardium, contrast agent wash-in and wash-out achieve constant enhancement within 2–3 minutes postinjection. During the initial phase of contrast wash-in, infarcted areas appear dark due to delayed uptake. However, approximately 10 minutes after injection, as contrast begins to wash out from normal myocardium, the infarcted regions become bright, and this hyperenhancement persists into the later stages of contrast wash-out.

Native T1 Mapping

The T1 mapping values increase both in acute infarcts and chronic fibrotic infarcts scar relative to normal myocardium, and therefore, increased T1 times may identify nonviable myocardium in acute or chronic, similar to LGE **(Figs. 3A and B)**. This approach has the advantage of not requiring the injection of contrast. The main disadvantage is the poor specificity for scars since increases in T1 mapping values are also seen in myocarditis, infiltrative disorders, etc.

VIABLE MYOCARDIUM IN ACUTE MYOCARDIAL INFARCTION

Primary percutaneous coronary intervention (PCI) is the preferred treatment for ST-elevation myocardial infarction (STEMI); however, in a subset of patients who present late or those with multivessel CAD, urgent CABG might be necessary. In these scenarios, assessing myocardial viability during the acute phase of MI is advisable before proceeding with such a significant procedure for these high-risk individuals.

Late Gadolinium Enhancement

The magnitude of infarction, as depicted by LGE-MRI, can forecast the potential for recovery of contractile function. In a study by Choi et al., it was found that the recovery of function at 2–3 months postinfarction was inversely proportional to the extent of myocardial damage as measured by LGE within 1 week of the acute event.[14] However, LGE imaging tends to overestimate the extent of MI during the early stage of STEMI. Thus, if a transmural threshold of ≤50% is applied to determine myocardial viability in acute MI, there is the possibility of overestimating the number of nonviable segments. The cutoff of ≤75% transmural extent was suggested by a study[15] on the acute scan with a very good sensitivity of 98% but a specificity of 66%.

T2–Late Gadolinium Enhancement Mismatch

There is an increased water content in acute infarct, leading to increased signal intensity on T2W images acquired within 10 days.

A mismatch where there is a high T2 signal without corresponding LGE, suggests areas of reversible injury or acute ischemia where the tissue might still be salvageable (ischemic area at risk). Combining T2 and LGE techniques may help to quantify the salvaged myocardium after reperfusion.

However, it is difficult to detect and precisely quantify the myocardial edema because of the poor contrast between normal and diseased myocardium and also due to artifacts of T2W images.

According to the Duke University study, there was no significant correlation ($p = 0.97$) between the extent of regions with high T2 signal and the area at risk for ischemia as the water content in reversibly injured heart tissue only rises by about 9% within the first 24 hours postevent. However, there was a robust correlation ($p < 0.0001$) with actual infarction, where the water content in the infarcted myocardium dramatically increased by 88%.[16] The standard errors in acquiring and interpreting T2W images are probably the reason for this. Thus, T2W imaging to quantify salvageable myocardium in acute MI is unreliable.

The emerging T2 mapping techniques could address the shortcomings associated with traditional T2W imaging.

VIABLE MYOCARDIUM IN CHRONIC MYOCARDIAL INFARCTION

Myocardial Wall Thickness

Chronic transmural infarcts are very thin due to remodeling. The end-diastolic wall thickness of >5.5 mm has >90% negative predictive value for transmural infarction, and in wall thickness <5.5 mm, the LGE images should be employed for detection of viable myocardium.

Contractile Reserve during Low-dose Dobutamine Infusion

Myocardial wall thickening in response to low-dose dobutamine infusion is also a marker for viability. Dobutamine CMR has an 89% sensitivity and a 94% specificity for predicting the recovery of function postrevascularization, using the recovery of wall thickening as the gold standard.[17]

Late Gadolinium Enhancement in Chronic Infarction

Late gadolinium enhancement-CMR not only helps quantify the infarct but also allows for differentiation between ischemic and nonischemic cardiomyopathy based on its location (subendocardial to transmural) and distribution (following coronary territory).

A ≤50% transmural extent of LGE is the cutoff used for defining viability in patients with stable CAD. Kim et al. showed that the likelihood of functional recovery is 10% of segments with 51–75% transmural extent of infarction after revascularization. Patients with >75% infarct extent and dysfunction did not recover after revascularization.[18]

COMPARISON OF DIFFERENT CARDIAC MAGNETIC RESONANCE IMAGING TECHNIQUES FOR MYOCARDIAL VIABILITY

A meta-analysis of 24 CMR studies involving 698 patients (11 studies employed LGE, 9 included dobutamine CMR, and 4 included wall thickness) concluded that LGE-CMR has the highest sensitivity and negative predictive value (95% and 90%, respectively) for predicting improvements in LV contractility postrevascularization.[19] End-diastolic wall thickness measurements were followed regarding sensitivity and negative predictive value, while low-dose dobutamine CMR was the least sensitive and had the lowest negative predictive value among the three. Conversely, for specificity and positive predictive value, low-dose dobutamine CMR led with 91% and 93%, respectively, followed by LGE-CMR, with end-diastolic wall thickness measurements showing the lowest values for these parameters.

Even with strong evidence backing the use of viability imaging to choose patients for revascularization, there is a significant reduction in the accuracy of predicting functional recovery after revascularization in patients with severe reduction of LV function (LVEF).

Research comparing LGE-CMR with a 25% transmurality threshold to low-dose dobutamine CMR (at 5 and 10 μg/kg/min) revealed that in patients with severely compromised ventricles, dobutamine CMR has lower sensitivity but maintains a high specificity of approximately 90%. LGE-CMR demonstrates superior accuracy for this group compared to dobutamine CMR.[20]

Late gadolinium enhancement-CMR has the advantage that it does not require pharmacologic stress and is also less observer-dependent for interpretation.

Both dobutamine and LGE-CMR can serve as complementary methods for assessing myocardial viability. The probability of seeing an improvement in contraction after administering dobutamine is most significant in heart segments with minor subendocardial scarring, lowest in those with complete transmural scarring, and moderate in segments with an intermediate scar extent. Kaandorp et al. suggest a combined LGE and dobutamine CMR algorithm to optimally predict outcomes in segments with an intermediate extent of scar **(Flowchart 1)**.[21]

Flowchart 1: Combined use of LGE and low-dose dobutamine CMR. Patients with <25% scar and >75% scar have low and high chances of recovery after revascularization, respectively. Patients who have intermediate probability (scar extent of 25–75% on LGE) should undergo low dobutamine CMR for better assessment of myocardial viability.

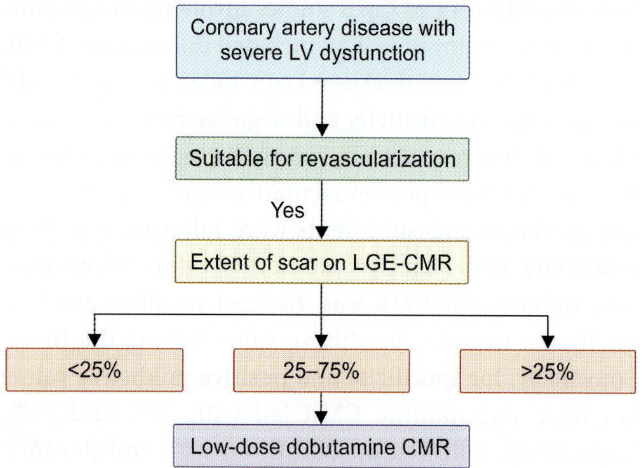

(CMR: cardiac magnetic resonance imaging; LGE: late gadolinium enhancement; LV: left ventricular)

CONCLUSION

Cardiac magnetic resonance imaging provides a thorough assessment of patients with ischemic heart disease, distinguishing it from nonischemic conditions, evaluating myocardial viability, quantifying scar tissue, and thereby aiding in prognosis. CMR's ability to characterize tissue helps identify microvascular obstruction and intramyocardial hemorrhage, which carry prognostic significance. Employing both dobutamine stress and LGE-CMR within the diagnostic framework can enhance the precision in detecting viable myocardium.

Although CMR-specific data remains limited, the STICH trial raised doubts about the clinical utility of viability imaging for enhancing patient outcomes. Future research with CMR could shed more light on the interplay between myocardial viability, ischemia, and their impact on patient management strategies.

REFERENCES

1. Velazquez EJ, Lee KL, Jones RH, Al-Khalidi HR, Hill JA, Panza JA, et al.; STICHES Investigators. Coronary-Artery Bypass Surgery in Patients with Ischemic Cardiomyopathy. N Engl J Med. 2016;374(16):1511-20.
2. Lawton JS, Tamis-Holland JE, Bangalore S, Bates ER, Beckie TM, Bischoff JM, et al. 2021 ACC/AHA/SCAI Guideline for Coronary Artery Revascularization: A Report of the American College of Cardiology/American Heart Association Joint Committee on Clinical Practice Guidelines. Circulation. 2022;145(3):e4-e17.
3. Allman KC, Shaw LJ, Hachamovitch R, Udelson JE. Myocardial viability testing and impact of revascularization on prognosis in patients with coronary artery disease and left ventricular dysfunction: a meta-analysis. J Am Coll Cardiol. 2002;39(7):1151-8.
4. Gerber BL, Rousseau MF, Ahn SA, le Polain de Waroux JB, Pouleur AC, et al. Prognostic Value of Myocardial Viability by Delayed-Enhanced Magnetic Resonance in Patients With Coronary Artery Disease and Low Ejection Fraction: impact of revascularization therapy. J Am Coll Cardiol. 2012;59(9):825-35.
5. Neumann FJ, Sousa-Uva M, Ahlsson A, Alfonso F, Banning AP, Benedetto U, et al.; ESC Scientific Document Group. 2018 ESC/EACTS Guidelines on myocardial revascularization. Eur Heart J. 2019;40(2):87-165.
6. Ito H, Tomooka T, Sakai N, Higashino Y, Fujii K, Katoh O, et al. Time course of functional improvement in stunned myocardium in risk area in patients with reperfused anterior infarction. Circulation. 1993;87(2):355-62.
7. Vanoverschelde JL, Wijns W, Depré C, Essamri B, Heyndrickx GR, Borgers M, et al. Mechanisms of chronic

regional postischemic dysfunction in humans. New insights from the study of noninfarcted collateral-dependent myocardium. Circulation. 1993;87(5):1513-23.

8. Flameng W, Suy R, Schwarz F, Borgers M, Piessens J, Thone F, et al. Ultrastructural correlates of left ventricular contraction abnormalities in patients with chronic ischemic heart disease: determinants of reversible segmental asynergy postrevascularization surgery. Am Heart J. 1981;102(5):846-57.
9. Reimer KA, Lowe JE, Rasmussen MM, Jennings RB. The wavefront phenomenon of ischemic cell death. 1. Myocardial infarct size vs duration of coronary occlusion in dogs. Circulation. 1977;56(5):786-94.
10. Jáuregui B, Soto-Iglesias D, Penela D, Acosta J, Fernández-Armenta J, Linhart M, et al. Follow-Up After Myocardial Infarction to Explore the Stability of Arrhythmogenic Substrate: The Footprint Study. JACC Clin Electrophysiol. 2020;6(2):207-18.
11. Kim RJ, Shah DJ. Fundamental concepts in myocardial viability assessment revisited: when knowing how much is "alive" is not enough. Heart. 2004;90(2):137-40.
12. Shah DJ, Kim HW, James O, Parker M, Wu E, Bonow RO, et al. Prevalence of Regional Myocardial Thinning and Relationship With Myocardial Scarring in Patients With Coronary Artery Disease. JAMA. 2013;309(9):909-18.
13. Baer FM, Theissen P, Schneider CA, Voth E, Sechtem U, Schicha H, et al. Dobutamine Magnetic Resonance Imaging Predicts Contractile Recovery of Chronically Dysfunctional Myocardium After Successful Revascularization. J Am Coll Cardiol. 1998;31(5):1040-8.
14. Choi KM, Kim RJ, Gubernikoff G, Vargas JD, Parker M, Judd RM. Transmural Extent of Acute Myocardial Infarction Predicts Long-Term Improvement in Contractile Function. Circulation. 2001;104(10):1101-7.
15. Bulluck H, Rosmini S, Abdel-Gadir A, Bhuva AN, Treibel TA, Fontana M, et al. Redefining viability by cardiovascular magnetic resonance in acute ST-segment elevation myocardial infarction. Sci Rep. 2017;7(1):14676.
16. Kim HW, Van Assche L, Jennings RB, Wince WB, Jensen CJ, Rehwald WG, et al. Relationship of T2-Weighted MRI Myocardial Hyperintensity and the Ischemic Area-At-Risk. Circ Res. 2015;117(3):254-65.
17. Baer FM, Voth E, Schneider CA, Theissen P, Schicha H, Sechtem U, et al. Comparison of Low-Dose Dobutamine–Gradient-Echo Magnetic Resonance Imaging and Positron Emission Tomography With [18F]Fluorodeoxyglucose in Patients With Chronic Coronary Artery Disease. A functional and morphological approach to the detection of residual myocardial viability. Circulation. 1995;91(4):1006-15.
18. Kim RJ, Wu E, Rafael A, Chen EL, Parker MA, Simonetti O, et al. The Use of Contrast-Enhanced Magnetic Resonance Imaging to Identify Reversible Myocardial Dysfunction. N Engl J Med. 2000;343(20):1445-53.
19. Romero J, Xue X, Gonzalez W, Garcia MJ. CMR Imaging Assessing Viability in Patients With Chronic Ventricular Dysfunction Due to Coronary Artery Disease: A Meta-Analysis of Prospective Trials. JACC Cardiovasc Imaging. 2012;5(5):494-508.
20. Wellnhofer E, Olariu A, Klein C, Gräfe M, Wahl A, Fleck E, et al. Magnetic resonance low-dose dobutamine test is superior to SCAR quantification for the prediction of functional recovery. Circulation. 2004;109(18):2172-4.
21. Kaandorp TAM, Bax JJ, Schuijf JD, Viergever EP, van Der Wall EE, de Roos A, et al. Head-to-head comparison between contrast-enhanced magnetic resonance imaging and dobutamine magnetic resonance imaging in men with ischemic cardiomyopathy. Am J Cardiol. 2004;93(12):1461-4.

Imaging in Valvular Heart Disease

Johann Christopher, Preeti Neve, Reefa Dsouza

INTRODUCTION

Valvular heart disease evaluation and treatment has made a marked resurgence in the last decade with the onset of structural heart intervention. Prior to this, the waning cases of rheumatic heart disease due to better socioeconomic conditions had pushed it into the background compared to coronary artery disease which has enjoyed the limelight.

The purpose of this review is to summarize the multimodality options that are currently available to evaluate cases of valvular heart disease.[1] We will approach imaging in valvular heart disease by looking at each of the valves individually and highlight the add on value of multimodality imaging over and above the industry standard, i.e., transthoracic echocardiogram (TTE).[2] The aim is to think beyond echocardiogram to an integrated approach to imaging in valvular heart disease.[3]

AORTIC VALVE DISEASE

Aortic Stenosis

Transthoracic echocardiography is the primary tool to evaluate the aortic valve in all its entirety. However, there are situations due to a poor echo window, prior to transcatheter aortic valve replacement (TAVR) procedure and where there is a discrepancy between clinical evaluation and echocardiogram finding where multimodality imaging will be utilized.

Cardiac MRI [cardiac magnetic resonance (CMR)] and cardiac CT [computed tomography angiography (CTA)] can be used interchangeably as the situation demands and the equipment and expertise of a particular center.

Etiology of Aortic Stenosis

- *Rheumatic aortic stenosis (AS):* Isolated AS 3rd most common valve lesion 73% associated mitral stenosis in most cases
- *Degenerative AS:* 65% most common cause; male preponderance rooted in all groups

Severity of Aortic Stenosis

- *Mild:* 1.5–2 cm^2
- *Moderate:* 1.5–1 cm^2
- *Severe:* <1 cm^2

Indications for Aortic Valve Replacement

Severe AS has an unoperated event free survival of 82%, 67%, and 33% at 1, 3, and 5 years.

- *Ib-symptomatic patient with severe AS with either:*
  - Decreased systole opening of a calcified stenotic aortic valve
  - Aortic velocity of 4 m/s or greater or mean pressure gradient 40 mm Hg or higher
  - Symptoms of congestive heart failure (CHF), syncope , edema , angina, or palpitation associated with moderate AS.
- Asymptomatic patients with severe AS and left ventricular ejection fraction (LVEF) <50% with decreased valve opening and an aortic valve velocity ≥4 m/s or mean pressure gradient of 40 mm Hg or higher.
- Severe AS when undergoing cardiac surgery for other indications when there is decreased systolic opening of a calcified aortic valve and an aortic velocity 4.0 m/s or greater or mean pressure gradient of 40 mm Hg or higher.

ROLE OF MULTIMODALITY IMAGING

Valve Area

- *Planimetry:* Cine CMR stack of thin perpendicular slices over the left ventricular outflow tract (LVOT) focusing on the aortic valve will give a series of valve orifices on which a planimetry can be performed[4] **(Figs. 1A and B)**. It can also be done by non-contrast CT (calcium scoring protocol) or by contrast CT where you can get valve morphology (bicuspid vs.

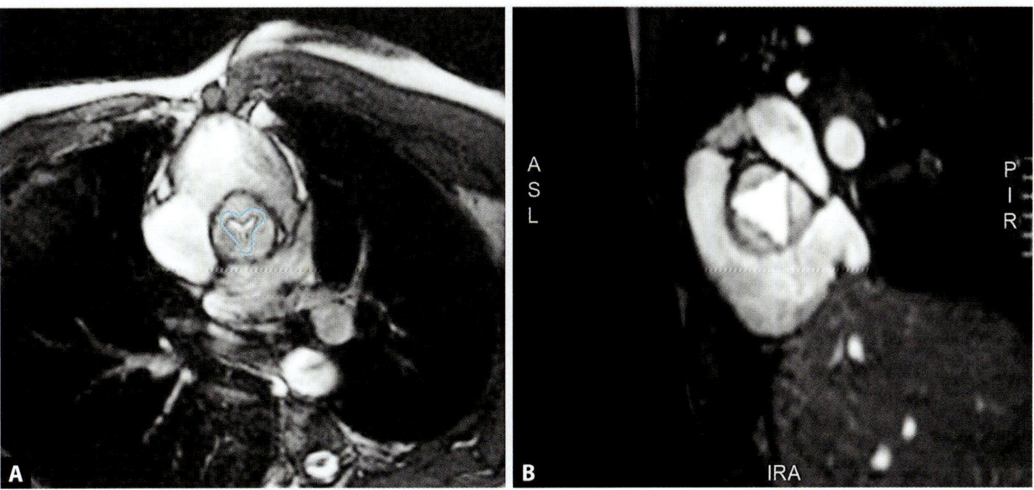

Figs. 1A and B: Aortic valve planimetry by cardiac magnetic resonance (CMR).

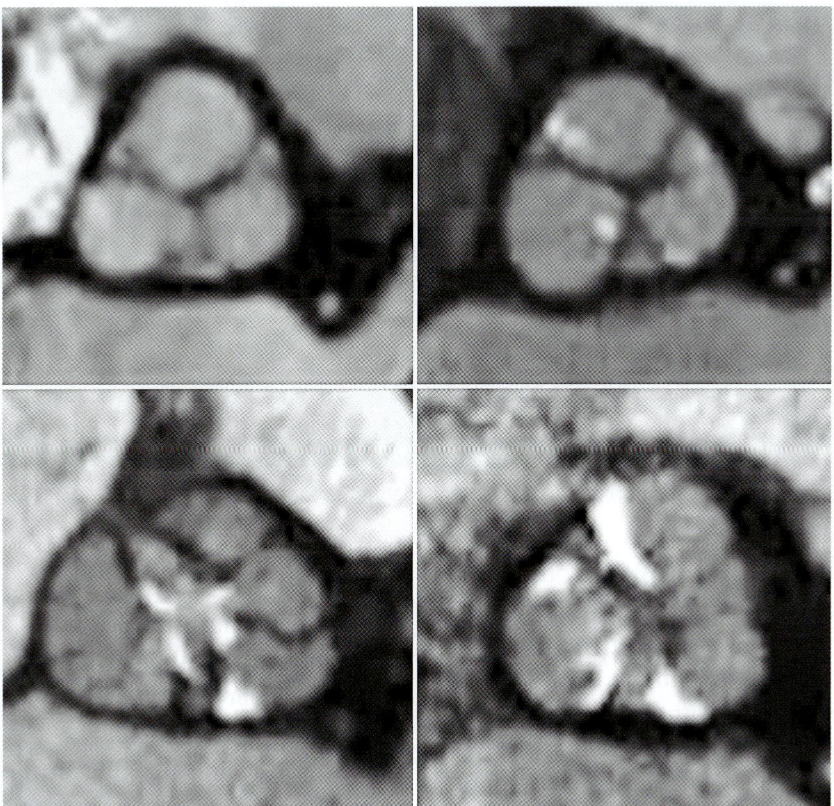

Fig. 2: Aortic valve evaluation by contrast computed tomography angiography (CTA).

tricuspid) and the distribution of calcium (leaflet vs. commissural) **(Fig. 2)**. The non-contrast protocol can give the calcium score which can distinguish a moderate over a severe stenosis (2,065 Agatston units in males and 1,275 Agatston units in females)[5] **(Fig. 3)**.

Positron emission tomography (PET) imaging of the valve with 18 F-fluoride can provide evidence of ongoing inflammation and calcification in the valve which can be a surrogate marker to the use of statin therapy for the stabilization of AS.[6]

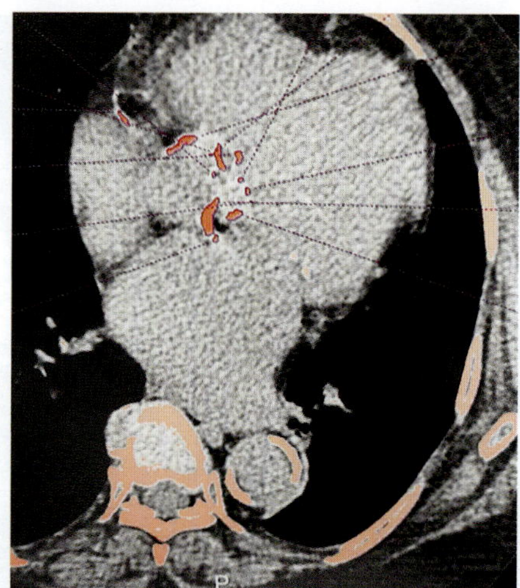

Fig. 3: Calcium scoring of aortic valve by non-contrast computed tomography angiography (CTA).

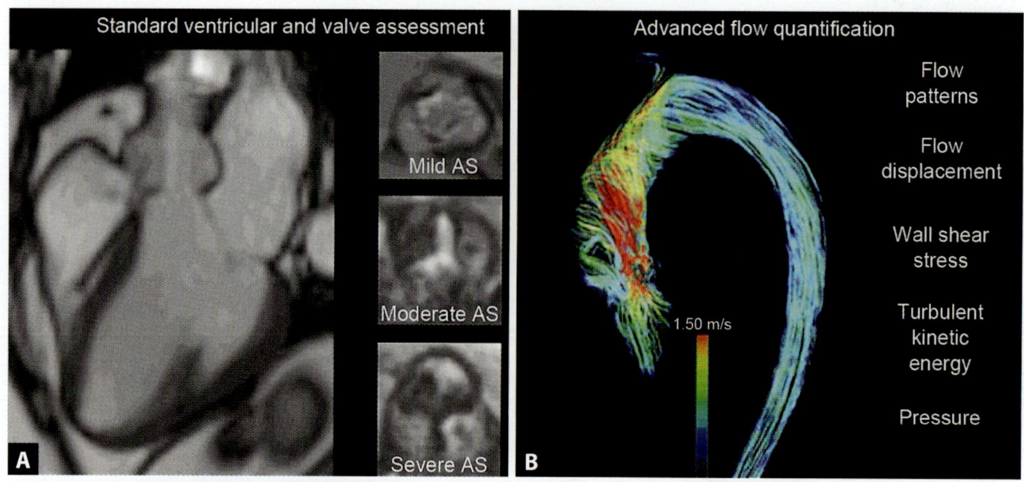

Figs. 4A and B: Aortic valve evaluation by (A) Cine cardiac magnetic resonance (CMR); (B) 4D CMR. (AS: aortic stenosis)

- *Gradient:* The TTE gives a standard peak transaortic velocity, mean gradient, and the effective orifice area. However, these measures give discordant results in certain clinical situations.[7] Transvalvular velocity can be measured with a velocity mapping technique (VENC) although peak velocity may be less accurate compared to continuous wave Doppler echocardiogram due to the small width of very high velocity jets (partial volume effects), lower temporal resolution and artifacts from turbulent jets[8] **(Figs. 4A and B)**. The continuity equation can be used with CMR for evaluation of gradients as direct evaluation of LVOT area which is an ellipsoid, would be more accurate than echo. Care must be taken to avoid aliasing by choosing the appropriate VENC value (150–350 cm/s).[9]

Valve Pathophysiology

Cardiac magnetic resonance and CTA are very exquisite in ascertaining the pathology in the valvular, supravalvular and subvalvular portion of the valve, especially if there is an associated root pathology.

The CMR cine imaging in the oblique plane can easily visualize the proximal ascending aorta and LVOT[10] **(Figs. 5A and B)**. The site of velocity acceleration can be accurately located by the in-plane velocity mapping. CMR can accurately evaluate the ascending aorta which may be dilated especially with an associated bicuspid aortic valve and may impact surgical planning for valve replacement by indicating additional root replacement. Except for linear, mobile masses such as vegetations (better visualized by

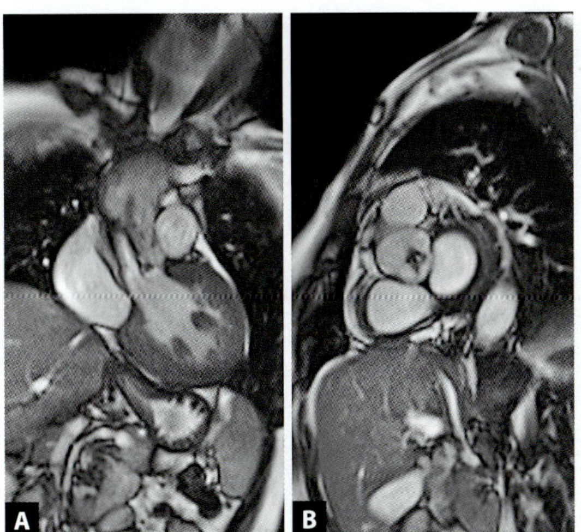

Figs. 5A and B: Qualitative aortic valve evaluation by cine cardiac magnetic resonance (CMR); (A) left ventricular outflow tract (LVOT) view; (B) Short axis (SAX) view.

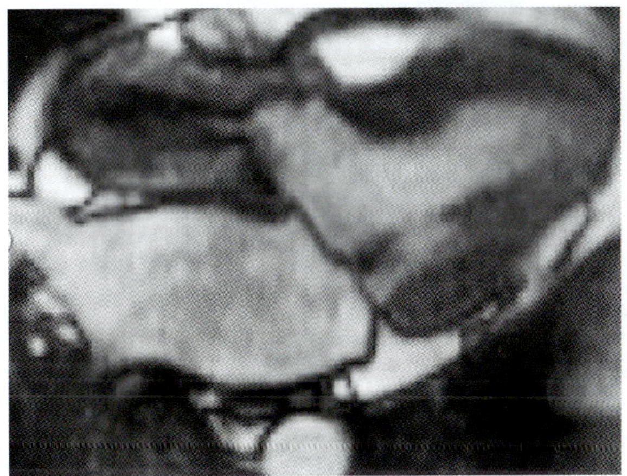

Fig. 6: Cine cardiac magnetic resonance (CMR) evaluation of a rheumatic aortic valve with severe aortic stenosis (AS).

TTE due to its superior temporal resolution) most other pathologies can be easily identified through a variety of sequences on CMR **(Fig. 6)**.

Left Ventricular Volumetry and Left Ventricular Mass Evaluation

Highly accurate left ventricular (LV) mass measurement provides a more precise and sensitive measure of the effect of AS on the LV rather than the measure of wall thickness alone. LV mass is a more reproducible measure for sequentially following up patients with AS. Volumetry involving nine slices of LV with 5 mm thickness is extremely accurate and reproducible for longitudinal follow-up compared to TTE.[11]

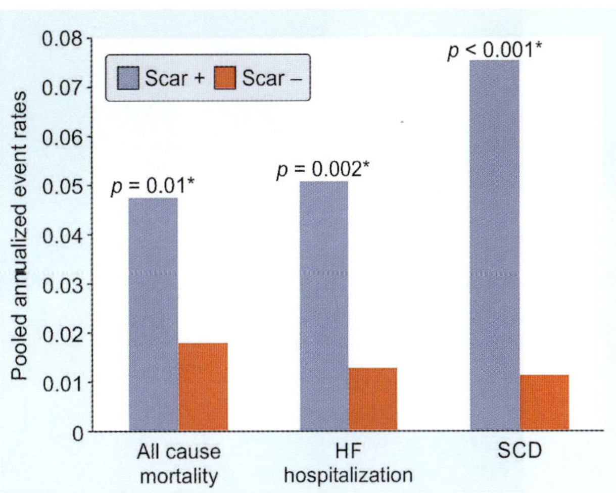

Fig. 7: Prognostic significance of late gadolinium enhancement (LGE).

*p-values are for the significance of annualized event rate difference between LGE + and LGE- subjects.

Source: Kuruvilla S, Adenaw N, Katwal AB, Lipinski MJ, Kramer CM, Salerno M. Late gadolinium enhancement on cardiac magnetic resonance predicts adverse cardiovascular outcomes in nonischemic cardiomyopathy: a systematic review and meta-analysis. Circ Cardiovasc Imaging. 2014;7:250-8.

Late Gadolinium Enhancement

Late gadolinium enhancement (LGE) imaging is performed 10 minutes after the injection of gadolinium to assess myocardial interstitial or replacement fibrosis. Patients with AS have shown midmyocardial LGE enhancement as opposed to subendocardial LGE in patients with ischemic heart disease (IHD), in up to a third of patients. Presence of LGE is an important prognostic marker in the natural history of AS. The mere presence of LGE should prompt early aortic valve replacement (AVR) in patients with even moderate AS while the absence of LGE ensures good postoperative recovery. Extensive LGE deposition signifies poor outcome even after AVR[12] **(Fig. 7)**.

Role of Computed Tomography Angiography in Transcatheter Aortic Valve Replacement Evaluation

Computed tomography angiography is already used in clinical practice if the ascending aorta is not well imaged on TTE or to check the aortic diameter when approaching a surgical threshold. It may be better to use CTA when considering referral for aortic valve surgery since this can also detect calcium in the ascending aorta and identify porcelain aorta as an indication for a transcatheter

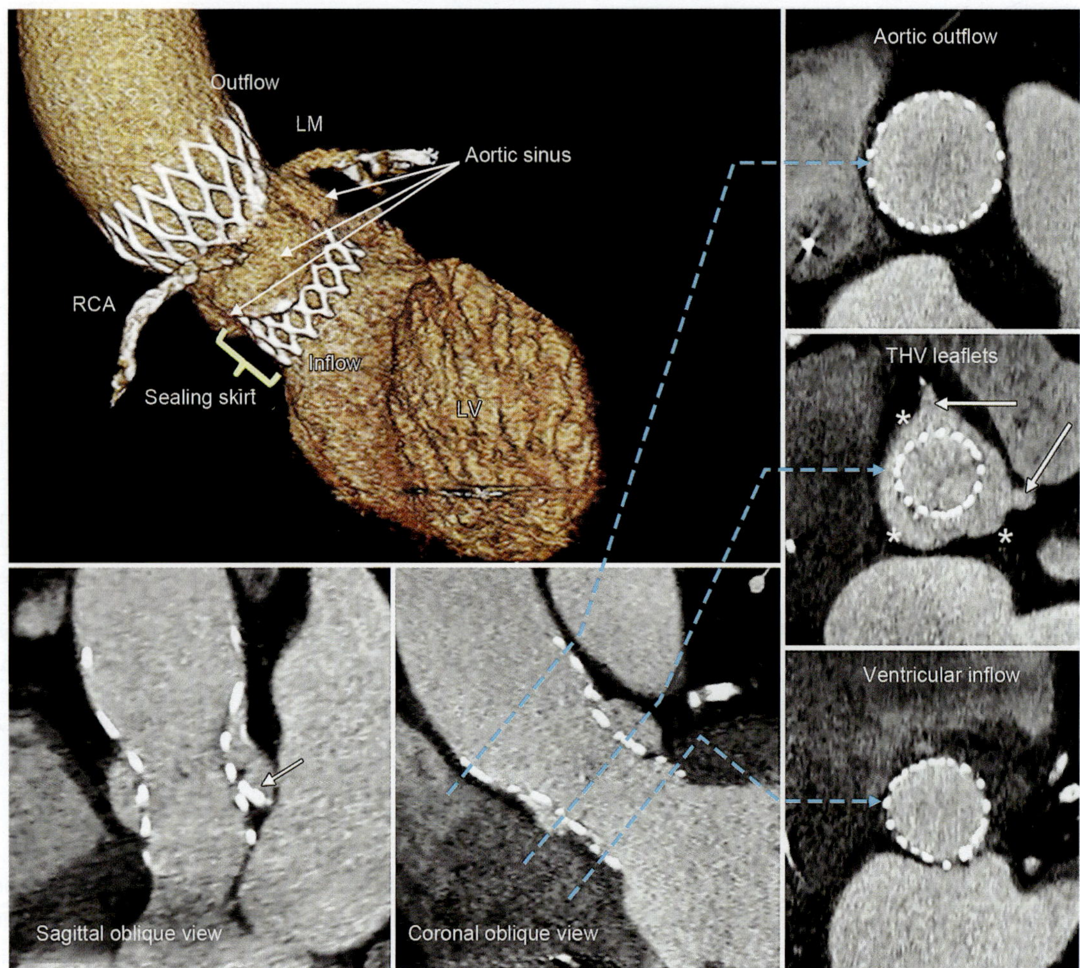

Fig. 8: *Aortic valve evaluation by computed tomography angiography (CTA):* Post-transcatheter aortic valve replacement (TAVR). (LM: left main; LV: left ventricular; RCA; right coronary artery; THV: TAVR valve)

procedure instead of conventional surgery. In those at no more than moderate coronary risk CTA can produce an assessment of the aortal and coronary arteries in one study. CTA is also useful in the workup toward intervention. It provides additional information over and above echo including accurate valve planimetry, degree of calcification of the leaflets, the distance to the coronary arteries and the caliber, tortuosity, and calcific burden of the peripheral vessels[13] **(Fig. 8)**.

Aortic Regurgitation

Regurgitation assessment is the forte of CMR in comparison to stenotic lesions. The estimation of AR using multiple echocardiographic modalities remains standard.[14] There are, however, certain situations like bicuspid valve eccentric jet which will be challenging to assess and follow up longitudinally on echocardiogram **(Fig. 9)**. This is an appropriate indication for CMR which can perform accurate quantification of aortic regurgitation fraction, provide complimentary information and identify patients at higher risk over and above what TTE can deliver.[15]

- *Aortic valve area [effective regurgitation orifice area (EROA)]:* The valve area is measured in diastole using perpendicular thin slice cine sequences on the LVOT oblique view to get an EROA[16] **(Fig. 10)**.
- *Aortic regurgitation fraction:* CMR can accurately quantify the amount of regurgitation using flow mapping and derived valves such as regurgitation fraction = (regurgitant volume/forward volume × 100%).[17] Qualitative measures including assessment of the venous contracta of the AR jet which gives a fair idea of the degree of regurgitation. Long axis LVOT view is the default view from which qualitative visualization

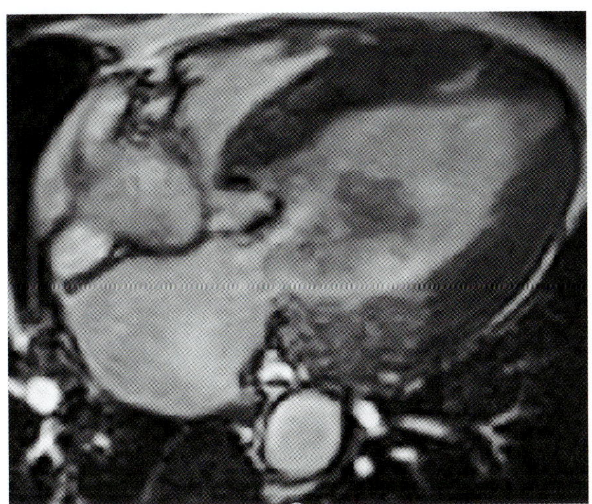

Fig. 9: Cine cardiac magnetic resonance (CMR) evaluation of a flail aortic valve leaflet with severe aortic regurgitation.

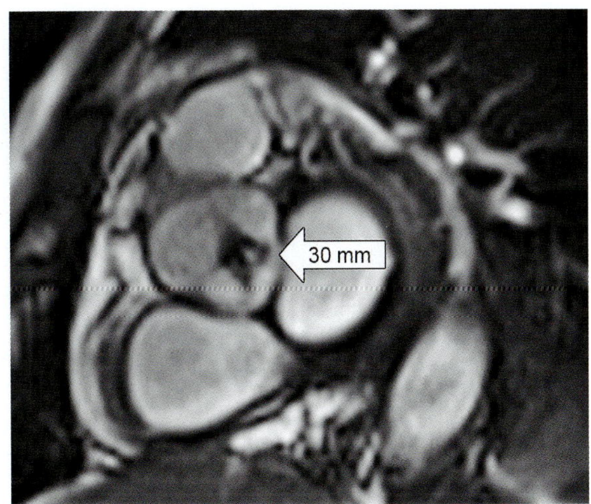

Fig. 10: Effective regurgitation orifice area (EROA) evaluation of aortic valve by cardiac magnetic resonance (CMR).

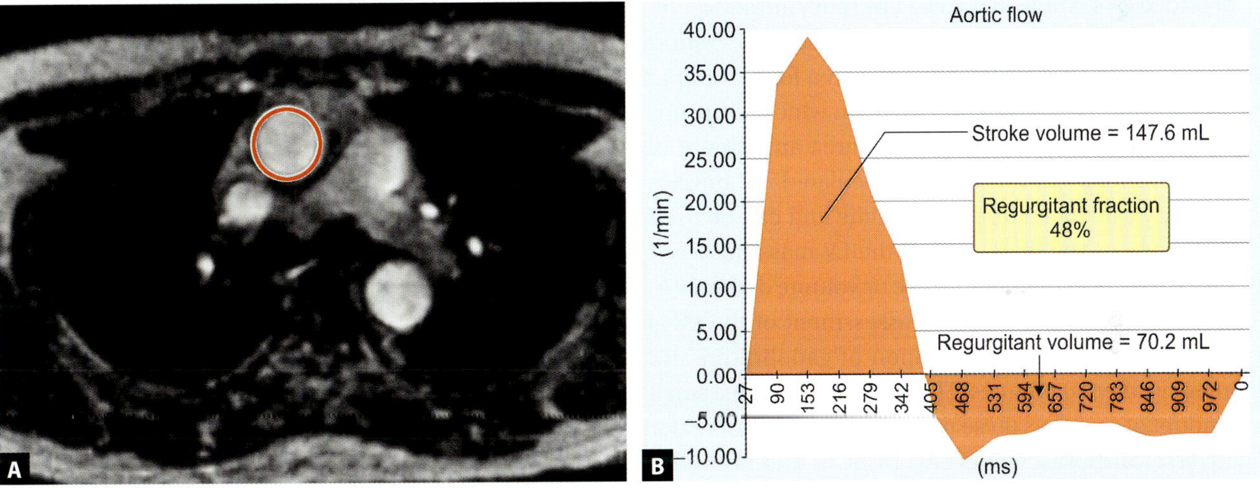

Figs. 11A and B: Velocity-encoded cine (VEC) imaging of aortic valve regurgitation by cardiac magnetic resonance (CMR).

of the regurgitation can be performed. Aortic flow is measured by placing the imaging slice for flow mapping above the aortic valve (1 cm) which will quantify the forward and regurgitant volume.[18] Care has to be taken to keep the imaging plane just above the valves to avoid turbulence but not far above to avoid omitting the volume of blood that would return to the ventricle in diastole. The through plane velocity mapping is extremely accurate vis-à-vis other competing techniques and is the only "true in vivo quantification of AR"[19] **(Figs. 11A and B)**. Reproducibility is excellent for intra and interobserver comparisons. Utmost care has to be used to ensure good technique including using non breath hold sequences, perpendicular slices and appropriate position of the imaging slice. Regurgitation fraction of 33% would be the optimal threshold for the identification of patients for early surgery **(Figs. 12A to D)**. Internal validation using the difference between the LV and right ventricular (RV) volumes to estimate regurgitation volume is also routinely performed as a quality parameter.[20]

- *Left ventricular volumetry:* Current thresholds for surgery in AR are based on LV diameter on the TTE, but these may not be reliable. The LV in severe AR becomes more spherical and a single linear dimension may not be representative. It is more likely that volumetry

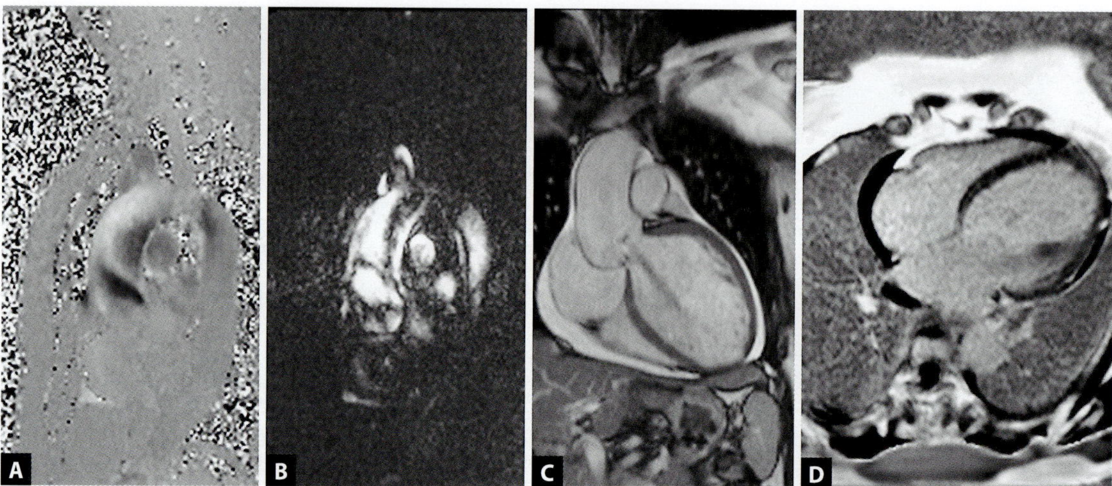

Figs. 12A to D: Cardiac magnetic resonance (CMR) evaluation of aortic valve regurgitation. (A) Phase contrast imaging; (B) Magnitude imaging; (C) CINE imaging of left ventricular outflow tract (LVOT); (D) Delayed enhancement imaging of myocardium.

provided by CMR which has a low inter/intraobserver variability will be a better threshold for surgery. A short axis stack taken from base to apex on a four-chamber (4C) view serves as the foundation on which Simpsons rule is applied and based on the area and height of each slice the volume of LV is calculated. LV mass is similarly calculated from the volume and can be used to document the regression of the LV mass post AVR which may be earlier than a size or volume decrease.[21]

- *Left ventricular fibrosis:* Scar assessment of the LV is best done by the administration of gadolinium and imaging after 10 minutes. The presence of even a small amount of scar puts these patients at high risk of major adverse cardiovascular events (MACE) and also poor prognosis post-AVR. It is most likely that myocardial fibrosis by CMR will be an important indicator for early surgery even in a moderate-to-severe AR but it is yet to make it into the guidelines. Scar pattern is also an indicator of the etiology of AR especially to distinguish between ischemic and non-ischemic etiologies of AR.[22]
- *Etiology:* CMR can distinguish common etiologic factors of AR.
  - *Aortic etiology:* CMR evaluation of the aortic root is unparalleled and quantitative evaluation of the root, annulus, ST function and ascending aorta can be done using cine sequences.
  - *Valvular etiology:* Pathologies intrinsic to the valve are not that easily ascertained compared to TTE since the imaging slices are 4–6-mm thick while the thin valve leaflets measure around (1–2 mm). However significant pathology such as large vegetations, abscess and thickened layouts can be easily visualized.

Conclusion

Aortic valve evaluation by CMR is a comprehensive, accurate, and reproducible technique. It can be done longitudinally with extremely low inter and intraobserver variability. It also correlates with MACE and regression of LV volume and mass after aortic valve replacement surgery.

TRICUSPID REGURGITATION

Cardiac magnetic resonance imaging plays an essential role in the assessment and management of tricuspid regurgitation (TR).[23] TTE is the primary tool for the evaluation of the tricuspid valve.[24] CMR is used in clinical situations of severe tricuspid or pulmonary regurgitation where decisions for surgery rest on an accurate assessment of RV volume, or a serial change in RV size or function.[25]

Anatomical Visualization

Detailed imaging: CMR provides high-resolution imaging of the heart structures, including the right atrium, right ventricle, and tricuspid valve. This detailed visualization helps in understanding the anatomy and any structural abnormalities that may contribute to TR. Steady-state free precession (SSFP) cine sequences are used to visualize the anatomy and function of the leaflets. The horizontal long axis view provides a good overview, but

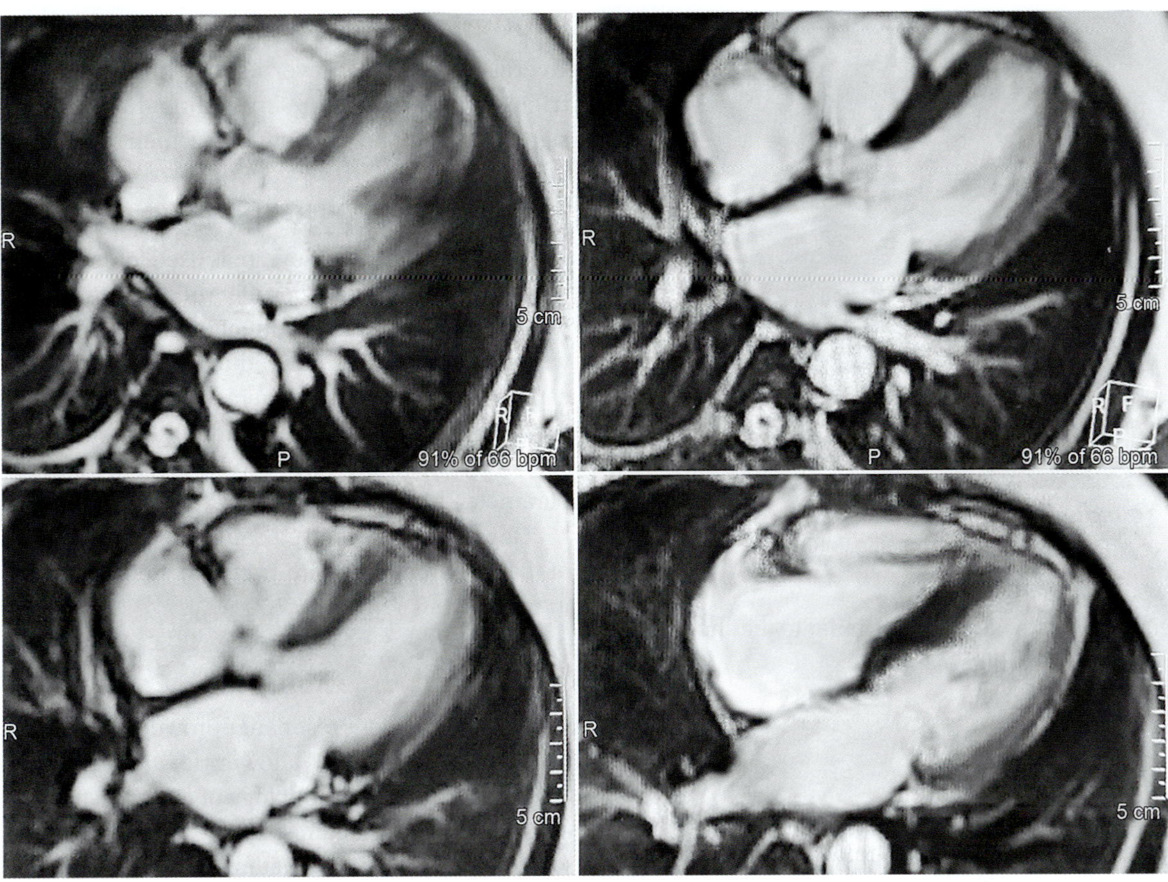

Fig. 13: Right ventricular (RV) function evaluation in a patient with tricuspid regurgitation.

multiple contiguous transverse images through the valve can often provide additional useful information, particularly for abnormal leaflet morphology such as in Ebstein's anomaly. Visualizing the jet is difficult on SSFP sequences due to the lower shear and turbulence. Wider jets (especially >7 mm at the vena contracta) suggest more severe tricuspid regurgitation. The regurgitant orifice can sometimes be assessed directly, in a similar fashion to mitral regurgitation, with a cine image through the leaflet tips in systole[24] **(Fig. 13)**.

Quantification of Tricuspid Regurgitation Severity

Regurgitant Volume and Fraction

Qualitative assessment of the TR jet can be achieved with in-plane velocity mapping in a long axis RV view. Through-plane velocity mapping in this plane can also aid in visualizing the size of the regurgitant orifice by visualizing the flow jet in cross-section. The "diameter" of the regurgitant orifice can be assessed but this is only an approximate guide. Quantification can be achieved using pulmonary flow measurement, combined with RV stroke volume to calculate the regurgitant volume (regurgitant volume = RV stroke volume – pulmonary forward flow) and the regurgitant fraction (TR/RV stroke volumes × 100%). Accuracy is impaired in arrythmias. Quantifying the TR can also be assessed using the difference in ventricular stroke volumes if only a single valve leak is present.[25]

Assessing Right Ventricular Function

Volume and Ejection Fraction

Cardiac magnetic resonance is excellent for assessing RV volumes and ejection fraction. RV function can be impaired in severe TR, and understanding this relationship helps in risk stratification and management. If there is difficulty of identifying the true ventricle on short axis images the long axis views can help in the identification of the valve position and an axial stack of RV images can

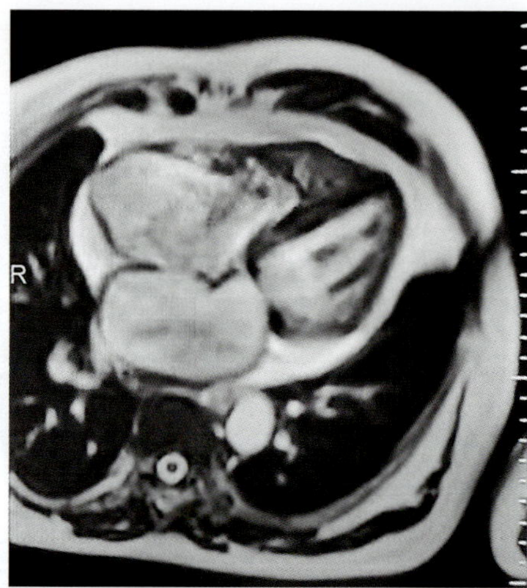

Fig. 14: Tricuspid regurgitation evaluation by cine magnetic resonance imaging (MRI).

be used to calculate EF which is similar to the short axis in terms of accuracy[26] **(Fig. 14)**.

Differentiating Causes of Tricuspid Regurgitation

Underlying Pathology

Cardiac magnetic resonance helps in identifying the underlying causes of TR, such as pulmonary hypertension, left-sided heart disease, or intrinsic valve pathology. This differentiation is critical for targeted intervention.[27]

Follow-up and Prognosis

Monitoring Disease Progression

Cardiac magnetic resonance is an excellent tool for follow-up assessments to monitor disease progression and the effectiveness of therapeutic interventions especially in regard to longitudinal EF and volumetry follow-up in cases of moderate TR prior to either surgical or interventional procedures due to its excellent accuracy, noninvasive nature, zero radiation risk, and low inter and intra observer variability.[28]

Guide Surgical Decisions

Surgical Planning

The detailed anatomical and functional information obtained from CMR, especially its ability to image the tricuspid valve in any desired imaging plane can assist in planning surgical interventions, such as tricuspid valve repair or replacement.[29]

Conclusion

Overall, CMR is a powerful tool in the evaluation of tricuspid regurgitation, providing insights that can significantly impact patient management and outcomes.

TRICUSPID STENOSIS

Transthoracic echocardiogram is used for initial diagnosis and will retain a first-line role into the future. Although extremely rare, and not routinely assessed with CMR, this valve lesion can be examined when required. Valve area can be measured by placement of an image slice through the valve tips in diastole, as for mitral stenosis, and forward velocity through the valve can be measured, though this parameter is perhaps less useful.

However, CMR is used routinely for the assessment of the RV in patients with tricuspid stenosis who require intervention.

Anatomical Visualization

- Cardiac magnetic resonance provides detailed imaging of cardiac structures, allowing for accurate assessment of the size and morphology of the tricuspid valve and surrounding structures.
- It helps identify any anatomical abnormalities such as valve calcification or associated congenital defects.[30]

Functional Assessment

- Cardiac magnetic resonance can evaluate right ventricular function, an important aspect in tricuspid stenosis. It assesses parameters such as ejection fraction and wall motion abnormalities.
- It measures right atrial pressure and volume, which can be increased due to tricuspid stenosis.

Quantification of Stenosis Severity

Cardiac magnetic resonance can quantify the severity of tricuspid stenosis through measurements of blood flow across the valve and pressure gradients, which can provide a more accurate assessment compared to Doppler echocardiography.[31]

Assessment of Associated Conditions

It helps in the detection of coexisting pathologies, such as pulmonary hypertension or right heart failure, that may be secondary to tricuspid stenosis.

Postoperative Evaluation

Cardiac magnetic resonance is useful for postoperative follow-up, helping evaluate the function of the tricuspid valve post-repair or replacement, as well as detecting potential complications.

Research and Future Directions

- Ongoing research is exploring the use of CMR techniques to better understand valvular heart diseases, including tricuspid stenosis, and how best to integrate these findings into clinical decision-making.[32]
- Overall, CMR offers a comprehensive approach to evaluate tricuspid stenosis, from anatomical details to functional impact, aiding in diagnosis, treatment planning, and management of this condition.

PULMONARY REGURGITATION

Cardiac magnetic resonance is an essential tool in the comprehensive evaluation of the pulmonary valve and its associated structures. Its ability to provide both anatomical and functional insights makes it invaluable in clinical decision-making regarding pulmonary valve disorders. The imprecise nature of echocardiogram in distinguishing moderate from severe pulmonary regurgitation, and imprecise RV function assessment make CMR an ideal method for assessment of the pulmonary valve and RV outflow tract.

Anatomical Assessment

- *Detailed imaging:* The pulmonary valve can sometimes be difficult to assess with echocardiogram, due to the location of the valve behind the sternum. CMR provides high-resolution images of the pulmonary valve anatomy, including the valve leaflets, annulus, and right ventricular outflow tract (RVOT) **(Fig. 15)** with its combination of free choice of imaging planes **(Fig. 16)**.
- *Congenital defects:* It is particularly useful in identifying congenital anomalies such as pulmonary valve stenosis, atresia, or transposition of great vessels.

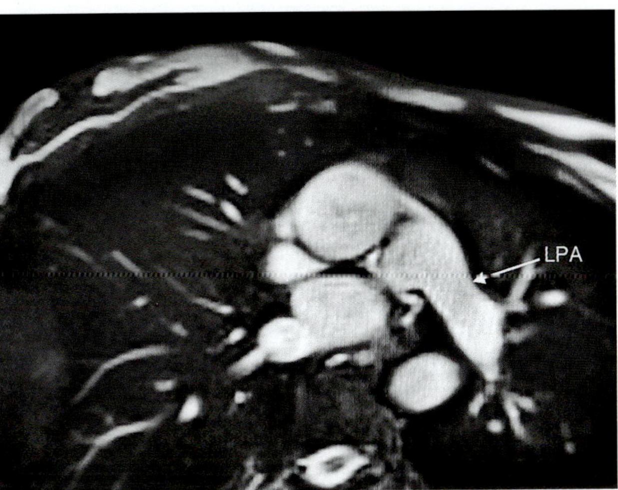

Fig. 15: Left pulmonary artery (LPA) view in a patient with pulmonary regurgitation.

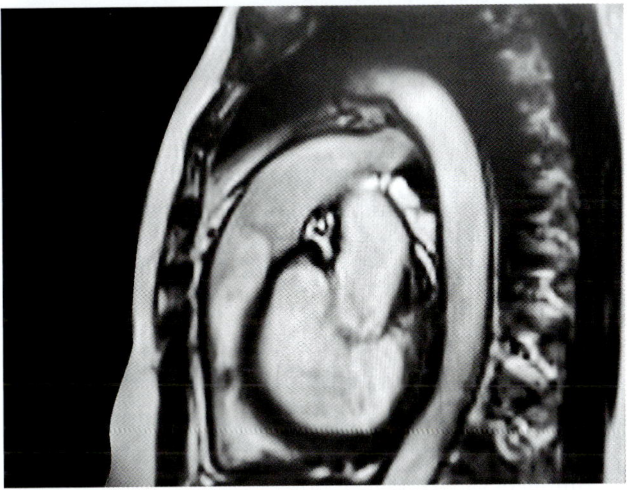

Fig. 16: Right ventricular outflow tract (RVOT) view in a patient with pulmonary regurgitation.

Functional Evaluation

- *Valvular function:* CMR allows for the assessment of pulmonary valve function, measuring parameters such as regurgitation fraction and valve area. CMR quantification of pulmonary regurgitation is achieved by through-plane velocity mapping just above the pulmonary valve. This compares well to quantification using ventricular stroke volumes[33] and correlates with echo parameters.[34] A regurgitant fraction ≥40% is considered severe[35] **(Fig. 17)**.
- *Dynamic function:* The imaging can evaluate how the valve performs during different phases of the cardiac cycle.

Quantification of Hemodynamics

- *Blood flow measurements:* CMR can quantify blood flow across the pulmonary valve, providing information on gradients and potential stenosis.

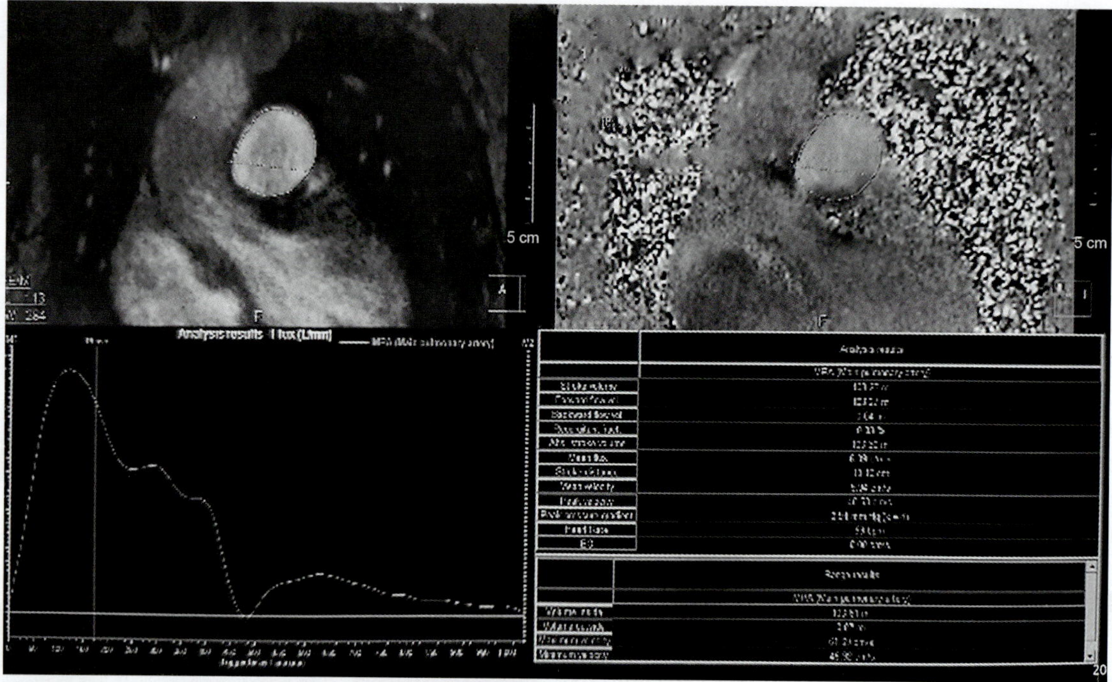

Fig. 17: Pulmonary regurgitation fraction evaluation.

- *Cardiac output:* It helps in evaluating cardiac output and assessing the impact of pulmonary valve diseases on right ventricular function.

Assessment of Surrounding Structures

- *Right ventricular morphology:* CMR assesses the right ventricular size and function, which can be affected by pulmonary valve disorders. Accurate measurement of RV volumes and function is crucial and can guide the timing of valve replacement.[36-38]
- *Pulmonary artery evaluation:* It also helps in evaluating the main and branch pulmonary arteries, detecting hypertensive changes, or lesions.

Post-intervention Evaluation

Follow-up examinations: CMR is valuable for post-surgical or post-interventional evaluations in patients who have undergone pulmonary valve repair or replacement, assessing the integrity and function of the valve over time.

Noninvasive Nature

Safety and comfort: As a noninvasive imaging modality, CMR poses minimal risk to patients compared to invasive procedures, making it a preferred choice in various clinical scenarios.

Pulmonary Stenosis

The excellent visualization of the RV outflow tract with CMR facilitates easy identification of the site and severity of pulmonary stenosis.[39] A qualitative assessment of severity can be made from the outflow tract views, by visualizing the valve motion and stenotic jet, and quantitative assessment is done by using direct planimetry of the orifice at the valve tips. Peak velocity can also be measured by in-plane velocity mapping which can identify the point of maximal velocity. Sub-valvular and supravalvular stenosis is evaluated from the outflow tract views. RV mass and function can be accurately assessed using the short axis cine stack. Pulmonary trunk or branch artery stenosis can also be identified with cine imaging, magnetic resonance angiography of the pulmonary arteries, or an anatomic image stack.[40]

MITRAL REGURGITATION

Multimodality cardiovascular imaging has a crucial role in the assessment of mitral valve disease. CMR provides accurate flow and volume quantification of the left and right ventricles with regional and global systolic function. Additionally, it allows assessment of the morphological and functional characteristics of mitral leaflets, annulus, and chordae tendineae with evaluation of the stenotic and

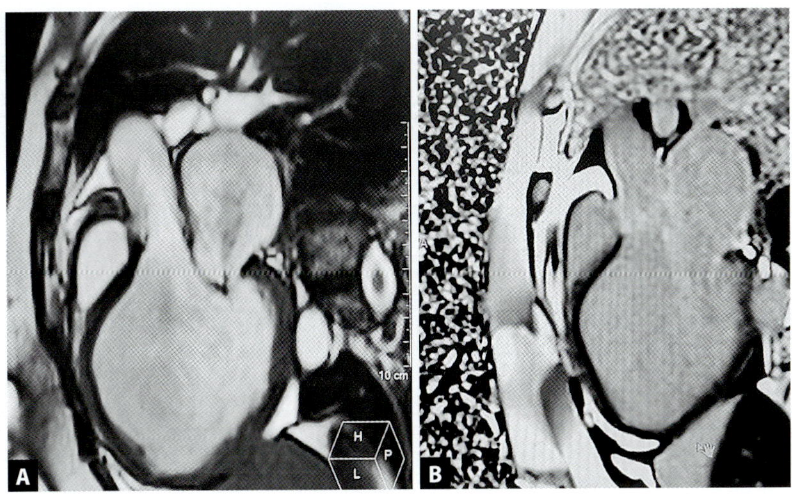

Figs. 18A and B: Mitral regurgitation flow void with delayed enhancement imaging.

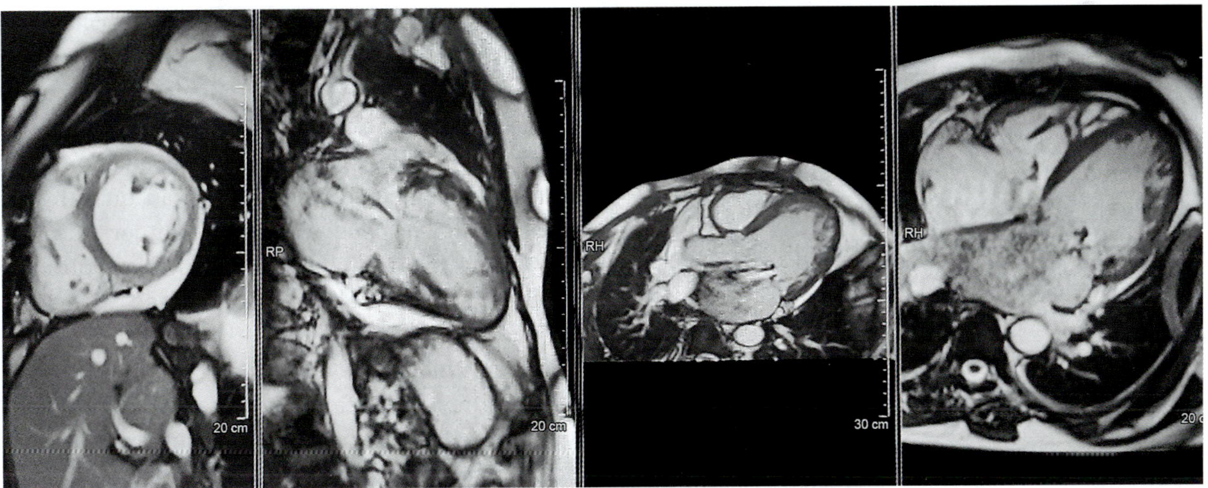

Fig. 19: Central jet of mitral regurgitation.

regurgitation jets. Direct visualization of mitral annulus and mitral leaflet scallops with assessment of valve coaptation can be done due to multiplanar capability of magnetic resonance imaging. Morphological leaflet lesions such as leaflet perforation, thickening/calcification commissural fusion, associated papillary muscle displacement or caudal tethering, and rupture of chordae tendineae are evaluated. CMR also evaluates ventricular remodeling and presence/absence of late gadolinium enhancement (LGE)—myocardial fibrosis **(Figs. 18A and B)**. CMR also evaluates degrees of left atrial dilatation and mitral regurgitation. Secondary causes of mitral regurgitation such as dilated cardiomyopathy—ischemic/nonischemic are also well evaluated[41] **(Fig. 19)**.

Anatomical Assessment

Mitral annulus is a fibromuscular ring separating the left atrium from the left ventricle. Anterior 1/3rd of the annulus is fibrous and contiguous with the aortic valve through the aortomitral continuity. Posterior 2/3rd of the annulus is predominantly muscular.

Mitral leaflets are approximately 5 mm in thickness. Anterior leaflet is attached to the anterior 1/3rd portion of the annulus. Anterior leaflet is longer than the posterior leaflet and has a normal length ranging from 1.8 to 2.5 cm. The posterior leaflet has a larger attachment. Both anterior and posterior leaflets are divided into three segments. Mitral subvalvular apparatus consists of thin fibrous filamentous chordae tendineae attached to the papillary muscles.[42]

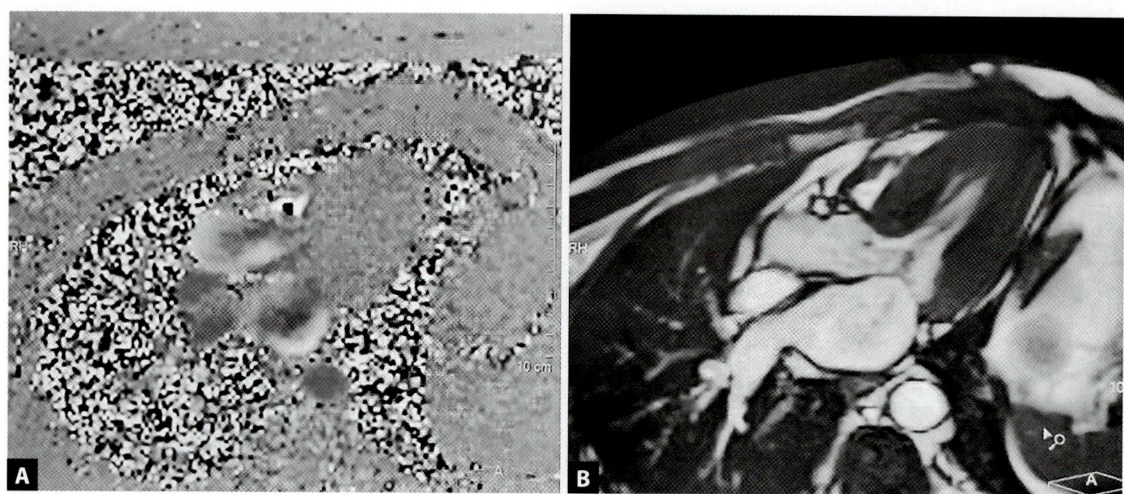

Figs. 20A and B: Mitral regurgitation evaluation by velocity encoding (VENC) imaging.

Functional Evaluation

Cardiac MRI has a role in mitral regurgitation, providing information on mechanism of regurgitation. Assessment of the myocardium with respect to viability and remodeling influences the surgical management.[43] Mitral regurgitation is visualized as a jet on the SSFP screening images. Location and direction of flow jet is visualized with evaluation of number of jets. Spoiled gradient recalled echo (SPGRE) sequences are more sensitive to flow turbulence and allow better visualization of regurgitation or stenotic jets. Velocity mapping remains the most sensitive imaging technique for visualization of mitral regurgitant jet[44] **(Figs. 20A and B)**. Cross-sectional thin images in a plane parallel to the leaflet plane ensure good views of the valve anatomy and morphology. Through plain evaluation also allows valve leaflet coaptation. A basal short axis inplane slice through the mitral commissure is used to then position three-chamber LVOT images perpendicular to the commissure for each of the three scallops. Systolic phase images in the three-chamber LVOT plane allow evaluation of all three anterior and posterior leaflet segments.

Quantification of Hemodynamics

Quantification of MR is performed by measurement of ventricular volumes. Indexed volumes for different body surface area (BSA) parameters allow better assessment of ventricular dilatation and guide regarding the impact of valve disease on ventricles. Chamber dilatation suggests chronic severe regurgitation.[45] MR quantification is performed using SSSP short axis stack to calculate the left ventricular stroke volume. The forward flow in aorta is calculated by phase contrast imaging. The regurgitant volume can then the calculated by substracting the aortic forward flow volume from the LV stroke volume. This is the most validated technique and can quantify mitral regurgitation irrespective of regurgitant jet morphology. Calculating the right ventricular stroke volume and pulmonary flow is also recommended with internal validation and quality cross check for all valves. Meyerson et al. recommended a regurgitant volume threshold of >55 mL and regurgitant fraction of >40% to quantify significant MR requiring mitral valve surgery for symptoms and disease progression. Combining regurgitant volume and left ventricular volume scan enhanced specificity and sensitivity to identify patients with poor outcome based on indexed left ventricular end-systolic volume of >35 mL per square meter.[46]

MITRAL VALVE PROLAPSE

Mitral valve prolapse is a single or bileaflet prolapse of mitral leaflets 2 mm beyond the long-axis annular plane, with or without mitral leaflet thickening. Mitral valve prolapse (MVP) is measured as the distance between the top of the prolapsed portion of the leaflet during peak systole to the mitral annulus plane, which is at the top of the basal-LV myocardium.[47]

MITRAL ANNULAR DISJUNCTION

Mitral annular disc junction is defined as atrial displacement of the hinge point of the mitral valve annulus into the atrium, away from the ventricular myocardium. Mitral annular disjunction (MAD) is most commonly associated with mitral valve prolapse, which is the expression of degenerative mitral valve disease characterized by abnormal displacement of the mitral valve leaflets above the mitral plane by >2 mm, causing poor coaptation of the valve scallops and mitral regurgitation. The thinned-out annulus paradoxically curls outward during ventricular systole. This increases the annulus diameter during systolic causing poor coarctation of the scallops. MAD is also implicated in myxomatous degeneration of the leaflets. Smaller length of mitral annular dysfunction in the range of 5–6 mm is generally incidentally seen. Longer disjunctions of >8.5 mm have been associated with a bad prognosis. Inferolateral wall is the most commonly affected segment in patients with mitral valve prolapse and myxomatous mitral valve disease and is also associated with life-threatening ventricular arrhythmias. MAD and arrhythmic MVP are related with the arrhythmic group having statistically significant higher MAD length, larger mitral annulus diameters, greater posterior annulus curling and posterobasal LV hypertrophy (basal to mid LV lateral wall thickness ratio 1.5). Presence of papillary muscle LG was more frequently seen in patients with ventricular arrhythmias.[48]

Miscellaneous Lesions of the Mitral Valve

Cardiac magnetic resonance allows evaluation of lesions along the mitral valve such as tumor and pseudo tumors. Commonly associated tumors are fibroelastoma and myxoma. Fibroelastomas show intense post-contrast enhancement on LGE images due to fibrous tissue. Myxomas are bright lesions attached to the distal interatrial septum and may prolapse into the ventricle through the mitral valve annulus. They show heterogeneous late gadolinium enhancement due to mixed composition. Enhancement of the pedicle attachment is a constant feature.

Mitral annular calcification is very commonly seen as a hypointense immobile mass restricting the mitral valve leaflet excursion. It appears hypointense on T1 and T2Wt images and may show peripheral rim LGE. Corresponding CT images show dense calcification along the mitral annulus.[48] In ischemic MR, the quantification of MR and myocardial infarct size with CMR can help for risk stratification in patients with advanced ischemic cardiomyopathy. In primary MR, especially MV prolapse, a high prevalence of focal replacement fibrosis, particularly in the segments adjacent to the posterior papillary muscle, can be observed. A recent parametric mapping technique (T1 mapping) allows for better characterization of global myocardial tissue composition by direct measurement of T1 relaxation times before and after contrast administration and by calculation of the extracellular volume (ECV). Diffuse interstitial fibrosis in primary MR may be more closely related to chronic LV volume overload than the etiology of MR.[49]

Comparison Between Transthoracic Echocardiogram and Cardiac Magnetic Resonance

Most studies have shown only limited agreement in the assessment of MR between CMR and echocardiography.[50] MR volume values truly differ among volumetric methods and the proximal isovelocity surface area (PISA) method. Therefore, using the same thresholds to define MR severity and the need for surgery may be inappropriate. The MR volume was similar using the volumetric method by 3D echocardiography and CMR. Recent reports have suggested that 3D-transthoracic echocardiography is less dependent on geometric assumptions and allows better visualization of the vena contracta regurgitant orifice. However, characterization of the Doppler jet is still challenging, with additional limitations of lower spatial and temporal resolution.[51]

Timing of Mitral Valve Surgery

Myerson et al.[52] on initially asymptomatic patients with moderate or severe MR followed up for up to 8 years, showed that MRvol and RF by CMR were the most discriminatory parameters to determine the need for surgery (symptoms or other indications for surgery), with cut-off thresholds of 55 mL for MRvol and 40% for RF, and an increasing risk with increasing values of the parameters. The RF cutoff for severe MR in this study was very similar to a recent study by Polte et al.[53] (RF >41%) and lower than echocardiographic criteria (RF ≥50%). As the MRvol is proportional to LV size in primary MR, for two patients with similar CMR MR volume, the patient with a smaller LV will have more severe MR; calculation of the RF may overcome this issue as it normalizes the MRvol to the size of the LV.

CONCLUSION

Cardiac magnetic resonance can be used to assess patients with multiple valve lesions, obtaining a detailed assessment of the severity of each component whether these occur in the same valve (i.e., mixed valve disease) or in different valves. As an extreme example, a patient with both mixed aortic and mixed mitral valve disease could have the opening area of each valve measured by direct planimetry with cine imaging to assess stenosis, the aortic regurgitation quantified from the diastolic (regurgitant) flow above the aortic valve and the mitral regurgitation quantified by subtracting the systolic (forward) flow above the aortic valve from the LV stroke volume. LV volumes and function would also be assessed. In this way, a comprehensive assessment can be undertaken.

REFERENCES

1. Walsh. Madame President. Journal of the American College of Cardiology. 2017;70:3195-8.
2. Baumgartner H, Hung J, Bermejo J, Chambers JB, Evangelista A, Griffin BP, et al. Echocardiographic assessment of valve stenosis: EAE/ASE recommendations for clinical practice. Eur J Echocardiogr. 2009;10:1-25.
3. Myerson SG. Heart valve disease: investigation by cardiovascular magnetic resonance. J Cardiovasc Magn Reson. 2012;14:7.
4. Westermann Y, Geigenmüller A, Elgeti T, Wagner M, Dushe S, Borges AC, et al. Planimetry of the aortic valve orifice area: comparison of multislice spiral computed tomography and magnetic resonance imaging. Eur J Radiol. 2011;77(3):426-35.
5. Clavel MA, Pibarot P, Messika-Zeitoun D, Capoulade R, Malouf J, Aggarval S, et al. Impact of aortic valve calcification, as measured by MDCT, on survival in patients with aortic stenosis: results of an international registry study. J Am Coll Cardiol. 2014;64:1202-13.
6. Dweck MR, Jones C, Joshi NV, Fletcher AM, Richardson H, White A, et al. Assessment of valvular calcification and inflammation by positron emission tomography in patients with aortic stenosis. Circulation. 2012;125:76-86.
7. L Sondergaard, P Hildebrandt, K Lindvig, C Thomsen, F Stahlberg, E Kassis, et al. Valve area and cardiac output in aortic stenosis: quantification by magnetic resonance velocity mapping. Am Heart J. 1993;126:1156-64.
8. P Reant, M Lederlin, S Lafitte, K Serri, M Montaudon, O Corneloup, et al. Absolute assessment of aortic valve stenosis by planimetry using cardiovascular magnetic resonance imaging: comparison with transesophageal echocardiography, transthoracic echocardiography, and cardiac catheterization. Eur J Radiol. 2006;59:276-83.
9. De Vecchi C, Caudron J, Dubourg B, Pirot N, Lefebvre V, Bauer F, et al. Effect of the ellipsoid shape of the left ventricular outflow tract on the echocardiographic assessment of aortic valve area in aortic stenosis. J Cardiovasc Comput Tomogr. 2014;8:52-7.
10. AJ Evans, RA Blinder, RJ Herfkens, CE Spritzer, DO Kuethe, EK Fram, et al. Effects of turbulence on signal intensity in gradient echo images. Invest Radiol. 1988;23;512-8.
11. Shah AS, Chin CW, Vassiliou V, Cowell SJ, Doris M, Kwok TC, et al. Left ventricular hypertrophy with strain and aortic stenosis. Circulation. 2014;130:1607-16.
12. Weidemann F, Herrmann S, Störk S, Niemann M, Frantz S, Lange V, et al. Impact of myocardial fibrosis in patients with symptomatic severe aortic stenosis. Circulation. 2009;120:577-84.
13. Achenbach S, Delgado V, Hausleiter J, Schoenhagen P, Min JK, Leipsic JA. SCCT Expert consensus document on computed tomography imaging before transcatheter aortic valve implantation (TAVI)/transcatheter aortic valve replacement (TAVR). J Cardiovasc Comput Tomogr. 2012;6:366-80.
14. Lancellotti P, Tribouilloy C, Hagendorff A, Moura L, Popescu BA, Agricola E, et al. European Association of Echocardiography recommendations for the assessment of valvular regurgitation. Part 1: aortic and pulmonary regurgitation (native valve disease). Eur J Echocardiogr. 2010;11:223-44.
15. Myerson SG, d'Arcy J, Mohiaddin R, Greenwood JP, Karamitsos TD, Francis JM, et al. Aortic regurgitation quantification using cardiovascular magnetic resonance: association with clinical outcome. Circulation. 2012; 126:1452-6.
16. Wagner S, Auffermann W, Buser P, Lim TH, Kircher B, Pflugfelder P, et al. Diagnostic accuracy and estimation of the severity of valvular regurgitation from the signal void on cine magnetic resonance images. Am Heart J. 1989;118:760-7.
17. Dulce MC, Mostbeck GH, O'Sullivan M, Cheitlin M, Caputo GR, Higgins CB. Severity of aortic regurgitation: interstudy reproducibility of measurements with velocity-encoded cine MR imaging. Radiology. 1992;185:235-40.
18. Chatzimavroudis GP, Oshinski JN, Franch RH, Pettigrew RI, Walker P1G, Yoganathan AP. Quantification of the aortic regurgitant volume with magnetic resonance phase velocity mapping: a clinical investigation of the importance of imaging slice location. J Heart Valve Dis. 1998;7:94-101.
19. Ichikawa Y, Sakuma H, Kitagawa K, Ishida N, Takeda K, Uemura S, et al. Evaluation of left ventricular volumes and ejection fraction using fast steady-state cine MR imaging: comparison with left ventricular angiography. J Cardiovasc Magn Reson. 2003;5:333-42.
20. Globits S, Frank H, Mayr H, Neuhold A, Glogar D. Quantitative assessment of aortic regurgitation by magnetic resonance imaging. Eur Heart J. 1992;13:78-83.

21. Myerson SG, d'Arcy J, Mohiaddin R, Greenwood JP, Karamitsos TD, Francis JM, et al. Aortic regurgitation quantification with cardiovascular magnetic resonance predicts clinical outcome. Heart. 2011;97:A93-4.
22. Dweck MR, Joshi S, Murigu T, Gulati A, Alpendurado F, Mohiaddin R, et al. Mid-wall fibrosis is an independent predictor of mortality in patients with aortic stenosis. Heart. 2011;58(12):1271-9.
23. Pype LL, Domenech-Ximenos B, Paelinck BP, Sturkenboom N, Van De Heyning CM. Assessment of tricuspid regurgitation by cardiac magnetic resonance imaging: current role and future applications. J Clin Med. 2024;13(15):4481. doi: 10.3390/jcm13154481. PMID: 39124748; PMCID: PMC11312898.
24. Wong TC, Chow CH, Go MCM, et al. Tricuspid regurgitation: diagnosis and management. J Am Coll Cardiol. 2018;71(12):1358-76.
25. Graham EE, Wang TKM, Rahmani B, Mirsadraee S, Newby DE, et al. Prognostic implications of tricuspid regurgitation: the role of cardiac MRI. Circulation Cardiovasc Imaging. 2019;12(2):e008499.
26. Aryal SR, Sharifov OF, Lloyd SG. Emerging role of cardiovascular magnetic resonance imaging in the management of pulmonary hypertension. Eur Respir Rev. 2020;29(156):190138.
27. Shah S, Jenkins T, Markowitz A, Gilkeson R, Rajiah P. Multimodal imaging of the tricuspid valve: normal appearance and pathological entities. Insights Imaging. 2016;7(5):649-67. doi: 10.1007/s13244-016-0504-7. Epub 2016 Jun 9. PMID: 27278389; PMCID: PMC5028338.
28. Muncunill J, Cibeira-Campos ML, Giraldo-Monterroso C, et al. Magnetic resonance imaging in the evaluation of tricuspid valve disease: a comprehensive review. Front Cardiovasc Med. 2020;7:10.
29. Mahle WT, Parks WJ, Fyfe DA, Sallee D. Tricuspid regurgitation in patients with repaired tetralogy of Fallot and its relation to right ventricular dilatation. Am J Cardiol. 2003;92:643-5.
30. Zaky SM, Ashamallah GA, El Bakry MA, et al. The role of CMR in assessing tricuspid valve performance and dysfunction. J Cardiovas Magnet Res. 2022;24(1):20.
31. Golebiowska, Jacek Habets, and Robin P.J. Budde. et al. Radiology - Heart Valve Imaging. Nat Rev Cardiol. 2019; 16(1):49-60.
32. Mc Carthy PM, Stewart DB. Innovations in imaging: The role of MRI in valvular heart disease. Trends Cardiovasc Med. 2018;28(7):435-42.
33. Puchalski MD, Askovich B, Sower CT, Williams RV, Minich LL, Tani LY. Pulmonary regurgitation: determining severity by echocardiography and magnetic resonance imaging. Congenit Heart Dis. 2008;3:168-75.
34. Beurskens NEG, Gorter TM, Pieper PG, Hoendermis ES, Bartelds B, Ebels T, et al. Diagnostic value of doppler echocardiography for identifying hemodynamic significant pulmonary valve regurgitation in tetralogy of Fallot: comparison with cardiac MRI. Int J Cardiovasc Imaging. 2017;33:1723-30.
35. Mercer-Rosa L, Yang W, Kutty S, Rychik J, Fogel M, Goldmuntz E. Quantifying pulmonary regurgitation and right ventricular function in surgically repaired tetralogy of Fallot: a comparative analysis of echocardiography and magnetic resonance imaging. Circ Cardiovasc Imaging. 2012;5:637-43.
36. Ammash NM, Dearani JA, Burkhart HM. Connolly Pulmonary regurgitation after tetralogy of Fallot repair: clinical features, sequelae, and timing of pulmonary valve replacement. Congenit Heart Dis. 2007;2:386-403.
37. Geva T. Indications and timing of pulmonary valve replacement after tetralogy of Fallot repair. Semin Thorac Cardiovasc Surg Pediatr Card Surg Annu (2006). pp. 11-22.
38. Oosterhof T, van Straten A, Vliegen HW, Meijboom FJ, van Dijk AP, Spijkerboer AM, et al. Preoperative thresholds for pulmonary valve replacement in patients with corrected tetralogy of Fallot using cardiovascular magnetic resonance. Circulation. 2007;116:545-51.
39. Costantini P, Perone F, Siani A, Groenhoff L, Muscogiuri G, Sironi S, et al. Multimodality imaging of the neglected valve: role of echocardiography, cardiac magnetic resonance and cardiac computed tomography in pulmonary stenosis and regurgitation. J Imaging. 2022;8(10):278.
40. Marchini F, Meossi S, Passarini G, Campo G, Pavasini R. Pulmonary Valve Stenosis: From Diagnosis to Current Management Techniques and Future Prospects. Vasc Health Risk Manag. 2023;19:379-90.
41. Zoghbi WA, Adams D, Bonow RO, Enriquez-Sarano M, Foster E, Grayburn PA, et al. Recommendations for noninvasive evaluation of native valvular regurgitation: a report from the American society of echocardiography developed in collaboration with the society for cardiovascular magnetic resonance. J Am Soc Echocardiogr. 2017;30:303-71.
42. Han Y, Peters DC, Salton CJ, Bzymek D, Nezafat R, Goddu B, et al. Cardiovascular magnetic resonance characterization of mitral valve prolapse. JACC Cardiovasc Imaging. 2008;1:294-303.
43. Fidock B, Archer G, Barker N, Elhawaz A, Al-Mohammad A, Rothman A, et al. Standard and emerging CMR methods for mitral regurgitation quantification. Int J Cardiol. 2021;331:316-21.
44. Blanken CPS, Westenberg JJM, Aben J-P, Bijvoet GP, Chamuleau SAJ, Boekholdt SM, et al. Quantification of mitral valve regurgitation from 4D Flow MRI using semiautomated flow tracking. Radiol Cardiothorac Imaging. 2020;2:e200004.
45. Lopez-Mattei JC, Ibrahim H, Shaikh KA, Little SH, Shah DJ, Maragiannis D, et al. Comparative assessment of mitral regurgitation severity by transthoracic echocardiography and cardiac magnetic resonance using an integrative and quantitative approach. Am J Cardiol. 2016;117:264-70.

46. Penicka M, Vecera J, Mirica DC, Kotrc M, Kockova R, Van Camp G. Prognostic implications of magnetic resonance-derived quantification in asymptomatic patients with organic mitral regurgitation: comparison with doppler echocardiography-derived integrative approach. Circulation. 2018;137:1349-60.
47. Groeneveld SA, Kirkels FP, Cramer MJ, Evertz R, Haugaa KH, Postema PG, et al. Prevalence of Mitral Annulus Disjunction and Mitral Valve Prolapse in Patients with Idiopathic Ventricular Fibrillation. J Am Heart Assoc. 2022;11(16):e025364.
48. Silva Ferreira MV, Soares CSP, Araujo-Filho JAB, Dantas RN Jr, Torres RVA, Morais TC, et al. Mitral Annular Disease at Cardiac MRI: What to Know and Look For. Radiographics. 2024;44(7):e230156.
49. Kitkungvan D, Nabi F, Kim RJ, Bonow RO, Khan MA, Xu J, et al. Myocardial fibrosis in patients with primary mitral regurgitation with and without prolapse. J Am Coll Cardiol. 2018;72:823-34.
50. Lancellotti P, Pibarot P, Chambers J, La Canna G, Pepi M, Dulgheru R, et al. Multi-modality imaging assessment of native valvular regurgitation: an EACVI and ESC council of valvular heart disease position paper. Eur Heart J Cardiovasc Imaging. 2022;23:e171-232.
51. Shanks M, Siebelink H-MJ, Delgado V, van de Veire NRL, Ng ACT, Sieders A, et al. Quantitative assessment of mitral regurgitation: comparison between three-dimensional transesophageal echocardiography and magnetic resonance imaging. Circ Cardiovasc Imaging. 2010;3:694-700.
52. Myerson SG, d'Arcy J, Christiansen JP, Dobson LE, Mohiaddin R, Francis JM, et al. Determination of clinical outcome in mitral regurgitation with cardiovascular magnetic resonance quantification. Circulation. 2016;133:2287-96.
53. Polte CL, Gao SA, Johnsson ÅA, Lagerstrand KM, Bech-Hanssen O. Characterization of chronic aortic and mitral regurgitation undergoing valve surgery using cardiovascular magnetic resonance. Am J Cardiol. 2017;119:2061-8.

CHAPTER 41

Cardiac Magnetic Resonance Imaging in Non-ischemic Cardiomyopathies

Nilay S Nimbalkar, Prajakta Kirdatpatil

INTRODUCTION

Cardiovascular diseases remain a leading cause of morbidity and mortality worldwide.[1] In spite of advances in medical therapies and diagnosis presently available, scientists and medical professionals are finding it hard to reduce the morbidity and mortality due to cardiovascular diseases and cardiomyopathies. Echocardiography (ECG), transesophageal echocardiogram (TEE), stress tests, and catheter coronary angiography act as primary modality of diagnosis and treatment. Last two decades have seen tremendous improvement in the scanning time, sensitivity, and innovations in cross-sectional cardiac imaging.[2]

Cardiac magnetic resonance imaging (CMR) has emerged as essential problem-solving tool in field of myocardial viability, myocardial fibrosis quantification, multiparametric imaging[2]. CMR has emerged as gold standard for LV, RV ejection fractions, and volume quantification.[3] Lack of visualization of cardiac apex and lack of sensitivity for RV wall evaluation on echocardiography and availability of 3D cine imaging and excellent spatial resolution with flow studies made CMR an important tool in cardiac imaging.[3] With availability of myocardial mapping with native T1, native T2 maps and extracellular volume (ECV) values, CMR can give positive feedback in tissue diagnosis and follow-up (e.g., amyloidosis, Fabry's disease, and iron quantification in cases of myocardial iron deposition)[4] **(Figs. 1A to F)**.

CARDIAC MAGNETIC RESONANCE IMAGING

Cardiac MRI is excellent for evaluation of cardiac morphology and signal intensity changes in different pathologies without radiation. The newer sequences giving excellent cine, 3D and flow imaging helps to evaluate morphology with function and flow analysis (e.g., Qp : Qs) making it gold standard for LV, RV functional analysis. Let us evaluate different indications of CMR.

Nonischemic cardiomyopathy is a primary myocardial disease caused by chronic injury, infiltration or abnormal storage diseases leading to signal intensity changes in the myocardium picked up with CMR with or without gadolinium-based contrast injections. CMR is widely accepted as non-invasive gold standard for quantifying biventricular volumes of myocardial mass as well as regional and global systolic function. Post contrast T1-weighted images help to identify scar infiltration and inflammation as well as intraventricular thrombus. Edema sensitive T2-weighted images help to identify acute injury and T2 star weighted imaging has proven useful in detection of myocardial hemorrhages and thrombus. Myocardial mapping allows direct measurement of changes of magnetic properties as expressed as negative T1, T2, T2* and ECV derived from postcontrast T1-weighted images.

Dilated cardiomyopathy (DCM) is characterized by ventricular dilatation, global systolic dysfunction and often accompanied by global myocardial fibrosis. In patients with DCM, late gadolinium enhancement (LGE) imaging can visualize regional fibrosis that allows for discriminating non-ischemic DCM from ischemic cardiomyopathy (mid myocardium vs. subendocardial LGE). A mid myocardial enhancing stripe typically involving basal anteroseptal segment is found in many patients of DCM and is predictor of sudden death and ventricular arrhythmia and helps in decision making for implantable cardioverter defibrillators (ICD). LGE and myocardial mapping are very useful in follow-up of patients with DCM. Negative T1 and ECV values can help in identifying interstitial fibrosis not seen on LGE[5] **(Figs. 2A to D)**.

Hypertrophic cardiomyopathy shows markers such as increased LV mass, asymmetric increase in wall

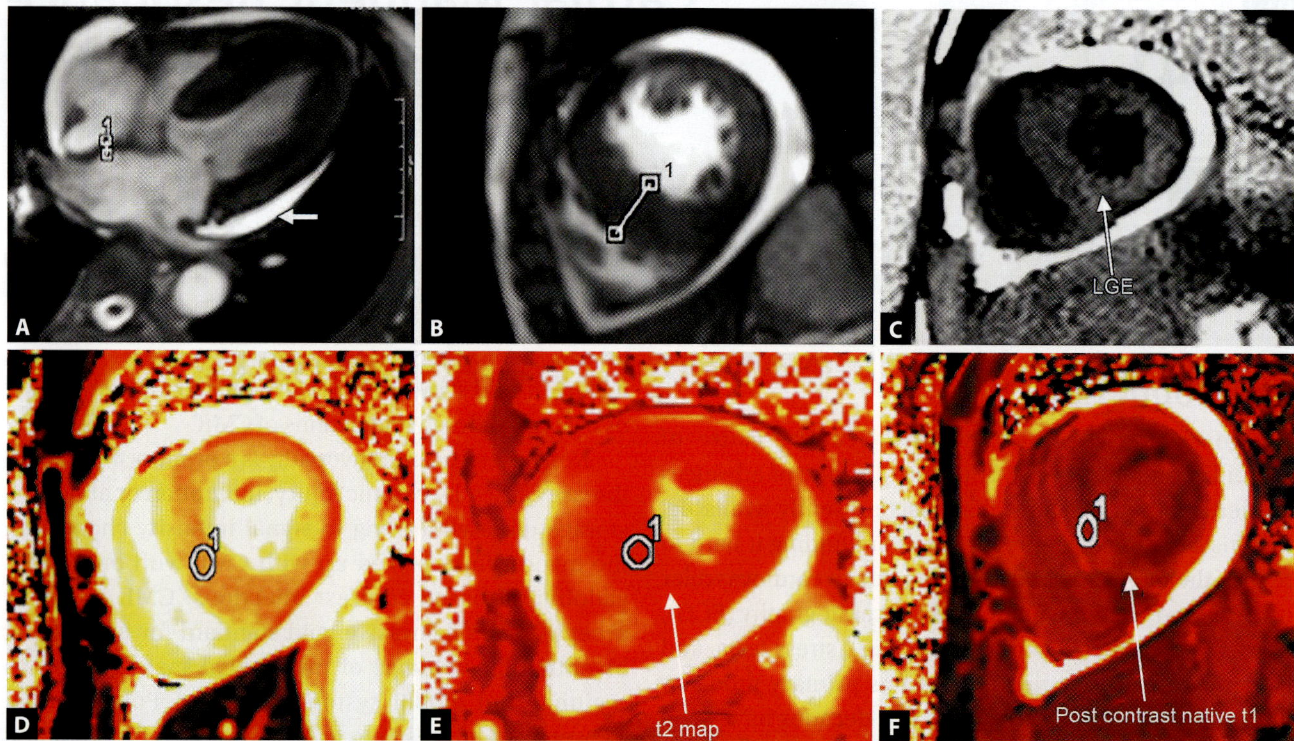

Figs. 1A to F: Cardiac MRI (CMR) demonstrated thickening of the interatrial septum (A), along with a circumferential pericardial effusion (indicated by the block arrow) on the four-chamber (4C) view; asymmetric left ventricular (LV) myocardial wall thickening was observed on short axis view steady-state free precession (SSFP) sequence (B), with diffuse late gadolinium enhancement (C); mapping sequences showed elevated native T1, T2, and extracellular volume (ECV) values (D to F); these findings were consistent with, and later confirmed to be, *cardiac amyloidosis*.

thickness, regional fibrosis and left ventricular outflow tract (LVOT) and LV cavity obstruction. All these markers can be quantitatively assessed by CMR. Presence of myocardial crypts, non-compaction can be assessed with LV planimetry evaluation can be easily done with CMR. Quantification of myocardial fibrosis is associated with risk for heart failure and sudden cardiac death. The fibrosis of >15% of LV myocardial volume can be taken as a marker for ICD placement. Another important aspect is differentiation between pathological hypertrophy and athletes' heart. Extracellular volume calculation (ECV) is increased in pathological hypertrophy and remains normal in cases of athletes heart[6] **(Table 1 and Figs. 3A to D)**.

Arrhythmogenic cardiomyopathy is a cause of sudden death especially in young people. Modified Task Force Criteria 2010 includes assessment of RV wall aneurysms/dyskinetic segments and RV functional abnormality in the form of significant increase in normalized end diastolic volume and reduction in RV ejection fraction. Padua criteria and recently published European Society of Cardiology Criteria have CMR as cornerstone of diagnosis. CMR is considered to be gold standard in RV volume measurements and hence significantly helpful in diagnosis of arrhythmogenic cardiomyopathy. Other abnormalities observed by CMR include irregular dilatation with trabecular hypertrophy of base of RV wall and dilatation of right ventricular outflow tract (RVOT)[7] **(Fig. 4)**.

Left ventricular non-compaction (LVNC) cardiomyopathy is characterized by LV dilatation, hypokinesis, and abnormally high proportion of trabecular non-compacted myocardium. Generally, a wall thickness ratio of non-compacted over compacted wall of 2.3 or higher was proposed to verify LVNC. A recent meta-analysis found that patients with LVNC without LGE have a better prognosis than those with LGE.

Anderson Fabry's disease is caused by a significant recognition of sphingolipids with symmetric hypertrophy. CMR's ability to detect fat on different sequences, especially native T1 allows diagnosis of Anderson Fabry's disease. Postcontrast images can show layers of LGE typically along

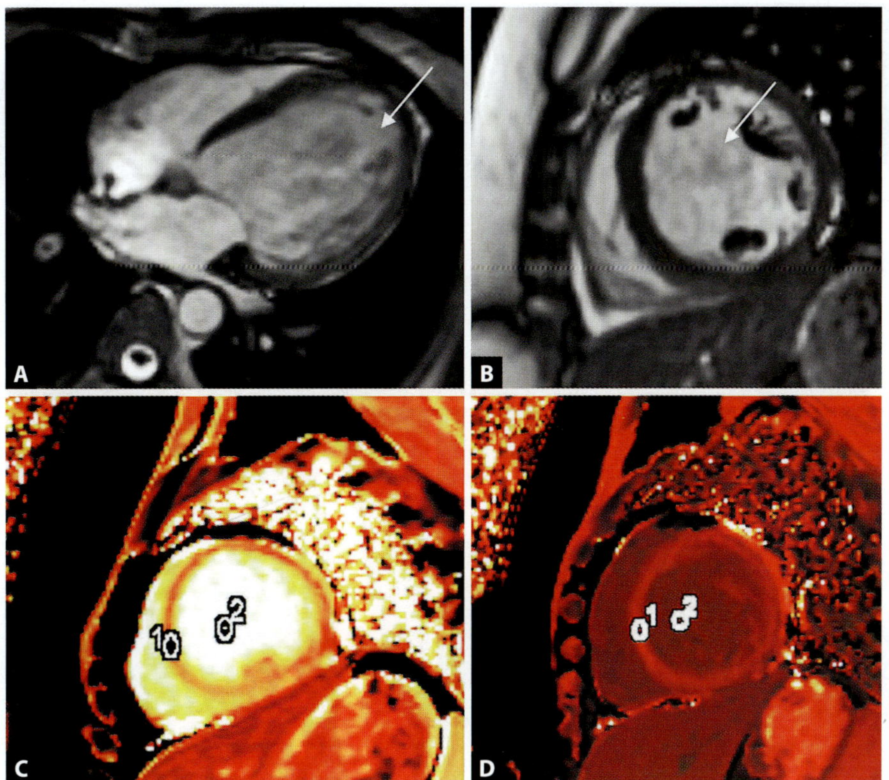

Figs. 2A to D: Cardiac MRI (CMR) in a patient with dilated cardiomyopathy (DCM) shows a dilated left ventricle (arrow) with myocardial wall thinning on the four-chamber (4C) view (A) and the short-axis (SA) view (B); Parametric mapping demonstrates elevated native T1, T2, and extracellular volume (ECV) values (C and D), suggesting interstitial fibrosis.

TABLE 1: Functional analysis on cardiac MRI (CMR) in same patient shows a significantly reduced left ventricular (LV) ejection fraction of 27%.

Left ventricle	
LV ejection fraction	27%
Stroke volume	29.1 mL
End-diastolic volume index	67.1 mL/m^2
End-systolic volume index	49.3 mL/m^2
End-diastolic volume	109 mL
End-systolic volume	80.3 mL
Heart rate	108 bpm
Mass ED	149 g
Peak filling rate	350 mL/s
Peak ejection rate	210 mL/s
Cardiac output	3.1 L/min
Cardiac index	1.93 L/min/m^2
Stroke volume Index	17.9 mL/m^2
Mass	153 g
Mass ES	165 g
End-diastolic epicardial volume	252 mL
End-systolic epicardial volume	237 mL
Standard deviation heart rate	2 bpm

Contd...

Contd...

the lateral wall. Decrease in native T1 and increased on T2 values with lateral wall enhancement can be characteristic for diagnosis of Anderson Fabry's disease.[7]

In cases of *cardiac sarcoidosis* CMR helps to exclude myocardial infiltration and associated inflammation. Cardiac sarcoidosis usually presents as global systolic dysfunction, LV dilatation and patterns of regional distribution of myocardial lesions may substantially vary

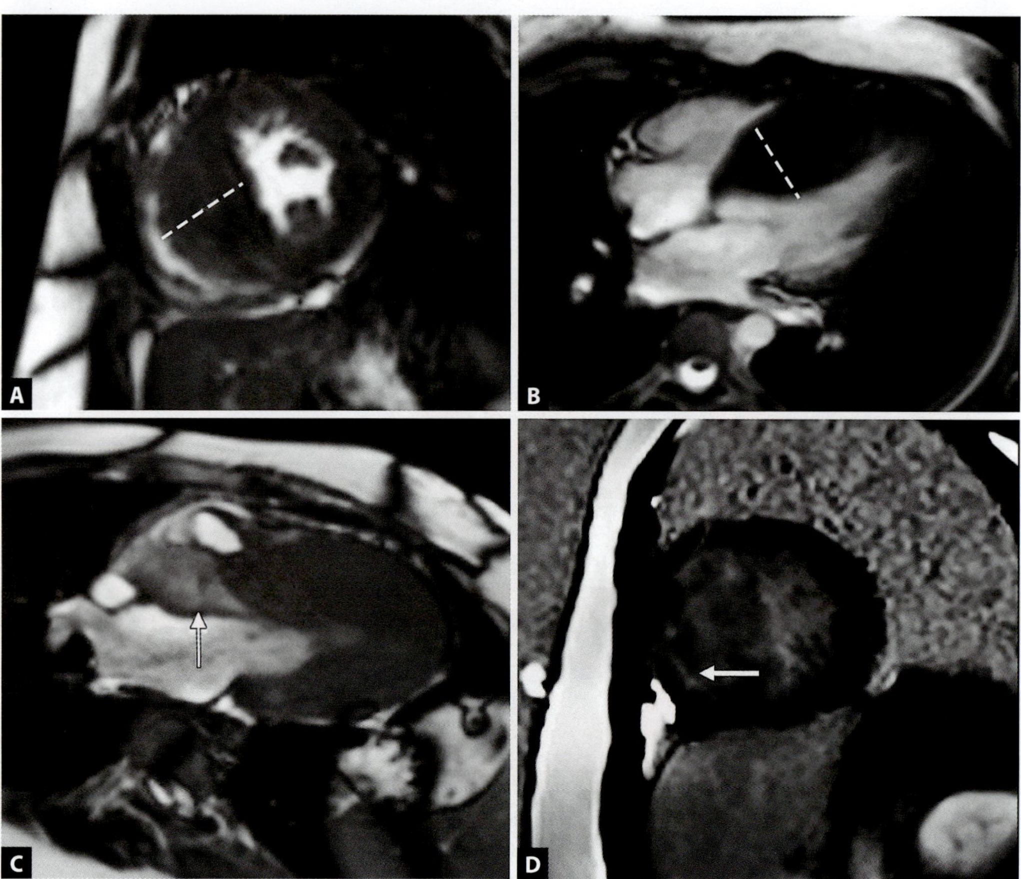

Figs. 3A to D: Cardiac MRI (CMR) demonstrates diffuse thickening of the left ventricular (LV) myocardium, predominantly involving the basal septal wall (dotted line), as seen on short-axis (SA) and four-chamber (4C) steady-state free precession (SSFP) images (A and B); the three-chamber (3C) view shows systolic anterior motion (SAM) of the mitral valve (arrow) resulting in left ventricular outflow tract (LVOT) obstruction (C); mid-myocardial late gadolinium enhancement (block arrow) is noted on the SA view (D); these findings are suggestive of hypertrophic obstructive cardiomyopathy (HOCM).

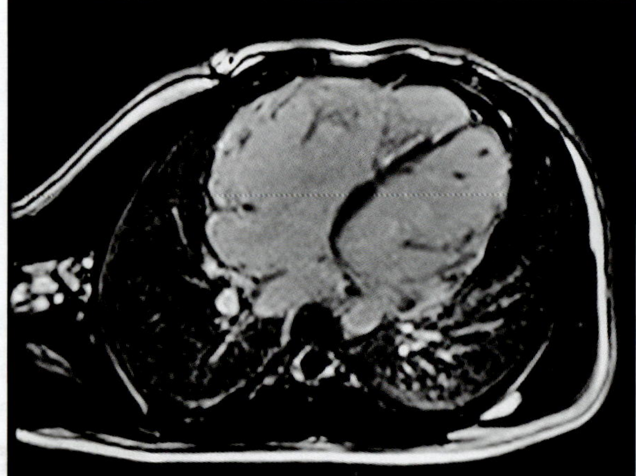

Fig. 4: Cardiac MRI (CMR) in a 20-year-old male patient with a history of syncope shows, on the four-chamber (4C) late gadolinium enhancement image, dilatation of both the right ventricle (RV) and left ventricle (LV); there is focal aneurysmal dilatation along the RV free wall, with areas of fibrosis involving both the RV and LV walls, suggesting biventricular involvement in a case of arrhythmogenic right ventricular dysplasia (ARVD) with associated left ventricular dysfunction (ALVD).

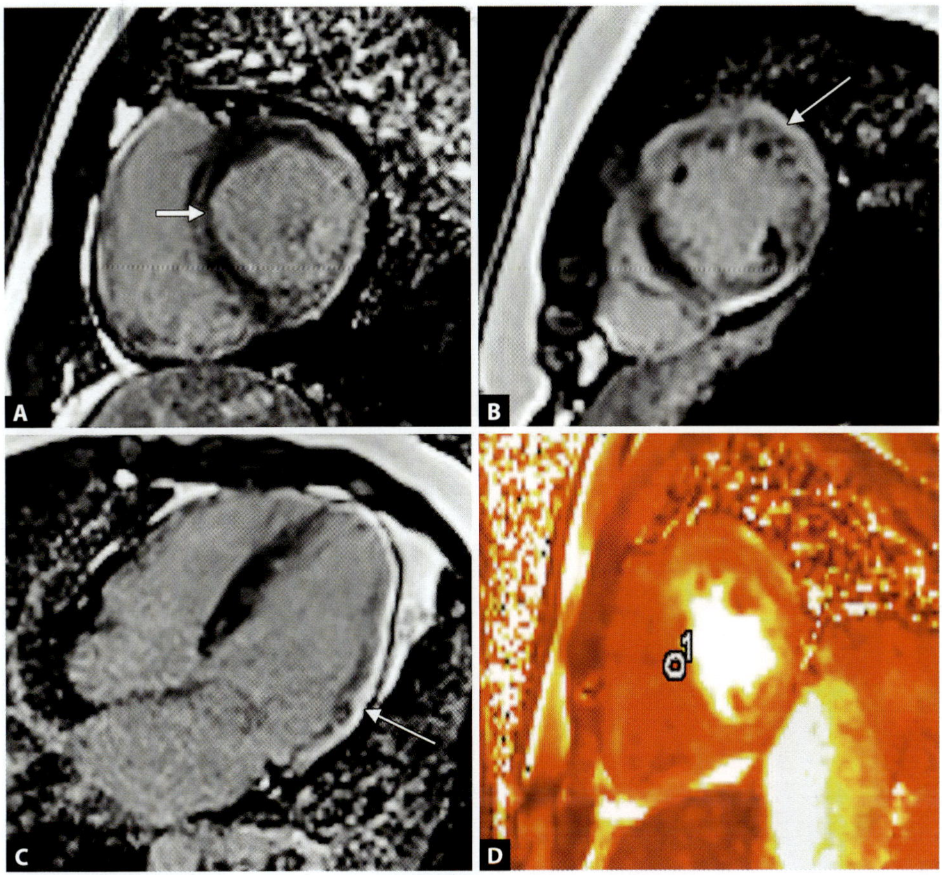

Figs. 5A to D: Cardiac MRI (CMR) in a biopsy proven case of sarcoidosis reveals a dilated left ventricle with late gadolinium enhancement showing sub-epicardial (arrow) and mid-myocardial (block arrow) areas of enhancement in the lateral segments of the basal and mid myocardium on the short-axis (SA) views (A and B) and the four-chamber (4C) view (C); T2 mapping shows elevated values (D), indicative of myocardial edema.

with areas of fibrosis in the transmural, mid-myocardial and some epicardial regions[5] **(Figs. 5A to D)**.

Stress-induced cardiomyopathy (Takotsubo) can show systolic ballooning of the LV. LGE is rarely observed. T2-weighted images show extensive myocardial edema with typical wall motion abnormality.[6]

Endomyocardial fibrosis on CMR shows typical small ventricular volumes with systolic dysfunction and typical pattern of LGE enhancement with apical clots **(Figs. 6A to D)**.

Myocardial iron overload: Myocardial Iron overload in patients undergoing repeated transfusion has become one of the most important applications of CMR. Its ability to detect presence of iron in myocardium by marked shortening effect on myocardial T2*. Corrective treatment is started in patients who have been shown to be at high risk, that is T2* of <10 ms.[5] It is a well-evaluated technique for follow-up for treatment evaluation[8] **(Fig. 7)**.

Myocarditis is non-ischemic myocardial inflammation and edema due to various causes from cardiotoxicity to viral myocarditis. Recently updated Lake Lewis criteria for CMR in non-ischemic myocardial inflammation recommend to assess myocarditis using native T1, native T2 markers that detect myocardial edema and myocardial injury with ECV measurements for increased extracellular space caused by necrosis or scar.[9] LGE has limited sensitivity to detect myocarditis and is not specific to the acuity of disease. When present LGE are typically present in non-ischemic regions of distribution **(Fig. 8 and Table 2)**.

Pericardial diseases: CMR has involved as one of the preferred modalities for pericardial imaging. Pericardial morphology evaluation in hemodynamic consequences

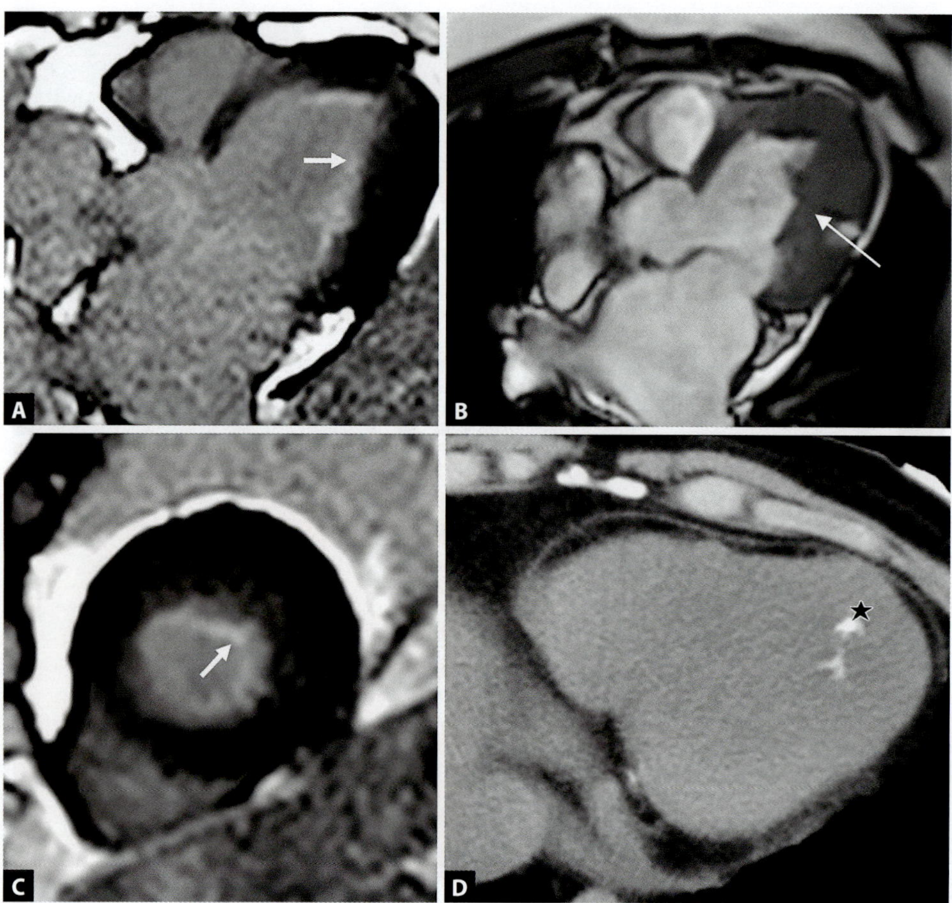

Figs. 6A to D: Multimodality imaging in this patient with endomyocardial fibrosis (EMF) demonstrates subendocardial late gadolinium enhancement (block arrows) on both the four-chamber (4C) view (A) and the short-axis (SA) view (B); asymmetric thickening of the lateral left ventricular (LV) wall with a thrombus is seen on steady-state free precession (SSFP) images (C); cardiac CT shows myocardial calcification (star) along the LV (D).

on heart and presence of concomitant or superimposed myocardial valvular disease can be well evaluated with CMR. It does not helps in evaluation of pericardial calcification which is best seen on CT. However, the balanced steady-state free precession (bSSFP) cine images allow evaluation of hemodynamic consequences such as cardiac tamponade and constriction. Complete morphological evaluation of pericardial and surrounding structures and cine free breathing sequences help in identifying constrictive pericarditis, pericardial inflammation, changes in the underlying myocardium, and even congenital abnormalities of pericardium **(Fig. 9 and Table 3)**.

Valve evaluation: TTE will likely remain the first line and most common imaging modality for assessing valve diseases. CMR is recommended when echocardiographic assessment is unable to provide sufficient information.[10] CMR can act as complimentary method in valve evaluation. It acts as class I indication for identification of sub and supravalvular stenosis, pulmonary stenosis, and pulmonary regurgitation **(Table 4)**.

Phase contrast velocity mapping delivers transvalvular velocity similar to echocardiogram with advantage of not relying on alignment of the flow jet with Doppler beam. The major advantage of this phase contrast imaging technique is to quantify flow. This facilitates true quantification of regurgitant valve lesions rather than quantitative grading based on arbitrary thresholds.

Flow quantification, planimetric valve area calculation, valve morphology evaluation, and evaluation of secondary changes on RV in LV myocardium as well as on the atria is comprehensively done with CMR. Evaluation of secondary fibrosis and remodeling in the ventricles is

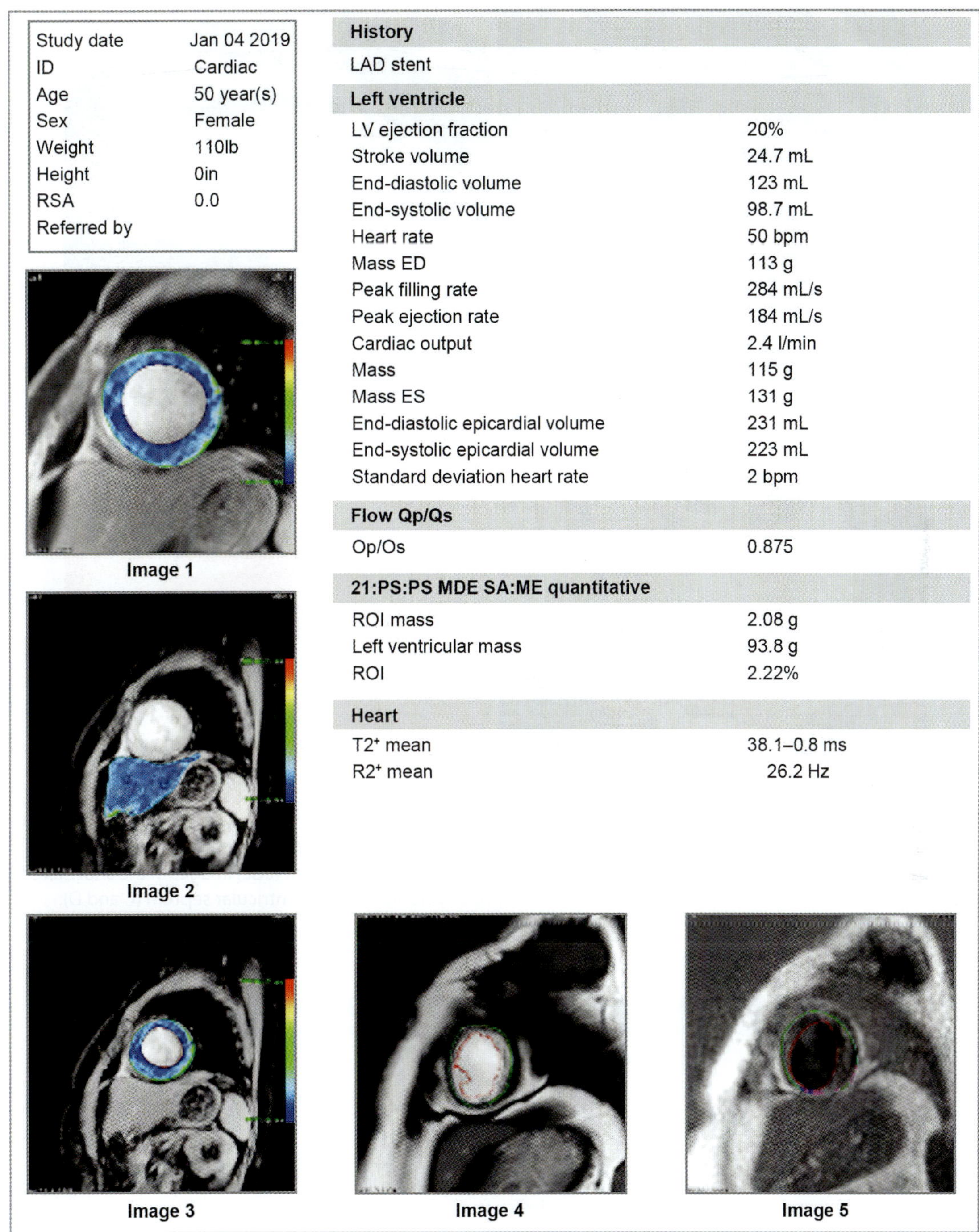

Study date	Jan 04 2019
ID	Cardiac
Age	50 year(s)
Sex	Female
Weight	110lb
Height	0in
RSA	0.0
Referred by	

History	
LAD stent	
Left ventricle	
LV ejection fraction	20%
Stroke volume	24.7 mL
End-diastolic volume	123 mL
End-systolic volume	98.7 mL
Heart rate	50 bpm
Mass ED	113 g
Peak filling rate	284 mL/s
Peak ejection rate	184 mL/s
Cardiac output	2.4 l/min
Mass	115 g
Mass ES	131 g
End-diastolic epicardial volume	231 mL
End-systolic epicardial volume	223 mL
Standard deviation heart rate	2 bpm
Flow Qp/Qs	
Op/Os	0.875
21:PS:PS MDE SA:ME quantitative	
ROI mass	2.08 g
Left ventricular mass	93.8 g
ROI	2.22%
Heart	
T2* mean	38.1–0.8 ms
R2* mean	26.2 Hz

Fig. 7: Cardiac MRI (CMR) comprehensive report giving information about LV volumes, QP: QS ratios, percentage fibrosis in the myocardium and myocardial and liver iron quantification.

best done with CMR. Negative T1 and ECV calculations can give ideas about interstitial fibrosis which may not be picked up with LGE. The diastolic and systolic volume calculations done with CMR with morphologic changes in the myocardium can predict optimal timing for valve replacement interventions or surgeries.

Virtually all prosthetic valve and rings are safe in both 1.5T and 3 T CMR scanners.

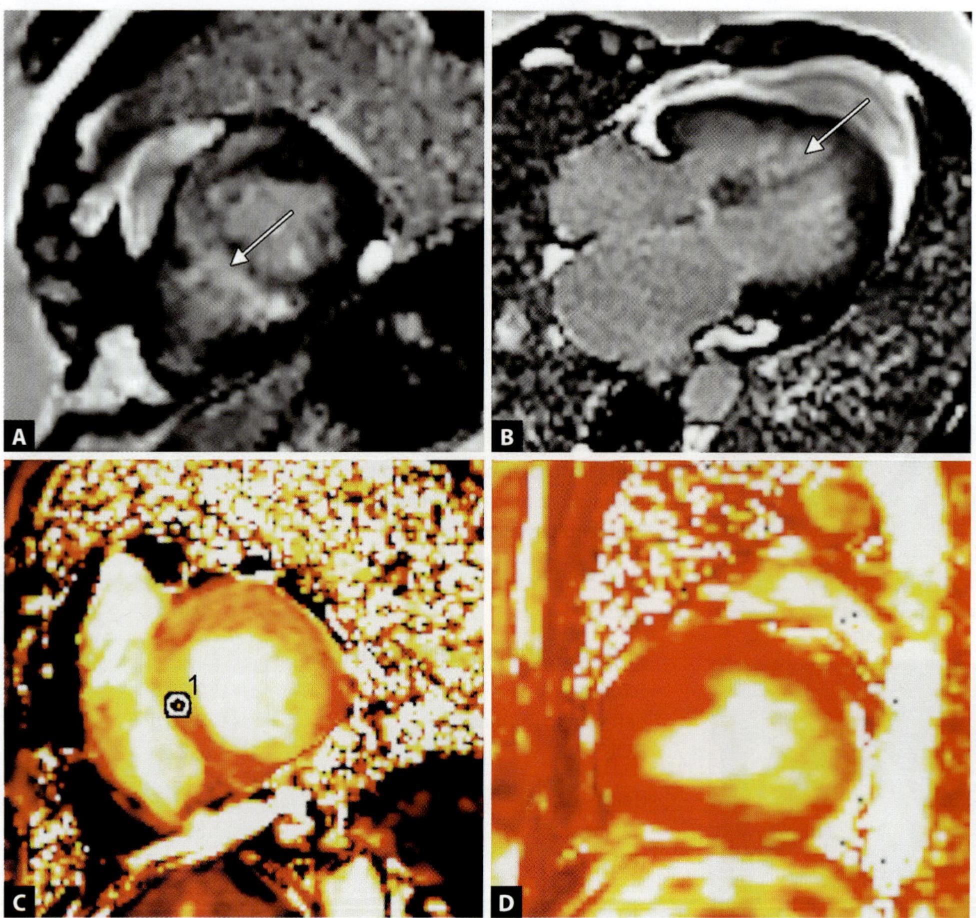

Figs. 8A to D: Cardiac MRI (CMR) reveals patchy areas of mid-myocardial and epicardial enhancement along the anterior and septal segments of the basal, mid, and apical myocardium (arrow) on late gadolinium enhancement (LGE) images in the short-axis (SA) view (A) and four-chamber (4C) view (B); T1 and T2 mapping show increased values along the interventricular septum (C and D).

TABLE 2: Indications of cardiac MRI (CMR) in cardiomyopathies.[11]

Level	*Indications*
I	• Dilated CM • Hypertrophic CM • Myocarditis • Arrhythmogenic CM • Cardiac amyloidosis • Myocardial iron overload • LV noncompaction • Fabry's disease • Cardiac sarcoidosis • Endomyocardial fibrosis (EMF) • Takotsubo CM
II	• Restrictive CM • Chemotherapy induced CM • Athletes' heart

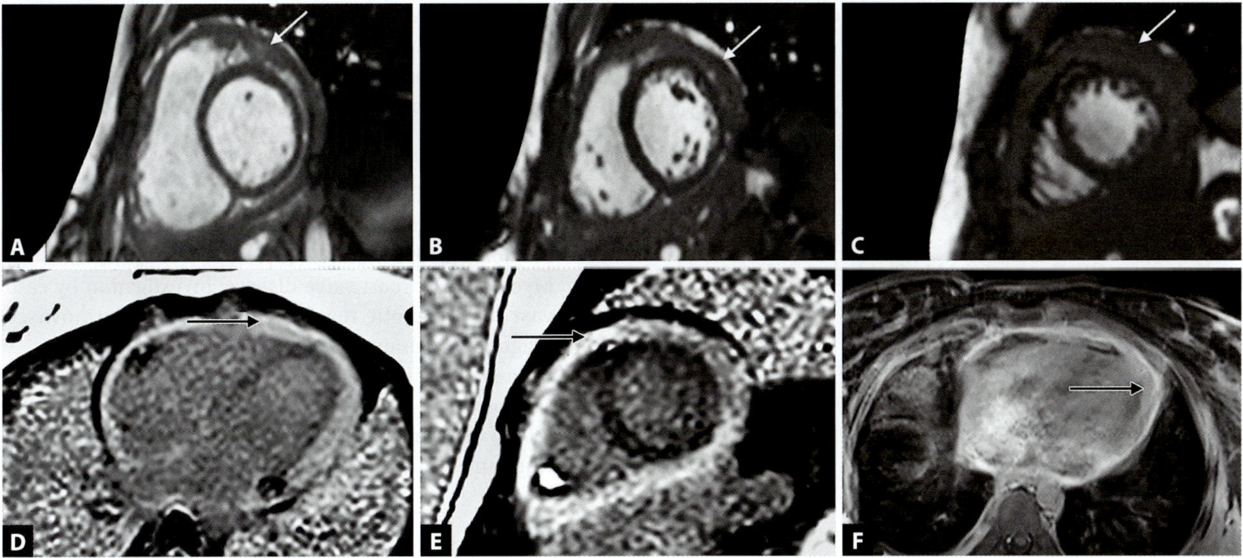

Figs. 9A to F: Cardiac MRI (CMR) in a patient with pericarditis demonstrates diffuse circumferential pericardial thickening (arrow) involving the basal (A), mid (B), and apical (C) levels of the myocardium on the short-axis (SA) view. Late gadolinium enhancement of the pericardium is seen on the four-chamber (4C) view (D), short-axis view (E), and post-contrast T1 imaging (F), as indicated by black arrows.

TABLE 3: Indications of cardiac MRI (CMR) in pericardial diseases[11]

Level	*Indications*
I	• Congenital anomalies of pericardium • Constrictive pericarditis • Pericardial inflammation
III	Pericardial effusion

TABLE 4: Indication of cardiac MRI (CMR) in valvular heart diseases[11]

Level	*Indications*
I	• Identification of sub and supravalvular stenosis • Pulmonary stenosis • Pulmonary regurgitation
II	• Aortic stenosis • Aortic regurgitation • Mitral regurgitation • Tricuspid regurgitation • Prosthetic valve disease
III	• Mitral stenosis • Tricuspid stenosis
IV	Ascending aortic flow patterns in aortic stenosis

CONCLUSION

Cardiac MRI acts as a solution or a guide in diagnosis and treatment follow-up in nonischemic cardiomyopathies. Newer genetic cardiomyopathies and metabolic cardiomyopathies can give appearances similar to one we have evaluated. Clinical background, distribution of LGE, and multiparametric mapping with native T1, T2, ECV, and T2* will help in better outcome in many patients.

REFERENCES

1. World Health Organization. (2024). Cardiovascular diseases (CVDs). [online] Available from https://www. who. int/news-room/fact-sheets/detail/cardiovascular-diseases-(cvds) [Last accessed September 2025].
2. Narula J, Chandrashekhar Y, Ahmadi A, Abbara S, Berman DS, Blankstein R, et al. SCCT 2021 expert consensus document on coronary computed tomographic angiography: a report of the society of cardiovascular computed tomography. Journal of cardiovascular computed tomography. 2020;15(3):192.
3. Grothues F, Smith GC, Moon JC, Bellenger NG, Collins P, Klein HU, et al. Comparison of interstudy reproducibility of cardiovascular magnetic resonance with two-dimensional echocardiography in normal subjects and in patients with heart failure or left ventricular hypertrophy. The American journal of cardiology. 2002;90(1):29-34.
4. Sado DM, White SK, Piechnik SK, Banypersad SM, Treibel T, Captur G, , et al. Identification and assessment

of Anderson–Fabry disease by cardiovascular magnetic resonance noncontrast myocardial T1 mapping. Circ Cardiovasc Imaging. 2013;6(3):392-8.

5. Ferreira VM, Schulz-Menger J, Holmvang G, Kramer CM, Carbone I, Sechtem U, et al. Cardiovascular magnetic resonance in nonischemic myocardial inflammation: Expert recommendations. J Am Coll Cardiol. 2018;72(24): 3158-3176.
6. Kotanidis CP, Bazmpani MA, Haidich AB, Karvounis C, Antoniades C, Karamitsos TD. Diagnostic accuracy of cardiovascular magnetic resonance in acute myocarditis: a systematic review and meta-analysis. J Am Coll Cardiol Cardiovasc Imaging. 2018;11(11):1583-90.
7. Meloni A, Pistoia L, Positano V, De Luca A, Martini N, Spasiano A, et al. Increased myocardial extracellular volume is associated with myocardial iron overload and heart failure in thalassemia major. Eur Radiol. 2023;33(2):1266-76.
8. Adam RD, Shambrook J, Flett AS. The prognostic role of tissue characterisation using cardiovascular magnetic resonance in heart failure. Cardiac Failure Review. 2017; 3(2):86.
9. Salcedo EE, Cohen GI, White RD, Davison MB. Cardiac tumors: diagnosis and management. Current problems in cardiology. 1992;17(2):77-137.
10. Myerson SG. Heart valve disease: investigation by cardiovascular magnetic resonance. Journal of Cardiovascular Magnetic Resonance. 2012;14(1):42.
11. Leiner T, Bogaert J, Friedrich MG, Mohiaddin R, Muthurangu V, Myerson S, et al. SCMR Position Paper (2020) on clinical indications for cardiovascular magnetic resonance. J Cardiovasc Magnet Res. 2020;22(1):76.

CHAPTER 42

Role of Cardiac Magnetic Resonance in Atrial Cardiomyopathy

Ruma Zaidi, Suraj Gowda, Richa Kothari

INTRODUCTION

Atria play an essential role in cardiac function, including hemodynamic regulation and endocrine function, and they host crucial parts of the conduction system such as pacemaker cells and the atrioventricular node. There are three main functional phases of the left atrium (LA): The reservoir phase during systole; collects blood from the pulmonary veins during left ventricular (LV) systole and isovolumetric diastole to maintain LV filling, the conduit phase in early diastole; passively pumping blood to the ventricle, and the booster pump phase in late diastole; the atrium actively contracts to pump the remaining blood into the LV.[1]

Atrial myocardium is susceptible to many cardiac and noncardiac conditions and can be more sensitive than ventricular myocardium.[2] Atrial cells, including cardiomyocytes and noncardiomyocyte elements such as fibroblasts, endothelial cells, and neurons, react briskly to pathological stimuli,[3] and are influenced by genetic factors.[4] Structural or architectural changes in the atrial myocardium may cause significant electrophysiological disturbances.

While most cardiomyopathies affect all parts of the heart, some target-specific chambers. The concept of atrial cardiomyopathy (ACM) first appeared in a study published in 1972, describing a familial syndrome affecting the atria and atrioventricular-conducting system.[5] More recently, Kottkamp proposed that "atrial fibrotic cardiomyopathy" is a common pathological denominator of all forms of atrial fibrillation (AF), caused by a primary cardiomyopathic process, independent of arrhythmia.[6] The clinical importance of left atrial cardiomyopathy (LACM) lies in its connection with AF and embolic strokes of unknown origins. Therefore, early identification of LACM could be crucial for stroke prevention.[7]

DEFINITION AND CLASSIFICATION

The European Heart Rhythm Association (EHRAS) consensus defines "atrial cardiomyopathy" as "any complex of structural, architectural, contractile, or electrophysiological changes affecting the atria with the potential to produce clinically relevant manifestations".[8]

ACM can be induced by various diseases, such as hypertension, heart failure, diabetes, and myocarditis, or conditions such as aging and endocrine abnormalities. These induced changes are often not disease-specific and tend to share many similarities. Pathological changes can vary over time and atrial location, leading to significant intraindividual and interindividual differences. While some pathological processes may selectively affect the atria (e.g., atrial fibrillation-induced remodeling), most cardiomyopathies impacting the atria also involve the ventricles to some extent.

EHRAS categorizes ACM into four classes[8] **(Table 1)**.

A limitation of this descriptive classification is that different atrial cardiomyopathies can exhibit features of

TABLE 1: Categorization of ACM into four classes by the EHRAS.

EHRAS class	*Histological characterization*
I	Primarily cardiomyocyte dependent with no significant fibrosis
II	Primarily fibroblast dependent with normal cardiomyocytes
III	Combination of I and II
IV	Primarily noncollagen deposits
IVa	Amyloid infiltration
IVf	Fatty infiltration
IVi	Inflammatory cells
IVo	Other interstitial changes

(ACM: atrial cardiomyopathy; EHRAS: the European Heart Rhythm Association)

multiple EHRAS classes.[8] The only exception is atrial amyloidosis, which falls exclusively into class IVa.

ETIOPATHOGENESIS

Table 2 provides a brief outlook on various etiopathogenesis of ACM.

DIAGNOSIS

To diagnose LACM accurately, a histological examination of the atrial myocardium is necessary, but due to the invasive nature of LA biopsies, this is rarely performed except in specific cases like mitral valve surgery. As an alternative, noninvasive methods like cardiac MRI (CMR), electro-anatomic mapping, and PET-CT are used to detect fibrosis or scars in the LA. Additionally, transthoracic echocardiography (TTE), CT, and MRI can identify mechanical dysfunctions, while ECG parameters can detect electrical dysfunctions resulting from LACM.[21] This chapter mainly focuses on the role of CMR in ACM.

Left Atrial Volume and Function Assessment

In the absence of mitral valve disease, an enlarged LA typically signifies elevated wall tension due to increased LA pressure, as well as LA dysfunction secondary to atrial myopathy. Enlarged LA is associated with a greater incidence of AF, stroke, and major cardiac events.[22-24] LA enlargement also marks the severity and chronicity of LV diastolic dysfunction.

Traditionally, atrial size was estimated using TTE-based linear long-axis LA diameters from two-dimensional (2D) images or M-mode tracings. However, due to the atrium's complex structure and nonuniform remodeling, this method often fails to provide an accurate assessment.[25] Thus, LA volume (LAV), indexed for body mass, is now preferred. The European Society of Cardiology considers an indexed LAV (LAVi) above 34 mL/m^2 as the threshold for LA enlargement.[26]

Although echocardiography is preferred for screening and monitoring abnormal LA morphology and function, it

TABLE 2: A brief outlook on various etiopathogenesis of atrial cardiomyopathy (ACM).

S. No.	Causative factors	Pathophysiology	EHARS class
1	Isolated atrial amyloidosis (IAA)	Atrial natriuretic peptide (ANP) is a fibrillogenic protein that forms IAA.[9] Resultant conduction blocks noted	IVa
2	Natriuretic peptide precursor A (NPPA) mutations	NPPA encodes prepro-ANP. Abnormal ANP is linked to familial atrial cardiomyopathy[10]	II
3	Hereditary muscular dystrophies	Myotonic dystrophy type I: Associated with atrial arrhythmias.[11] Emery–Dreifuss and Limb–Girdle IB: extensive atrial fibrosis[12]	Any
4	ACM due to congestive heart failure (CHF)	CHF induces atrial fibrosis and atrial hypocontractility[13]	II and III
5	Obstructive sleep apnea (OSA)	OSA prolongs atrial conduction times and reduces atrial electrogram voltages[14]	II
6	AF-induced atrial remodeling	AF causes Ca^{2+} loading and atrial contractile dysfunction,[15] leading to atrial fibrosis	I and III
7	Myocarditis	Infiltration of inflammatory cells causes architectural remodeling interfering with atrial conduction[16]	IVi
8	Aging	Various conduction abnormalities seen with progressive age[17]	II
9	Hypertension	Slowed global and regional conduction with LA enlargement, reduced LA emptying fraction and atrial fibrosis[18]	I–III
10	Obesity	Increase in the left atrial epicardial fat, a global reduction in atrial conduction velocity, LA dilatation and dysfunction[19]	IVf and III
11	Diabetes mellitus	Insulin resistance is associated with increased left atrial size and structural heterogeneity[20]	I, III, and IV
12	ACM due to valvular heart disease	Mitral and aortic stenoses have been associated with atrial structural remodeling and a propensity for AF	III

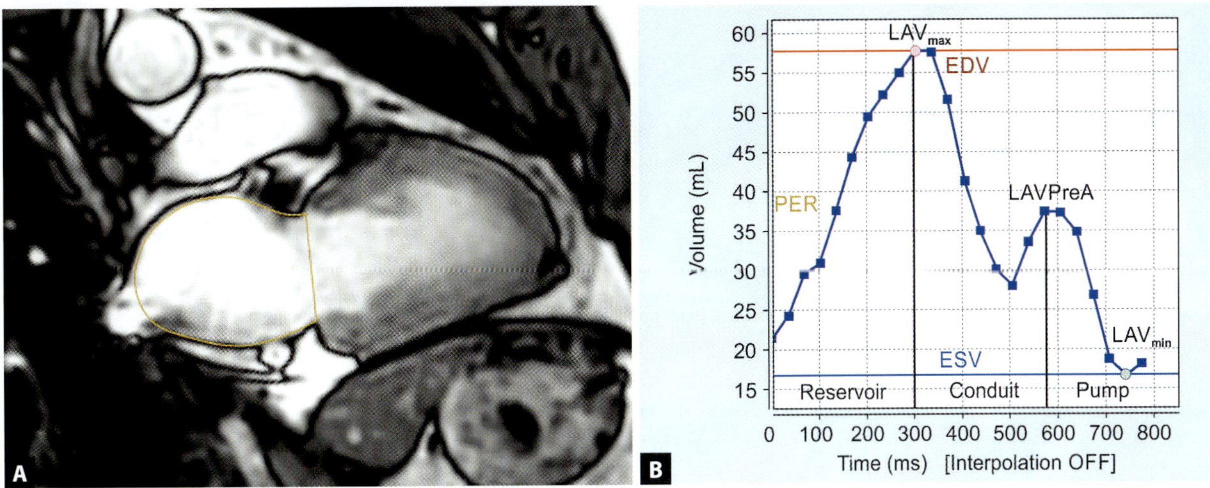

Figs. 1A and B: Normal LA volume measurement depicted on CMR feature tracking using two-chamber cine SSFP sequence (A). LAV_{max}, LAV_{min}, and LAVPreA measure 57 mL, 16 mL and 37 mL, respectively (B). LA ejection fractions can be calculated using these parameters. (CMR: cardiac magnetic resonance; LA: left atrium; LAV: left atrium volume; SSFP: steady-state free precession)

can underestimate LAV due to geometric assumptions and LA cavity foreshortening in apical views. Additionally, the long axis of the LV differs from the LA, leading to potential underestimation when compared with three-dimensional (3D) echocardiography and CMR.[26]

In recent years CMR feature-tracking (CMR-FT) has been increasingly used to evaluate a number of novel parameters for more detailed assessment of passive and active emptying volumes and fractions **(Figs. 1A and B)**. Steady-state free precession (SSFP) cine sequences are typically used to obtain LA strain and volume quantification from baseline four-chamber and two-chamber cine CMR images by drawing contours along LA endocardium and epicardium. The CMR-FT software then tracks endocardial and epicardial borders in subsequent frames.[27]

Measured LA volumes and derived LA functions are tabulated in **Tables 3 and 4**.

In volumetric method, total, passive and active left atrium emptying fractions (LAEF) are surrogates of reservoir, conduit, and booster pump functions respectively.[28]

The LA volume was 17% larger in patients with incident AF compared with control group ($LAVI_{max}$: 41 ± 15 mL/m^2 versus 35 ± 10 mL/m^2).[29] A cut-off of active LAEF ≤20% has a sensitivity and specificity of 88% and 81%, respectively for new onset AF.[30]

TABLE 3: Left atrial volume quantification.

LA volumes	*Definition*
Maximum LA volume (LAV_{max})	LA volume at end-systole before mitral valve opening
Minimum LA volume (LAV_{min})	LA volume at end-diastole right after mitral valve closure
Preatrial contraction LA volume (LAVPreA)	LA volume before atrial contraction

(LA: left atrium; LAV: left atrium volume)

TABLE 4: Left atrial function calculation.

LA function	*Formula*	*Surrogate marker of*
Passive LA emptying fraction (passive LAEF)	(LAV_{max} – LAVPreA)/ LAV_{max}	LA conduit function
Active LA emptying fraction (active LAEF)	(LAVPreA – LAV_{min})/ LAVPreA	LA booster pump function
Total LA emptying fraction (total LAEF)	(LAV_{max} – LAV_{min})/ LAV_{max}	LA reservoir function

(LA: left atrium; LAEF: left atrium emptying fractions; LAV: left atrium volume)

Strain Analysis

Cardiac magnetic resonance feature-tracking and post-processing software are used to measure LA strain and strain rate parameters. Due to the unique fiber orientation and thin atrial wall, only the longitudinal strain of the atria

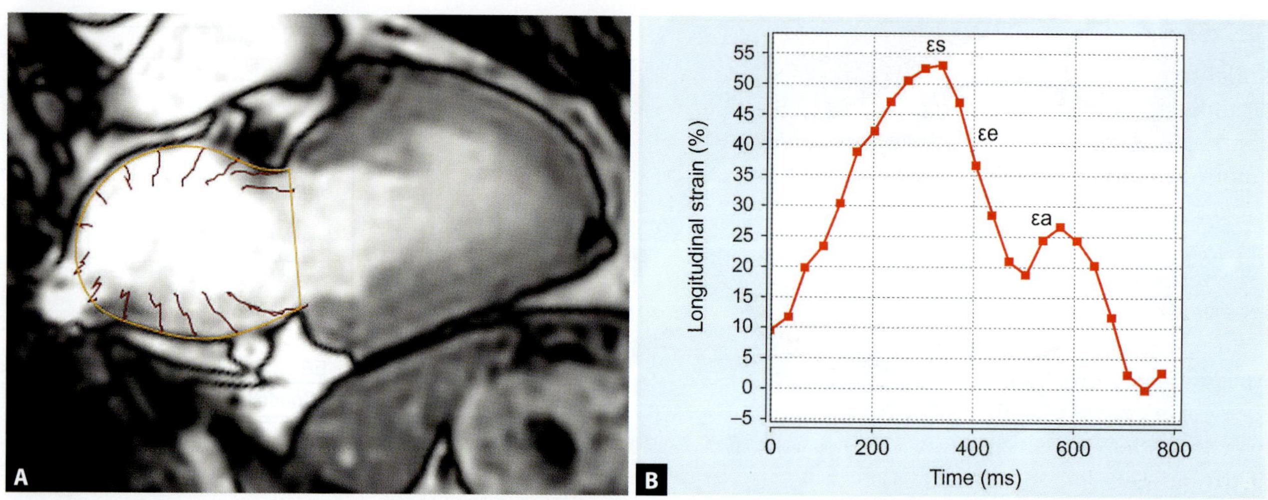

Figs. 2A and B: Normal LA longitudinal strain parameters using two-chamber cine SSFP sequence (A). εs, εe, and εa are depicted on the graph (B). (LA: left atrium; SSFP: steady-state free precession)

is typically measured.[31] CMR-derived LA strain and strain rate can assess atrial function in three phases, including reservoir strain (LA εs), peak positive strain rate (SRs), conduit strain (LA εe), peak early negative strain rate (SRe), booster strain (LA εa), and peak late negative strain rate (SRa) **(Figs. 2A and B)**.[32]

Currently, atrial strain measurements using CMR-FT are primarily a research tool. The variability and lack of standardized LA strain parameter values across different postprocessing software hinder its broader use, and normal reference values should be used cautiously in clinical settings.[31]

Studies have shown that LA strain can identify microscopic pump dysfunction in patients with paroxysmal AF; LA εa reduces before the decrease in LAEF booster.[33] LA εs (≤18%) and LA εa (≤8%) were associated with a nearly three- and fourfold increased risk of new-onset AF, respectively.[34] The main effect of AF is on atrial compliance, thereby impairing LA εs and LA εe.[35] AF with extensive LA fibrosis records lower LA εs and LA εe and conduit function (LA εe) correlates most strongly with the degree of LA fibrosis.[36] Peak LA longitudinal strain is used as a representative of LA reservoir function.[28]

Tissue Characterization

Delayed-enhancement MRI

Assessment of atrial fibrosis from CMR images can be performed using late gadolinium enhancement (LGE) images with a high intra- and interobserver correlation. Furthermore, the total volume of fibrotic tissue can be calculated as a percentage of the LA wall volume and subsequently categorized into stages.

LGE images are acquired 15 minutes after the contrast injection (0.1 mmol/kg) using 3D inversion recovery, ECG-gated gradient-echo pulse with fat saturation. The optimal inversion time is identified with an inversion time scout scan to maximize nulling of the LA myocardium. ECG gating is used to acquire views during the diastolic phase of LA cardiac cycle (LV systole). It is advised to image patients with AF after restoration of sinus rhythm.

For fibrosis quantification, the epicardial and endocardial contours are drawn and analyzed by software. The extent of fibrosis in the LA wall is quantified using a threshold-based algorithm. Fibrosis can be classified according to the Utah stage model: Stage I (mild) with <15% LA wall enhancement, stage II (moderate) with 15–35% LA wall enhancement, and stage III (extensive) with >35% LA wall enhancement.[37]

LGE-fibrosis correlates with decreased LA function and shows inverse relation with LA strain and strain rate parameters.[38] Rising Utah stage is associated with increased risk of major cardiovascular events, predominantly due to the increased risk of stroke or transient ischemic attack (TIA).[39]

Although CMR offers excellent spatial resolution for identifying the endocardial atrial wall borders, its ability to distinguish between the atrial myocardial and epicardial walls is limited. This is because the imaging signal of the LA wall may be affected by partial volume effects due to the thinness of the atrial wall compared to the LGE-CMR voxel size.[40]

T1 Mapping

Cardiac magnetic resonance (CMR) T1 mapping is a newly developed technique used to measure contrast-enhanced T1 relaxation times in targeted tissues. It has been demonstrated that there is an inverse linear correlation between contrast-enhanced LV myocardial T1 time and the extent of global myocardial fibrosis.[41]

A modified Look-Locker inversion recovery sequence in the vertical long-axis view is used for imaging. Regions of interest (ROIs) are placed on the LA posterior wall myocardium across all phases of the Look-Locker sequence **(Fig. 3)**. The median LA T1 relaxation time is significantly lower in patients with AF (364–428 ms) compared to healthy individuals (418–532 ms).[42] Recent studies suggest that quantifying fibrosis could help to identify patients who are most likely to benefit from AF ablation.[43]

Four-dimensional Flow by Cardiac Magnetic Resonance

Four-dimensional (4D) **(Figs. 4A and B)** flow CMR provides comprehensive quantification of time-resolved, three-directional blood flow velocities with full volumetric coverage of the LA with the potential to comment on global and regional peak velocities, stasis, and time to peak. Significant reduction in peak LA appendage velocity is noted in AF patients compared to those in sinus rhythm, a marker to predict thromboembolism.[44] Higher prevalence of LA flow stasis (voxels with velocity <0.1 m/s) is found among AF patients versus healthy controls.[45] However, data acquisition using 4D flow is time-consuming with scan time dependent on breathing patterns of the subject, limiting the applicability of this method in a clinical setting.

Epicardial Adipose Tissue: CMR and CT

Epicardial adipose tissue (EAT) is located between the epicardium and pericardium. EAT is associated with the presence, severity, and recurrence of AF, but the exact mechanism is unclear and thought to involve adipokines and inflammatory cytokines. CMR effectively visualizes and measures EAT without using radiation or contrast agents. EAT is a risk factor and independent predictor of AF development and recurrence after ablation.[46]

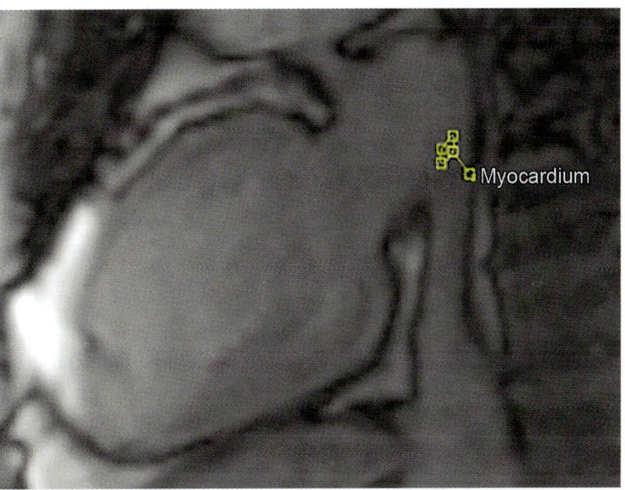

Fig. 3: Vertical long-axis modified Look-Locker inversion-recovery sequence. The region of interest (yellow) has been placed on the posterior LA wall. (LA: left atrium)

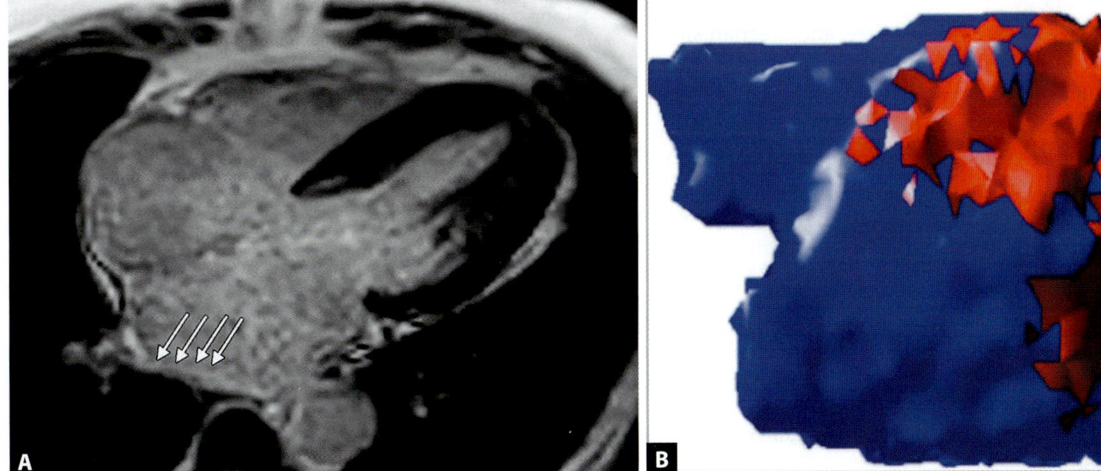

Figs. 4A and B: Four-chamber PSIR LGE sequence demonstrated left atrial wall enhancement (arrows) in this patient with AF (A). Three-dimensional (3D) segmentation of atrial LGE is represented in image B. (AF: atrial fibrillation; PSIR LGE: phase-sensitive inversion recovery late gadolinium enhancement)

LIMITATIONS

Currently, there are no established guidelines for clinically diagnosing LACM, and the existing classifications lack therapeutic and preventative guidance.[8] It is important to note that most studies generally equate left atrial myopathy with ACM, but the characteristics of right ACM may differ from those of LACM, warranting further research. Additionally, many LACM studies focus solely on atrial fibrosis, but fibrosis can also arise from aging, degenerative processes, and other comorbidities. It is probable that LACM is a multifaceted condition.

CONCLUSION

We have the tools to evaluate electrical, mechanical, and structural problems in the left atrium, but no single test can definitively diagnose ACM. Patients with AF show greater structural and functional changes in the left atrium compared to healthy individuals. Given the difficulty in diagnosing ACM, it is best to look for a combination of indicators linked to the condition.

REFERENCES

1. Thomas L, Marwick TH, Popescu BA, Donal E, Badano LP. Left atrial structure and function, and left ventricular diastolic dysfunction: JACC state-of-the-art review. J Am Coll Cardiol. 2019;73:1961-77.
2. Burstein B, Libby E, Calderone A, Nattel S. Differential behaviors of atrial versus ventricular fibroblasts: a potential role for platelet-derived growth factor in atrial-ventricular remodeling differences. Circulation. 2008;117:1630-41.
3. Andrade J, Khairy P, Dobrev D, Nattel S. The clinical profile and pathophysiology of atrial fibrillation: relationships among clinical features, epidemiology, and mechanisms. Circ Res. 2014;114:1453-68.
4. Tucker NR, Ellinor PT. Emerging directions in the genetics of atrial fibrillation. Circ Res. 2014;114:1469-82.
5. Nagle RE, Smith B, Williams DO. Familial atrial cardiomyopathy with heart block. Br Heart J. 1972;34:205.
6. Kottkamp H. Fibrotic atrial cardiomyopathy: a specific disease/syndrome supplying substrates for atrial fibrillation, atrial tachycardia, sinus node disease, AV node disease, and thromboembolic complications. J Cardiovasc Electrophysiol. 2012;23:797-9.
7. Hart RG, Diener HC, Coutts SB, Easton JD, Granger CB, O'Donnell MJ, et al. Embolic strokes of undetermined source: the case for a new clinical construct. Lancet Neurol. 2014;13:429-38.
8. Goette A, Kalman JM, Aguinaga L, Akar J, Cabrera JA, Chen SA, et al. EHRA/HRS/APHRS/SOLAECE expert consensus on atrial cardiomyopathies: definition, characterization, and clinical implication. Heart Rhythm. 2017;14:e3-40.
9. Johansson B, Wernstedt C, Westermark P. Atrial natriuretic peptide deposited as atrial amyloid fibrils. Biochem Biophys Res Commun. 1987;148:1087-92.
10. Postma AV, van de Meerakker JB, Mathijssen IB, Barnett P, Christoffels VM, Ilgun A, et al. A gain-of-function TBX5 mutation is associated with atypical Holt-Oram syndrome and paroxysmal atrial fibrillation. Circ Res. 2008;102:1433-42.
11. Bhakta D, Shen C, Kron J, Epstein AE, Pascuzzi RM, Groh WJ. Pacemaker and implantable cardioverter-defibrillator use in a US myotonic dystrophy type 1 population. J Cardiovasc Electrophysiol. 2011;22:1369-75.
12. Wallace GQ, McNally EM. Mechanisms of muscle degeneration, regeneration, and repair in the muscular dystrophies. Annu Rev Physiol. 2009;71:37-57.
13. Yeh YH, Wakili R, Qi XY, Chartier D, Boknik P, Kääb S, et al. Calcium-handling abnormalities underlying atrial arrhythmogenesis and contractile dysfunction in dogs with congestive heart failure. Circ Arrhythm Electrophysiol. 2008;1:93-102.
14. Dimitri H, Ng M, Brooks AG, Kuklik P, Stiles MK, Lau DH, et al. Atrial remodeling in obstructive sleep apnea: implications for atrial fibrillation. Heart Rhythm. 2012;9:321-7.
15. Wakili R, Voigt N, Kääb S, Dobrev D, Nattel S. Recent advances in the molecular pathophysiology of atrial fibrillation. J Clin Invest. 2011;121:2955-68.
16. Corradi D. Atrial fibrillation from the pathologist's perspective. Cardiovasc Pathol. 2014;23:71-84.
17. Kistler PM, Sanders P, Fynn SP, Stevenson IH, Spence SJ, Vohra JK, et al. Electrophysiologic and electroanatomic changes in the human atrium associated with age. J Am Coll Cardiol. 2004;44:109-16.
18. Medi C, Kalman JM, Spence SJ, Teh AW, Lee G, Bader I, et al. Atrial electrical and structural changes associated with longstanding hypertension in humans: implications for the substrate for atrial fibrillation. J Cardiovasc Electrophysiol. 2011;22:1317-24.
19. Abed HS, Samuel CS, Lau DH, Kelly DJ, Royce SG, Alasady M, et al. Obesity results in progressive atrial structural and electrical remodeling: implications for atrial fibrillation. Heart Rhythm. 2013;10:90-100.
20. Shigematsu Y, Norimatsu S, Ogimoto A, Ohtsuka T, Okayama H, Higaki J. The influence of insulin resistance and obesity on left atrial size in Japanese hypertensive patients. Hypertens Res. 2009;32:500-4.
21. Kreimer F, Gotzmann M. Left Atrial Cardiomyopathy—A Challenging Diagnosis. Front Cardiovasc Med. 2000,9:942385.
22. Di Tullio MR, Sacco RL, Sciacca RR, Homma S. Left atrial size and the risk of ischemic stroke in an ethnically mixed population. Stroke. 1999;30:2019-24.
23. Tsang TS, Barnes ME, Bailey KR, Leibson CL, Montgomery SC, Takemoto Y, et al. Left atrial volume:

important risk marker of incident atrial fibrillation in 1655 older men and women. Mayo Clin Proc. 2001;76:467-75.
24. Bouzas-Mosquera A, Broullón FJ, Álvarez-García N, Méndez E, Peteiro J, Gándara-Sambade T, et al. Left atrial size and risk for all-cause mortality and ischemic stroke. CMAJ. 2011;183:E657-64.
25. Vyas H, Jackson K, Chenzbraun A. Switching to volumetric left atrial measurements: impact on routine echocardiographic practice. Eur J Echocardiogr. 2011;12:107-11.
26. Lang RM, Badano LP, Mor-Avi V, Afilalo J, Armstrong A, Ernande L, et al. Recommendations for cardiac chamber quantification by echocardiography in adults: an update from the American society of echocardiography and the European association of cardiovascular imaging. J Am Soc Echocardiogr. 2015;28:1-39.
27. Hudsmith LE, Cheng AS, Tyler DJ, Shirodaria C, Lee J, Petersen SE, et al. Assessment of left atrial volumes at 1.5 Tesla and 3 Tesla using FLASH and SSFP cine imaging. J Cardiovasc Magn Reson. 2007;9:673-9.
28. Hoit BD. Left atrial size and function: role in prognosis. J Am Coll Cardiol. 2014;63:493-505.
29. Habibi M, Samiei S, Ambale Venkatesh B, Opdahl A, Helle-Valle TM, Zareian M, et al. Cardiac Magnetic Resonance-Measured Left Atrial Volume and Function and Incident Atrial Fibrillation: Results From MESA (Multi-Ethnic Study of Atherosclerosis). Circ Cardiovasc Imaging. 2016;9:10.
30. Hirose T, Kawasaki M, Tanaka R, Ono K, Watanabe T, Iwama M, et al. Left atrial function assessed by speckle tracking echocardiography as a predictor of new-onset non-valvular atrial fibrillation: results from a prospective study in 580 adults. Eur Heart J Cardiovasc Imaging. 2012;13:243-50.
31. Buggey J, Hoit BD. Left atrial strain: measurement and clinical application. Curr Opin Cardiol. 2018;33:479-85.
32. Zhao Y, Song Y, Mu X. Application of left atrial strain derived from cardiac magnetic resonance feature tracking to predict cardiovascular disease: A comprehensive review. Heliyon. 2024;10(7):e27911.
33. Yamada A, Hashimoto N, Fujito H, Hatta T, Saito Y, Otsuka N, et al. Comprehensive assessment of left atrial and ventricular remodeling in paroxysmal atrial fibrillation by the cardiovascular magnetic resonance myocardial extracellular volume fraction and feature tracking strain. Sci Rep. 2021;11:10941.
34. Raman B, Smillie RW, Mahmod M, Chan K, Ariga R, Nikolaidou C, et al. Incremental value of left atrial booster and reservoir strain in predicting atrial fibrillation in patients with hypertrophic cardiomyopathy: a cardiovascular magnetic resonance study. J Cardiovasc Magn Reson. 2021;23:109.
35. Hsu PC, Lee WH, Chu CY, Lee HH, Lee CS, Yen HW, et al. Prognostic role of left atrial strain and its combination index with transmitral E-wave velocity in patients with atrial fibrillation. Sci Rep. 2016;6:17318.
36. Hopman LHGA, Mulder MJ, van der Laan AM, Demirkiran A, Bhagirath P, van Rossum AC, et al. Impaired left atrial reservoir and conduit strain in patients with atrial fibrillation and extensive left atrial fibrosis. J Cardiovasc Magn Reson. 2021;23:131.
37. Oakes RS, Badger TJ, Kholmovski EG, Akoum N, Burgon NS, Fish EN, et al. Detection and quantification of left atrial structural remodelling with delayed enhancement magnetic resonance imaging in patients with atrial fibrillation. Circulation. 2009;119:1758-67.
38. Kuppahally SS, Akoum N, Burgon NS, Badger TJ, Kholmovski EG, Vijayakumar S, et al. Left atrial strain and strain rate in patients with paroxysmal and persistent atrial fibrillation: relationship to left atrial structural remodeling detected by delayed-enhancement MRI. Circ Cardiovasc Imaging. 2010;3:231-9.
39. King JB, Azadani PN, Suksaranjit P, Bress AP, Witt DM, Han FT, et al. Left atrial fibrosis and risk of cerebrovascular and cardiovascular events in patients with atrial fibrillation. J Am Coll Cardiol. 2017;70:1311-21.
40. Hopman LHGA, Bhagirath P, Mulder MJ, Eggink IN, van Rossum AC, Allaart CP, et al. Quantification of left atrial fibrosis by 3D late gadolinium-enhanced cardiac magnetic resonance imaging in patients with atrial fibrillation: impact of different analysis methods. Eur Heart J Cardiovasc Imaging. 2022;23:1182-90.
41. Iles L, Pfluger H, Phrommintikul A, Cherayath J, Aksit P, Gupta SN, et al. Evaluation of diffuse myocardial fibrosis in heart failure with cardiac magnetic resonance contrast-enhanced T1 mapping. J Am Coll Cardiol. 2008;52:1574-80.
42. Beinart R, Khurram IM, Liu S, Yarmohammadi H, Halperin HR, Bluemke DA, et al. Cardiac magnetic resonance T1 mapping of left atrial myocardium. Heart Rhythm. 2013;10:1325-31.
43. Akoum N, Daccarett M, McGann C, Segerson N, Vergara G, Kuppahally S, et al. Atrial fibrosis helps select the appropriate patient and strategy in catheter ablation of atrial fibrillation: a DE-MRI guided approach. J Cardiovasc Electrophysiol. 2011;22:16-22.
44. Goldman ME, Pearce LA, Hart RG, Zabalgoitia M, Asinger RW, Safford R, et al. Pathophysiologic correlates of thromboembolism in nonvalvular atrial fibrillation: I. Reduced flow velocity in the left atrial appendage (the stroke prevention in atrial fibrillation [SPAF-III] study). J Am Soc Echocardiogr. 1999;12:1080-7.
45. Markl M, Lee DC, Ng J, Carr M, Carr J, Goldberger JJ. Left atrial 4-dimensional flow magnetic resonance imaging: Stasis and velocity mapping in patients with atrial fibrillation. Invest Radiol. 2016;51:147-54.
46. Wong CX, Ganesan AN, Selvanayagam JB. Epicardial fat and atrial fibrillation: current evidence, potential mechanisms, clinical implications, and future directions. Eur Heart J. 2017;38:1294-302.

Coronary Computed Tomography in Coronary Artery Disease: Recent Guidelines, Case Examples

Parul Samir Garde, Aparna Mukund Patankar

INTRODUCTION

Computed tomography (CT) coronary angiography has emerged as a crucial tool for evaluating coronary artery disease (CAD). Due to its noninvasive nature and comprehensive anatomical details, there is increasing use of CT coronary angiography in both stable and unstable angina. The advantage of coronary computed tomography angiography (CCTA) is that it not only quantifies the degree of stenosis like a conventional angiogram but also characterizes and quantifies the plaque burden. Plaque characterization helps in further prognostication and navigating treatment protocols. However, a very high coronary calcium burden limits the positive predictive value of this test. Also, performing CCTA in symptomatic patients with high pretest probability can be counterproductive. Hence, it is essential to understand the recommended guidelines for the appropriate use of CCTA.

DISCUSSION WITH REVIEW OF LITERATURE

Multiple trials and studies published in the last decade have appropriated the use of CT coronary angiography, especially in patients with stable angina with intermediate pretest probability.

The update to the United Kingdom National Institute for Health and Care Excellence (NICE) guidelines published in 2017 was among the first societies to recommend that cardiac CT is the first-line investigation for patients presenting with new-onset chest pain due to suspected CAD.[1] These were followed by the 2019 European Society of Cardiology guidelines for the diagnosis and management of chronic coronary syndromes.[2]

The Society of Cardiovascular Computed Tomography (SCCT) has published an expert consensus document for the use of CT coronary angiography for patients with stable angina and those presenting with acute chest pain to the emergency department in the year 2021 and 2022, respectively.[3,4]

The SCCT expert consensus recommendations for coronary CT angiography have been discussed in this chapter.

Evaluation of Stable CAD

- It is appropriate to perform computed tomography angiography (CTA):
  - As the first-line test for evaluating patients *with no known CAD* who present with stable typical or atypical chest pain, or other symptoms which are thought to represent a possible anginal equivalent.
  - As a first-line test for evaluating patients *with known CAD* who present with stable typical or atypical chest pain, or other symptoms which are thought to represent a possible anginal equivalent (e.g., dyspnea on exertion and jaw pain).
  - Following a nonconclusive functional test, in order to obtain more precision regarding diagnosis and prognosis for subsequent patient management.
- It may be appropriate to perform CTA in selected asymptomatic high-risk individuals, especially in those who have a higher likelihood of having a large amount of noncalcified plaque.
- It is rarely appropriate to perform CCTA:
  - In very low-risk symptomatic patients, e.g., <40 years of age with noncardiac symptoms (chest wall pain, pleuritic chest pain)
  - In low- and intermediate-risk asymptomatic patients

Evaluation of Stable CAD: CCTA Post-revascularization

- It is appropriate to perform CCTA in symptomatic patients with an intracoronary stent diameter ≥3.0 mm.

- It may be appropriate to perform CCTA in symptomatic patients with stents <3.0 mm, especially those known to have thin stent struts (<100 mm) in proximal, nonbifurcation locations.
- It is appropriate to perform CTA for the evaluation of patients with prior CABG, particularly if graft patency is the primary objective.
- It is appropriate to perform CTA to visualize grafts prior to redo cardiac bypass surgery.

Evaluation of Stable CAD: CCTA with Fractional Flow Reserve or Computed Tomography Perfusion (CTP)

It may be appropriate to perform CT-derived fractional flow reserve (FFR) and CT myocardial perfusion imaging to evaluate the functional significance of intermediate stenoses on CTA (30–69% diameter stenosis), particularly in the setting of multivessel disease, to help guide invasive coronary angiography (ICA) referral and revascularization treatment planning.

Evaluation of Stable CAD: CCTA in Other Conditions

- It is appropriate to perform CCTA:
  - Prior to noncoronary cardiac surgery as an equivalent alternative to invasive angiography in selected patients, e.g., low-intermediate probability of CAD, and younger patients with primarily nondegenerative valvular conditions.
  - As an alternative to other noninvasive tests for the evaluation of selected patients prior to noncardiac surgery.
  - To exclude CAD in patients with suspected nonischemic cardiomyopathy.
  - Suspected coronary artery anomalies
- It may be appropriate to perform CCTA:
  - As part of the triple rule-out study for evaluation of aortic dissection, the coronary arteries, and pulmonary arteries.

Society of Cardiovascular Computed Tomography Guidelines for Evaluation of Acute Chest Pain

In the emergency department setting, the high accuracy of CCTA is driven by its high sensitivity and negative predictive value for detecting or excluding obstructive CAD, particularly in patients with low-to-intermediate pretest risk for acute coronary syndrome (ACS) **(Table 1)**.[3,5-8]

CASE EXAMPLES

Case 1

- *Clinical presentation:* A 44-year-old male with dyslipidemia and vague chest pain. Calcium score: 10
- *CCTA findings:* Type A significant stenosis in proximal left anterior descending (LAD) artery **(Figs. 1A and B)**

TABLE 1: Guidelines for CCTA for the evaluation ACS.

High risk for ACS: Normal or nonischemic ECG, high pretest risk for ACS, and • Normal or equivocal baseline Tn, or • hs-cTn <99th percentile	CCTA is an alternative to functional testing or invasive angiography
Low-to-intermediate risk for ACS: Normal or nonischemic ECG, low-to-intermediate risk for ACS, and • Normal or equivocal baseline Tn, or • hs-cTn <99th percentile • Inadequate or mildly abnormal functional test during index ED visit or within the previous 1 year	CCTA is most effective in ruling out ACS

(ACS: acute coronary syndrome; CCTA: coronary computed tomography angiography; ECG: electrocardiogram; ED: emergency department; hs-cTn: high-sensitivity cardiac troponin; Tn: troponin)

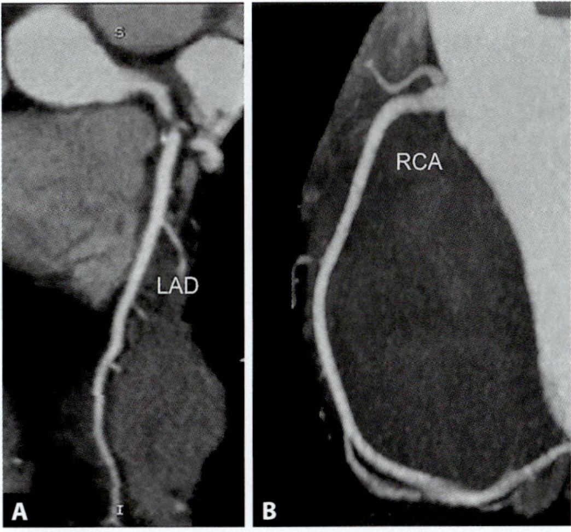

Figs. 1A and B: (A) Significant short-segment stenosis in proximal LAD with (B) no significant disease in RCA. (LAD: left anterior descending artery; RCA: right coronary artery)

- *Management:* Underwent ICA with angioplasty and stent placement
- *Guidelines relevance:* It is in keeping with recommendations as a first-line test for evaluating patients *with no known CAD*, who present with stable, typical, or atypical chest pain

Case 2

- *Clinical presentation:* A 45-year-old asymptomatic diabetic male with a high calcium score of 705
- *CCTA findings:* Scattered calcified and partially calcified plaques in proximal and mid LAD and in proximal right coronary artery (RCA) with <50% stenosis **(Figs. 2A to C)**

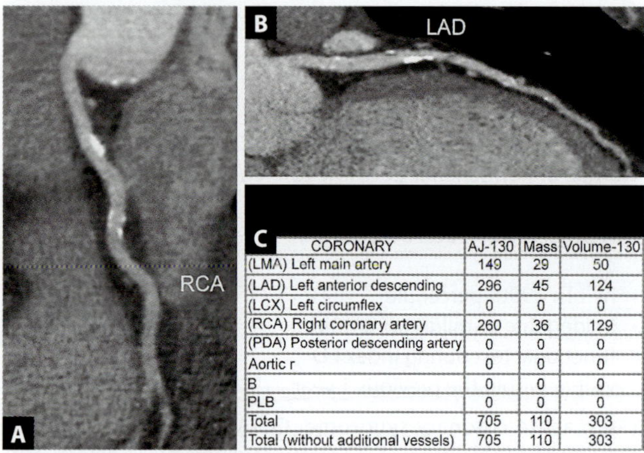

CORONARY	AJ-130	Mass	Volume-130
(LMA) Left main artery	149	29	50
(LAD) Left anterior descending	296	45	124
(LCX) Left circumflex	0	0	0
(RCA) Right coronary artery	260	36	129
(PDA) Posterior descending artery	0	0	0
Aortic r	0	0	0
B	0	0	0
PLB	0	0	0
Total	705	110	303
Total (without additional vessels)	705	110	303

Figs. 2A to C: (A) and (B) Scattered calcified plaques in proximal RCA and in proximal and mid LAD with <50% stenosis; (C) A high calcium score. (AJ: Agatston-Janowitz; PLB: posterolateral branch)

- *Management:* Aggressive medical management and lifestyle changes
- *Guidelines relevance:* It is appropriate to perform CTA in selected asymptomatic high-risk individuals, especially in those who have a higher likelihood of having a large amount of noncalcified plaque.

Case 3

- *Clinical presentation:* A 72-year-old male with dyslipidemia and glycated hemoglobin (HbA1c) of 7.7, with a recent history of one episode of chest pain on exertion. Stress test equivocal for inducible ischemia
- *CCTA findings:* Partially calcified plaques in ostioproximal LAD, resulting in a variable degree of stenosis ranging from 50% to >75%. Partially calcified plaques also seen in proximal left circumflex artery (LCX) with <25% stenosis **(Figs. 3A and B)**
- *Management:* Underwent ICA with LAD angioplasty and stenting
- *Guidelines relevance:* It is appropriate to perform CCTA following a nonconclusive functional test, in order to obtain more precision regarding diagnosis and prognosis for subsequent patient management.

Case 4

- *Clinical presentation:* A 67-year-old male who underwent angioplasty in 2019, with new onset of shortness of breath on walking. More than 3 mm-sized stents were placed in the RCA.

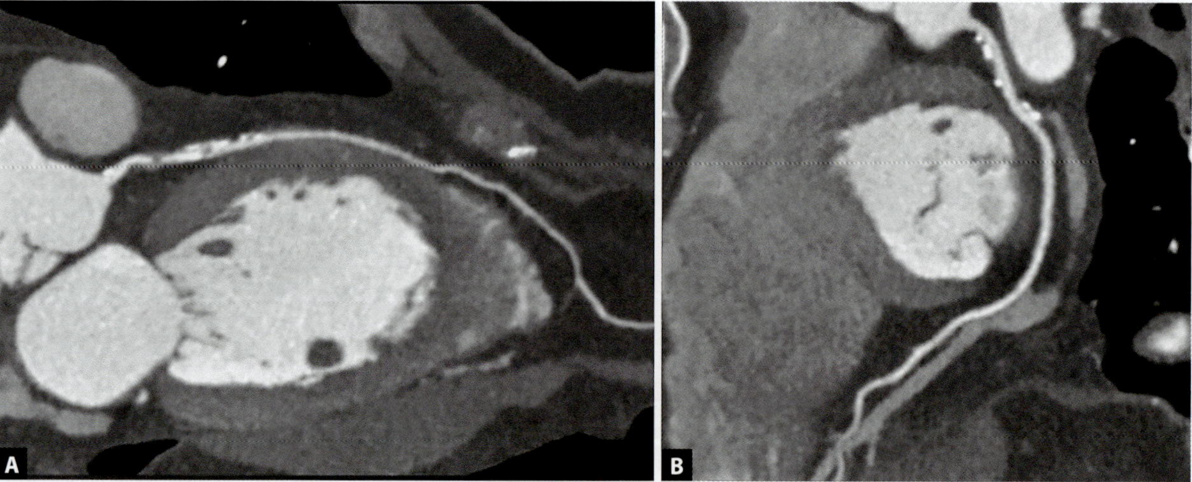

Figs. 3A and B: (A) Partially calcified plaque in ostioproximal LAD, resulting in a variable degree of stenosis ranging from 50% to >75%; (B) Partially calcified plaques in proximal LCX with <25% stenosis. (LAD: left anterior descending artery; LCX: left circumflex artery)

- *CCTA findings:* Two stents in situ in the RCA with in-stent restenosis **(Figs. 4A and B)**
- *Management:* Underwent bypass surgery with right internal mammary artery (RIMA) graft to posterior descending artery (PDA)
- *Guidelines relevance:* It is in keeping with appropriate to perform CCTA in symptomatic patients with an intracoronary stent diameter >3.0 mm.

Case 5

- *Clinical presentation:* A 68-year-old male, 15 years post bypass surgery, with anginal pain.
- *CCTA findings:* Patent left internal mammary artery (LIMA) to LAD and radial artery (RA) to first diagonal branch of left anterior descending artery (D1) grafts; however, total occlusion of the RA graft to first obtuse marginal artery (OM1). There was significant stenosis in the proximal LCX secondary to predominantly noncalcified plaque. **(Figs. 5A and B)**
- *Management:* Underwent stenting for proximal circumflex significant stenosis.
- *Guidelines relevance:* It is in keeping with appropriate to perform CTA for the evaluation of patients with prior CABG, particularly if graft patency is the primary objective.

Case 6

- *Clinical presentation:* In a known case of aortic valve stenosis, a catheter angiogram done before valve replacement could not demonstrate the RCA, hence CCTA was done.
- *CCTA findings:* High take-off of RCA from >1 cm above the sinotubular junction and anterior wall of the ascending aorta **(Fig. 6)**
- *Management:* No action taken as the anomaly was not hemodynamically significant.

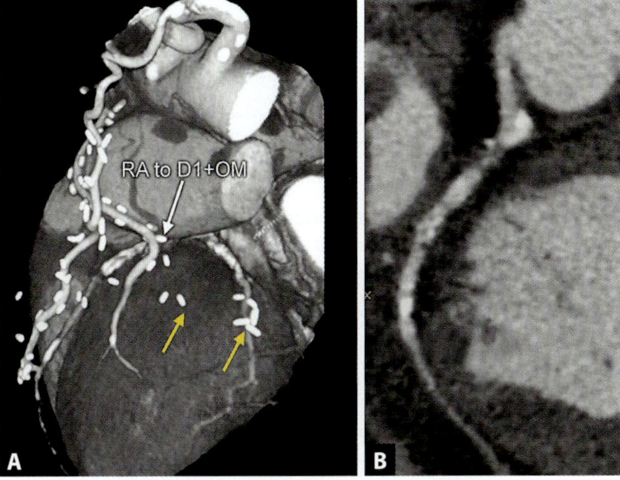

Figs. 5A and B: (A) Patent LIMA to LAD and RA to D1 grafts; however, total occlusion of the RA graft to OM1; (B) Significant stenosis in proximal LCX secondary to predominantly noncalcified plaque. (LAD: left anterior descending artery; LIMA: left internal mammary artery; LCX: left circumflex artery; D1: first diagonal branch of left anterior descending artery; OM1: first obtuse marginal artery; RA: radial artery)

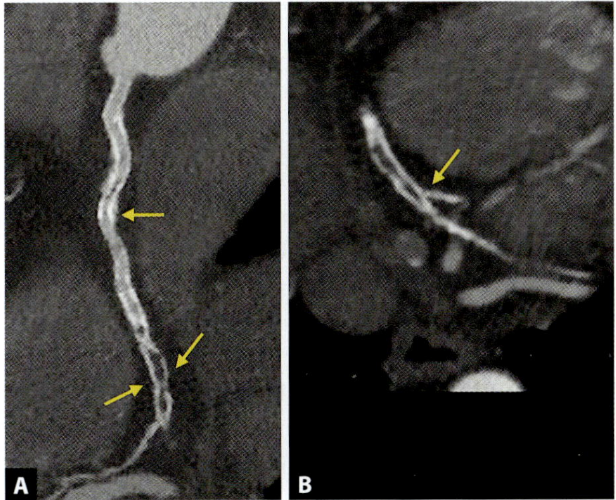

Figs. 4A and B: Two long stents in situ in the RCA with significant in-stent restenosis and significant plaque burden in the rest of the coronary arteries. (RCA: right coronary artery)

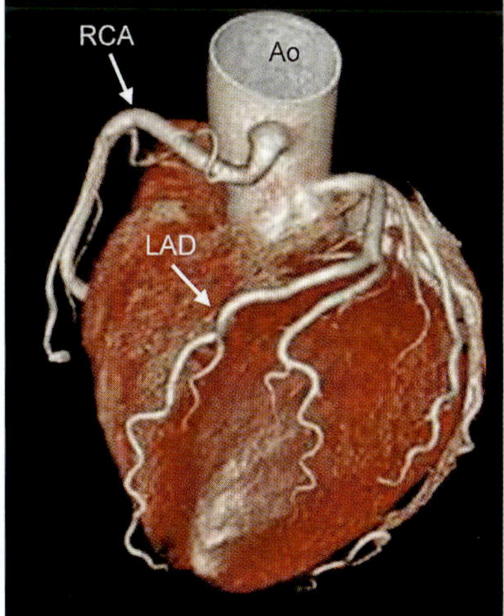

Fig. 6: A volume-rendered image revealing high take-off of RCA from the anterior wall of the ascending Ao, >1 cm above the sinotubular junction. (Ao: aorta; LAD: left anterior descending artery; RCA: right coronary artery)

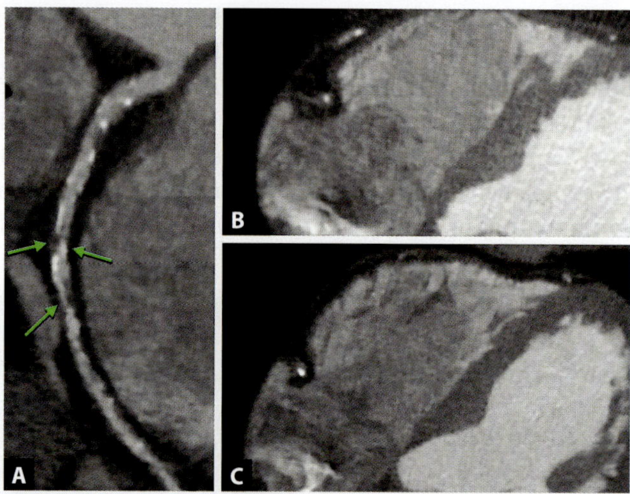

Figs. 7A to C: Two tandem lesions with >70% stenosis in mid RCA, just before the bend. (RCA: right coronary artery)

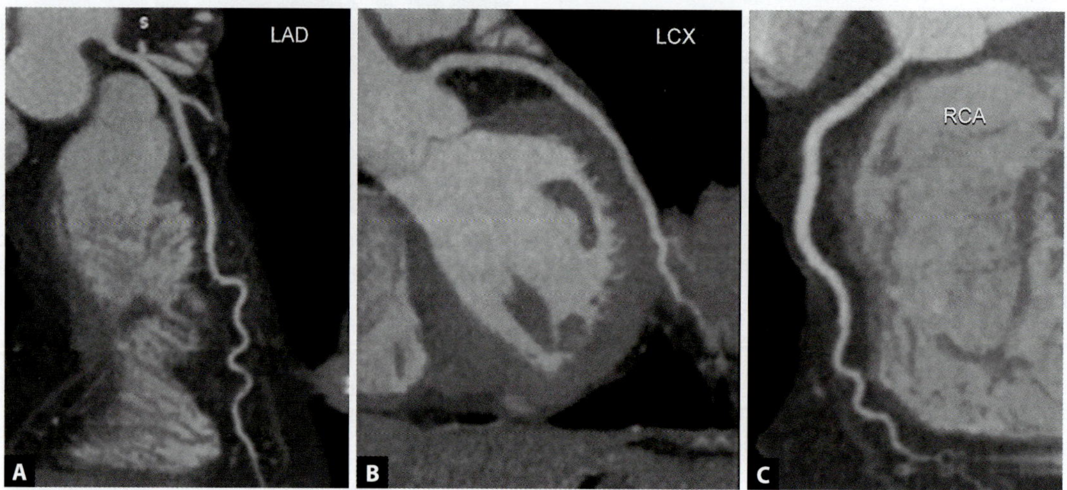

Figs. 8A to C: No significant disease in (A) LAD; (B) LCX; and (C) RCA. (LAD: left anterior descending artery; LCX: left circumflex artery; RCA: right coronary artery)

- *Guidelines relevance:* Appropriate to perform CCTA in suspected coronary artery anomalies

Case 7

- *Clinical presentation:* A 57-year-old diabetic male with retrosternal tightness, with equivocal cardiac enzymes with no ST-T changes on electrocardiogram (ECG).
- *CCTA findings:* Calcium score of 989. Two tandem lesions with >70% stenosis in mid RCA, just before the bend **(Figs. 7A to C)**
- *Management:* Angioplasty with long stent in RCA
- *Guidelines relevance:* High pretest risk for ACS, unstable angina-like symptoms, and equivocal troponins. Alternative for functional test or ICA.

Case 8

- *Clinical presentation:* A 40-year-old male with no comorbidities presented with acute left-sided chest pain, especially on deep inspiration. Cardiac enzymes were normal, and the ECG was normal.
- *CCTA findings:* No abnormality of coronary arteries with no calcium burden **(Figs. 8A to C)**
- *Management:* To evaluate for noncardiac causes of chest pain and treat accordingly.
- *Guidelines relevance:* It is rarely appropriate to perform CCTA in very low-risk symptomatic patients.

CONCLUSION

CCTA should be the investigation of choice in patients with chronic stable chest pain with intermediate-to-high pretest probability. In addition, it is an appropriate investigation in majority of postrevascularized symptomatic patients and in cases of suspected anomalous origin and course of coronary arteries. In the setting of acute chest pain, it is appropriate to perform CCTA in patients with high pretest probability but equivocal cardiac enzymes and no ST-T changes on ECG, and in patients with low-to-intermediate pretest probability as it has a high negative predictive value.

REFERENCES

1. Moss AJ, Williams MC, Newby DE, Nicol ED. The Updated NICE Guidelines: Cardiac CT as the First-line Test for Coronary Artery Disease. Curr Cardiovasc Imaging Rep. 2017;10(5):15.
2. Knuuti J, Wijns W, Saraste A, Capodanno D, Barbato E, Funck-Brentano C, et al; ESC Scientific Document Group. 2019 ESC Guidelines for the diagnosis and management of chronic coronary syndromes. Eur Heart J. 2020;41(3):407-7.
3. Maroules CD, Rybicki FJ, Ghoshhajra BB, Batlle JC, Branch K, Chinnaiyan K, et al. 2022 use of coronary computed tomographic angiography for patients presenting with acute chest pain to the emergency department: an expert consensus document of the Society of Cardiovascular Computed Tomography (SCCT): Endorsed by the American College of Radiology (ACR) and North American Society for Cardiovascular Imaging (NASCI). J Cardiovascr Comput Tomogr. 2023;17(2):146-63.
4. Narula J, Chandrashekhar Y, Ahmadi A, Abbara S, Berman DS, Blankstein R, et al. SCCT 2021 Expert Consensus Document on Coronary Computed Tomographic Angiography: a report of the Society of Cardiovascular Computed Tomography. J Cardiovasc Comput Tomogr. 2021;15(3):192-217.
5. Hulten E. Pickett C, Bittencourt MS, Villines TC, Petrillo S, Di Carli MF, et al. Outcomes after coronary computed tomography angiography in the emergency department: a systematic review and meta-analysis of randomized, controlled trials. J Am Coll Cardiol. 2013;61(8):880-92.
6. Knuuti J, Ballo H, Juarez-Orozco LE, Saraste A, Kolh P, Rutjes AWS, et al. The performance of non-invasive tests to rule-in and rule-out significant coronary artery stenosis in patients with stable angina: a meta-analysis focused on post-test disease probability. Eur Heart J. 2018;39(35):3322-30.
7. Samad Z, Hakeem A, Mahmood SS, Pieper K, Patel MR, Simel DL, et al. A meta-analysis and systematic review of computed tomography angiography as a diagnostic triage tool for patients with chest pain presenting to the emergency department. J Nucl Cardiol. 2012;19(2):364-76.
8. Staniak HL, Bittencourt MS, Pickett C, Cahill M, Kassop D, Slim A, et al. Coronary CT angiography for acute chest pain in the emergency department. J Cardiovasc Comput Tomogr. 2014;8(5):359-67.

Cardiac Computed Tomography in Preoperative Evaluation of Transcatheter Aortic Valve Replacement/Transcatheter Mitral Valve Replacement

Zeeshan Sakina A Lakhani, Tosha J Desai

INTRODUCTION

Transcatheter aortic valve replacement (TAVR) is a minimally invasive alternative to valvular surgery for severe symptomatic aortic stenosis. According to the 2021 European Society of Cardiology (ESC)/European Association for Cardio-Thoracic Surgery (EACTS) valvular heart disease (VHD) Guidelines, candidates for TAVR should be those older than 75 years or with high-risk (STS-Prom/Euro SCORE >8) in the European guidelines, or those older than 80 years or with life expectancy <10 years in the American guidelines.[1] CT is the mainstay for annular sizing, risk determination of annular injury or coronary occlusion, coplanar fluoroscopic angle prediction and peripheral access measurements prior to the procedure. Transcatheter mitral valve replacement (TMVR) is an emerging procedure for patients with severe native mitral regurgitation that failed goal-directed medical therapy, poor surgical candidates, with unfavorable anatomy for transcatheter mitral valve repair, calcific mitral stenosis, and failed mitral valve rings or bioprosthetic valves.[2]

PREPROCEDURAL IMAGING OF TRANSCATHETER AORTIC VALVE REPLACEMENT

Anatomy: Valve Morphology

The aortic root comprises the annulus, sinuses of Valsalva (SOV), the fibrous interleaflet triangles and the valvular cusps and sinotubular junction (STJ). The aortic annulus is defined as the luminal contour within a virtual plane aligned with the most basal attachment points of the three aortic valve cusps (referred to as the 'basal hinge points')[3] **(Fig. 1)**. Bicuspid aortic valves (BAV) account for nearly half of TAVR referrals due to aortic stenosis and is associated with procedural complexity. transcatheter aortic valve implantation (TAVI)/TAVR-based classification for BAV morphologies are: (1) Tricommissural, in clinical routine often referred to as "functional" or "acquired" BAV (not part of Sievers classification); (2) bi-commissural raphe-type (equivalent to Sievers Type 1); and (3) bicommissural nonraphe-type (equivalent to Sievers Type 0). Accurate aortic root measurement is important and is depicted below **(Figs. 1A to G)**.

With regard to the mechanism of valve expansion, transcatheter heart valves (THVs) can be classified into self-expanding valves (SEV) and balloon-expandable valves (BEV). The evolute FX (Medtronic, Minneapolis, MN, USA) is the latest core valve self-expanding valve. Hydra (Sahajanand Medical Technologies Limited, Mumbai, India) has optimal alignment and conformability to aorta and easier coronary access. Sapien 3, Sapien 3 Ultra, and Sapien 3 Ultra Resilia (Edwards Lifesciences, Irvine, CA, USA) are the third, fourth, and fifth iterations within the BEV Sapien family. MyVal and MyVal Octacor (Meril, Vapi, Gujarat, India) BEV allow implantation across a wide range of annular dimensions[4] **(Figs. 2A to D)**.

CT Data Acquisition and Reconstruction

The key component of all approaches is an ECG-synchronized computed tomographic angiography (CTA) data set that covers at least the aortic root in order to provide artifact free anatomical information of the aortic root, followed by a non-ECG synchronized CTA data acquisition of the aorto-/iliofemoral vasculature/proximal arch branches for assessment of the access vasculature. Ideally, both acquisitions are combined in a comprehensive scanning protocol with a single dose of contrast administration[5] **(Table 1)**.

Landing Zone Calcifications[6]

Calcification at the device landing zone *[annular and subannular/left ventricular outflow tract (LVOT)]* is an important predictor of procedural outcome and

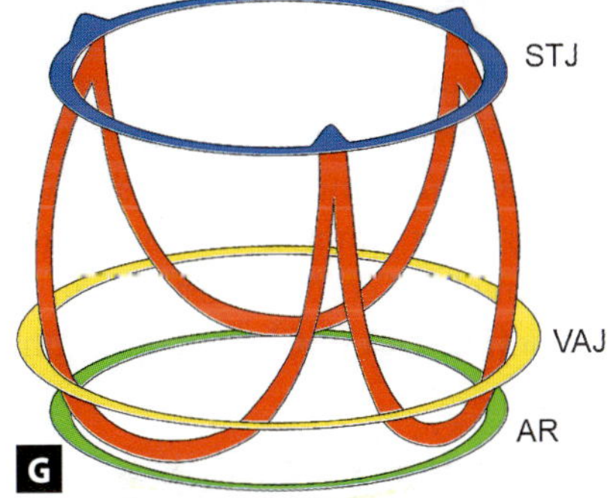

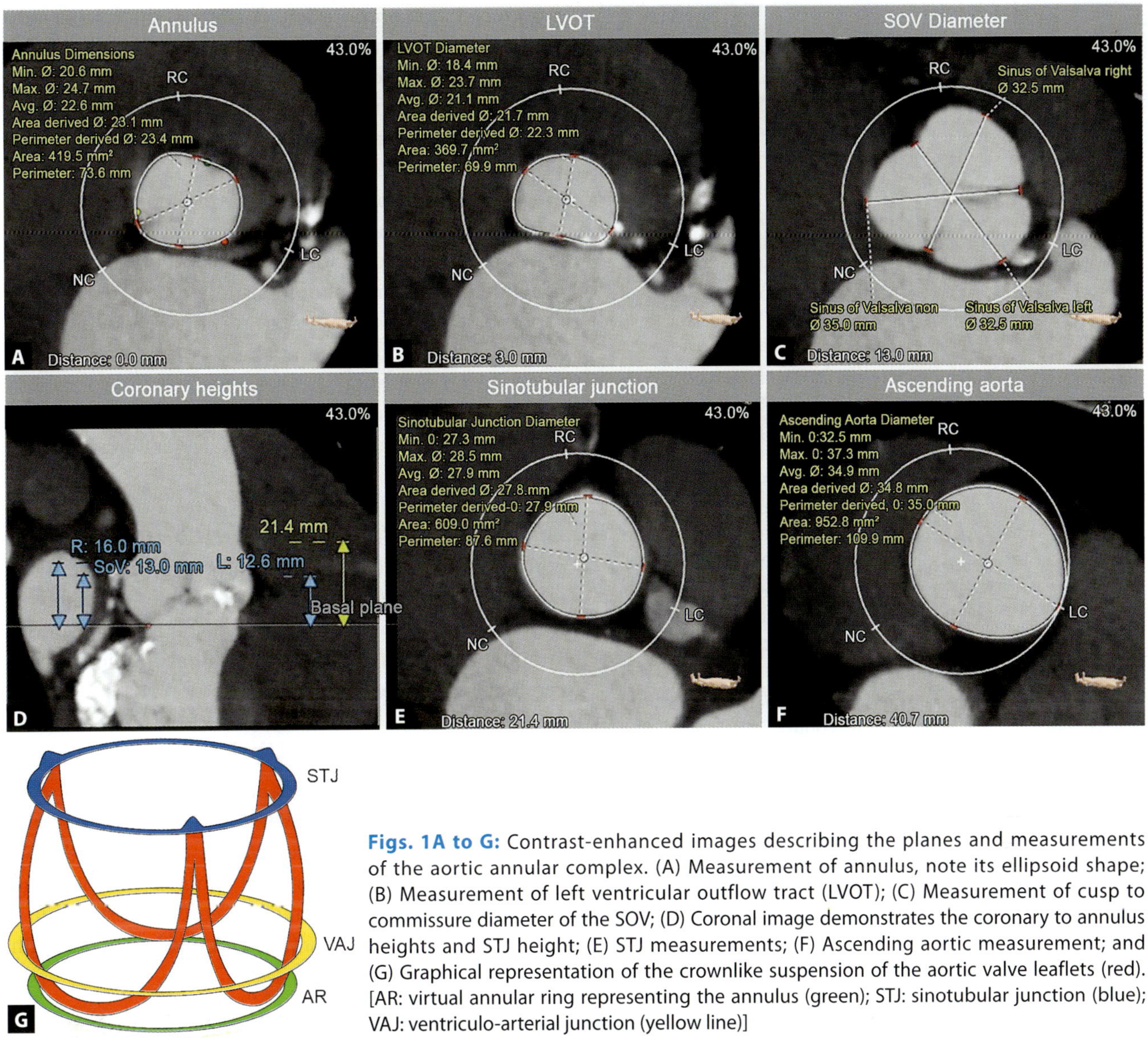

Figs. 1A to G: Contrast-enhanced images describing the planes and measurements of the aortic annular complex. (A) Measurement of annulus, note its ellipsoid shape; (B) Measurement of left ventricular outflow tract (LVOT); (C) Measurement of cusp to commissure diameter of the SOV; (D) Coronal image demonstrates the coronary to annulus heights and STJ height; (E) STJ measurements; (F) Ascending aortic measurement; and (G) Graphical representation of the crownlike suspension of the aortic valve leaflets (red). [AR: virtual annular ring representing the annulus (green); STJ: sinotubular junction (blue); VAJ: ventriculo-arterial junction (yellow line)]

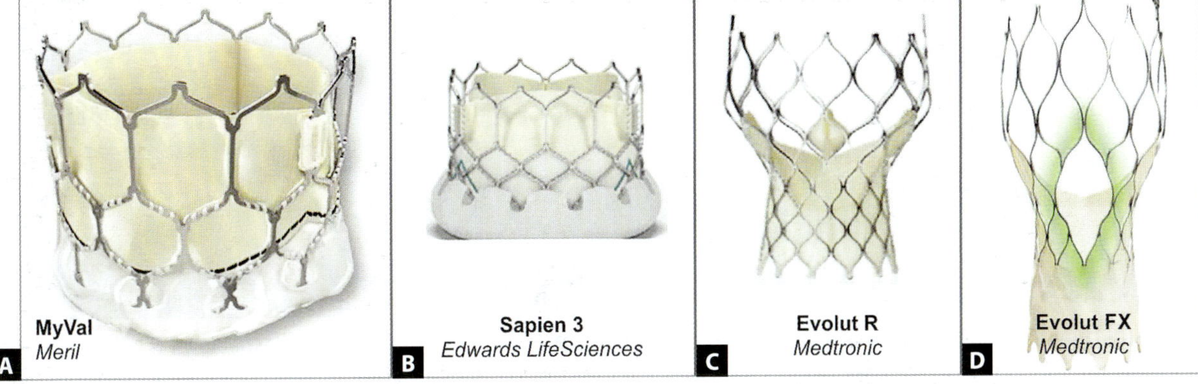

Figs. 2A to D: MyVal and Sapien 3 (balloon expandable). Evolut R and Evolut FX (self-expandable) transcatheter heart valves (THVs).

TABLE 1: Acquisition and reconstruction technique for preprocedural transcatheter aortic valve implantation (TAVI).

ECG-synchronized CTA of heart	Scan coverage should include aortic root completely though addition of entire heart and image acquisition during entire cardiac cycle is beneficial. Especially, systolic phase image reconstruction is recommended
Non-ECG-gated CTA of the aorta and access vessels	Scan should extend from upper thoracic aperture to the lesser trochanter to include the thoracic and abdominal aorta, iliac arteries, and common femoral arteries, can be extended cephalad to fully include subclavian arteries and mid common carotid arteries
Radiation parameters and consideration	• Tube potential of 100 kV for patients weighing ≤90 kg/BMI ≤30 kg/m^2 and 120 kV for >90 kg and with BMI >30 kg/m^2 • Prospectively triggered acquisitions focusing on systole can be considered a reasonable alternative particularly in patients with lower and regular heart rate
Contrast administration	*Total contrast volume:* ~50–100 cc, *flow rate:* 4–6 mL/sec, *IV access:* Antecubital vein with at least 20-gauge intravenous access, *Timing:* Bolus tracking to allow for peak contrast in the proximal ascending aorta
Patient preparation	Adequate pre-examination hydration status. Routine heart rate control with β-blockers is not recommended. Sublingual nitrates in severe aortic stenosis are contraindicated
Reconstruction technique	Postprocessing is done on dedicated software. Identification of annular plane is done either manually or using semiautomated/facilitated workflow followed by quantification of annular dimensions

(BMI: body mass index; CTA: computed tomographic angiography)

periprocedural complication. Grading of the calcification as none, mild, moderate, and severe based on the calcification extent, depth, and thickness of calcification extending into the LVOT. Calcification can also be described as crescent/flat/adherent or protruding. Large protruding nodules of calcification increase the risk of annular rupture particularly with balloon expandable valves **(Figs. 3B and C)**. Calcification along membranous septum can cause atrioventricular block. The degree of raphe calcification should also be reported as severe raphe calcification may relate to higher likelihood of paravalvular regurgitation. There is increased risk of paravalvular regurgitation when calcium protrudes into the LVOT. The region below the noncoronary and the left coronary cusps, including the intervalvular fibrosa, is most frequently affected.

CT additionally establishes the morphology of *noncalcific aortic valve stenosis* characterized by continuous and diffuse low-intensity thickening of leaflets on axial images and a ≥50% ratio of the height of hypoattenuating opacities to the distance between the annulus and tip of the valve, which has implications in cerebral ischemic lesions post-TAVR.[7]

Risk of Coronary Ostial Obstruction

Displacement of the native aortic-valve leaflets during deployment of the THV in patients with low coronary ostial height (<10 mm) from the annulus and sinus of Valsalva mean diameter <30 mm carries a minimal but important risk of subsequent occlusion of the coronary ostia, with a reported mortality of >50% **(Figs. 3A to C)**. Leaflet length

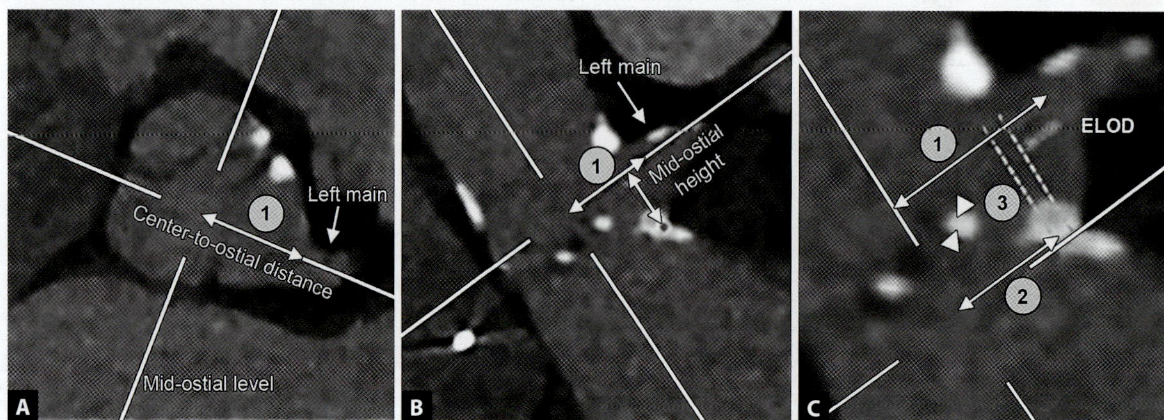

Figs. 3A to C: Double-oblique CT image (A) depicts the measurement of center to ostium at mid-ostial level (1); (B) Calculation of mid-ostial height; (C) Center to annulus distance (2) and leaflet thickness (3). Calculation of expected leaflet-to-ostium distance (ELOD): 1-(2 + 3).

greater than the mid-ostial height with the Expected Leaflet-to-ostium Distance (ELOD) <2 mm (measured by subtracting the sum of leaflet thickness and center to annular distance from center to ostial distance) is a very high risk for coronary ostial obstruction in TAVR in native valve.[8] However, the derived values for coronary height and sinus of Valsalva width should be interpreted in the context of annular dimensions, overall root dimensions and the anticipated THV size **(Figs. 3A to C)**.

Aortoventricular Angle and Optimal Projection Curve

The aortic angle is defined as the angle between the horizontal (axial) and aortic annular planes in the coronal section. Increased angulation or unfolding of the aortic root and ascending aorta, often referred to as a "horizontal aorta" (aortic angle $\geq$48°) is an anatomical challenge particularly for the transfemoral approach for TAVI. A horizontally oriented aortic root may hamper valve crossing, impair THV delivery, prevent optimal positioning and coaxial alignment of the THV, particularly high-frame SE valves, within the aortic annulus. Each type of transcatheter prosthetic valve has a maximum aorto-ventricular angle for successful valve deployment, typically 70° for the iliofemoral approach and 30° for the subclavian approach.[9] Recent advances in postprocessing software enable a comprehensive analysis of landing zone characteristics—landing zone identification on aortic center line, aortic root length, STJ plane angulation, proximal and distal landing zone plane angulation with reference to aortic angulation and thus quantification of the cumulative absolute curvature of the aortic centerline on the aortic root and landing zone regions.[10]

Use of CT-derived angulations [reported as degrees (°) LAO or RAO with the corresponding values for cranial or caudal angulation] allow optimization of initial predeployment fluoroscopic angulation, reducing the need for repeat predeployment root shots thereby reducing radiation exposure, contrast usage, and procedural time[11] **(Figs. 4A to E)**.

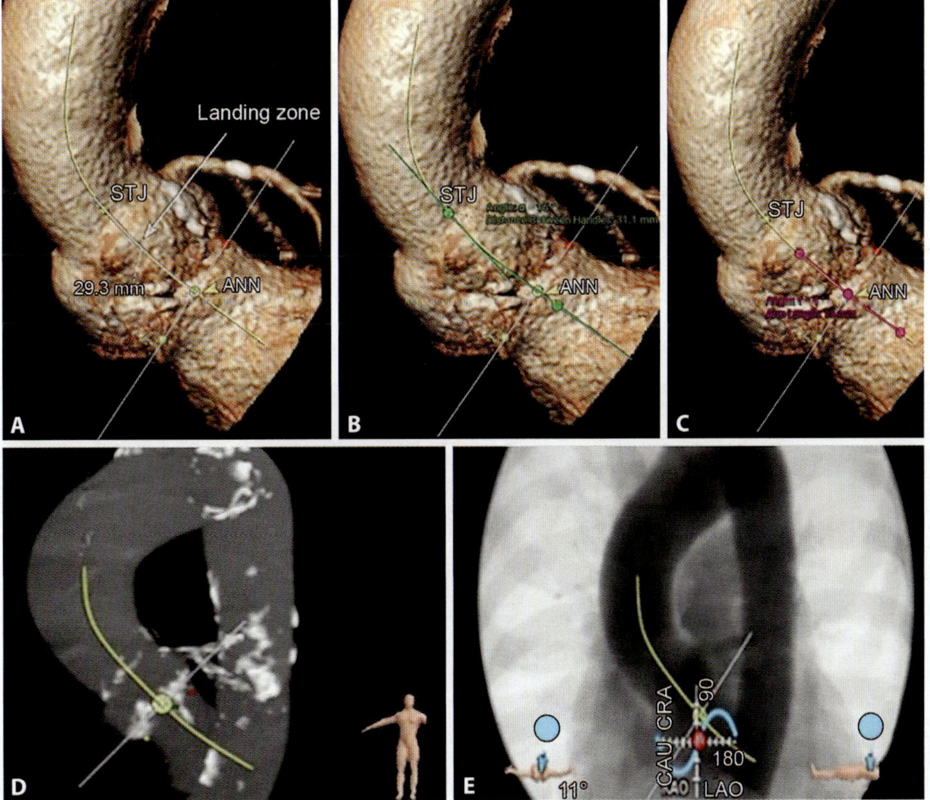

Figs. 4A to E: Landing zone analysis (A) Identification of the landing zone on the aortic center line for a SE valve (B) the proximal LZ angulation and (C) distal landing zone angulation with respect to the plane of aortic annulus demonstrates CT-based desired plane for coplanar fluoroscopic angles. (D and E) The angulation (LAO 11°/cranial 3°) was used during the TAVI procedure as the C-arm angulation for the first aortogram.

Sizing Considerations and Implantation Depth

Oversizing: The term "oversizing" has been introduced to help to describe when a THV is deployed that is larger than the native annulus. In clinical practice, balloon expandable devices are largely sized on the basis of annular area, with self-expandable devices relying on perimeter. Owing to vendor specific device properties, sizing of THV valves remains a multifactorial and multimodality process.[11]

Implantation depth: A suboptimal distance between membranous septum (MS) length and implantation depth (ID) may cause compression of the conduction tissue by TAVR prosthesis. The difference between MS length measured in the coronal view of pre-TAVR CT and ID (Coronal ΔMSID) is the most powerful independent predictor of permanent pacemaker implantation post-TAVR. Ying-Hwa Chen et al. established coronal ΔMSID ≤3.2 mm and an infra-annular ΔMSID ≤–0.2 mm as the optimal cutoff points, which could help to determine the optimal ID in preprocedural planning to mitigate conduction disturbances following TAVR.[12]

Vascular Access

CT is useful to evaluate the size of vessel, vascular calcification, and tortuosity of the entire aorta, iliofemoral, and arch vessels **(Figs. 5A and B)**. A vascular caliber ≥6-mm is required for both the CoreValve and Sapien devices.[13] Mild tortuosity is not a limiting factor; however, significant angulations >90° in the iliofemoral vessels may hinder large caliber catheter insertion. In addition, findings like dissection/thrombus or ulcerated/vulnerable plaques may result in difficult access.

The final CT report should be comprehensive and concise and should leave no room for any discrepancy from radiological perspective **(Table 2)**.

Transcatheter Aortic Valve Replacement in Bicuspid Aortic Valves

Bicuspid aortic valves account for nearly half of the candidates for aortic valve replacement due to aortic stenosis and are associated with faster valvular remodeling, degeneration, and procedural complexity.[14] TAVI/TAVR-directed simplified classification for bicuspid aortic valves yields three broad morphologies: (1) Tricommissural, often referred to as "functional" or "acquired" BAV (not part of Sievers classification); (2) bicommissural raphe-type (equivalent to Sievers Type 1); and (3) bicommissural nonraphe-type (equivalent to Sievers Type 0). Meticulous valve sizing is imperative for apt selection of bioprosthesis. In BAV cases, the smallest and most appropriate point for the implantation of the bioprosthesis may be higher than the anatomical annulus. The aortic anatomic subtypes defined on CT are: Tubular or flared (regular annulus perimeter/area to be used for sizing) or tapered (the supra-annular perimeter/area 4 mm above the anatomical annulus to be used). Another method for sizing incorporates the level of implantation at the raphae (LIRA) plane. Calcium load and its distribution, raphae type, and length are important factors for sizing.[15]

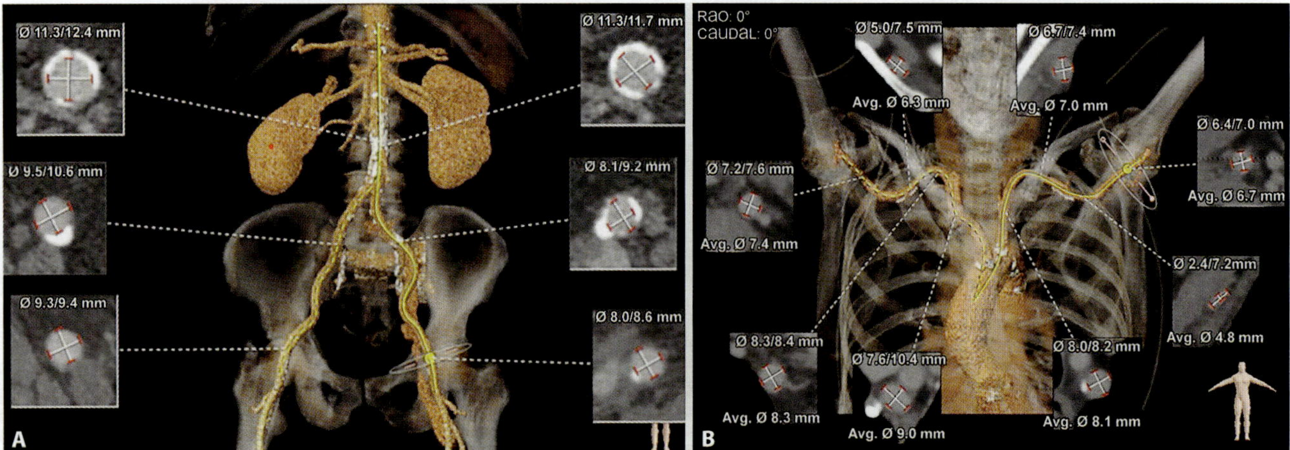

Figs. 5A and B: Three-dimensional (3D) valve replacement (VR) CT reconstruction (central image) demonstrating aorta and both iliac arteries (A) and aortic arch and arch branches (B). The side panels shows contrast-enhanced true axial images used for measuring minimal luminal diameters at various levels.

TABLE 2: Overview of required measurements.

Anatomy	*Component*	*Characteristics*
Aortic valve	• Cuspidity • Valvular calcifications • Subvalvular calcifications • Quantification of valve leaflet calcification • Leaflet length • Leaflet thickness	• Bicuspid/tricuspid/undefinable • Amount (absent to severe)/location/distribution • Present or not, location, amount • Use the Agatston method, only indicated in discrepant • Doppler echocardiography results • *Leaflet length:* Distance between the tip and the hinge point to the aortic annulus of the corresponding aortic valve leaflet
Aortic annulus	• Short- and long-axis diameter • Perimeter • Area • Center to annular distance • Pre-deployment fluoroscopic angle	Systolic measurements preferred, ensure correct double-oblique annular plane orientation
Aortic sinus	• Height • Width • Coronary height • Mid-ostial height • Center-to-ostial distance • Diameter of sinotubular junction	• Requirements differ from type of transcatheter heart valves and manufacturer • *Coronary height:* Distance from annular plane to the lower margin of coronary ostia • *Mid-ostial height:* Shortest distance between the mid-level of the ostium and the hinge point of the corresponding aortic cusp
Aorta	• Aortic angle • Maximum cross-sectional diameter of ascending aorta • Cross-sectional diameter at different levels • Wall characteristics	Amount and distribution of calcification, thrombus, ulcerative plaques, other findings
Membranous interventricular septum (MS)	• Coronal MS length • Infra-annular MS length	• *Coronal MS length:* Distance from the aortic annular plane to the most superior portion of the muscular septum in the coronal view • *Infra-annular MS length:* Distance from the vertex of the muscular septum and the annular plane measured on stretched vessel image
Access route	• Diameter subclavian and common carotid arteries • Diameter of brachiocephalic trunk • Diameter of common and external iliac arteries • Diameter of common femoral arteries • Wall characteristics • Left ventricular apex • Ascending aorta	• Minimal luminal diameters are required • Amount and distribution of calcification, thrombus, ulcerative plaques, other findings • Myocardium characteristics, presence of thrombus, other findings • Wall characteristics, especially anterior and antero-lateral wall for transaortic access

Valve-in-valve Prosthesis

The term valve-in-valve (ViV) TAVR includes TAVR-in-SAVR, TAVR-in-TAVR and even TAVR-in-TAVR-in-SAVR. Initial assessment of the indwelling bioprosthetic surgical valve comprising of its size, type, leaflet orientation via CT need to be weighed in the choice of transcatheter valve. Measurements pertaining to annular plane, coronary artery heights, STJ height, and SOV dimensions followed by implantation of a "virtual valve" to estimate valve-to-coronary (VTC) and valve-to-STJ (VTSTJ) distances are imperative. The VTC, VTSTJ, leaflet lengths and relationship of the leaflet tips of the existing surgical valve to the coronary ostia and STJ will help to determine the risk for coronary obstruction. A VTC <3–4 mm and VTSTJ <2 mm is considered high risk for coronary obstruction in the setting of ViV TAVR calling for further complex procedural planning[16] **(Figs. 6A and B)**.

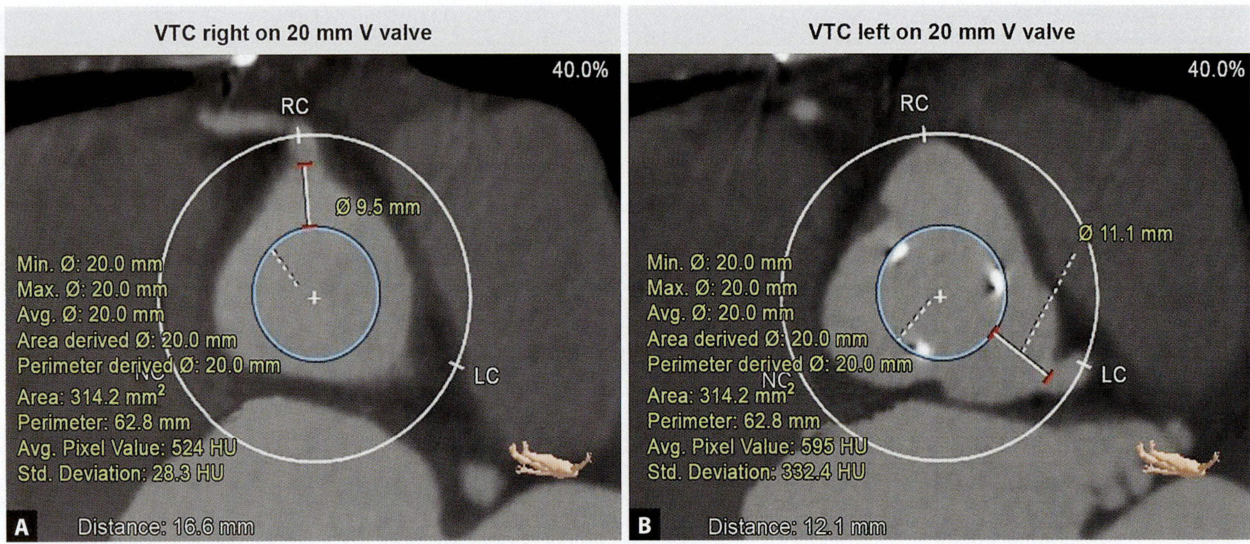

Figs. 6A and B: Valve-to-coronary (VTC) measurements for right coronary artery ostium (A) and left main coronary artery ostium (B) for ViV TAVR.

PREPROCEDURAL IMAGING OF TRANSCATHETER MITRAL VALVE REPLACEMENT

CT Protocol

Similar to the CT, TAVR trigger is placed in LV and a high KVp protocol is used to negate the artifacts caused by the metallic ring of the mitral prosthesis/annuloplasty ring/MAC. Coverage extends from the carina to the diaphragm, and the field of view includes the adjacent chest wall. ECG gating is retrospective and data from both systolic and diastolic images are used for assessment.

Critical CT Preprocedural Parameters[17]

CT plays a crucial role in planning of TMVR: Performed using dedicated software with the semiautomated method.

Annular segmentation and sizing: Defined by connecting 16 seed points deposited at the base of the MV leaflets. For prosthesis ring and annulus tracing is along the inner rim of the metallic ring. Native MV annulus is saddle-shaped, truncation of the anterior horn with a straight-line connecting the two trigones resulting in D shaped annulus. This is more reproducible for device sizing.

Neo-LVOT assessment: Post-TMVR the anterior deflection of the AML results in elongation and narrows the LVOT, referred to as the neo-LVOT. Neo-LVOT obstruction is a potentially fatal complication of TMVR. 3D-CT datasets are used to estimate the size of the anticipated neo-LVOT following placement of simulated virtual prostheses a neo-LVOT of >200 mm^2 is considered adequate **(Figs. 7A and B)**.

TMVR access planning: Cardiac MDCT can help to identify the optimal access location to achieve the perpendicular coaxial trajectory to the mitral annulus by aligning fluoroscopic projections with key anatomical landmarks. Transseptal and transapical are the two main access routes used for TMVR. The three main MDCT-derived coplanar fluoroscopic projections used for THV navigation and deployment are named based on the directions of mitral annular measurements: Septal-lateral (SL), trigone-to-trigone (TT), or intercommisural (IC). A compromise view between IC and SL views is usually provided due to C-arm angulation constraints to achieve an IC or TT view.

TMVR for Valve-in-valve, Valve-in-ring, and Valve-in-mitral Annular Calcifications

Cardiac MDCT has been an integral component for preprocedural ViV, ViR, ViMAC planning by providing (1) anchoring parameters (MAC distribution and characteristics), (2) landing zone and oversizing dimensions, (3) neo-LVOT area and other predictors of LVOTO.

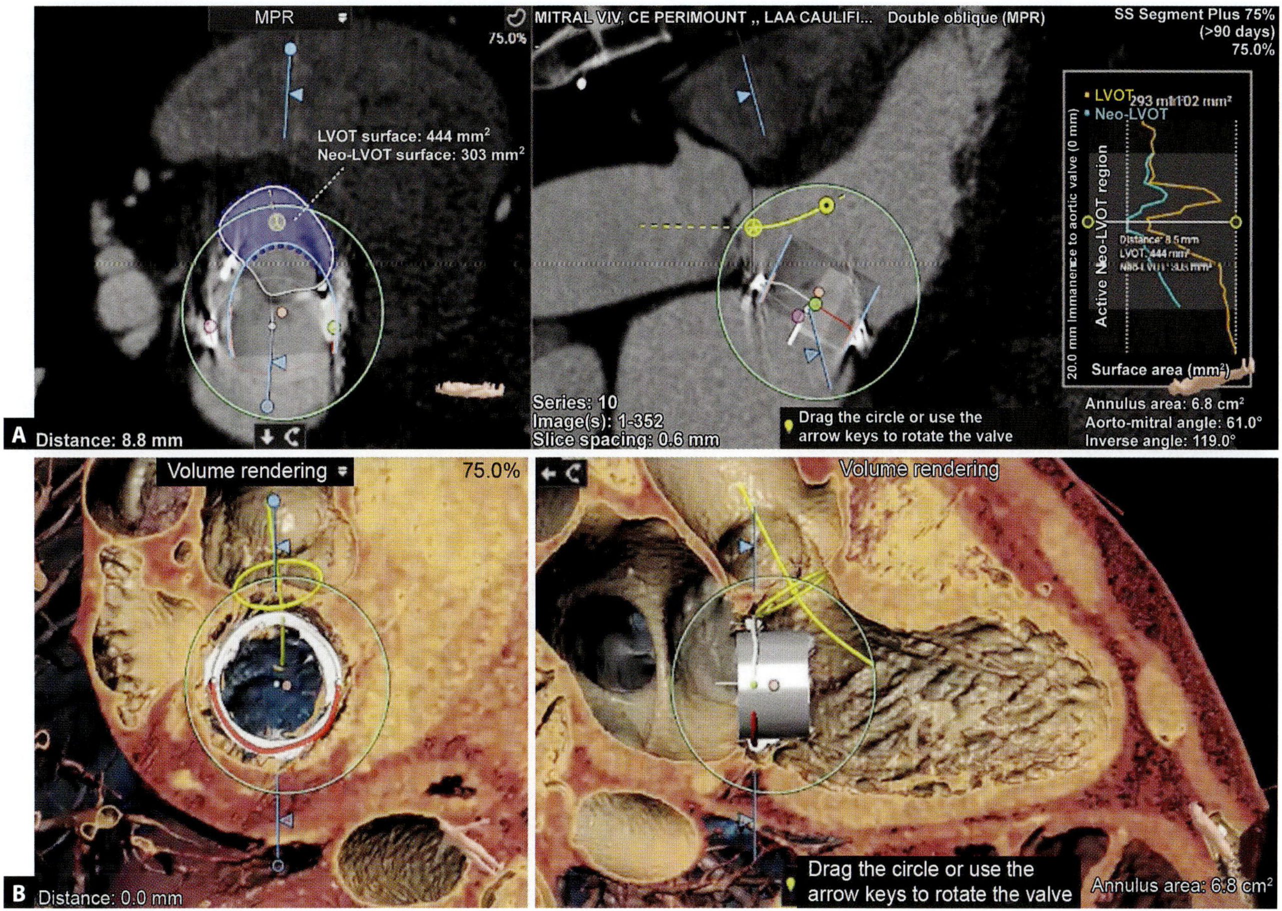

Figs. 7A and B: Short axis and three chamber images (A) and 3D VR CT images (B) demonstrate segmentation of neo-LVOT following virtual implantation of TMVR device. The smallest neo-LVOT area is measured.

CONCLUSION

Cardiac MDCT is a fundamental diagnostic imaging tool for TAVR and TMVR planning, enabling comprehensive evaluation of patient's cardiac anatomy and function, which informs patient suitability, device selection, and risk of potential complications. The knowledge continues to evolve in this dynamic field, and constant developments require training and immersion from imagers involved to gain expertise in the planning of these procedures.

REFERENCES

1. Vahanian A, Beyersdorf F, Praz F, Milojevic M, Baldus S, Bauersachs J, et al. 2021 ESC/EACTS Guidelines for the management of valvular heart disease: Developed by the Task Force for the management of valvular heart disease of the European Society of Cardiology (ESC) and the European Association for Cardio-Thoracic Surgery (EACTS). Eur heart j. 2022;43(7):561-632.
2. Ranganath P, Moore A, Guerrero M, Collins J, Foley T, Williamson E, et al. CT for pre- and postprocedural evaluation of transcatheter mitral valve replacement. Radiographics. 2020;40(6):1528-53.
3. Schwarz F, Lange P, Zinsser D, Greif M, Boekstegers P, Schmitz C, et al CT-Angiography-Based Evaluation of the Aortic Annulus for Prosthesis Sizing in Transcatheter Aortic Valve Implantation (TAVI)-Predictive Value and Optimal Thresholds for Major Anatomic Parameters. PLoS One. 2014;9(8):e103481.
4. Vinayak M, Leone PP, Tanner R, Dhulipala V, Camaj A, Makhija RRK, et al. Transcatheter aortic valve replacement: current status and Future Indications. J Clin Med. 2024; 13(2):373.
5. Francone M, Budde RP, Bremerich J, Dacher JN, Loewe C, Wolf F, et al. CT and MR imaging prior to transcatheter aortic valve implantation: standardisation of scanning protocols, measurements and reporting—a consensus document by the European Society of Cardiovascular Radiology (ESCR). Eur Radiol. 2020;30:2627-50.

6. Blanke P, Weir-McCall JR, Achenbach S, Delgado V, Hausleiter J, Jilaihawi H, et al. Computed tomography imaging in the context of transcatheter aortic valve implantation (TAVI)/transcatheter aortic valve replacement (TAVR) an expert consensus document of the Society of Cardiovascular Computed Tomography. JACC Cardiovasc Imaging. 2019;12(1):1-24.
7. Liu X, Zhou D, Fan J, Dai H, Zhu G, Chen J, et al. Cerebral Ischemic Lesions after Transcatheter Aortic Valve Implantation in Patients with Non-Calcific Aortic Stenosis. J Clin Med. 2022;11(21):6502.
8. Oh JH, Kobayashi Y, Kang G, Nishi T Willemink MJ, Fearon WF, et al. Distance between valvular leaflet and coronary ostium predicting risk of coronary obstruction during TAVR. IJC Heart Vascul. 2021;37:100917.
9. Medranda GA, Musallam A, Zhang C, Rappaport H, Gallino PE, Case BC, et al. The impact of aortic angulation on contemporary transcatheter aortic valve replacement outcomes. Cardiovasc Intervent. 2021;14(11):1209-15.
10. Gorla R, Oliva OA, Arzuffi L, Milani V, Saitta S, Squillace M, et al. Angulation and curvature of aortic landing zone affect implantation depth in transcatheter aortic valve implantation. Sci Reports. 2024;14(1):10409.
11. Binder RK, Leipsic J, Wood D, Moore T, Toggweiler S, Willson A, et al. Prediction of optimal deployment projection for transcatheter aortic valve replacement: angiographic 3-dimensional reconstruction of the aortic root versus multidetector computed tomography. Circ Cardiovasc Intervent. 2012;5(2):247-52.
12. Chen YH, Chang HH, Liao TW, Leu HB, Chen IM, Chen PL, et al. Membranous septum length predicts conduction disturbances following transcatheter aortic valve replacement. J Thorac Cardiovasc Surg. 2022;164(1):42-51.
13. Zamorano JL, Gonçalves A, Lang R. Imaging to select and guide transcatheter aortic valve implantation. Eur Heart J. 2014;35(24):1578-87.
14. Kalra A, Das R, Alkhalil M, Dykun I, Candreva A, Jarral O, et al. Bicuspid aortic valve disease: classifications, treatments, and emerging transcatheter paradigms. Struct Heart. 2024;8(1):100227.
15. Nikas DN, Lakkas L, Naka KK, Michalis LK. Transcatheter Aortic Valve Implantation (TAVI) in Bicuspid Anatomy. J Clin Med. 2025;14(3):772.
16. Perdoncin E, Paone G, Byku I. Valve-in-valve transcatheter aortic valve replacement for failed surgical valves and adjunctive therapies. US Cardiol Rev. 2022;16:e09.
17. Hashimoto G, Lopes BB, Sato H, Fukui M, Garcia S, Gössl M, et al. Computed Tomography Planning for Transcatheter Mitral Valve Replacement. Struct Heart. 2022;6(1):100012.

Role of Computed Tomography in Congenital Heart Disease

Nilay S Nimbalkar, Shruthi Kalyan

INTRODUCTION

Congenital heart disease (CHD) refers to structural abnormalities in the heart and blood vessels that develop during fetal growth. It is the most prevalent type of birth defect, impacting 8–9 out of every 1,000 children.

With advances in medical imaging, the ability to diagnose, classify, and plan interventions for CHD has significantly improved. Among the available modalities, computed tomography (CT) has emerged as a powerful tool, offering high spatial resolution, rapid acquisition, and detailed anatomical visualization.

Traditionally, echocardiography and cardiac catheterization were the mainstays for CHD assessment. However, the advent of advanced CT techniques, including electrocardiogram (ECG)-gated acquisitions, high-pitch helical scans, and low-dose protocols, has expanded its role. CT is particularly valuable for evaluating complex vascular anomalies, extra cardiac structures, and surgical planning, often supplementing or even replacing invasive angiography.

This chapter explores the evolving role of CT in CHD, highlighting its strengths, limitations, and clinical applications. From preoperative planning to postoperative assessment, CT plays a crucial role in improving patient outcomes. By integrating modern imaging protocols with three-dimensional (3D) reconstructions, CT provides a comprehensive roadmap for cardiologists, radiologists, and surgeons involved in managing congenital heart defects.

TECHNIQUES AND PARAMETERS OF PEDIATRIC THORACIC COMPUTED TOMOGRAPHY ANGIOGRAPHY

Performing computed tomography angiography (CTA) in pediatric patients requires careful consideration of various technical aspects to optimize image quality while minimizing potential risks associated with ionizing radiation.

Technical Factor

Multidetector computed tomography (MDCT) 64 slice or higher detector scanners preferred (the higher the detector collimation the larger coverage per rotation time).

Higher rotation speed and dual energy source preferred for better temporal resolution.

Radiation safety is achieved by adjusting the exposure parameters according to the patient's age and weight. Iterative reconstruction technology and automated low-dose software further help in keeping a check on the radiation dose used.

Technique

- *IV-line access:* Peripheral upper or lower limb line secured.
- *Size:* 24–20-gauge cannula depending upon the age and access site.

Sedation

Often feeding and wrapping methods should suffice for neonates, if needed oral/IV sedation could be used.

- Older kids may need good counseling to avoid sedation.
- In young children who may not cooperate during the procedure, sedation or general anesthesia is frequently required. The choice of sedation method should be based on the child's age, clinical condition, and the length of the procedure.
- For infants <4 months of age, the "feed and swaddle" technique can often be utilized. Sedation may still be required to minimize motion, slow the heart rate, and control respirations if detailed evaluation is needed of very small structures such as coronary arteries or severely hypoplastic branch pulmonary arteries.

Iodinated contrast agent used: Non-ionic (low osmolar/iso-osmolar) agent

- *Dose: Contrast:* 1–2 mL/kg body weight
- *Saline chase:* 1–2 mL/kg body weight up to about 20 mL

Injection Rate

- Hand injection in smaller children may be required with difficult access.
- Dual head power injector for older kids. Injection rate varies between 1.5 and 3 mL/s depending upon the age and gauge of access line used.
- *Power injector limit (psi):* Adjusted to about 100–175 for pediatric age group.

Timing of Acquisition

- Test bolus injection or bolus tracking of which latter is preferred.
- Computed tomography angiography image acquisition planned when maximum contrast density reaches RV/pulmonary artery (slower scanner) or LA (faster scanners).

Computed Tomography Angiography Protocol

Electrocardiogram gated versus non-ECG gated:

- Electrocardiogram gated gives better images with reduced cardiac motion artefacts, but there is increased radiation exposure.
- A dual-run study with one being ECG gating and the other being non-gated study should help for more detail.
- *Coverage:* Thoracic inlet to the diaphragm, the field of view (FOV) should be tailored to the size of the patient, with the aim of covering only the relevant anatomical structures to minimize unnecessary radiation exposure.
- *Positioning:* The patient should be positioned supine on the CT table, with the arms placed overhead to reduce attenuation from the upper limbs.

IMAGING PARAMETERS

- *Scanner type:* MDCT scanners are typically used for pediatric thoracic CTA. These scanners allow for fast image acquisition, high spatial resolution, and improved 3D rendering, which are essential for visualizing the complex anatomy of pediatric patients with congenital heart disease.
- *Scan coverage and FOV:* The scan should cover the entire thoracic cavity, from the thoracic inlet (above the clavicles) to the diaphragm, to fully assess the heart and great vessels.
- *Slice thickness and reconstruction parameters:* Slice thickness is typically set between 0.6 and 1.5 mm for pediatric thoracic CTA. Thin slices are preferred for better resolution, particularly when assessing small vascular structures. Thin slices also improve the quality of 3D reconstructions, which are essential for surgical planning and interventional procedures.
- *Pitch and rotation time:* The pitch is typically set between 0.5 and 1.0 in pediatric CTA studies. A lower pitch results in higher image quality but increases the radiation dose, while a higher pitch reduces the dose but may lead to motion artifacts or a decrease in image quality. The rotation time is generally set to 0.4–0.5 seconds for optimal temporal resolution, which is important for capturing high-quality images of the heart and great vessels during the scan.

RADIATION DOSE REDUCTION STRATEGIES

Given the concerns regarding radiation exposure, particularly in pediatric patients, minimizing radiation dose is a key priority in pediatric thoracic CTA. Several strategies are employed to reduce the dose while maintaining diagnostic image quality:

- *Low-dose protocols:* Modern CT scanners allow for the use of low-dose protocols that adjust radiation dose based on the patient's size and age. Pediatric protocols are specifically designed to deliver lower radiation doses compared to adult protocols.
- *Prospective gating:* In some cases, prospective ECG gating is used to minimize radiation exposure. This method allows the scanner to capture images only during specific phases of the cardiac cycle (e.g., diastole), reducing the number of unnecessary scans and minimizing radiation dose.
- *Iterative reconstruction algorithms:* Advanced image reconstruction techniques, such as iterative reconstruction, can improve image quality at lower radiation doses. These algorithms reduce noise and enhance image clarity, especially in cases where radiation dose reduction is necessary.
- *Minimizing scan length:* Optimizing scan coverage to avoid unnecessary imaging of non-essential regions can help further minimize radiation exposure. The scan should be tailored to the patient's anatomy to reduce the volume of radiation delivered.

POSTPROCESSING AND 3-DIMENSIONAL RECONSTRUCTION

- *Image reconstruction:* After the scan is completed, the acquired raw data is processed to create high-resolution images. These images are then reconstructed into multiple planes (axial, coronal, and sagittal) to allow for thorough assessment of the anatomy.
- *3D imaging and visualization:* Multidetector CTA allows for the creation of 3D reconstructions that provide excellent visualization of complex anatomical structures such as congenital heart defects, vascular malformations, and coronary artery anomalies.
- *Postprocessing software:* Advanced software tools for post-processing and visualization, such as volume rendering, maximum intensity projection (MIP), and multiplanar reconstruction (MPR), are often used to enhance the diagnostic value of the images and provide clearer depictions of complex anatomy **(Figs. 1A to D)**.

ROLE OF COMPUTED TOMOGRAPHY ANGIOGRAPHY IN COMPLEX CARDIAC ANOMALIES

Detailed Visualization of Cardiac Anatomy

- *Assessment of heart chambers and vessels:* CT provides detailed images of the heart chambers, valves, and vessels, allowing for an assessment of congenital defects such as ventricular septal defects (VSDs), atrial septal defects (ASDs), and atrioventricular septal defects. It helps define the size and location of the defect, which is important for surgical planning or other interventions **(Figs. 2 and 3)**.
- *Complex congenital heart defects:* For conditions such as tetralogy of Fallot, transposition of the great arteries, or double-outlet right ventricle, CT can visualize the abnormal connections between the heart chambers and the great vessels, assisting in

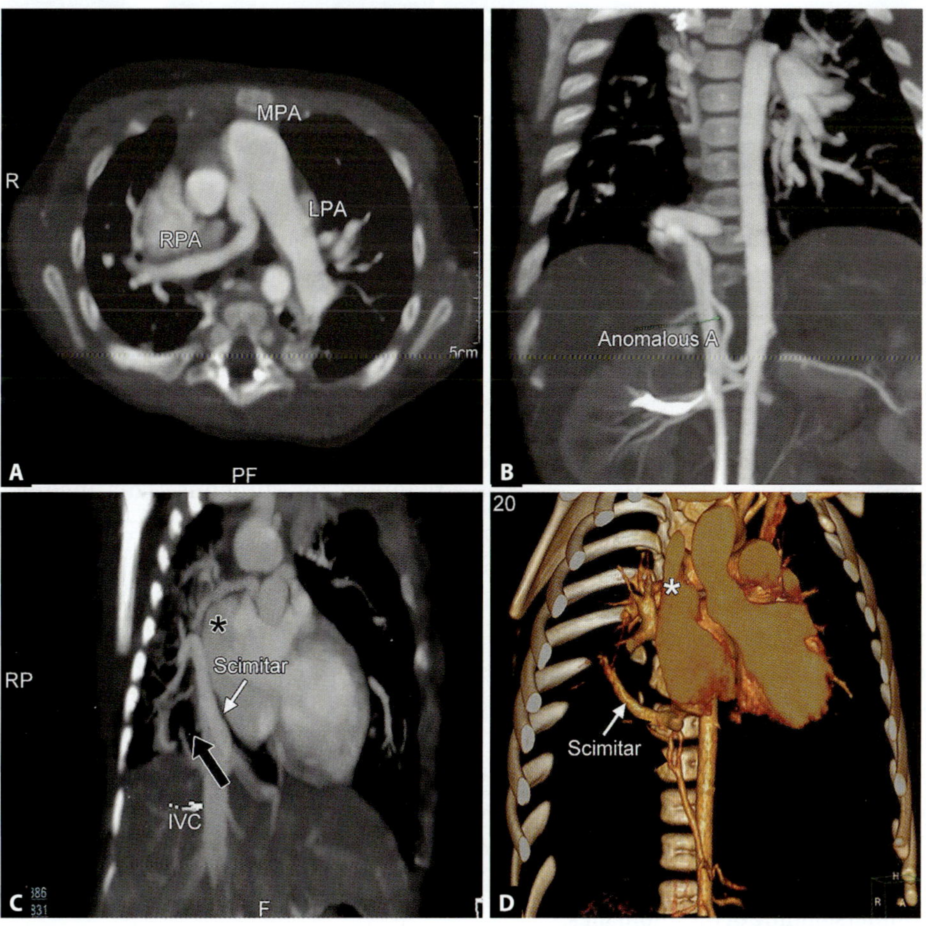

Figs. 1A to D: Maximum intensity projection (MIP) computed tomography angiography (CTA) axial MIP (A), coronal MIP (B and C), and three-dimensional volume rendering technique (3D VRT) images (D) of scimitar syndrome.

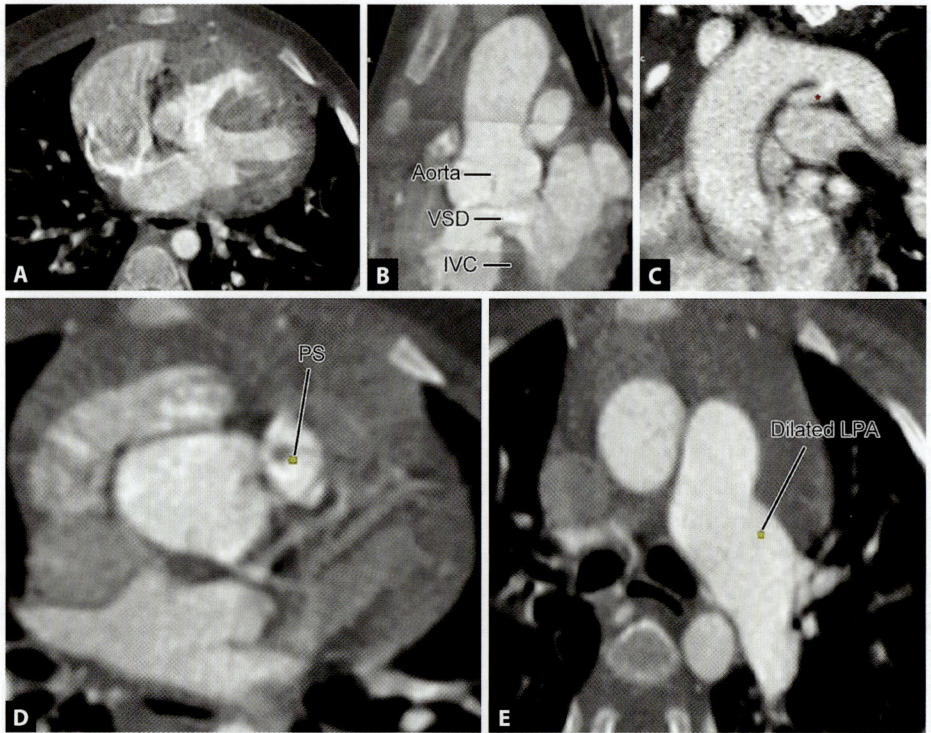

Figs. 2A to E: Case of tetralogy of Fallot (TOF); (A) Thickened interventricular septum with large membranous ventricular septal defects (VSDs) with overriding of the aorta and RV wall thickening; (B) Oblique coronal image showing overriding of aorta and VSD; (C) Demonstrating large patent ductus arteriosus (PDA)(*); (D) Severe pulmonary stenosis; (E) Dilatation of left pulmonary artery. (IVC: inferior vena cava)

defining the exact anatomical relationship and the pathophysiology of these defects.

Computed Tomography Angiography for Vascular and Coronary Assessment

One of the significant roles of CT in congenital heart disease is the evaluation of coronary arteries. In some congenital conditions, such as anomalous coronary arteries, CTA can provide high-resolution imaging of coronary anatomy, helping to identify the presence of coronary artery anomalies that may require surgical or interventional treatment or may cause issues in surgical approach to right ventricular outflow tract (RVOT) [e.g., aberrant origin of left anterior descending (LAD) which passes along the surface of RVOT].

For congenital defects such as pulmonary artery stenosis, pulmonary atresia, or anomalous pulmonary venous return, CT angiography is a valuable tool to visualize the pulmonary vasculature in three dimensions, facilitating better understanding of the anomalies.

Computed tomography angiography also helps in assessing the aorta's anatomy, particularly in cases of coarctation of the aorta, where the narrowing of the aorta needs to be accurately visualized to plan interventions such as balloon angioplasty or surgery.

Three-dimensional Imaging and Surgical Planning

Three-dimensional CT imaging can provide a detailed roadmap for surgeons. This includes understanding the anatomy of the heart, great vessels, and associated structures, allowing for better surgical planning, particularly for open-heart surgeries or catheter-based interventions such as stenting or device placements. For patients with intricate anomalies involving multiple structures, such as univentricular hearts, hypoplastic left heart syndrome, or conotruncal anomalies, CT allows for the reconstruction of these anomalies in 3D as well 3D model printing, helping guide decision-making for corrective surgery or palliation.

Assessment of Postsurgical Outcomes

After surgeries such as Fontan procedure or arterial switch operation, CT is used to assess the anatomical

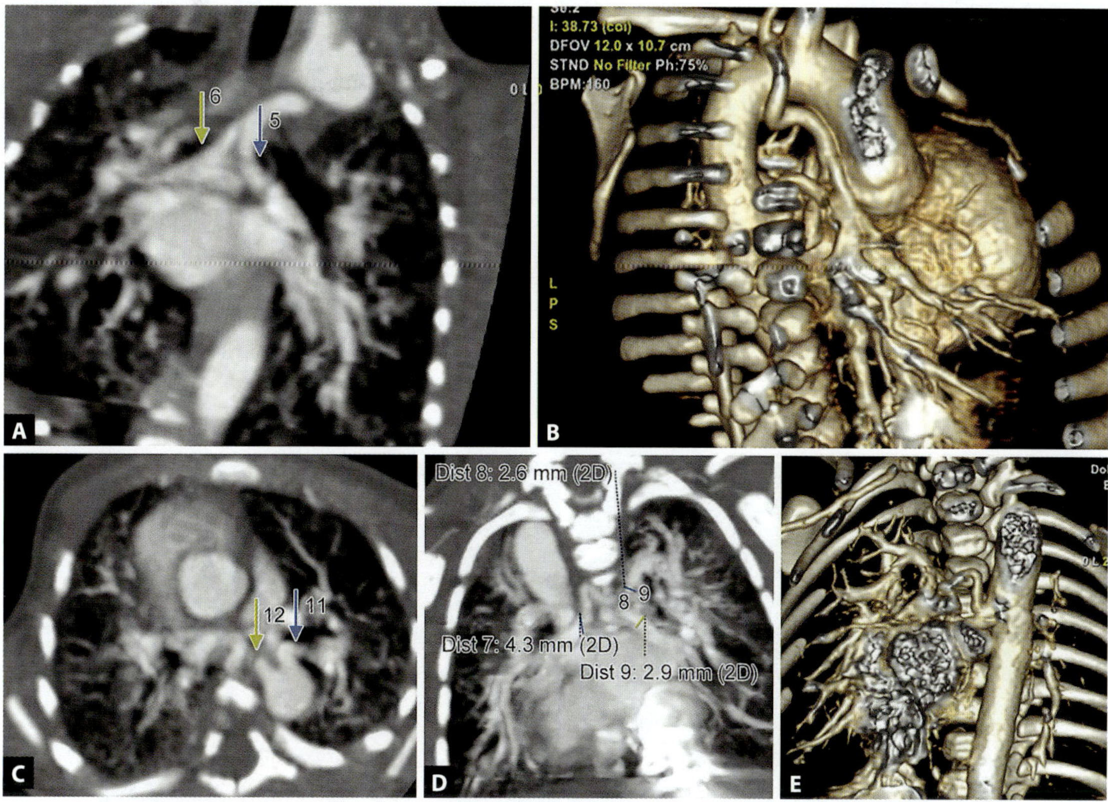

Figs. 3A to E: Known case of tetralogy of Fallot (TOF) with pulmonary atresia; (A) Coronal maximum intensity projection (MIP); (B) Volume rendering (VR) image showing indirect MAPCA (major aortopulmonary collateral arteries) from left subclavian artery branches; (C to E) Large direct MAPCAs from descending thoracic aorta supplying right and left pulmonary artery circulation. (arrow 5 and 6 showing small right and left pulmonary arteries, 7,8.9 showing sizes for MAPCAs,11 and 12 showing MAPCAS from aorta)

changes and evaluate potential complications, such as stenosis or recurrent defects. It can help detect changes in the pulmonary arteries, cardiac chambers, and great vessels. CT is useful for monitoring post-surgical complications, including stenosis of the pulmonary arteries, aortic dilation, or the development of collateral vessels, all of which may impact the long-term function of the heart.

Assessment of Pulmonary Circulation and Lung Vascularization

In congenital heart disease, especially when there are pulmonary venous anomalies, CT angiography provides a clear picture of pulmonary vascular structures, evaluating the blood flow and the degree of pulmonary hypertension. In congenital anomalies such as pulmonary sequestration or bronchopulmonary malformations, CT helps assess the relationship between the heart and the lungs, determining if these anomalies contribute to heart failure or increased cardiac workload.

Detection of Associated Abnormalities

Many congenital heart defects are associated with extracardiac anomalies, such as diaphragmatic hernia, kidney malformations, or spinal deformities. CT can help in identifying these associated anomalies and guide the overall management approach. In some cases of complex congenital anomalies, such as those involving ectopic or accessory cardiac tissue, CT may help locate these areas and decide whether they require surgical intervention.

CONGENITAL PULMONARY VENOUS ANOMALIES

Computed tomography plays a critical role in the diagnosis, assessment, and management of pulmonary venous anomalies. These anomalies can involve abnormal connections, malformations, or developmental defects in the pulmonary veins. CT, particularly CTA, offers detailed imaging to evaluate the complex anatomical features of the pulmonary venous system and associated structures.

Identification of Pulmonary Venous Malformations

- *Total or partial pulmonary venous return anomalies:* CT is crucial in diagnosing total anomalous pulmonary venous return (TAPVR), where the pulmonary veins drain abnormally into systemic veins or other parts of the circulatory system instead of returning to the left atrium. CT can help identify the abnormal venous connections, such as drainage into the superior vena cava (SVC), inferior vena cava (IVC), or right atrium **(Figs. 4 and 5)**.
- *Partial anomalous pulmonary venous connection (PAPVC):* This type of anomaly can be harder to detect without detailed imaging, but CT provides clear visualization of how the veins connect, aiding in diagnosis **(Figs. 6A and B)**.
- *Pulmonary venous obstruction:* CT can also detect obstruction or stenosis of the pulmonary veins, which can be congenital or develop later due to scarring or surgical interventions. This is critical for assessing conditions such as pulmonary vein stenosis, which can lead to pulmonary hypertension and respiratory distress **(Figs. 7A and B)**.

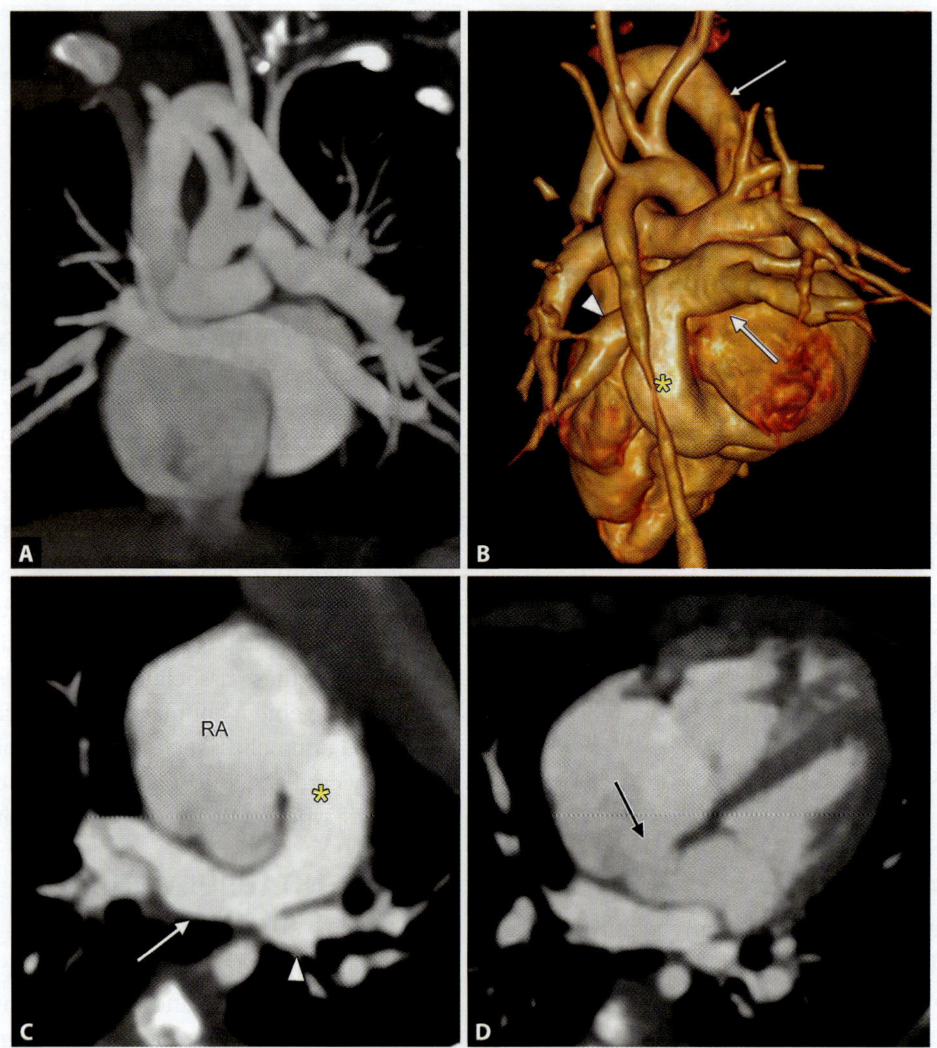

Figs. 4A to D: Three-dimensional (3D), maximum intensity projection (MIP) computed tomography angiography (CTA) images of mixed total anomalous pulmonary venous connection (TAPVC)—right upper pulmonary vein (RUPV) and right lower pulmonary vein (RLPV) join to form a common trunk of right pulmonary veins (white arrow) which joins the left pulmonary vein (white arrowhead) and drain into the coronary sinus (yellow asterisk), left upper pulmonary vein (thin white arrow) drains into the left innominate vein to superior vena cava (SVC). Note atrial septal defect (ASD) (black arrow) in this patient.

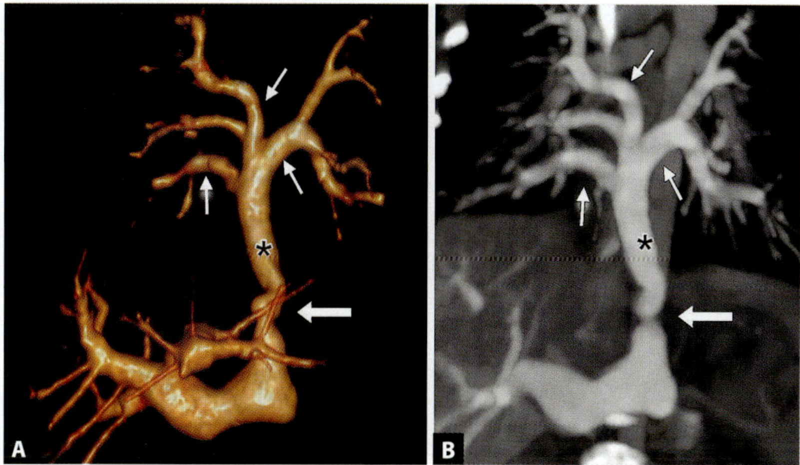

Figs. 5A and B: Maximum intensity projection (MIP), 3D volume-rendered computed tomography angiography (CTA) images of infracardiac obstructive total anomalous pulmonary venous connection (TAPVC). All pulmonary veins (thin white arrows) join to form a descending vertical vein (black asterisk); (A) Note narrowing of a vertical vein just at hiatus level (thick white arrow) which passes below the diaphragm and drain into the portal vein (B).

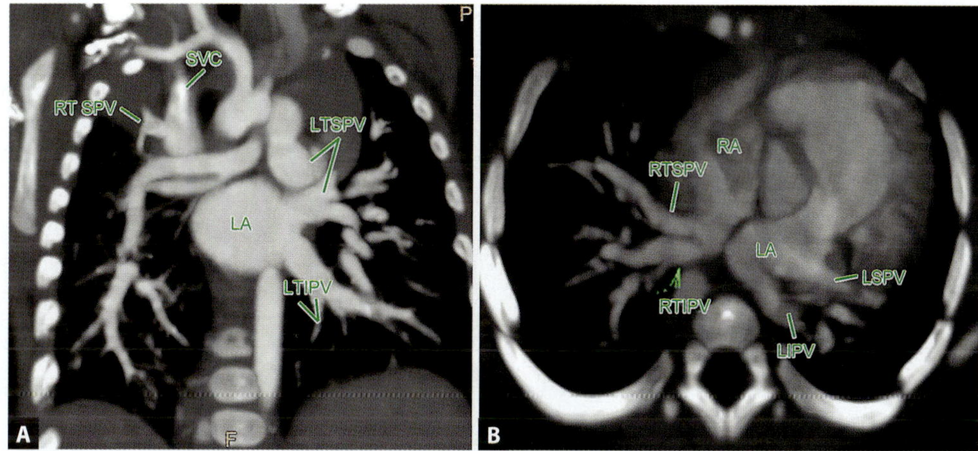

Figs. 6A and B: Partial anomalous pulmonary venous connection (PAPVC); (A) Maximum intensity projection (MIP) computed tomography angiography (CTA) image shows right superior pulmonary vein (RTSPV) draining into superior vena cava (SVC) and left pulmonary veins draining into LA; (B) Right-sided PV's draining into right atrium and left-sided PV's into left atrium. (RA: right atrium; LA: left atrium; RTIPV: right inferior pulmonary vein; LSPV: left superior pulmonary vein; LIPV: left inferior pulmonary vein)

3-dimensional Imaging and Surgical Planning

Computed tomography provides 3D imaging, allowing for the creation of a detailed anatomical model of the pulmonary veins, their connections, and the surrounding structures. This is particularly useful in surgical planning for conditions such as *TAPVR* and *pulmonary vein stenosis*, where precise visualization of the venous.

Assessment of Pulmonary Veins and Left Atrium

Computed tomography provides clear visualization of the pulmonary veins entering the left atrium. This is important when there is a need to evaluate the connections and check for any abnormalities, such as multiple pulmonary veins draining into a single chamber or vascular malformations.

Postsurgical Follow-up and Complications

- *Postoperative assessment*: After surgery to correct pulmonary venous anomalies (such as repair of TAPVR), CT is used to assess the success of the operation. It can identify complications such as stenosis or recurrent drainage issues, ensuring that the veins are adequately connected to the left atrium and there is no abnormal obstruction.

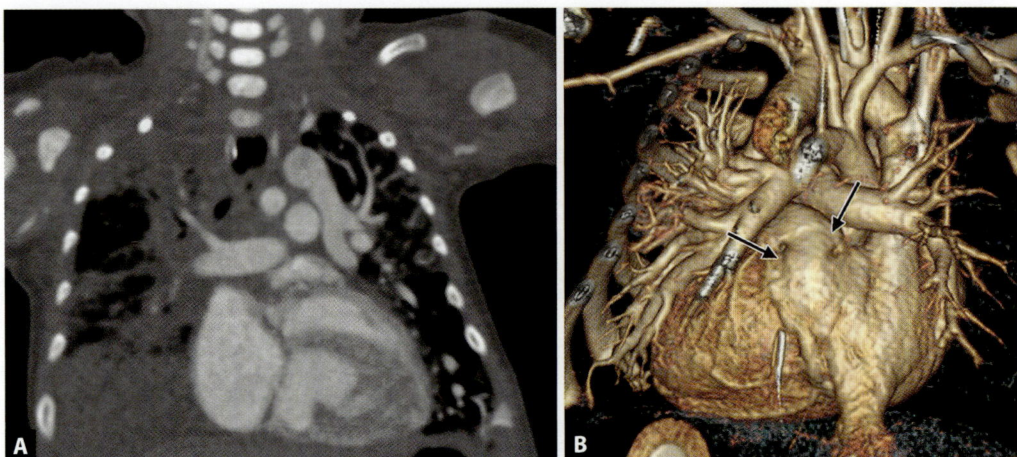

Figs. 7A and B: Case of partial anomalous pulmonary venous drainage of left upper pulmonary vein and rest of the pulmonary veins showing venous atresia; (A) Coronal maximum intensity projection (MIP) image showing partial anomalous venous drainage of left upper lobe pulmonary vein into the innominate vein with areas of ground-glass opacities in the visualized right lung parenchyma and non-opacification of rest of the pulmonary veins; (B) Volume rendered image showing small size left atrium with arrows showing markings of nonopacified pulmonary veins from left lower and right lung parenchyma.

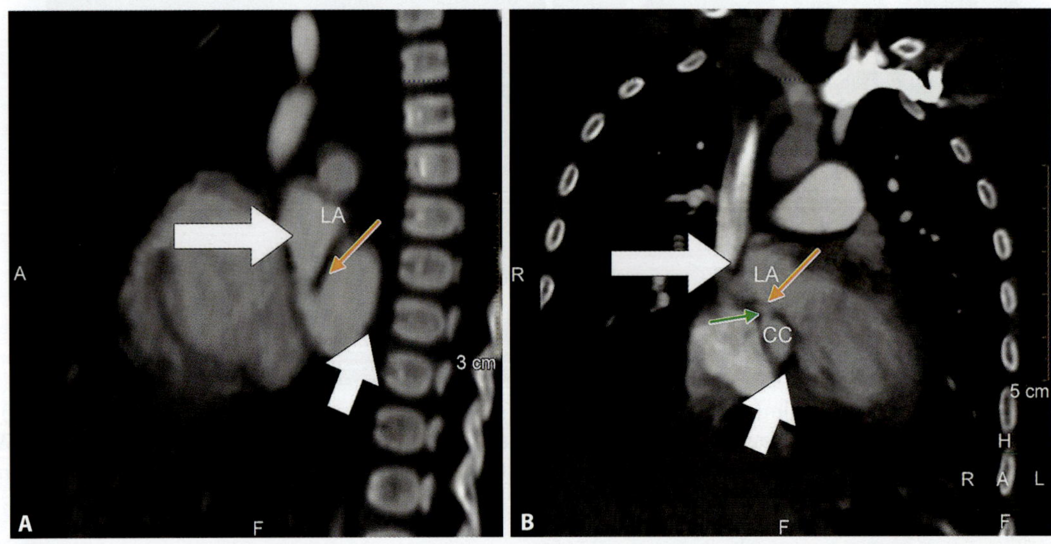

Figs. 8A and B: Maximum intensity projection (MIP) computed tomography angiography (CTA) images of postoperative total anomalous pulmonary venous connection (TAPVC) shows stenosis at the anastomosis site (orange thin arrow) of common confluence (arrowhead) to LA (long arrow).

- *Monitoring of pulmonary vein stenosis:* After surgical or interventional procedures, CT is useful for detecting the early development of pulmonary vein stenosis, which is a potential complication after surgery for anomalies such as TAPVR. Early detection can prevent long-term issues such as pulmonary hypertension and heart failure **(Figs. 8A and B)**.

Evaluation of Associated Cardiac Anomalies

Pulmonary venous anomalies, particularly TAPVR, often occur in conjunction with other congenital heart defects, such as ASDs, VSDs, or patent ductus arteriosus (PDA). CT can evaluate these associated defects simultaneously, providing a comprehensive view of the heart and vascular anatomy.

Evaluation of Congenital and Acquired Malformations

Computed tomography is effective in diagnosing congenital abnormalities, such as pulmonary venous diverticula, venous duplication, or persistent left superior vena cava (LSVC).

ROLE OF COMPUTED TOMOGRAPHY IN CORONARY ARTERY ANOMALIES

Coronary artery anomalies (CAAs) refer to congenital or acquired conditions where the coronary arteries do not follow the typical course or origin. These anomalies can lead to ischemic heart disease, sudden cardiac arrest, or even death in some cases. Here is how CT plays a role.

Computed tomography is invaluable for visualizing anomalous coronary arteries, such as an artery arising from the wrong sinus of Valsalva (e.g., left coronary artery arising from the right sinus of Valsalva or right coronary artery arising from the left sinus of Valsalva).

In some cases, CT identifies the origin of a coronary artery in an unusual location, such as from the pulmonary artery, a condition referred to as anomalous origin of the coronary artery from the pulmonary artery (ALCAPA), which is a rare but life-threatening condition.

Computed tomography can reveal abnormal connections between coronary arteries and other vascular structures, such as veins or the right atrium, which may lead to an increased workload on the heart.

Computed tomography is highly effective in detecting coronary artery aneurysms or dilatations that may arise as a result of congenital conditions, trauma, or infectious processes (e.g., Kawasaki disease).

ROLE OF COMPUTED TOMOGRAPHY IN PULMONARY ARTERY ANOMALIES

These anomalies may include conditions such as pulmonary artery stenosis, pulmonary artery hypoplasia, and anomalous origin of the pulmonary arteries, all of which can lead to significant cardiopulmonary complications.

Computed tomography angiography is highly effective in identifying pulmonary artery stenosis, where the pulmonary artery narrows and limits blood flow to the lungs, or pulmonary artery atresia, where the artery is absent or blocked. These conditions are often congenital and require early diagnosis and intervention **(Figs. 2 and 3)**.

Computed tomography angiography can also identify anomalous origins of the pulmonary arteries, such as a right pulmonary artery originating from the left pulmonary artery (or vice versa), or from aorta in cases of truncus arteriosus or abnormal connections between the pulmonary arteries and systemic veins or other vascular structures **(Figs. 9 and 10)**.

Computed tomography angiography can detect dilatation of the pulmonary arteries, which can occur in

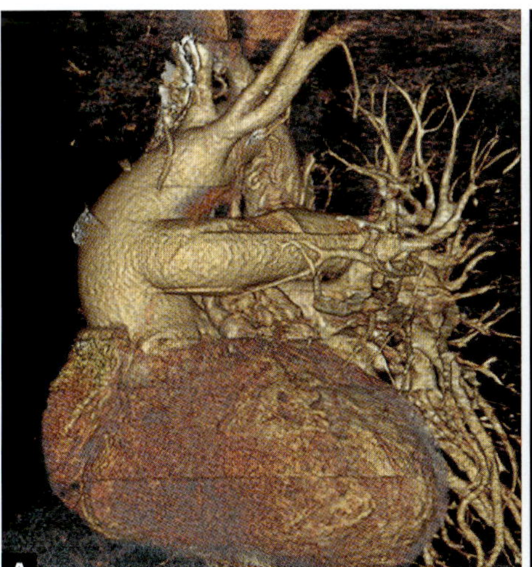

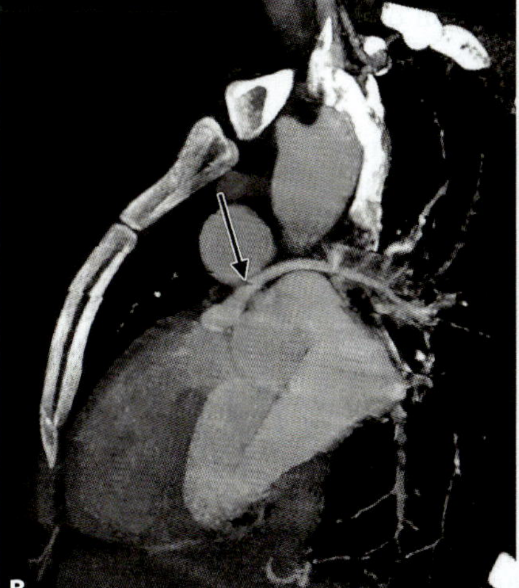

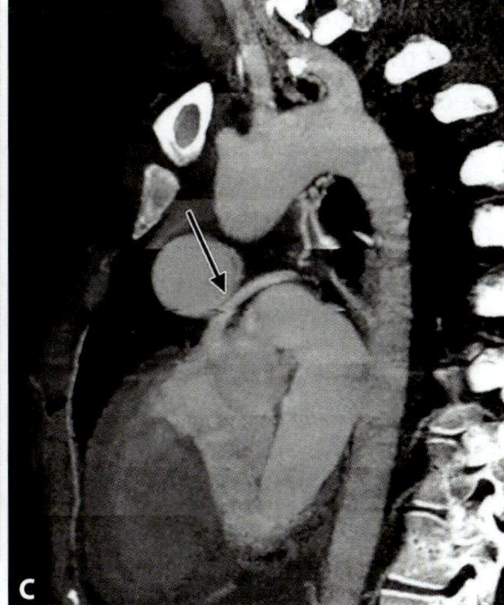

Figs. 9A to C: Case of hemi truncus with the origin of left pulmonary artery from ascending aorta and small sized right pulmonary artery from right ventricular outflow tract (RVOT). Normal branching of left pulmonary artery is seen. Small-sized right pulmonary artery (arrows) also show normal branching.

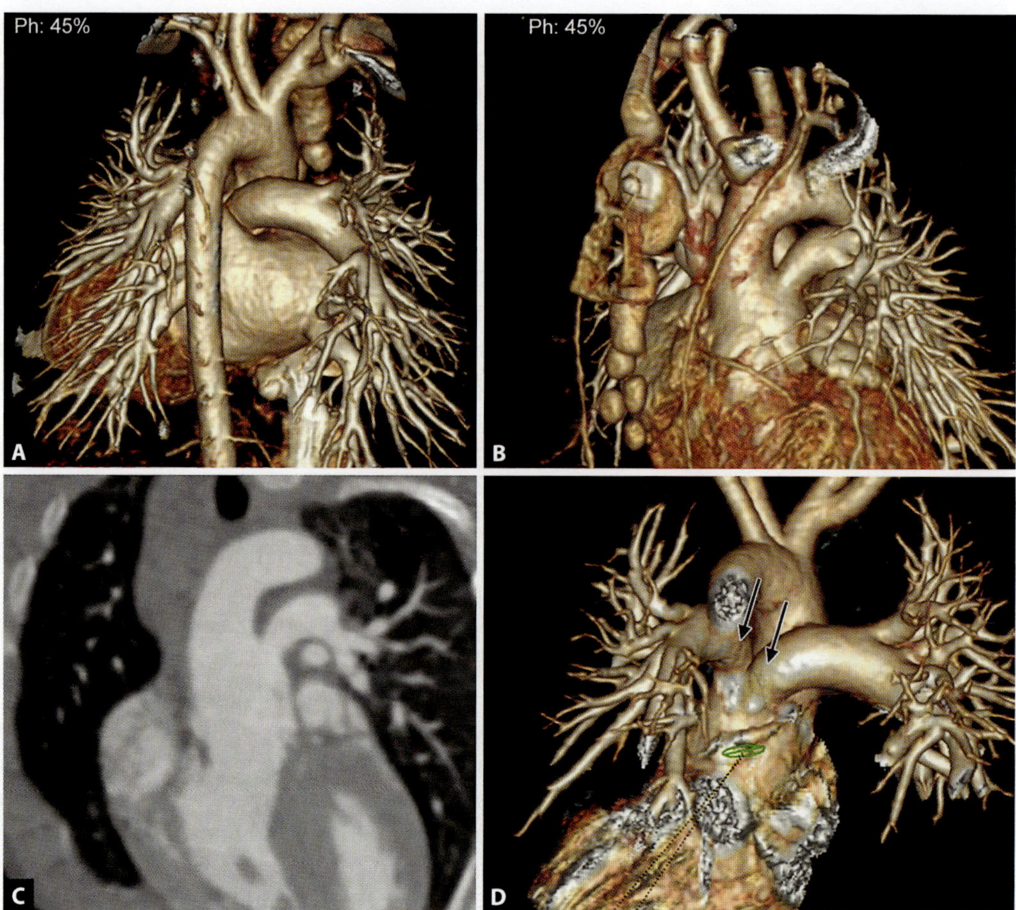

Figs. 10A to D: Volume-rendered images and oblique coronal maximum intensity projection (MIP) images showing common truncus with right and left pulmonary arteries arising from the posterior aspect of the truncus close to one another and showing normal pulmonary artery branching, suggesting type II of truncus arteriosus (TA).

conditions such as pulmonary hypertension or in cases where there is volume overload due to congenital heart defects.

For congenital heart conditions such as tetralogy of Fallot or pulmonary sequestration, CT can map the branching patterns of the pulmonary arteries to identify malformations in the major pulmonary branches and evaluations of MAPCAs (major aortopulmonary collateral arteries) aiding in surgical planning or intervention **(Figs. 3A to E)**. After surgical correction of pulmonary artery anomalies (such as pulmonary artery reconstruction in congenital heart disease), CT is used to monitor for complications, including restenosis, pulmonary artery dilation, or thrombus formation. It can also help assess the success of surgeries, such as Fontan surgery or arterial switch surgery, which may affect pulmonary artery function **(Figs. 11A and B)**.

ROLE OF COMPUTED TOMOGRAPHY IN POSTOPERATIVE CONGENITAL CARDIAC ANOMALIES

Computed tomography plays a crucial role in the postoperative management and follow-up of congenital cardiac diseases. CT provides detailed, non-invasive imaging that helps evaluate the success of the surgery, detect complications early, and monitor the patient's long-term outcomes.

After corrective surgeries or palliative procedures (e.g., Fontan procedure, arterial switch surgery, atrial septal defect closure), CT plays a key role in evaluating the effectiveness of the repair.

Computed tomography provides detailed images to ensure that the heart's anatomy has been correctly restored after surgery. This includes checking the

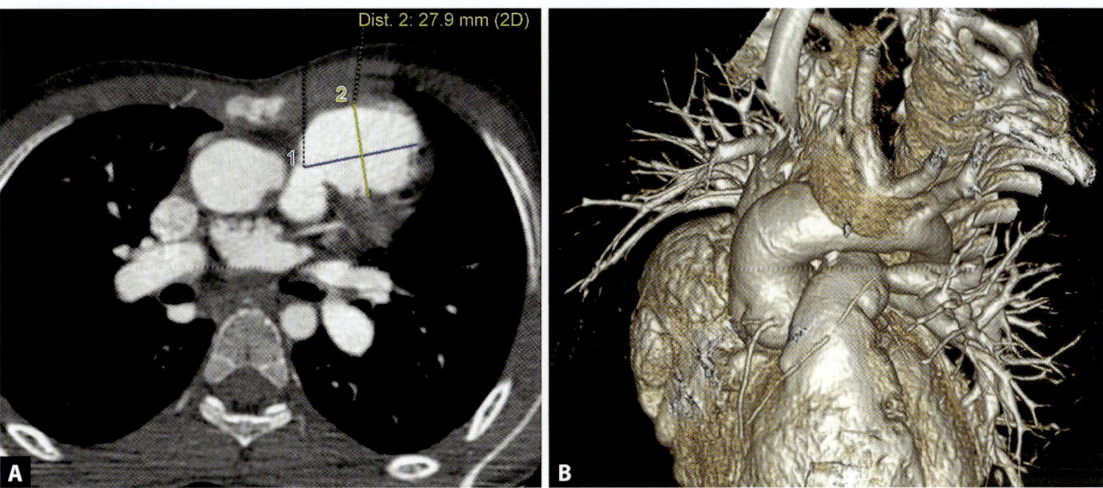

Figs. 11A and B: Known case of tetralogy of Fallot (TOF), postintracardiac repair follow-up CT; (A) Axial maximum intensity projection (MIP); (B) Volume rendering (VR) image showing aneurysmal dilatation of right ventricular outflow tract (RVOT) as one of the postoperative complications.

position of the repaired or reconstructed vessels, heart chambers, and valves.

In cases of complex congenital heart defects such as hypoplastic left heart syndrome or tetralogy of Fallot, CT helps verify the success of surgeries such as Fontan or corrective repairs, ensuring that the heart and great vessels are correctly restructured and if there are any residual defects or surgical site.

Postoperative complications are common after congenital heart surgeries. CT plays a vital role in identifying these issues early.

In cases of postsurgical pulmonary stenosis or dilatation, CT can detect narrowing or blockages in the pulmonary arteries, which could lead to pulmonary hypertension and require further intervention. Postarterial switch operations for transposition of the great arteries, CT can assess for aortic stenosis. CT is particularly effective in detecting complications such as vascular obstructions, pseudoaneurysms, or vascular injuries that can result from surgical procedures. These can be life-threatening and often require early intervention.

ROLE OF COMPUTED TOMOGRAPHY IN THORACIC AORTIC CONGENITAL ANOMALIES

One of the most common congenital anomalies involving the thoracic aorta is aortic coarctation, which involves narrowing of the aorta, usually distal to the left subclavian artery. CT angiography can accurately identify the location and severity of the narrowing, providing essential information for surgical or interventional planning **(Figs. 12A and B)**.[12]

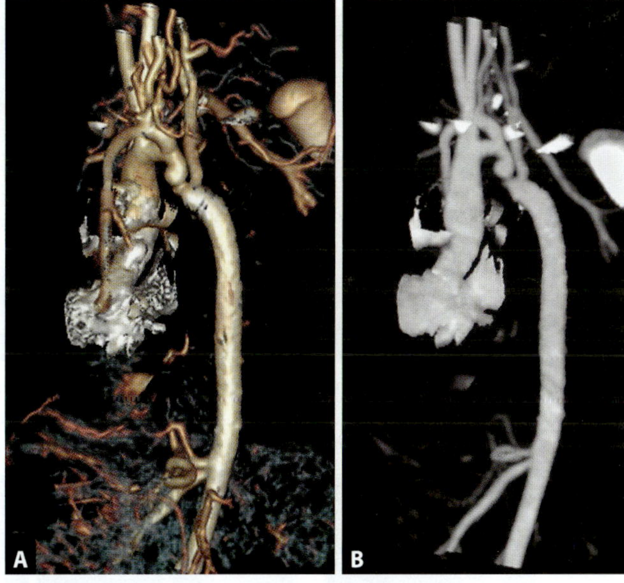

Figs. 12A and B: Volume rendering (VR) and maximum intensity projection (MIP) coronary images of computed tomography angiography (CTA) shows severe coarctation of aorta in the distal arch.

In congenital conditions such as Marfan syndrome and Loeys-Dietz syndrome, aortic root dilation or ascending aorta abnormalities are common. CT is excellent at visualizing the aortic root and its relationship with the aortic valve, helping to detect dilation or aneurysms in these regions.

In cases where a PDA persists beyond infancy, CT can evaluate its size and the effects it may have on the aorta, as it may cause abnormal blood flow and lead to dilatation of the aortic vessels **(Figs. 13A and B)**.

Computed tomography angiography is highly effective in detecting an aberrant subclavian artery, a condition where the subclavian artery arises from the descending aorta instead of the normal position at the aortic arch. This anomaly can lead to dysphagia (difficulty swallowing) or vascular compression. CT provides clear visualization of the anatomy and helps plan surgical or interventional management **(Figs. 14A and B)**.

Double aortic arch is a rare congenital anomaly where two aortic arches form, encircling the trachea and esophagus, which can lead to compression of these structures. CT imaging allows for precise identification of both arches and their relationships with the trachea and esophagus, guiding the treatment plan. A right-sided aortic arch is another congenital anomaly where the aorta arches to the right rather than the left. It may or may not be associated with other defects such as ductus arteriosus or vascular rings.

Computed tomography provides a clear image of the arch's course and its branches, which is essential for planning surgery or monitoring potential complications **(Figs. 13A and B)**.

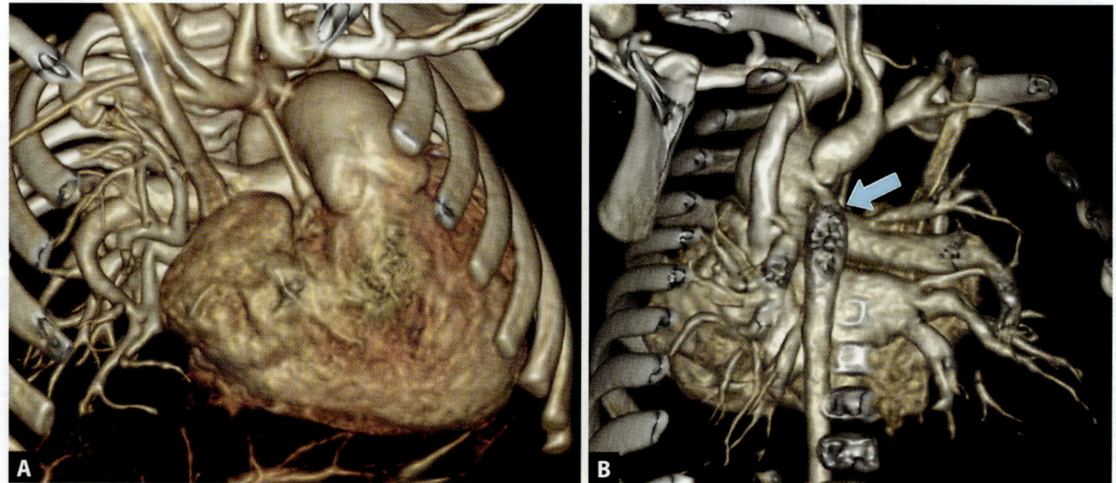

Figs. 13A and B: Volume rendering (VR) images showing interrupted aortic arch with large patent ductus arteriosus (PDA) (arrow) supplying distal thoracic aorta.

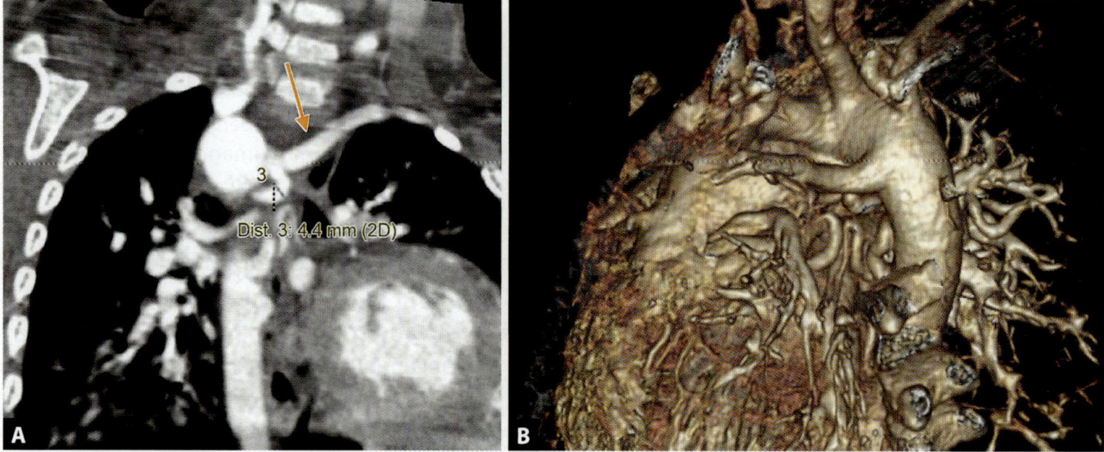

Figs. 14A and B: Coronal maximum intensity projection (MIP) and volume rendering (VR) images showing aberrant origin of left subclavian artery (SCA) from right-sided descending thoracic aorta and large direct major aortopulmonary collateral arteries (MAPCA) (2D measurement).

Assessment of Postoperative Changes and Complications

- *Postoperative aortic dilatation:* For congenital aortic anomalies, such as aortic coarctation repair or aortic arch reconstruction, CT is essential for long-term monitoring to detect any postoperative aortic dilatation or restenosis at the surgical site. This helps in timely intervention to prevent complications such as aortic dissection or rupture.
- *Aortic valve assessment:* After surgeries such as aortic valve replacement or repair of aortic root dilation, CT can evaluate the function of the aortic valve and check for leakage or stenosis that may require further intervention.
- *Aortic pseudoaneurysm:* Postoperative complications, such as the development of a pseudoaneurysm at the site of an aortic repair or surgical anastomosis, can be detected using CT. This can help in early intervention to prevent rupture.
- *Surgical graft patency:* After procedures such as aortic bypass surgery or grafting of the aorta, CT angiography is used to assess the patency of the graft and ensure there is no occlusion or other complications that could lead to reduced blood flow.

CONCLUSION

Computed tomography imaging is now an integral part of the evaluation of CHD because of its high-detail anatomical information, rapid image acquisition, and comprehensive assessment of both intracardiac and extracardiac structure, with excellent image quality with minimal radiation exposure.

However, CT imaging does have some limitations, and alternative imaging modalities such as echocardiography and MRI should be considered, especially when functional assessment or serial follow-ups may be necessary. Collaboration among radiologists and treating physicians is necessary for optimizing imaging protocols to ensure optimal diagnosis and surgical planning.

FURTHER READING

1. 2018 AHA/ACC Guideline for the Management of Adults With Congenital Heart Disease. Circulation. 2018
2. ACR Appropriateness Criteria: Congenital Heart Disease (Pediatric and Adult; Interventional Planning and Follow-up). American College of Radiology.
3. Banderker E, Pretorius E, de Decker R, (2015). The role of cardiac CT angiography in the pre- and postoperative evaluation of tetralogy of Fallot. South African Journal of Radiology, 19(2), 9 pages.
4. Baz RO, Refi D, Scheau C, Savulescu-Fiedler I, Baz RA, Niscoveanu C. Coronary Artery Anomalies: A Computed Tomography Angiography Pictorial Review. J Clin Med. 2024 Jul 4;13(13):3920.
5. Bean MJ, Pannu H, Fishman EK. Three-dimensional computed tomographic imaging of complex congenital cardiovascular abnormalities. J Comput Assist Tomogr. 2005;29(6):721-4.
6. Escalon JG, Browne LP, Bang TJ, Restrepo CS, Ocazionez D, Vargas D. Congenital anomalies of the pulmonary arteries: an imaging overview. Br J Radiol. 2019;92(1093): 20180185.
7. Hollingsworth CL, Yoshizumi TT, Frush DP, Chan FP, Toncheva G, Nguyen G, et al. Pediatric cardiac-gated CT angiography: assessment of radiation dose. AJR Am J Roentgenol. 2007;189(1):12-8.
8. Kumar P, Bhatia M. Role of CT in the Pre- and Postoperative Assessment of Conotruncal Anomalies. Radiol Cardiothorac Imaging. 2022 Jun 30;4(3):e210089.
9. Leschka S, Oechslin E, Husmann L, Desbiolles L, Marincek B, Genoni M, et al. Pre- and postoperative evaluation of congenital heart disease in children and adults with 64-section CT. Radiographics. 2007;27(3):829-46.
10. Lyen S, Wijesuriya S, Ngan-Soo E, et al. Anomalous pulmonary venous drainage: a pictorial essay with a CT focus. J Congenit Heart Dis 1,7(2017).
11. van der Linde D, Konings EE, Slager MA, Witsenburg M, Helbing WA, Takkenberg JJ, et al. Birth prevalence of congenital heart disease worldwide: a systematic review and meta-analysis. J Am Coll Cardiol. 2011;58(21):2241-7.
12. Wang J, et al. (2020). Journal of Cardiovascular Development and Disease, 7(1), 8.

CHAPTER 46

Computed Tomography-derived Fractional Flow Reserve: Ready for Prime-time Use

Supreetha Hegde A, Suraj Gowda, Richa Kothari

INTRODUCTION

Computed tomographic coronary angiography (CTCA) is a non-invasive test for coronary artery disease (CAD), offering high sensitivity and negative predictive value for obstructive CAD. However, the relationship between stenosis severity and ischemia in intermediate stenoses is complex. *Invasive angiography* (IA) with fractional flow reserve (FFR) is the gold standard for evaluating lesion significance, but its invasive nature and risks limit its clinical adoption.[1]

Computed tomography-derived fractional flow reserve (CT FFR) uses computational fluid dynamics (CFD) and machine learning to simulate FFR, combining anatomical and hemodynamic assessment in a single non-invasive test. Studies show that CT FFR enhances CTCA accuracy, reduces unnecessary invasive procedures, and avoids pharmacologic vasodilation.[2] While strict study protocols may not reflect real-world conditions, data suggest CT FFR leads to fewer invasive tests and revascularizations, reducing healthcare costs, complications, and improving patient satisfaction.[3]

Non-invasive functional evaluations such as nuclear myocardial perfusion imaging (SPECT—single photon emission CT) and stress cardiac magnetic resonance imaging have their limitations, such as low resolution or high cost.[4] Amongst the various CT-based techniques for assessing stenosis significance, CT FFR is amongst the most studied.

Invasive FFR measures the ratio of maximum achievable blood flow to a stenosed myocardial area during maximal hyperemia compared to the maximum achievable blood flow in the same vessel in the absence of the blockage. This is done by measuring the pressure ratio measured distal and proximal to the area of stenosis, using a pressure sensor. FFR is used to evaluate the significance of coronary artery stenoses and guide revascularization decisions. An FFR ≤0.80 indicates ischemia-causing lesions, while an FFR >0.80 typically defers revascularization, improving clinical outcomes and reducing costs. Revascularization for FFR ≤0.80 reduces the risk of death and myocardial infarction.[5]

COMPUTED TOMOGRAPHY-DERIVED FRACTIONAL FLOW RESERVE

Computed tomography-derived fractional flow reserve combines patient-specific imaging, physiological models and CFD in five key steps:[6,7]

- *Creating 3D anatomic models*: CTCA data generates a detailed 3D model of coronary arteries, capturing vessel dimensions and stenosis features.
- *Quantifying baseline coronary flow*: This is done by considering blood pressure and scaling laws to estimate coronary flow.
- *Determining microcirculatory resistance*: Resistance is calculated based on vessel area, accounting for flow in coronary arteries and their microcirculation.
- *Simulating hyperemia*: Increased blood flow is modelled computationally to assess resistance changes during hyperemia without vasodilators.
- *Applying CFD methods*: CFD and Navier-Stokes equations model blood flow, pressure, and velocity in coronary arteries during rest and hyperemia.

Computed tomography-derived fractional flow reserve offers a comprehensive assessment of pressure and flow across the coronary tree, unlike invasive FFR, which is limited to directly interrogated vessels.[8]

HeartFlow is currently the most widely used and the only US Food and Drug Administration-approved technique for assessing CT FFR using off-site supercomputers. It creates a patient-specific 3D coronary artery model through semiautomatic contouring and segmentation, incorporates hemodynamic conditions using CFD principles to calculate FFR from CTCA data.[5]

Hybrid models for on-site, faster computation and deep learning-based approaches for estimating CT FFR are promising ongoing advancements.[5] These techniques are focused on improving accuracy and efficiency; however, they are limited by challenges in small vessel assessment and complex coronary geometries.

INDICATION

Computed tomography-derived fractional flow reserve is recommended for patients with intermediate stenosis or lesions with <50% stenosis in proximal coronary artery segments, especially in moderate-to-severe or multivessel disease. It helps guide revascularization decisions and should be assessed on a case-by-case basis.

RISK CATEGORIES

- *Low risk:* Stenosis <30%
- *Intermediate risk:* Stenosis 30–69%
- *High risk:* Left main disease, three-vessel disease, or stenosis ≥70%

Computed tomography-derived fractional flow reserve values:

- *>0.80:* Not significant
- *0.76–0.80:* Borderline significance
- *≤0.75:* Significant

Computed tomography-derived fractional flow reserve interpretation:[7,9]

- For *focal* lesions, measurements are taken 10–20 mm distal to the stenosis.
- *Diffuse* disease is suggested when there is no focal lesion, but the terminal vessel FFRCT is ≤0.80.
- *Sequential* lesions are assessed by evaluating CT FFR distal to each lesion.

The threshold of 0.80 shows strong agreement with invasive FFR. Clinical decisions for values between 0.76 and 0.80 should consider other factors. In small vessel or distal lesions, optimal medical therapy may be preferred.[10] A 3D color-coded map offers additional insights into lesion impact.

Post-test risk stratification: CT FFR results should be interpreted with clinical context, including symptoms, patient preferences, and revascularization potential. The report should highlight pressure-loss lesions, their location, and small vessel occlusions. Results should indicate the likelihood of hemodynamic significance (low, borderline, or high), emphasizing lesions with significant impact, including distal coronary disease.[6,8]

CASE ILLUSTRATION

See **Figure 1**.

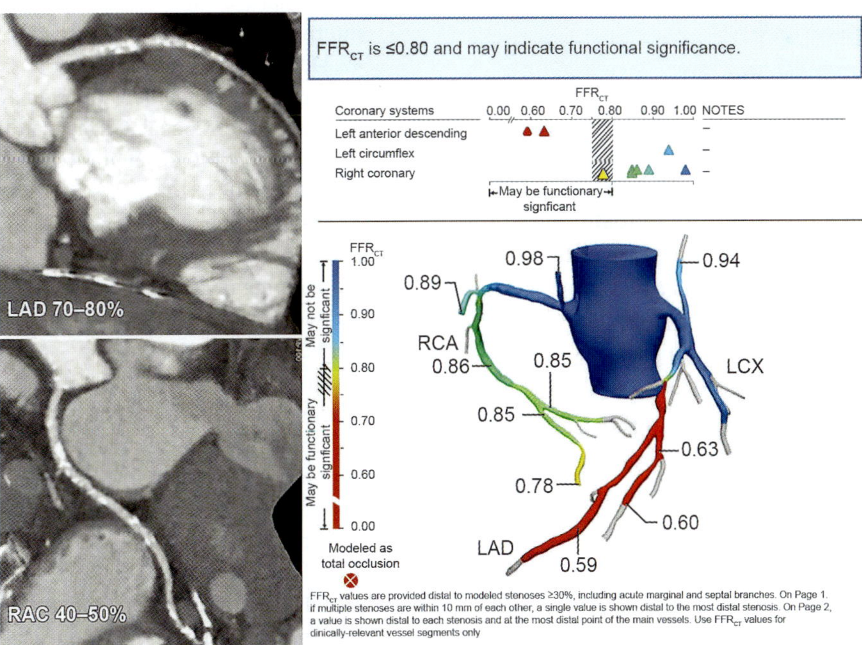

Fig. 1: Computed tomography (CT) angiographic images (left) and fractional flow reserve computed tomography (FFR CT) model (right) shows severe disease in left anterior descending (LAD) and intermediate disease in right coronary artery (RCA) with anatomically and functionally significant obstructive disease of LAD but no functionally significant disease in RCA.
Courtesy: Bhavana Nagabhushana Reddy, Consultant at University Hospitals Sussex NHS Foundation Trust

STRENGTHS OF COMPUTED TOMOGRAPHY-DERIVED FRACTIONAL FLOW RESERVE [4,11]

- *Clinical validation:* Studies, including the DISCOVER-FLOW trial, show CT FFR's high accuracy, with improved specificity and diagnostic accuracy compared to CTCA alone.
- *Non-invasive and fast:* CT FFR offers a non-invasive, efficient alternative to invasive FFR, providing similar diagnostic power without the need for catheterization.
- *Clinical benefits:* It helps identify functionally significant coronary lesions, aiding treatment decisions and potentially reducing unnecessary procedures.

CHALLENGES AND LIMITATIONS[12]

- *Availability and cost:* CT FFR requires advanced computational resources, limiting its availability and increasing its cost compared to other non-invasive tests.
- *Image quality requirements:* Suboptimal CTCA data quality, such as motion artifacts, can affect CT FFR accuracy.
- *Time for calculation*: While improvements are ongoing, CT FFR calculations can take hours, though future advances may reduce this time.

CONCLUSION

Since its introduction, CT FFR has shown promise in assessing CAD, particularly for evaluating ischemic lesions. The DISCOVER-FLOW trial demonstrated CT FFR's comparable sensitivity to CTCA and significant improvements in specificity and diagnostic accuracy.[1] However, a recent real-world multicenter audit showed that FFR-CT had a low positive predictive value evaluated against invasive FFR, thus making its use less cost-effective compared to conventional functional imaging methods.[13] While CT FFR offers good diagnostic performance, its broader adoption depends on addressing cost, availability, and imaging quality issues.[13] Despite challenges, ongoing advancements may bring CT FFR closer to becoming a standard tool in CAD management.

REFERENCES

1. Tesche C, De Cecco CN, Albrecht MH, Duguay TM, Bayer RR 2nd, Litwin SE, et al. Coronary CT angiography-derived fractional flow reserve. Radiology. 2017;285(1):1-10.
2. Becker LM, Peper J, Verhappen BJLA, Swart LA, Dedic A, van Dockum WG, et al. Real world impact of added FFR-CT to coronary CT angiography on clinical decision-making and patient prognosis - IMPACT FFR study. Eur Radiol. 2023;33: 5465-75.
3. Nørgaard BL, Fairbairn TA, Safian RD, Rabbat MG, Ko B, Jensen JM, et al. Coronary CT angiography-derived fractional flow reserve. Radiol Cardiothorac Imaging. 2019;1(5): e190050.
4. Min JK, Taylor CA, Achenbach S, Koo BK, Leipsic J, Nørgaard BL, et al. Noninvasive fractional flow reserve derived from coronary CT angiography: Clinical data and scientific principles. JACC Cardiovasc Imaging. 2015;8(10): 1203-16.
5. Zhang D, Lv S, Song X, Yuan F, Xu F, Zhang M, et al. Fractional flow reserve versus angiography for guiding percutaneous coronary intervention: a meta-analysis. Heart. 2015;101:518-24.
6. Peters B, Paul JF, Symons R, Franssen WMA, Nchimi A, Ghekiere O. Invasive fractional-flow-reserve prediction by coronary CT angiography using AI vs computational fluid dynamics software in intermediate-grade stenosis. J Cardiovasc Imaging. 2024;12(7):800-11.
7. Weir-McCall JR, Fairbairn TA. Fractional flow reserve derived from CT: The state of play in 2020. Radiol Cardiothorac Imaging. 2020;2(1):e190153
8. Rajiah P, Cummings KW, Williamson E, Young PM. CT Fractional Flow Reserve: A Practical Guide to application, interpretation and problem solving. Radiographics. 2022; 42:340-58.
9. Soschynski M, Scheffler R, Birkemeyer C, Hagar MT, Faby S, Schwemmer C, et al. CT myocardial perfusion & CT-FFR vs invasive FFR for hemodynamic relevance of CAD. Radiology. 2024;312(2):e233234.
10. Andreini D, Mushtaq S, Conte E, Mei M, Nicoli F, Melotti E, et al. The usefulness of cardiac CT integrated with FFRCT for planning myocardial revascularization in complex CAD: a lesson from SYNTAX studies. Cardiovasc Diagn Ther. 2019;9(6):738-48
11. Chen J, Wetzel LH, Pope KL, Meek LJ, Rosamond T, Walker CM. FFRCT: Current Status. Coronary artery disease, fractional flow reserve, fractional flow reserve derived from coronary CT angiography. AJR. 2021;216:640.
12. Packard RR, Karlsberg RP. Integrating FFRCT into routine clinical practice: A solid PLATFORM or slippery slope? J Am Coll Cardiol. 2016;68(5):446-9.
13. Mittal TK, Hothi SS, Venugopal V, Taleyratne J, O'Brien D, Adnan K, et al. The use and efficacy of FFR-CT: Real-world multicenter audit of clinical data with cost analysis. J Am Coll Cardiol Intv. 2023;15(10):1491-502.

SECTION 6

Miscellaneous

CHAPTER 47

Gold Standard Positron Emission Tomography Imaging: A Game Changer in the Assessment of Cardiovascular Disease

GN Mahapatra

INTRODUCTION

Positron emission tomography (PET) imaging is one of the novel diagnostic modalities of investigation in the diagnosis and assessment of patients suffering from coronary and noncoronary artery disease (CAD). PET has contributed significantly with a higher diagnostic accuracy in the assessment of CAD and non-CAD patients, has been reported to be superior to other noninvasive test like stress ECG, two-dimensional (2D) echocardiography, multidetector computed tomography (MDCT) and MRI study with their well-known limitations with a sensitivity of 93% and specificity of 95%. Additionally, the diagnostic accuracy of myocardial perfusion by PET has been reported to be superior and a game changer to single photon emission computed tomography (SPECT).

Positron emission tomography is the gold standard nuclear imaging and it is a noninvasive, nonpainful technique for measuring the metabolic activity of cardiac cells/myositis in CAD and non-CAD.

The following are various PET methods for diagnosing and assessing cardiovascular disease process.

- Stress PET myocardial perfusion study
- Stress PET myocardial perfusion study with coronary blood flow quantitation/coronary flow reserve (CBF/CFR)
- Resting SPECT study with F-18 fluorodeoxyglucose (FDG) study for the assessment of myocardial viability
- F-18 FDG/F-sodium fluoride (NaF) study for detection of unstable atheromatous plaque (vulnerable plaque) in coronary arteries as well as in large vessel atherosclerosis.
- F-18 FDG/F-18 florbetaben/F-18 florbetapir/Ga-68 Dotatate for detection, monitoring the progression or regression of infiltrative cardiac disease such as sarcoidosis, amyloidosis and other inflammatory cardiac disease.
- F-18 FDG tracer for detection of inflammation/infection of prosthetic valve, bacterial endocarditis, other inflammation of cardiac muscles, pacemaker lead, and large vessel vasculitis.
- F-18 FDG/I-123 metaiodobenzylguanidine (MIBG) tracer/C-11-hydroxyephedrine (C11-HED) for imaging sympathetic denervation following MI to select patient for cardiac resynchronization therapy (CRT) by implanting cardioverter defibrillation therapy (DCD).
- Ga-86 fibroblast activation protein inhibitor (FAPI) for imaging myofibroblast in the infarcted myocardium as well as focal vessel wall lesion in big arteries to detect atherosclerosis/fibrosis.
- Ga-68 Pentixafor/Ga-68 dotatate for targeting inflammatory *CXCR4* in large vessel inflammation/infection.

STRESS POSITRON EMISSION TOMOGRAPHY MYOCARDIAL PERFUSION STUDY

N13-Ammonia/O-15 Labeled Water/F-18 Flurpiridaz

Myocardial perfusion PET has a superior diagnostic accuracy, lower radiation dose and absolute quantification of myocardial blood flow (coronary flow reserve, CFR) as compared to SPECT myocardial perfusion. N-13 ammonia is a radiopharmaceutical commonly used for stress positron emission tomography-myocardial perfusion imaging (PET-MPI) offering several advantages over other techniques like SPECT. N-13 ammonia is injected intravenously at rest and again during pharmacological stress like IV adenosine or regadenoson. This protocol is faster than SPECT and it needs to be separated by about 50 minutes but looking at short half-life of 10 minutes it can be performed one after the other meaning first rest study of 12 minutes duration of 2 minutes for myocardial blood

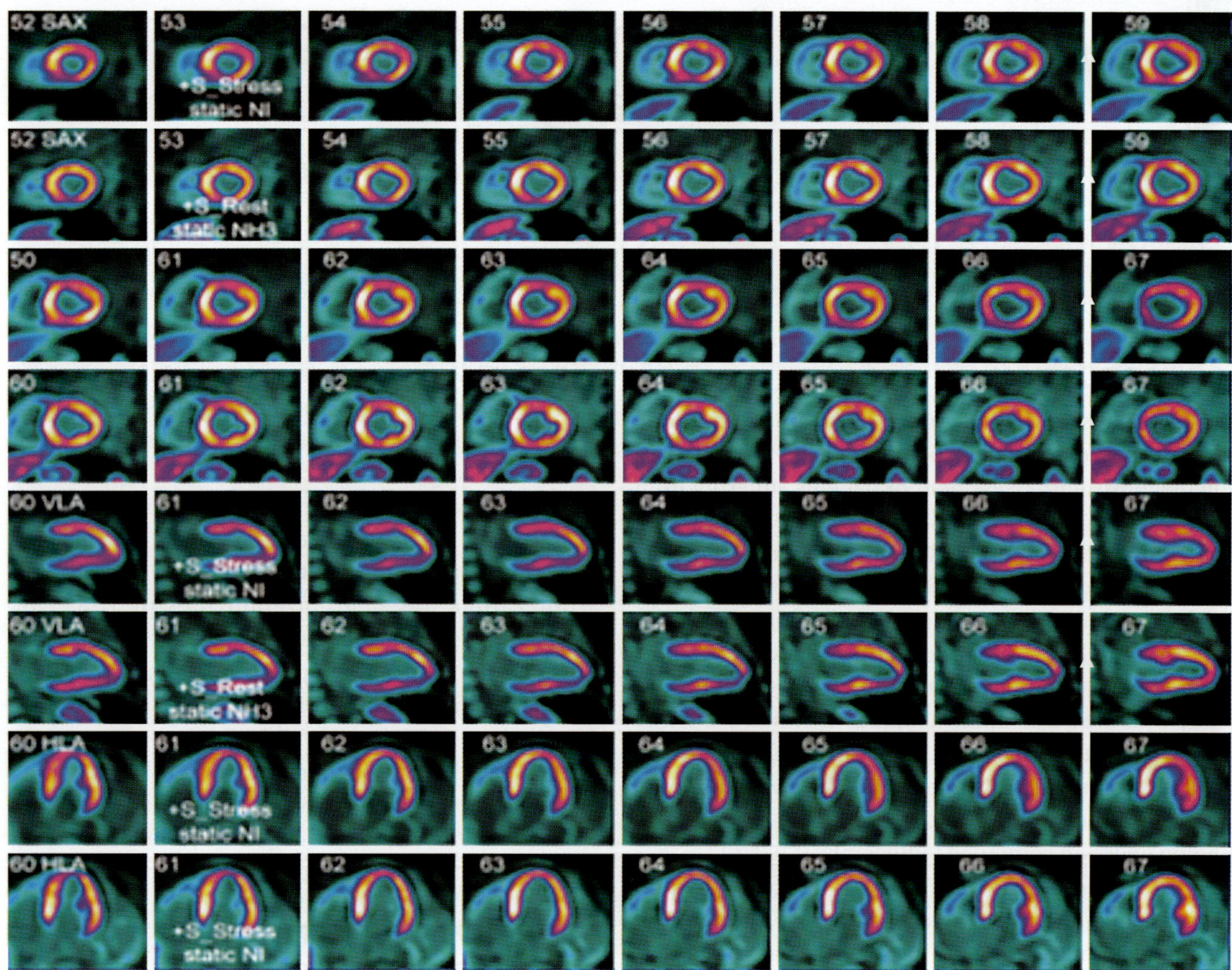

Fig. 1: Stress 13-N ammonia positron emission tomography (PET) myocardial perfusion study showing uniform perfusion pattern involving all the defined myocardial segments.

flow quantitation followed by 10 minutes of myocardial perfusion. Following which one can inject 2–3 times of resting doses of N-13 ammonia (7–8 mCi) where the stress doses amount to be 18–20 mCi of N-13 ammonia at pharmacological stress study with IV adenosine which completes stress study including 1st 2 minutes of stress study for blood flow quantitation and 10 minutes for myocardial perfusion.

Overall, 13-N-ammonia PET-MPI is a powerful tool for diagnosing and managing CAD offering high diagnostic accuracy, lower radiation exposure and the ability to quantify CBF/CFR along with stress and rest myocardial perfusion slices.

This study requires onsite cyclotron as 13N-NH3 has a relatively short half-life (approximately 10 minutes) for its availability which can impact the cost and logistical feasibility for some imaging centers **(Figs. 1 and 2)**.

Advantages of 13N-Ammonia Positron Emission Tomography Imaging

- *High sensitivity and accuracy:* 13N-ammonia provides excellent image quality and a high extraction rate leading to more accurate assessment of blood flow and CAD detection.
- *Lower radiation dose:* PET scan generally involves lower radiation exposure compared to SPECT MPI.
- *Improved image resolution and attenuation correction:* PET offers better image resolution and incorporates intrinsic attenuation correction, minimizing artifacts and provides clearer images.

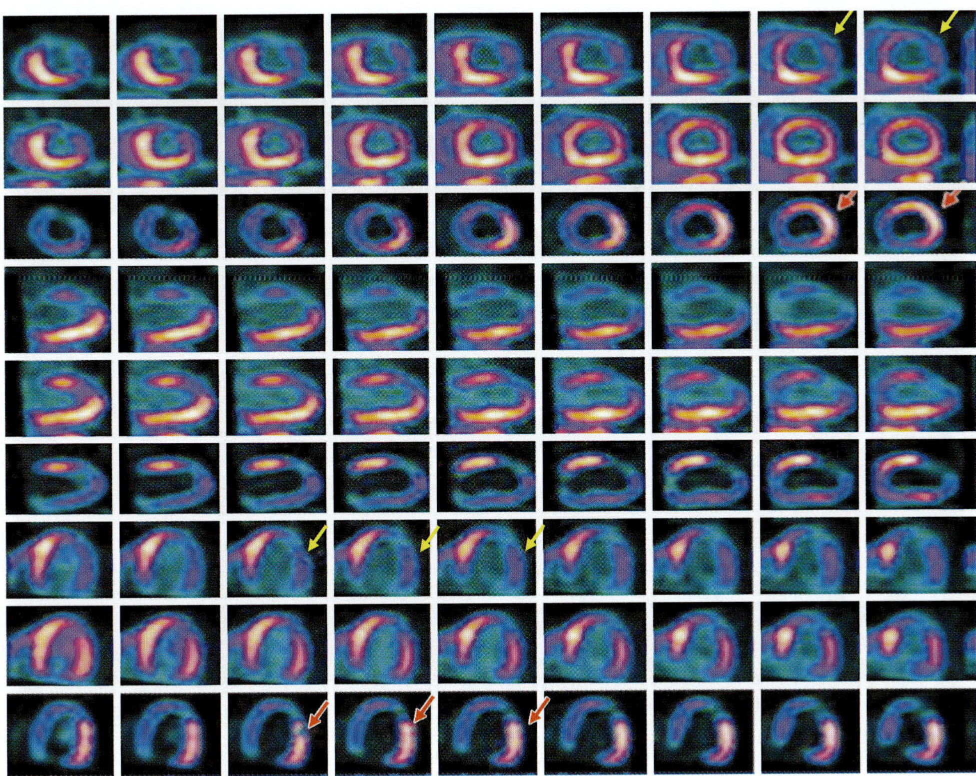

Fig. 2: Stress N-13 ammonia positron emission tomography (PET) myocardial perfusion study reveals a sizeable perfusion defect involving anterolateral segments with evidence of reversible ischemia.

- *Quantitative blood flow measurement (MBF/CFR):* N-13 ammonia allows for the absolute quantification of myocardial blood flow (MBF) providing more comprehensive understanding of cardiac function and enabling the calculation of myocardial flow reserve (MFR). MFR helps to identify the culprit lesion in triple vessel disease to reclassify the myocardial ischemia, heart failure with preserved ejection fraction (HFpEF), subclinical CAD, and balanced ischemic patients whose artery to be intervened.
- *Assessment in difficult patient population:* PET-MPI with N-13 NH3 is particularly a valuable diagnostic tool for obese individuals, women, and suspected patients having multivessel disease.

F-18 Flurpiridaz as Stress Positron Emission Tomography-Myocardial Perfusion Imaging Tracer along with Absolute Quantitation of Myocardial Blood Flow/Coronary Flow Reserve

F-18 flurpiridaz is a novel PET-MPI tracer labeled with radiotracer fluorine-18 (F-18) which has a high myocardial extraction across a wide range of MBF values superior in the upper range of flow compared with other tracers and can be produced as a unit dose from a regional cyclotron preventing the need for an onsite cyclotron. Various phase trial studies show that flupiridaz is clinically safe, has acceptable clinical dosimetry, and provides high-quality images in conjunction with exercise treadmill and pharmacological stress testing demonstrating improved CAD diagnostic performance, image quality and confidence of interpretations with coronary myocardial blood flow (MBF-CFR) of the individual artery left anterior descending (LAD)/circumflex (Cx)/left main (LM)/right coronary artery (RCA) over Tc99-m leveled single photon emission computed tomography (SPECT) **(Figs. 3 and 4)**.

RESTING TC-99M SESTAMIBI WITH F18-FLUORODEOXYGLUCOSE STUDY FOR THE GOLD STANDARD ASSESSMENT OF MYOCARDIAL VIABILITY

Detection and quantitative abnormalities of ischemic/viable/hibernating myocardium in patients having CAD or history of past myocardial infarction would

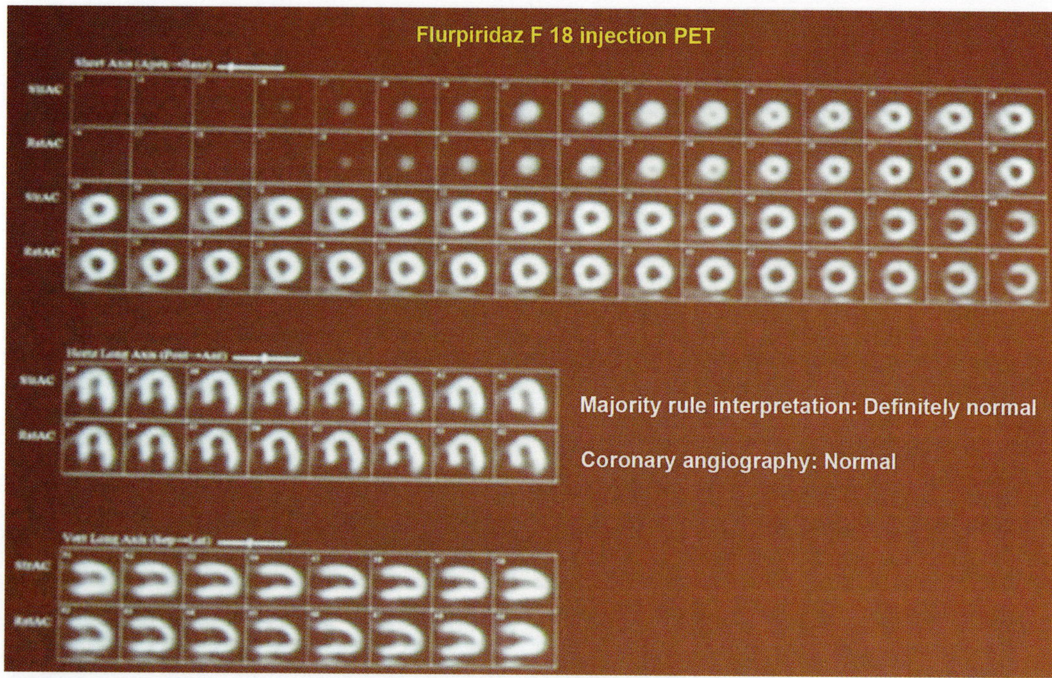

Fig. 3: F-18 flurpiridaz stress myocardial positron emission tomography (PET) imaging showing uniform perfusion pattern involving all the defined myocardial segments.
Source: Maddahi J et al. Eur Heart J 2011;13:A45

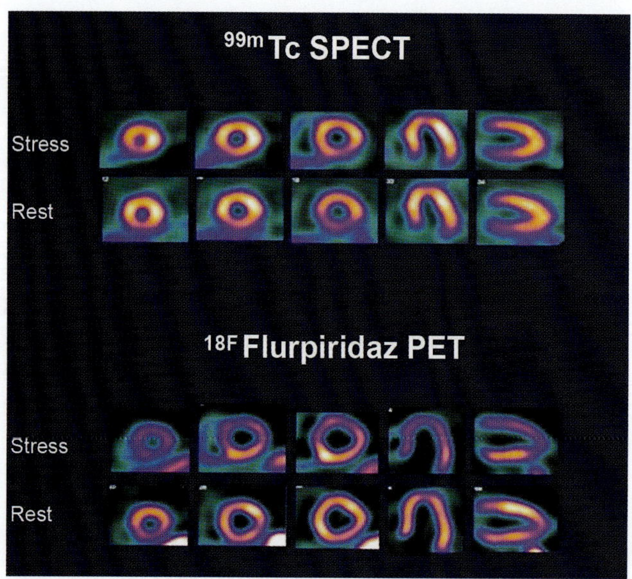

Fig. 4: A patient having left main disease where single photon emission computed tomography (SPECT) study reveals uniform perfusion pattern involving all the defined myocardial segments whereas the same patient showing stress perfusion defects with reversible ischemia confined to anterior, septal, apical myocardial segments using F-18 flurpiridaz positron emission tomography (PET) perfusion imaging study suggestive of increase sensitivity and specificity over SPECT perfusion study.

benefit from revascularization whereas scar tissue is unlikely to show functional recovery. Because viability directed revascularization would improve cardiovascular outcomes, reduces heart failure symptoms thereby reducing frequent admission to the hospital improving the quality of life. The calculated amount of viable myocardium above the threshold of 20% would likely benefit from revascularization. This quantitative parameter is only available with PET/SPECT myocardial perfusion imaging and viability study. Various metabolic tracers such as F18-FDG, rubidium-82, N13-ammonia, and F18-flurpiridaz are available in day-to-day practice and more commonly F18-PET tracers along with Tc-99m sestamibi-myoview myocardial resting perfusion scan **(Figs. 5 and 6)**.[1-3,10]

F-18 Fluorodeoxyglucose/F-18 Sodium Fluoride/Ga-68 Dotatate to Detect Atheromatous Plaque Along with its Vulnerable Nature

The complex nature of formation of atherogenesis leading to plaque formation may be exploited as targets for imaging and to differentiate between stable and unstable plaques to be diagnosed and assessed with novel PET tracers.

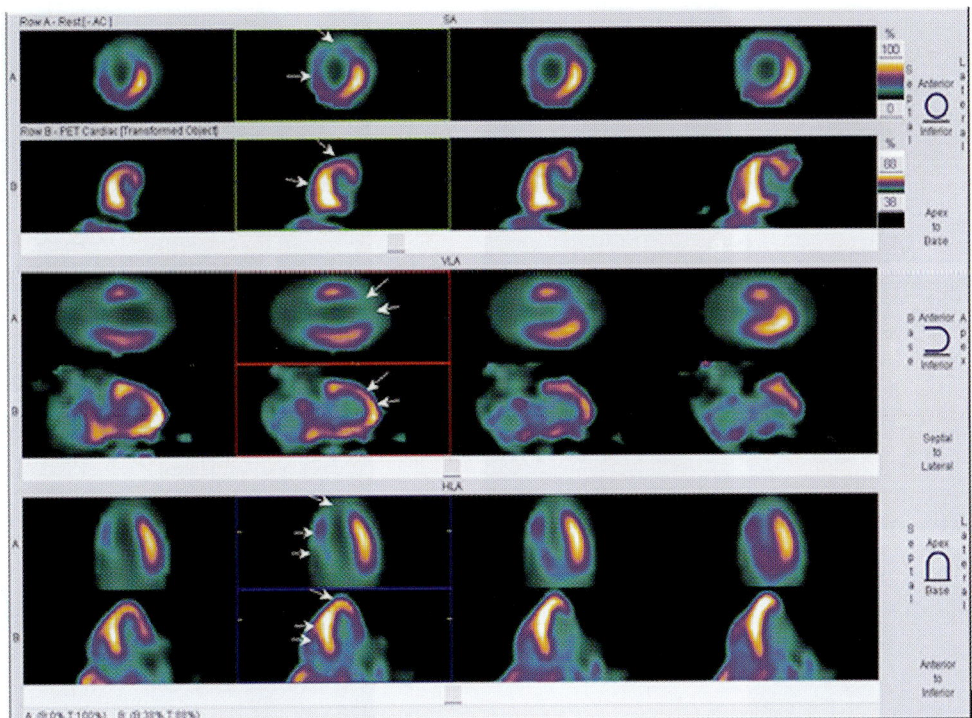

Fig. 5: Resting positron emission tomography (PET) myocardial perfusion study reveals multiple areas of perfusion defects involving anteroseptal and apical myocardial showing the adequate fluorodeoxyglucose (FDG) uptake pattern involving anteroseptal and apical myocardial segments suggestive of hibernating ischemic myocardium where patient would get benefit out of revascularization.

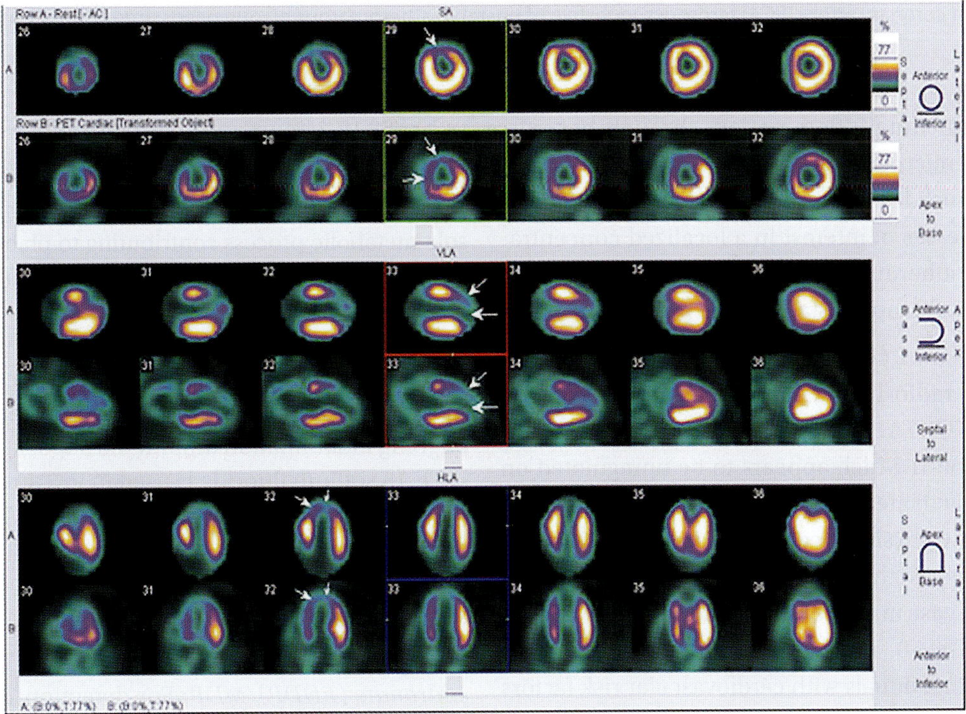

Fig. 6: Resting single photon emission computed tomography (SPECT) study showing multiple areas of perfusion defects involving anterior, part of septal and apical segments which do not show any significant fluorodeoxyglucose (FDG) uptake pattern in the segments mentioned suggestive of match pattern of having scarred myocardium would not get benefit out of revascularization.

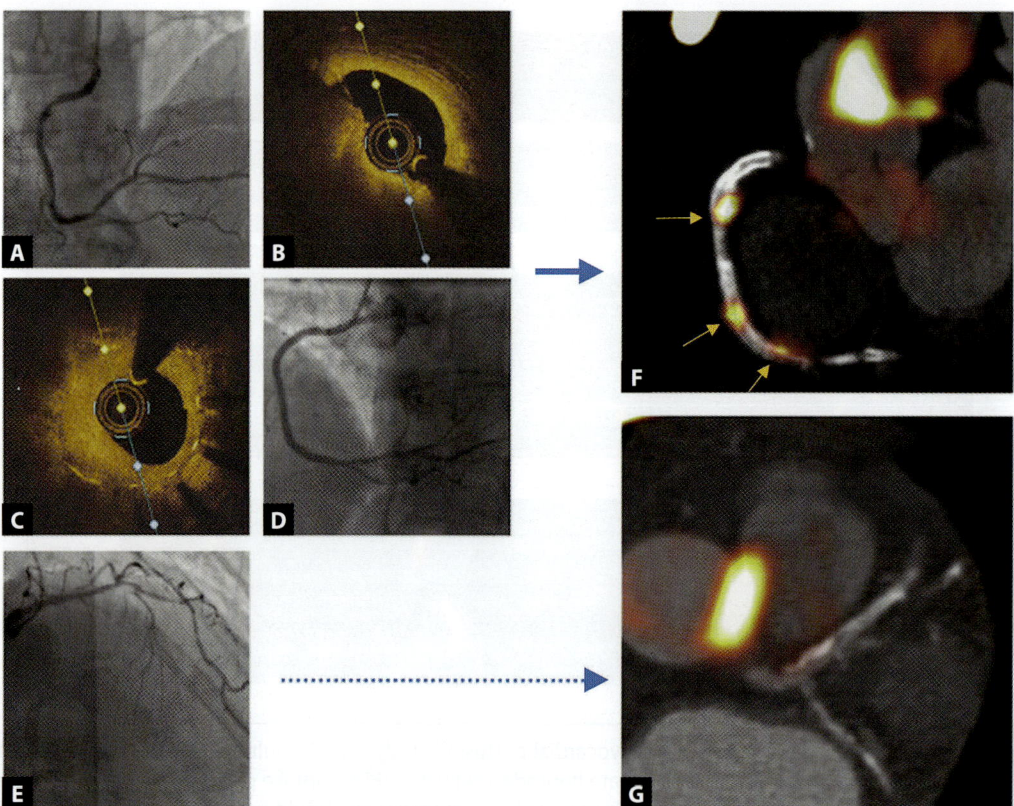

Figs. 7A to G: Ga-68 dotatate plaque imaging showing multiple focal areas of increased tracer uptake involving proximal and distal right coronary artery (RCA) territory suggestive of unstable atheromatous plaque needs urgent stabilization.

These targets include inflammation, through hypoxia, apoptosis, and microcalcification. PET utilizes positron-emitting radionuclides that accumulated at these different biological processes of interest in a localized concentration inside the atheromatous plaque thereby advocating aggressive statin therapy to stabilize the plaque.

Ga-68 dotatate and Cu-64 dotatate: Another clinically available PET radio-ligand for use in atherosclerosis imaging is *DOTATATE* which binds to somatostatin receptor subtype-II which appears to be upregulated on the surface of activated macrophages inside the wall of arteries. The low physiological expression of SST2 by the myocardium suggest that this tracer may be advantageous for targeting disease in the coronary arteries.[6]

Vascular Ga-68 *DOTATATE* uptake imaged in asymptomatic individuals with cardiovascular risk factors and coronary calcification.

Cu-64-DOTATATE has also been investigated for use in carotid imaging because of longer half-life of 68 minutes vs. Ga-68 12.7 hours and shorter maximum positron range **(Figs. 7A to G)**.

F-18 sodium fluoride (F-18 NaF): Inflammation is not the sole metabolic process contributing to plaque vulnerability as inflammation within the atheroma can promote microcalcification, the formation of deposit of calcium inside the plaque is smaller than 50 μ^3. Microcalcification may predispose to plaque rupture either through mechanical disruption to the fibrous cap or provoking ongoing inflammation around the deposit.[4]

F-18 sodium fluoride is used in PET imaging is to avail to identify areas of microcalcification in vivo because the radiolabeled fluoride is taken up at sites of microcalcification where it replaces the hydroxyl group of hydroxyl appetite **(Fig. 8)**.[5]

F-18 FDG/F-18 florbetaben/Ga-68 DOTATATE/Tc99m etidronate (EHDP)/MDP: For detection, monitoring the progression or regression of infiltrative cardiac disease such as sarcoidosis, amyloidosis, and other inflammatory cardiac diseases.

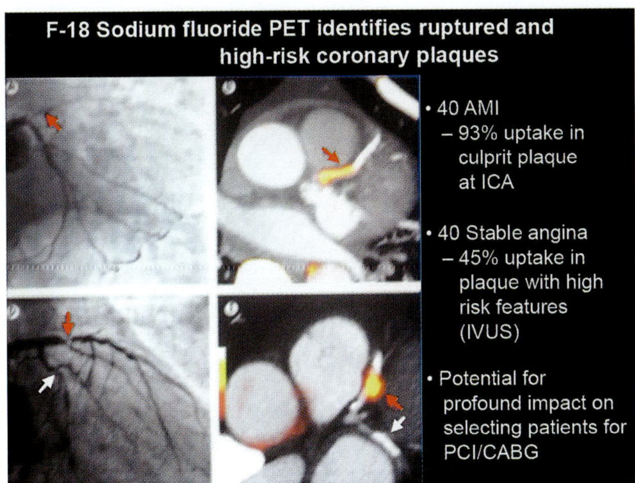

Fig. 8: F-18 sodium fluoride plaque shows focal increase radiotracer uptake involving proximal segment of the left anterior descending (LAD) suggestive of unstable atheromatous plaque needs urgent stabilization of plaque by intensive intake of statins.

- *Amyloidosis:* It is not so rare systemic diseases characterized by the interstitial deposition of insoluble protein fibrils that affect tissue structure and function. Cardiac involvement may occur in light-chain amyloidosis (LA) and in transthyretin-associated amyloidosis (ATTR) and limits patient prognosis.

  It is stabilized that seeking radiopharmaceuticals identify cardiac involvement in amyloidosis contributing to significant causes of heart failure with reduced ejection fraction (HFrEF). The usefulness of bone seeking radiotracers in diagnosing cardiac ATTR emphasizing early diagnosis of cardiac involvement in transthyretin gene carries or subjects with proven systemic ATTR and new onset of cardiac symptoms. The largest role, however, is in the workup of subjects with newly diagnosed heart failure for which echocardiography and cardiac MRI shows findings suggestive of cardiac amyloidosis (AL and ATTR varieties) which fails to diagnose between these two. In this setting, a bone scan using Tc99m MDP/Tc99m EHDP can differentiate whether it is ATTR showing increased uptake in the cardiac muscle without showing any uptake in AL variety and thereby decision can be best on the bone scan having moderate or strong cardiac uptake.[7-9]

  The transthyretin stabilizes tafamidis which can be prescribed with positive bone seeking agent in myocardium showing beneficial effects on surviving hospitalization rate and quality of life.

  Additionally, PET techniques are emerging in amyloidosis. Although the role of bone seeking agent F-18-NaF is still under debate because of low signal intensity.

  The original C-11 labeled Pittsburgh compound B as well as the F-18 labeled florbetaben bind to both ATTR and light chain amyloidosis (LA) in the heart where they allow quantification of cardiac amyloid burden. Importantly amyloid targeted PET also provides quantitative information about whole body amyloid distribution.

  A potential area of growth for amyloid PET is in monitoring treatment efficacy in the light chain amyloidosis and ATTR. Ultimately, the available and increasing use of bone seeking agents such as Tc99m MDP/Tc99m EHDP to stabilized molecular phenotypes of patients which will help in early identification of cardiac amyloidosis guiding patients toward early and effective molecular treatments **(Figs. 9 and 10)**.
- *Sarcoidosis:* Sarcoidosis is a systemic granulomatous disease wherein cardiac involvement may occur and contribute to adverse outcome. Like amyloidosis, cardiac sarcoidsis is traditionally underdiagnosed and this underdiagnosis has been a trigger for increasing implementation of normal reliable tools. Presently a combination of F-18 FDG-PET after preparing the patient under high fat and low carbohydrate diet for 15 days (2 weeks) and on the day of the test injection of unfractionated heparin (to increase free fatty acid) to suppress myocardial physiological glucose uptake along with resting myocardial perfusion imaging is recommended by expert consensus. Focal or multifocal sites with increased glycolytic activity are indicators of cardiac involvements suggesting of active sarcoid involving with perfusion-metabolism mismatch pattern in which reduced perfusion identifies tissue damage. Nonetheless focally increased F-18 FDG uptake may not necessarily be specific for sarcoid and has been reported in other inflammatory processes such as Chagas disease particularly. Late gadolinium enhancement cardiac MRI studies also identify cardiac sarcoid but fails to differentiate scar or active disease process in the cardiac muscle as well as caution to be exercised in patients with impaired renal function or implantable metal devices. Advantage of PET as a whole-body technique readily identifies extracardiac conduction abnormalities

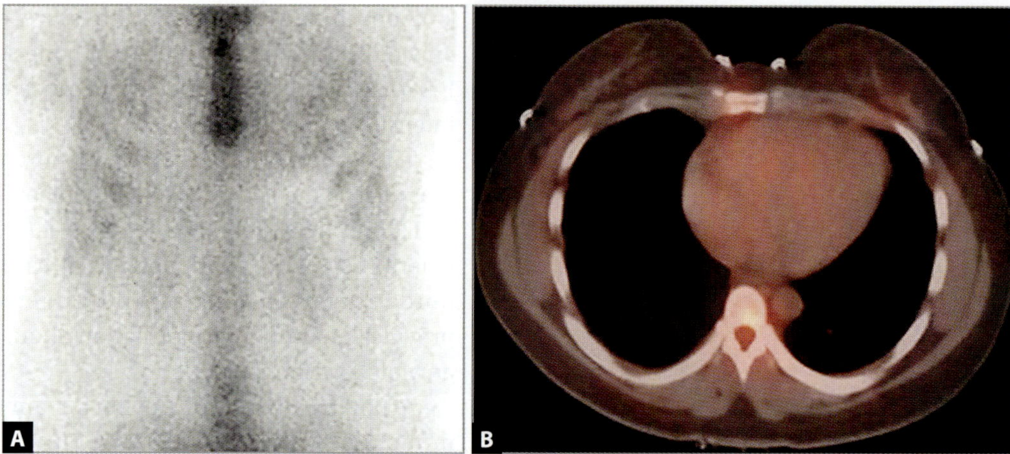

Figs. 9A and B: Tc99m etidronate (EHDP) bone seeking agent showing no significant myocardial uptake suggestive of absence of active amyloidosis of transthyretin-associated amyloidosis (ATTR) variety.

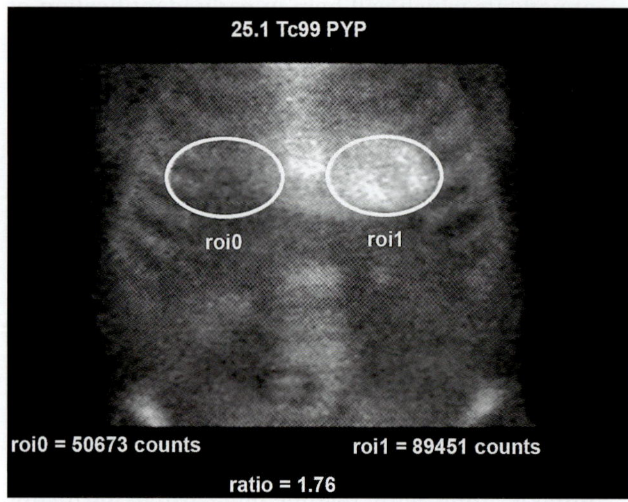

Fig. 10: Tc99m etidronate (EHDP) bone seeking agent showing multiple focal areas of myocardial uptake suggestive of presence of active transthyretin-associated amyloidosis (ATTR) variety of amyloid.

(2nd or 3rd degree atrioventricular block or idiopathic sustained ventricular tachycardia). Additionally, F-18-FDG sarcoid study can pinpointly diagnose active sarcoidosis with tissue damage or scar tissue, where therapeutic monitoring is essential and proved to be the best modality option.[11-13]

Corticosteroids remain the first line of therapy in sarcoidosis as well as its monitoring. Steroid sparing agents such as antimetabolites (methotrexate, azathiaprine, and leflunomide) are also embedded in therapeutic algorithm in refractory disease. The therapeutic armamentarium has been further expanded by several drugs targeting T-cell activation pathways **(Figs. 11 and 12)**.

F-18 Fluorodeoxyglucose Tracer for Detection of Inflammation/Infection of Prosthetic Valve, Bacterial Endocarditis, Other Inflammation of Cardiac Muscle, Pacemaker Lead, and Large Vessel Vasculitis

Infective endocarditis (IE) is associated with significant morbidity and mortality. Diagnosis of IE is usually accomplished through the use of the modified duke criteria. FDG-PET has been shown to be a useful imaging modality for the assessment of the prosthetic valve IE with high sensitivity of 100% and specificity of 100% than leukocyte scintigraphy. Infarct inclusion of FDG-PET positivity as a major criteria has been shown to significantly improve sensitivity of the modified duke criteria. In addition, extracardiac metastatic manifestation of IE identified on FDG-PET-CT can significantly affect management and prognosis of patients with IE extracardiac findings include septic emboli found in 30–55% of cases where an FDG-PET scan is performed for the suspected endocarditis. Whole body FDG-PET image allows detection of septic emboli a finding highly suggestive for the diagnosis of infectious endocarditis **(Fig. 13)**.

- *Native valve endocarditis:* The use of FDG-PET for the assessment of native valve IE has been less widely studied than for prosthetic valve IE. Inclusion of FDG-PET positivity results in an increase in sensitivity as in the case of prosthetic valve. Limitations include physiological myocardial uptake which be usually do

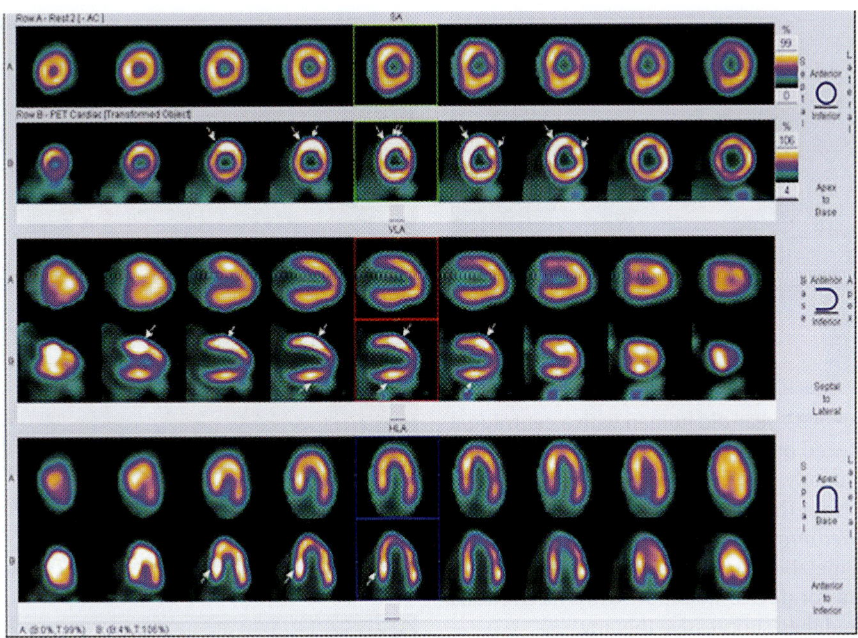

Fig. 11: Tc99m single photon emission computed tomography (SPECT) myocardial perfusion study and F18-FDG-PET study reveals focal areas of presence of active sarcoids seen involving anterior and inferior myocardial segments as compared to almost uniform perfusion pattern involving the rest SPECT study suggestive of no myocardial damage.

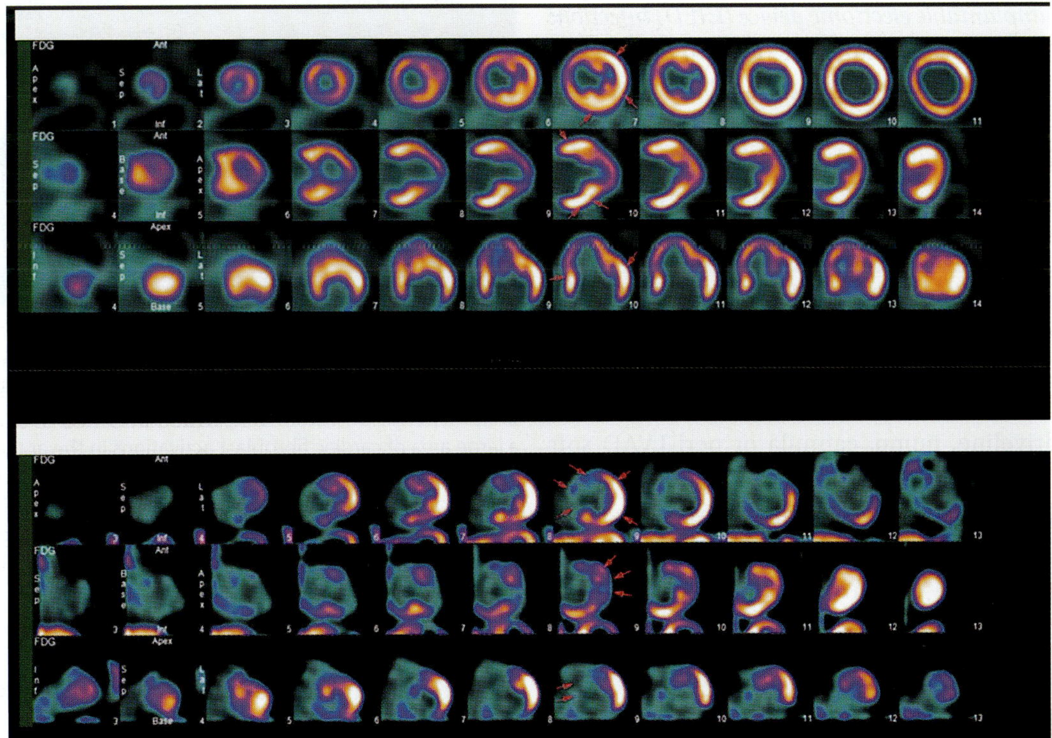

Fig. 12: F18-fluorodeoxyglucose (FDG) positron emission tomography (PET) study of the myocardium involving its anterior, lateral, and septal as well as inferior myocardial segments involvements suggestive of active sarcoid following which the treatment of steroid got started and there is significant response seen in the form of absence of FDG uptake involving anterior, septal and small part of inferior myocardial segments.

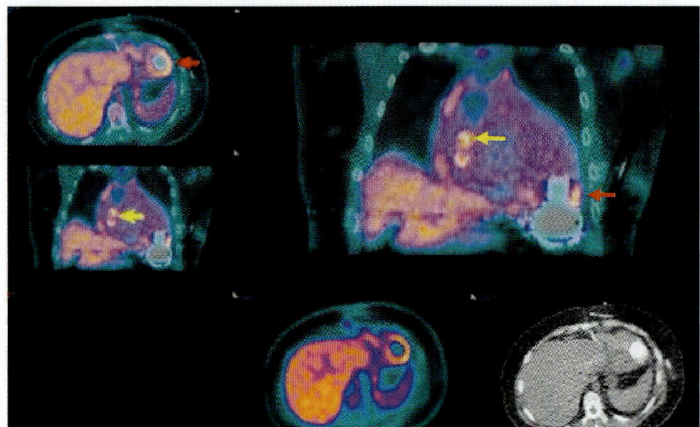

Fig. 13: The positive scan: A 33-year-old human with a centrifugal flow left ventricular-assisted device who presented with fatigue and fevers, and subsequently was found to have *Streptococcus anginosus* bacteremia. Note the increased radiolabeled uptake along the device pump *(red arrows)* and tricuspid valve ring *(yellow arrows)*, indicating high metabolic activity and possible infection. The patient was treated for device infection with intravenous antibiotics for 6 weeks and then suppressive therapy.

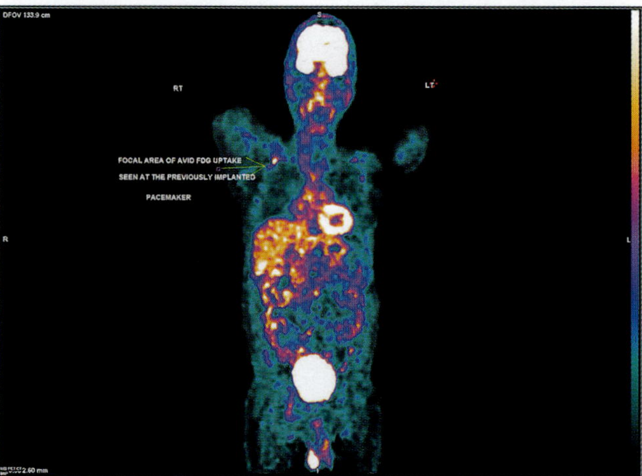

Fig. 14: Focal area of increased fluorodeoxyglucose (FDG) activity in the right side of the axilla suggestive of focal inflammation involving the pacemaker region which was previously implanted.

a suppression while doing the PET scanning, previous antibiotic therapy, cardiac motion, and in small vegetations.

- *Cardiac implantable electronic device (CIED) infection:* CIED infections can occur at the level of the pocket, leads or both. Management, usually, dependent on the severity and location of the infection within either deep pocket infection or involvement of the leads requiring surgical extraction of the device while more superficial infections can typically be treated with antibiotic therapy. FDG-PET has been shown to be accurate in the diagnosis of CIED infections **(Fig. 14)**.
- *LVAD infection:* Left ventricular-assisted devices are increasingly being used in patients with heart failure. Unfortunately, a complication of LVAD is concomitant of the driveline, pump, cannula or peri-LVAD soft tissues. It has been shown that FDG-PET can be useful for the diagnosis of early LVAD infection.

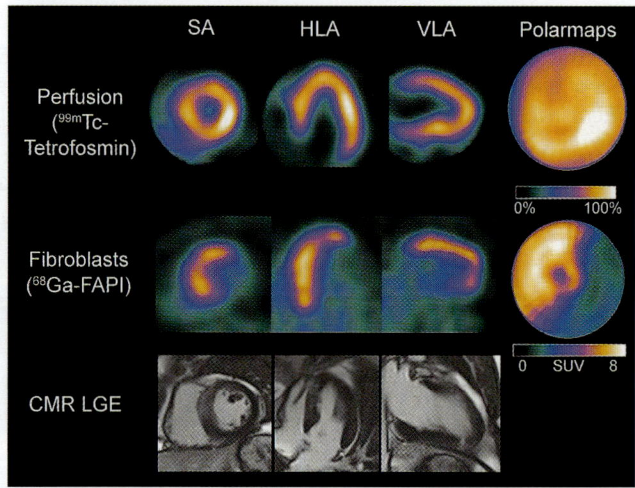

Fig. 15: Images showing reperfusion therapy following acute myocardial infarction (MI). The first row depicts single photon emission computed tomography (SPECT) images at resting phase uniform perfusion pattern followed by second row image showing a large area of cardiac fibroblast activations in the anteroseptal and apical wall. The 3rd row of the image shows absence of LGE in the corresponding myocardial images. (CMR: cardiovascular magnetic resonance; HLA: horizontal long axis; LGE: late gadolinium enhancement; LV: left ventricle; SA: short axis; VLA: vertical long axis)

Ga-68 Fibroblast Activation Protein Inhibitor for Imaging Myofibroblast (Fibroblast Imaging) in the Infarcted Myocardium as well as Focal Vessel Wall Lesion in Big Arteries to Detect Atherosclerosis/Fibrosis

It is known that after acute inflammation/infarction in the myocardium following which repair is characterized by activated fibroblasts along with aggregation of structural proteins shaping the extracellular matrix (ECM). This activation triggers an excessive accumulation of those proteins leading to fibrosis, stiffness, and finally heart failure.[15]

PET proves targeting fibroblast which is frequently used for various applications in oncology and, in recent years,

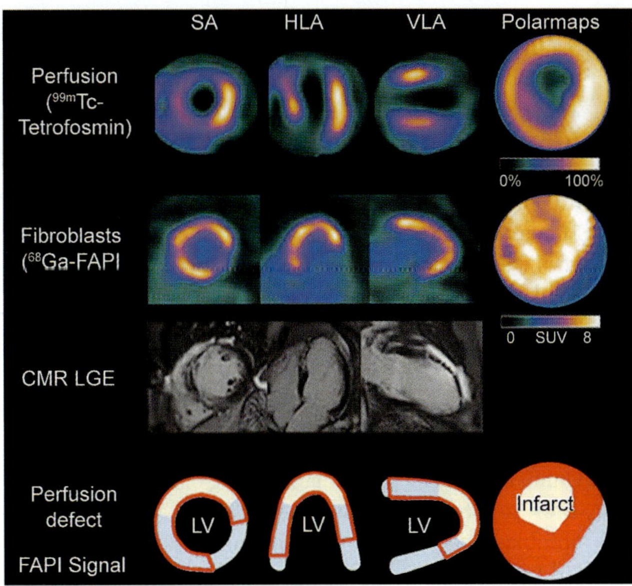

Fig. 16: Multiple areas of perfusion defects on the first row showing anteroseptal, apical, and part of inferior segment following postmyocardial infarction, where Ga-68 fibroblast activation protein inhibitor (FAPI) myocardial imaging shows presence of active increased Ga-68 FAPI tracer involving anteroseptal, apical, and part of inferior segments suggestive of presence active fibrosis going for ventricular remodeling where cardiologist can increase the dose of angiotensin-converting enzyme (ACE) inhibitors which can prevent this remodeling of the ventricle. (CMR: cardiovascular magnetic resonance; FAPI: fibroblast activation protein inhibitor; HLA: horizontal long axis; LGE: late gadolinium enhancement; SA: short axis; VLA: vertical long axis)

the clinical spectrum has been expanded toward cardiovascular medicines, e.g., after myocardial infarction. There is an increase uptake of Ga-68 FAPI from day-6 to day-11 showing persistent activation of interstitial fibrosis following MI leading to cardiac remodeling suggestive of bad prognosis and the treating cardiac physician should start immediately ACE-inhibitor to prevent cardiac remodeling **(Figs. 15 and 16)**.[14]

CONCLUSION

Nuclear cardiology procedures are no doubt the state-of-the-art procedures in the present-day clinical practice in diagnosis, prognosis, and guidance of therapy in CAD and non-CAD patients. The appropriate use of multimodality screening depends on clinical history, other risk factors so as to determine the correct order to conduct such tests to maximize clinical utility and cost effectiveness. The field of cardiovascular atherosclerosis imaging is rapidly expanding with increasing availability of noninvasive tools of PET, CT, and MR imaging. PET has emerged as a predominant noninvasive imaging tool using state-of-the-art radiotracers like F-18 sodium fluoride, Ga-68 dotatate/Cu-64 dotatate, and F-18 FDG for characterizing plaque morphology and in its disease activity for detecting vulnerability in various types of atheromatous plaque thereby aggressive pharmacotherapy can be started immediately to stabilize the plaque. Hybrid imaging platforms combined these modalities CT or MR with PET. Newer more specific radioligands and the increasing availability of PET/MRI or PET/CT is likely to hold promise in detecting and characterizing vulnerable plaque so that immediate starting of pharmacotherapy to stop the dislodging of the unstable plaque. Similarly, calculation of coronary flow reserve (CFR), particularly in patients of subclinical CAD, asymptomatic diabetic patients having endothelial dysfunction and microvascular disease can pinpoint the various involved coronary artery so that proper treatment can be instituted.

REFERENCES

1. Greenland P, Alpert JS, Beller GA, Benjamin EJ, Budoff MJ, Fayad ZA, et al. 2010 ACCF/AHA guideline for assessment of cardiovascular risk in asymptomatic adults: Executive summary: A report of the American College of Cardiology Foundation/American Heart Association Task Force on practical guidelines. Circulation. 2010;122(25):2748-64.
2. Shclendorf KH, Nasir K, Blmenhal RS. Limitations of the Framingham risk score are now much clearer. Prev Med. 2009;48(2):115-6.
3. Silverman MG, Blaha MJ, Krumholz HM, Budoff MJ, Blankstein R, Sibley CT, et al. Impact of coronary artery calcium or coronary heart disease events in individuals at the extremes of traditional risk factor burden: The multi-ethnic study of artherosclerosis. Eur Heart J. 2014;35(33):2232-41.
4. Divakaran S, Cheezum MK, Hulten EA, Bittencourt MS, Silverman MG, Nasir K, et al. Use of cardiac CT and calcium scoring for detecting coronary plaque: Implications on prognosis and patient management. Br J Radiol. 2015;88(1046):20140594.
5. Mojtahedi A, Alavi A, Thamake S, Amerinia R, Ranganathan D, Tworowska I, et al. Assessment of vulnerable atherosclerotic and fibrotic plaques in coronary arteries using (68) Ga-DOTATATE PET/CT. Am J Nuc Med Mol Imaging. 2015;5(1):65-71.
6. Irkle A, Vesey AT, Lewis DY, Skepper JN, Bird JL, Dweck MR, et al. Identifying active vascular microcalcification by (18) F-sodium fluoride positron emission tomography. Nat Common. 2015;6:7495.
7. Joshi NV, Vesey AT, Williams MC, Shah AS, Calvert PA, Craighead FH, et al. 18F-fluoride positron emission

tomography for identification of ruptured and high-risk coronary atherosclerotic plaques: a prospective clinical trial. Lancet. 2014;383(9918):705-13.

8. Kang X, Berman DS, Lewin H, Miranda R, Erel J, Friedman JD, et al. Comparative ability of myocardial perfusion single-photon emission computed tomography to detect coronary artery disease in patients with and without diabetes mellitus. Am Heart J. 1999;137(5):949-57.
9. Rajagopalan N, Miller TD, Hodge DO, Frye RL, Gibbons RJ. Identifying high-risk asymptomatic diabetic patients who are candidates for screening stress single photon emission tomography Imaging. J Am Coll Cardiol. 2005;45(1):43-9.
10. Wackers FJ, Chyun DA, Young LH, Heller GV, Iskandrian AE, Davey JA, et al. Resolution of asymptomatic myocardial ischemia in patients with type 2 diabetes in the detection of ischemia in Asymptomatic Diabetics (DIAD) study. Diabetes Care. 2007;30(11):2892-8.
11. Kay J, Dorbala S, Goyal A, Fazel R, Di Carli MF, Einstein AJ, et al. Influence of sex on risk stratification with stress myocardial perfusion Rb-82 positron emission tomography: results from the PET (Positron Emission Tomography) Prognosis Multicenter Registry. J Am Coll Cardiol. 2013;62(20):1866-76.
12. Di Carli MF, Hachamovitch R. Should PET replace SPECT for evaluating CAD? The end of the beginning. J Nucl Cardiol. 2006;13(1):2-7.
13. Matter MA, Paneni F, Libby P, Frantz S, Stähli BE, Templin C, et al. Inflammation in acute myocardial infarction, the good, the bad and the ugly. Eur Heart J. 2024;45(2):89-103.
14. Tillmanns J, Hoffmann D, Habbaba Y, Schmitto JD, Sedding D, Fraccarollo D, et al. Fibroblast activation protein alpha expression identifies activated fibroblasts after myocardial infarction. J Mol Cell Cardiol. 2015;87:194-204.
15. Varasteh Z, Mohanta S, Robu S, Braeuer M, Li Y, Omidvari N, et al. Molecular imaging of fibroblast activity after myocardial infarction using a (68)Ga-labeled fibroblast activation protein inhibitor, FAPI-04. J Nucl Med. 2019;60(12):1743-9.

CHAPTER 48

Diabetes and Hypertension: What is New and Most Recent?

Ashok Das, Alok Modi, Bharat Saboo, Harsh Hirani

INTRODUCTION

Diabetes mellitus and hypertension constitute two converging epidemics with profound clinical, societal, and economic impact. Globally, over half a billion people live with diabetes, while hypertension affects nearly 1.3 billion adults, often coexisting in the same individual.[1-25] The synergistic effect of these conditions amplifies cardiovascular risk, accelerates renal impairment, and drives premature mortality.[24] Despite decades of research, achieving durable glycemic and blood pressure control in real-world settings remains elusive, underscoring the urgent need for innovation.

Recent years have marked a turning point. Updated *American Diabetes Association Standards of Care (2025)* and the *latest European and Japanese hypertension guidelines (2025)* emphasize individualized targets, risk-based therapy, and the integration of multidisciplinary strategies. These recommendations reflect the dynamic landscape of treatment, where precision medicine and digital technologies are beginning to supplement traditional approaches.

Diagnostic innovations are particularly noteworthy. Continuous glucose monitoring (CGM), wearables, and AI-based predictive algorithms are enhancing early detection of dysglycemia, nocturnal hypoglycemia, and blood pressure variability.[22] Similarly, biomarkers and imaging modalities are refining stratification for microvascular and macrovascular complications. Such progress allows earlier, more precise intervention.

Equally transformative are therapeutic advances. Novel incretin-based therapies such as dual agonists, outcome-driven antihypertensive regimens, and pharmacogenomic-guided drug selection are redefining standards.[1-25] AI-based drug response prediction further personalizes therapy, minimizing trial-and-error prescribing and optimizing safety and efficacy.[22]

Digital therapeutics, mobile health platforms, and remote monitoring tools have become integral extensions of care. Systematic reviews confirm their effectiveness in lowering HbA1c, improving adherence, and supporting lifestyle interventions.[25] ChatGPT-like large language models and AI-enabled decision support are now being piloted in hypertension and diabetes clinics, with potential to scale globally.[24]

The objective of this review is to synthesize the *most recent and impactful updates in diabetes and hypertension management*, focusing on diagnostic advances, therapeutic developments, and the transformative role of AI and digital technologies. In doing so, it highlights both opportunities and challenges, with an eye toward their integration into routine clinical practice and future global health strategies **(Figs. 1 and 2)**.

ADVANCES IN DIAGNOSTIC APPROACHES

Accurate diagnosis and timely risk stratification remain central to the management of diabetes and hypertension. The *2025 ADA Standards of Care* emphasize annual screening for type 2 diabetes in high-risk adults and universal screening beginning at age 35, with fasting plasma glucose, oral glucose tolerance tests, and HbA1c as primary tools.[1] While HbA1c remains the cornerstone, its limitations in populations with hemoglobinopathies, anemia, or chronic kidney disease have led to the recommendation of complementary measures, including fasting and postprandial glucose.[2]

Continuous glucose monitoring has now become integral to diabetes care. The 2025 guidelines advocate CGM use across both type 1 and type 2 diabetes, underscoring *time in range (TIR)* and *time below range (TBR)* as more meaningful clinical outcomes than HbA1c alone.[6] Real-world data confirm that these parameters are strongly linked with microvascular and macrovascular

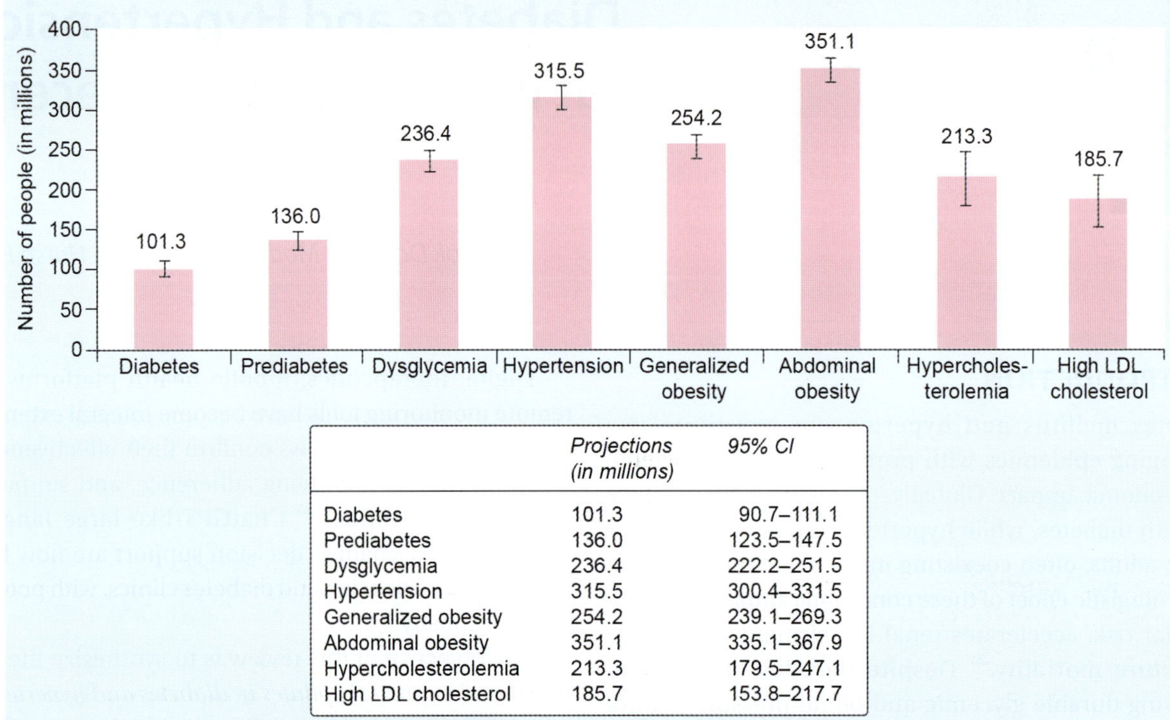

	Projections (in millions)	*95% CI*
Diabetes	101.3	90.7–111.1
Prediabetes	136.0	123.5–147.5
Dysglycemia	236.4	222.2–251.5
Hypertension	315.5	300.4–331.5
Generalized obesity	254.2	239.1–269.3
Abdominal obesity	351.1	335.1–367.9
Hypercholesterolemia	213.3	179.5–247.1
High LDL cholesterol	185.7	153.8–217.7

Fig. 1: Projections for metabolic prevalence in India.[26] (CI: confidence interval)

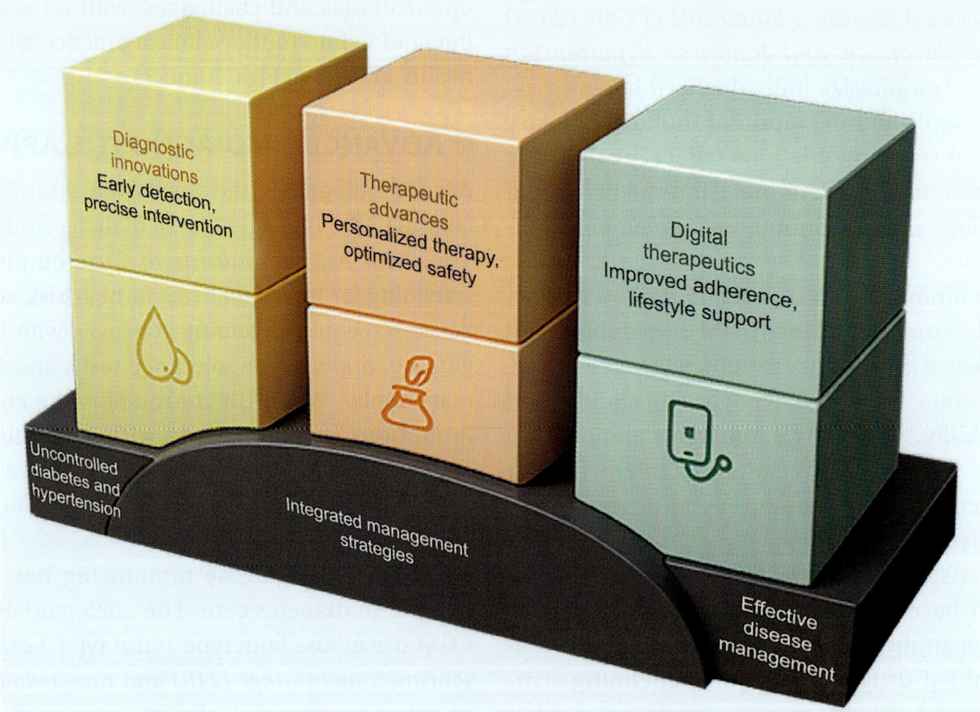

Fig. 2: Conceptual framework for transforming diabetes and hypertension management. Diagnostic innovations, therapeutic advances, and digital therapeutics function as complementary pillars, integrated through management strategies to transition from uncontrolled disease toward effective long-term control.

TABLE 1: Emerging diagnostic innovations in diabetes and hypertension from ADA 2025 Standards and contemporary hypertension guidelines, including AI applications.

Diagnostic domain	*Traditional approach*	*Recent advances (2025)*	*Clinical impact*
Diabetes – glycemia	HbA1c, FPG, OGTT[2]	CGM metrics (*time in range, variability*)[6,7]	Earlier detection, links to complications
Complications	Urinary ACR, fundus exam, monofilament[10-12]	Retinal imaging, vascular stiffness, automated screening[12]	Risk stratification, early intervention
Hypertension	Office BP alone[18]	ABPM, HBPM, nocturnal dipping and morning surge[18,19]	More accurate diagnosis, outcome prediction
AI Models	Limited regression approaches	EHR/phenotype clustering, ECG-based risk prediction[22]	Phenotype-specific precision diagnostics
Special Populations	FPG/HbA1c thresholds[14,15]	Tailored youth/pregnancy thresholds, CGM use in T1DM[6]	Improved maternal and pediatric outcomes

(ABPM: ambulatory blood pressure monitoring; ACR: albumin-to-creatinine ratio; CGM: continuous glucose monitoring; HBPM: home blood pressure measurement; FPG: fasting plasma glucose; OGTT: oral glucose tolerance test)

complications.[6] Importantly, CGM is no longer restricted to insulin-treated patients but increasingly considered for broader populations, reflecting its role in early detection of glycemic variability.[7]

In hypertension, the *European and Japanese 2025 guidelines* highlight the superiority of out-of-office blood pressure monitoring—home blood pressure measurement (HBPM) and ambulatory blood pressure monitoring (ABPM)—over clinic values for predicting target organ damage.[18,19] These recommendations aim to overcome "white-coat" and "masked" hypertension, common pitfalls in routine diagnosis. The emphasis on 24-hour profiles, nocturnal dipping patterns, and morning surges reflects the recognition of blood pressure variability as a predictor of cardiovascular events.[19]

Risk assessment is further enhanced by comorbidity-focused evaluations. The ADA 2025 chapters on cardiovascular disease, kidney disease, and complications such as retinopathy and neuropathy recommend routine use of urinary albumin-to-creatinine ratio, eGFR, retinal imaging, and monofilament testing for early detection of complications.[10-12] Importantly, these evaluations serve not just to diagnose comorbidities but to refine global cardiovascular and renal risk in diabetic and hypertensive patients.

In children, adolescents, and pregnancy, tailored diagnostic thresholds are now emphasized. Screening of overweight youth with additional risk factors is strongly advised, while in pregnancy, early testing for preexisting diabetes and mid-gestational screening for gestational diabetes are mandatory to improve outcomes.[14,15]

Collectively, diagnostic strategies have shifted from static to dynamic, from isolated measurements to continuous monitoring, and from single disease focus to *integrated cardiometabolic risk profiling*. See **Table 1** for a comparative summary of diagnostic advances in diabetes and hypertension based on ADA 2025 and ESC/JSH 2025 guidelines.

DEVELOPMENTS IN THERAPEUTICS

Therapeutics for diabetes and hypertension have entered a new era defined by outcome-driven targets and multidimensional strategies. The *2025 ADA Standards* endorse a patient-centered approach that prioritizes not just glycemic reduction but also cardiovascular, renal, and weight benefits.[9]

In diabetes, incretin-based therapies lead this transformation. *GLP-1 receptor agonists* and the newer *dual GIP/GLP-1 receptor agonists* offer robust glycemic control alongside reductions in weight and cardiovascular risk.[9] *SGLT2 inhibitors* are now strongly recommended for patients with diabetes and established cardiovascular disease, chronic kidney disease, or heart failure, irrespective of baseline HbA1c levels.[11] Their role extends beyond glucose lowering to organ protection, marking a major paradigm shift.

The ADA 2025 guidelines integrate these advances by recommending therapy sequencing according to comorbidities rather than glucose thresholds alone. For example, patients with heart failure with preserved ejection fraction (HFpEF) or reduced ejection fraction (HFrEF) benefit from early initiation of SGLT2 inhibitors, while GLP-1 receptor agonists are prioritized in those with established atherosclerotic cardiovascular disease.[10,11] **Table 2** summarizes the major therapeutic innovations introduced in the ADA 2025 and ESC/JSH 2025 guidelines.

Table 3 outlines the leading antihypertensive drug classes emphasized in ESC 2025 and JSH 2025 guidelines, with relevance for patients with diabetes.

Hypertension therapies have also been modernized. The *ESC 2025* and *JSH 2025 guidelines* advocate initiating

TABLE 2: Therapeutic innovations in diabetes and hypertension integrating cardiovascular, renal, and metabolic outcomes.

Therapeutic area	*Traditional strategy*	*Recent advances (2025)*	*Evidence/guidelines*
Type 2 diabetes	Metformin, sulfonylureas[9]	GLP-1 RA, Dual GIP/GLP-1, SGLT2i for HF/CKD/ASCVD[9-11]	ADA SOC 2025
Obesity	Lifestyle ± bariatric referral[8]	Pharmacologic obesity drugs with glycemic benefit[8]	ADA SOC 2025
Hypertension	Stepwise monotherapy[18]	Early combination: RAS blocker + CCB/thiazide[18,19]	ESC/JSH 2025
Resistant HTN	Escalation with beta-blockers	Mineralocorticoid receptor antagonists[19]	JSH 2025
CRM integration	Separate management	Combined GLP-1 RA + SGLT2i in high-risk groups[8,10,11]	ADA SOC 2025
Inpatient/pregnancy	Insulin protocols[15,16]	Structured basal–bolus, tighter GDM criteria[15,16]	ADA SOC 2025

(ASCVD: atherosclerotic cardiovascular disease; CCB: calcium channel blocker; CKD: chronic kidney disease; GLP: glucagon-like peptide-1; SGLT2i: sodium-glucose cotransporter-2 inhibitor)

TABLE 3: Top eight drug classes in hypertension management (2025), integrating evidence from ESC 2025 and JSH 2025 guidelines, with emphasis on diabetes comorbidity.

Rank	*Drug/class*	*Example(s)*	*Mechanism of action*	*Key 2025 highlights*
1	ACE inhibitors	Ramipril, Perindopril	Inhibit angiotensin-converting enzyme → ↓ RAAS	First-line in diabetes with HTN; CV/renal protection
2	ARBs	Telmisartan, Olmesartan	Block AT1 receptor	Preferred in CKD, DM with albuminuria; better tolerability
3	Calcium channel blockers (CCB)	Amlodipine, Cilnidipine	Block L-type calcium channels	Effective in Asians; lower stroke risk
4	Thiazide(-like) diuretics	Indapamide, chlorthalidone	Inhibit Na/Cl reabsorption in DCT	Strong outcome evidence; guideline-recommended in combos
5	Beta-blockers	Bisoprolol, Nebivolol	Block β-adrenergic receptors	Indicated in CAD, arrhythmias, post-MI patients
6	Mineralocorticoid receptor antagonists	Spironolactone, Eplerenone	Block aldosterone receptors	Key role in resistant HTN; CV risk reduction
7	ARNI (sacubitril/valsartan)	Entresto	Neprilysin inhibitor + ARB	Expanding role in HTN with heart failure
8	Direct renin inhibitor	Aliskiren	Inhibits renin	Niche use; not first-line but option in resistant cases

(CAD: coronary artery disease; CKD: chronic kidney disease; RAAS: renin-angiotensin-aldosterone system)

TABLE 4: Top eight glucose-lowering drugs in 2025, prioritized by ADA Standards of Care 2025 with integration of cardio-renal-metabolic benefits.

Rank	*Drug/class*	*Example(s)*	*Mechanism of action*	*Key 2025 highlights*
1	Metformin	Metformin	↓ Hepatic gluconeogenesis	Remains cornerstone; weight-neutral, safe, low cost
2	SGLT2 inhibitors	Empagliflozin, dapagliflozin	Inhibit renal glucose reabsorption	CV, renal, HF benefit; used independent of HbA1c
3	GLP-1 receptor agonists	Semaglutide, liraglutide	Incretin mimetic; enhances insulin, satiety	Strong CV risk reduction, weight loss
4	Dual GIP/GLP-1 agonist	Tirzepatide	Dual incretin agonism	Superior HbA1c and weight reduction
5	Insulin (next-generation analogs)	Insulin degludec, glargine U300	Long-acting basal analogs	Improved safety, ↓ hypoglycemia
6	DPP-4 inhibitors	Linagliptin, Sitagliptin	Inhibit DPP-4 enzyme	Moderate efficacy; safe in CKD
7	Thiazolidinediones	Pioglitazone	PPAR-γ agonist	Insulin sensitizer; role in MASLD/MASH
8	Fixed-dose combinations (FDCs)	Metformin + SGLT2i or GLP-1 RA	Multi-target synergy	Enhances adherence, improves outcomes

treatment with *combination therapy*—typically an angiotensin receptor blocker or ACE inhibitor plus either a calcium channel blocker or thiazide diuretic.[18,19] This strategy reflects evidence that most patients require at least two agents to achieve targets and that early combination improves adherence and efficacy. Resistant hypertension pathways highlight the role of mineralocorticoid receptor antagonists and newer non-steroidal agents.[19]

The pharmacologic landscape is increasingly shaped by the integration of *cardiorenal-metabolic care*. ADA 2025 guidance underscores the synergistic use of GLP-1 receptor agonists and SGLT2 inhibitors in patients with overlapping risk factors, offering dual benefits for glycemia, weight, kidney function, and cardiovascular protection.[8,10]

Obesity management has also advanced. The ADA 2025 section on obesity emphasizes pharmacologic therapies with dual glycemic and weight benefits, reinforcing their role in preventing diabetes onset and progression.[8]

Therapeutic goals are now individualized. Glycemic targets are tailored based on age, comorbidities, and hypoglycemia risk, with less stringent HbA1c goals for older adults and those with advanced complications.[13] Similarly, blood pressure thresholds are stratified by global cardiovascular risk, with stricter targets for high-risk individuals such as those with diabetes.[18,19]

In pregnancy, insulin remains first-line, but growing evidence supports adjunctive strategies for optimizing maternal and fetal outcomes.[15] For hospitalized patients, the ADA recommends structured insulin protocols and highlights the risks of therapeutic inertia in acute care settings.[16]

These therapeutic advances reflect a decisive movement toward *precision, integration, and prevention*. Where once glucose and blood pressure control alone dominated, the new paradigm prioritizes reducing cardiovascular events, preserving renal function, optimizing weight, and tailoring treatment to life stage and comorbidity. **Table 4** lists the highest-priority antihyperglycemic agents in 2025 according to ADA guidance.

DIGITAL THERAPEUTICS AND AI IN PATIENT MANAGEMENT

The incorporation of digital therapeutics (DTx) and artificial intelligence (AI) into diabetes and hypertension care represents one of the most significant paradigm shifts of recent years. The *2025 ADA Standards* explicitly recognize the role of diabetes technology, including CGM, insulin pumps, and decision-support platforms, in improving outcomes across diverse populations.[7] These tools not only enhance glucose control but also reduce hypoglycemia risk and improve quality of life.[6,7]

TABLE 5: AI and digital health tools supporting personalized management in diabetes and hypertension.

Domain	*Application*	*Evidence/benefit*
Digital therapeutics	Smartphone apps, wearables, lifestyle coaching	HbA1c ↓ 0.54%, BMI ↓ 0.84 in RCTs[25]
Remote monitoring	CGM, cuffless BP, telemedicine[7,23]	Reduced hypoglycemia, improved BP control
Drug response prediction	AI models using EHR, genomics[22]	Optimized drug selection, reduced inertia
Patient engagement	ChatGPT-like conversational AI[24]	Medication adherence, lifestyle reinforcement
Health systems integration	Hybrid models combining DTx + clinician oversight[7,23]	Cost-effective, scalable

Digital therapeutics extend this vision by offering software-driven, evidence-based interventions delivered via smartphones and connected devices. A 2025 meta-analysis of randomized controlled trials confirmed that DTx significantly reduce HbA1c (–0.54%), fasting blood glucose, and BMI in adults with diabetes, particularly type 2 diabetes.[25] Such platforms facilitate self-monitoring, lifestyle modification, and real-time feedback, bridging the gap between clinic visits and daily self-care. Importantly, they demonstrate scalability and cost-effectiveness, making them relevant for both high- and low-resource settings.[25] **Table 5** summarizes key domains of digital therapeutics and AI-driven management, integrating evidence from ADA 2025, RCT meta-analyses, and real-world studies.

AI-driven applications provide an additional layer of personalization. Machine learning models applied to electronic health records, pharmacogenomic data, and real-world registries can predict drug response, enabling clinicians to select therapies most likely to succeed in a given patient.[22] For diabetes, this includes predicting responses to metformin, GLP-1 receptor agonists, or SGLT2 inhibitors, while in hypertension, models can stratify patients likely to respond to ACE inhibitors, calcium channel blockers, or diuretics.[18,22] This predictive capability reduces therapeutic inertia and improves efficiency of care.

Remote monitoring has been revolutionized by AI-enabled devices. Wearables now capture continuous blood pressure, glucose, sleep, and activity data, feeding into integrated platforms that provide real-time alerts to both patients and providers.[6,23] In hypertension, AI-powered cuffless monitoring and retinal image analysis can detect subclinical damage, while in diabetes, predictive alerts from CGM prevent severe hypoglycemia episodes.[7,23]

The role of conversational AI, including large language models, has also emerged in patient education and support. ChatGPT-based interfaces have shown potential in assisting with medication reminders, answering patient queries, and delivering behavior change interventions.[24] These systems improve accessibility, particularly in populations with limited health literacy, and offer continuous, low-cost engagement.

Integration of these technologies into routine care is not without challenges. Barriers include variable patient engagement, disparities in digital literacy, and questions around long-term adherence. Yet, combined with traditional therapy, digital tools are transforming patient management into a *hybrid model* where human clinicians are supported by real-time, AI-enhanced insights.

CHALLENGES, ETHICAL CONSIDERATIONS, AND FUTURE DIRECTIONS

Despite the promise of novel therapeutics and digital solutions, several challenges must be addressed before widespread adoption.

First, *data privacy and security* remain paramount. The ADA and international guidelines emphasize strict compliance with data protection frameworks, as the increasing use of CGM, remote monitoring, and AI-driven platforms involves sensitive health data.[6,7] Breaches or misuse could erode trust and slow adoption.

Second, *algorithmic bias* is a concern. AI models trained predominantly on Western datasets may not generalize to populations in Asia, Africa, or Latin America, risking inequitable recommendations.[22,23] Ensuring diversity in training datasets and transparent validation is essential for global applicability.

Third, *regulatory frameworks* lag behind innovation. While agencies such as the FDA and EMA have begun

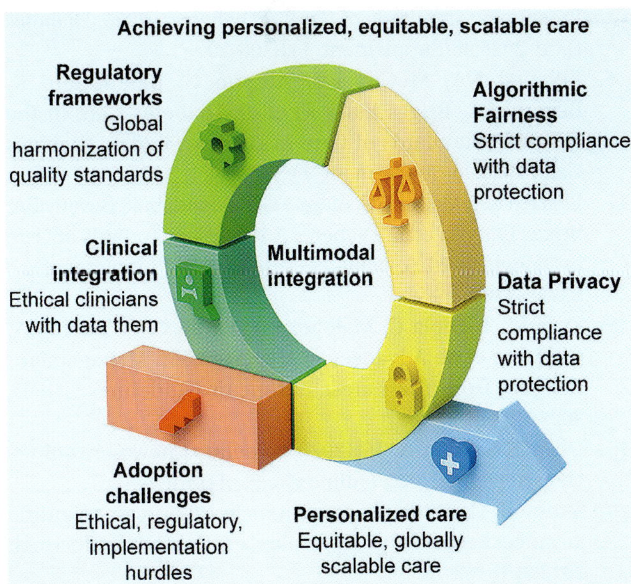

Fig. 3: Multimodal integration framework for achieving personalized, equitable, and scalable care in diabetes and hypertension. Key enablers include regulatory frameworks, clinical integration, algorithmic fairness, data privacy, and strategies to overcome adoption challenges, converging toward globally scalable personalized care.

approving DTx products, global harmonization of definitions, reimbursement, and quality standards remains incomplete.[25] Without clear guidelines, uptake may be inconsistent.

Clinical integration is another hurdle. Physicians often face "alert fatigue" from digital systems, while patients may disengage if platforms are overly complex. Embedding AI into workflows in ways that augment rather than burden clinicians will be critical.[7,23]

Looking ahead, the future lies in *multimodal integration*: combining pharmacologic innovation (e.g., GLP-1/GIP agonists, SGLT2 inhibitors), guideline-driven hypertension therapy, and AI-powered DTx into unified care pathways. Real-world evidence, pragmatic trials, and cross-disciplinary collaborations will be needed to validate and refine these models.[18,20,22]

Ultimately, by addressing ethical, regulatory, and implementation challenges, digital and therapeutic advances can achieve their full potential: *personalized, equitable, and globally scalable care for diabetes and hypertension* **(Fig. 3)**.

CONCLUSION

Diabetes and hypertension, two intertwined global health burdens, are entering a transformative era. The *2025 ADA Standards of Care* and contemporary *European and Japanese hypertension guidelines* reflect a decisive move toward individualized, outcome-based management, emphasizing prevention of cardiovascular and renal complications as much as control of glucose and blood pressure.[1-20] Advances in diagnostics, including CGM-derived metrics, out-of-office blood pressure monitoring, and integrated complication screening, now allow earlier and more precise risk stratification.[6,12,18,19]

Therapeutics have expanded beyond glucose and pressure lowering to encompass organ protection, weight reduction, and improved quality of life. GLP-1 receptor agonists, dual incretin agonists, and SGLT2 inhibitors are reshaping standards, while hypertension management increasingly relies on early combination therapy and resistant hypertension protocols.[8-11,18,19]

Complementing pharmacology, *AI and digital therapeutics* are redefining patient engagement and precision medicine. Predictive models for drug response, app-based self-management, and AI-driven decision support hold promise for equitable, scalable care.[22-25]

Yet, challenges of data privacy, algorithmic bias, and regulatory clarity remain. Addressing these issues will be essential to realize the full potential of this new paradigm: *integrated, personalized, and technology-enabled care for diabetes and hypertension worldwide.*

REFERENCES

1. ElSayed NA, McCoy RG, Aleppo G, Balapattabi K, Beverly EA, Briggs Early K, et al. Improving Care and Promoting Health in Populations: Standards of Care in Diabetes—2025. Diabetes Care. 2025;48(Supplement_1):S14-S26.
2. ElSayed NA, McCoy RG, Aleppo G, Balapattabi K, Beverly EA, Briggs Early K, et al. Diagnosis and Classification of Diabetes: Standards of Care in Diabetes—2025. Diabetes Care. 2025;48(Supplement_1):S27-S49.
3. ElSayed NA, McCoy RG, Aleppo G, Balapattabi K, Beverly EA, Briggs Early K, et al. Prevention or Delay of Diabetes and Associated Comorbidities: Standards of Care in Diabetes—2025. Diabetes Care. 2025 Jan 1; 48(Supplement_1):S50-8.
4. ElSayed NA, McCoy RG, Aleppo G, Bajaj M, Balapattabi K, Beverly EA, et al. Comprehensive Medical Evaluation and Assessment of Comorbidities: Standards of Care in Diabetes—2025. Diabetes Care. 2025;48(Supplement_1): S59-S85.
5. ElSayed NA, McCoy RG, Aleppo G, Balapattabi K, Beverly EA, Briggs Early K, et al. Facilitating Positive Health Behaviors and Well-being to Improve Health Outcomes:

Standards of Care in Diabetes—2025. Diabetes Care. 2025; 48(Supplement_1):S86-S127.

6. ElSayed NA, McCoy RG, Aleppo G, Balapattabi K, Beverly EA, Briggs Early K, et al. Glycemic Goals and Hypoglycemia: Standards of Care in Diabetes—2025. Diabetes Care. 2025; 48(Supplement_1):S128-S145.
7. ElSayed NA, McCoy RG, Aleppo G, Balapattabi K, Beverly EA, Briggs Early K, et al. Diabetes Technology: Standards of Care in Diabetes—2025. Diabetes Care. 2025; 48(Supplement_1):S146-S166.
8. ElSayed NA, McCoy RG, Aleppo G, Balapattabi K, Beverly EA, Briggs Early K, et al. Obesity and Weight Management for the Prevention and Treatment of Type 2 Diabetes: Standards of Care in Diabetes-2025. Diabetes Care. 2025;48(Supplement_1):S167-80.
9. ElSayed NA, McCoy RG, Aleppo G, Bajaj M, Balapattabi K, Beverly EA, et al. Pharmacologic Approaches to Glycemic Treatment: Standards of Care in Diabetes—2025. Diabetes Care. 2025;48(Supplement_1):S181-S206.
10. ElSayed NA, McCoy RG, Aleppo G, Balapattabi K, Beverly EA, Briggs Early K, et al. Cardiovascular Disease and Risk Management: Standards of Care in Diabetes—2025. Diabetes Care. 2025;48(Supplement_1):S207-S238.
11. ElSayed NA, McCoy RG, Aleppo G, Balapattabi K, Beverly EA, Briggs Early K, et al. Chronic Kidney Disease and Risk Management: Standards of Care in Diabetes—2025. Diabetes Care. 2025;48(Supplement_1):S239-S251.
12. ElSayed NA, McCoy RG, Aleppo G, Balapattabi K, Beverly EA, Briggs Early K, et al. Retinopathy, Neuropathy, and Foot Care: Standards of Care in Diabetes—2025. Diabetes Care. 2025;48(Supplement_1):S252-S265.
13. ElSayed NA, McCoy RG, Aleppo G, Balapattabi K, Beverly EA, Briggs Early K, et al. Older Adults: Standards of Care in Diabetes—2025. Diabetes Care. 2025; 48(Supplement_1):S266-82.
14. ElSayed NA, McCoy RG, Aleppo G, Balapattabi K, Beverly EA, Briggs Early K, et al. Children and Adolescents: Standards of Care in Diabetes—2025. Diabetes Care. 2025; 48(Supplement_1):S283-S305.
15. ElSayed NA, McCoy RG, Aleppo G, Balapattabi K, Beverly EA, Briggs Early K, et al. Management of Diabetes in Pregnancy: Standards of Care in Diabetes—2025. Diabetes Care. 2025;48(Supplement_1):S306-20.
16. ElSayed NA, McCoy RG, Aleppo G, Balapattabi K, Beverly EA, Briggs Early K, et al. Diabetes Care in the Hospital: Standards of Care in Diabetes—2025. Diabetes Care. 2025;48(Supplement_1):S321-34.
17. ElSayed NA, McCoy RG, Aleppo G, Balapattabi K, Beverly EA, Briggs Early K, et al. Diabetes Advocacy: Standards of Care in Diabetes—2025. Diabetes Care. 2025; 48(Supplement_1): S335-S336.
18. Zuin M, Tognola C, Maloberti A, Parati G, Di Fusco SA, Gil Ad V, et al. Advances in Hypertension Management: Insights from the Latest European Guidelines. JCDD. 2025;12(4):155.
19. Ohya Y, Sakima A. JSH2025 guidelines new viewpoints. Hypertens Res. 2025. Online ahead of print.
20. Shomali M. Diabetes treatment in 2025: can scientific advances keep pace with prevalence?. Ther Adv Endocrinol. 2012;3(5):163-73.
21. Zhang K, Qi Y, Wang W, Tian X, Wang J, Xu L, et al. Future horizons in diabetes: integrating AI and personalized care. Front Endocrinol. 2025;16:1583227.
22. Garg S, Kitchen R, Gupta R, Pearson E. Applications of AI in Predicting Drug Responses for Type 2 Diabetes. JMIR Diabetes. 2025;10:e66831.
23. Bae YS, Park S, Noh C, Choi B, Yi SA, Kim SE, et al. A comprehensive digital medicine platform for hypertension and diabetes care in primary care: A real-world feasibility test. Digit Health. 2025;11:20552076251344375.
24. Layton AT. A Heart-to-Heart With ChatGPT: AI Applications in Hypertension. Am J Hypertens. 2025;38(9): 621-7.
25. Li M, Chen Y, Chen X, Yao H, You L. Impact of Digital Therapeutics for the Management of Adult Patients With Diabetes: Systematic Review and Meta-Analysis of Randomized Controlled Trials. J Med Internet Res. 2025;27: e70428.
26. Anjana RM, Unnikrishnan R, Deepa M, Pradeepa R, Tandon N, Das AK, et al. Metabolic non-communicable disease health report of India: the ICMR-INDIAB national cross-sectional study (ICMR-INDIAB-17). Lancet Diab Endocrinol. 2023;11(7):474-89.

Diabetic Cardiomyopathy: Contemporary Understanding, Clinical Evaluation, and Therapeutic Advances

Ashok Das, Sureshkumar Vellingiri, Viswanathan Venkatachalam, RM Anitha, Bhargav Kiran Gaddam

INTRODUCTION

Diabetic cardiomyopathy is a heart condition that develops in people with diabetes, causing the heart muscle to weaken and not work properly, even in the absence of high blood pressure or blocked arteries.[1] It affects around 1 in 100 people in the general population and can be seen in 12–67% of individuals with diabetes, depending on how it is diagnosed. New treatments, such as SGLT2 inhibitors and glucagon-like peptide-1 (GLP-1) receptor agonists, have shown remarkable heart-protective benefits and are reshaping how doctors manage this condition. Still, there are major gaps when it comes to clear diagnostic tools, reliable biomarkers, and more precise treatment strategies, making it crucial to focus on personalized care and collaborative research effort.[2]

Background and Clinical Significance

Diabetic cardiomyopathy, first described in 1972 by Rubler and colleagues, is recognized as a separate condition marked by structural and functional changes in the heart muscle of diabetic patients in the absence of coronary artery disease, hypertension, or significant valvular problems.[3] With diabetes now affecting more than 450 million people globally, DCM has become a significant cardiovascular complication and a leading contributor to heart failure in this population.[4]

The importance of DCM lies not just in how common it is, but in the fact that it is a potentially preventable cause of heart-related illness and death. Studies show that people with diabetes are 2–3 times more likely to develop heart failure than those without diabetes, with DCM playing a major role in this increased risk.[2] The condition typically advances in stages, beginning with early diastolic dysfunction and eventually leading to full-blown heart failure, which makes timely detection and intervention essential for improving patient outcomes.[5]

Scope and Objectives

This detailed review is designed to offer doctors and researchers an up-to-date overview of dilated cardiomyopathy (DCM). It covers the latest insights into the disease's underlying mechanisms, modern methods for diagnosis, current treatment options, and directions for future research. Drawing on findings from major clinical studies, cutting-edge biomarker discoveries, and new therapeutic developments, this article aims to support evidence-based medical care while highlighting important gaps in knowledge that need further study.

DEFINITION AND PATHOPHYSIOLOGY

Definition and Diagnostic Criteria

Diabetic cardiomyopathy is currently defined as structural and functional changes in the heart muscle of diabetic patients, occurring independently of coronary artery disease or high blood pressure. The 2024 European Society of Cardiology (ESC) Position Paper describes it as the presence of systolic and/or diastolic dysfunction in individuals with diabetes mellitus.[6] However, the criteria used for diagnosing this condition vary widely among studies, leading to reported prevalence rates ranging from about 12 to 67%, depending on how strictly the criteria are applied.[7] This reflects ongoing challenges in reaching a standardized diagnosis for DCM in clinical practice.

Modern diagnostic methods emphasize echocardiographic evaluation, particularly assessing left ventricular diastolic dysfunction. According to the 2016 guidelines from the American Society of Echocardiography and the European Association of Cardiovascular Imaging, diastolic dysfunction is diagnosed when at least three of the following criteria are met: a septal e' velocity below 7 cm/s or lateral e' velocity below 10 cm/s, a peak tricuspid regurgitation velocity greater than 2.8 m/s, an E/e' ratio exceeding 14, and a left atrial volume index over 34 mL/m^2. These criteria help clinicians identify subtle changes in heart function in diabetic patients before symptoms become apparent. This approach provides a standardized and evidence-based framework for early detection of cardiac involvement in diabetes.[8]

Pathophysiological Mechanisms

The development of DCM involves a complex network of mechanisms primarily triggered by high blood sugar levels and insulin resistance. Key metabolic disturbances include reduced glucose utilization, increased fatty acid breakdown, and the accumulation of advanced glycation end products (AGEs). These changes cause mitochondrial dysfunction, elevated production of harmful reactive oxygen species, and activation of damaging signaling pathways such as protein kinase C and the polyol pathway.[3] Collectively, these processes contribute to structural and functional impairments of the heart muscle seen in diabetes. This multifactorial pathophysiology underpins the progressive cardiac abnormalities characterizing DCM.[9]

In type 2 diabetes, insulin resistance results in high blood sugar levels and excessive lipid buildup, which leads to lipotoxicity and damage to heart muscle cells. The increased production of AGEs and angiotensin II causes metabolic changes, mitochondrial dysfunction, and oxidative stress.[7] These harmful processes eventually contribute to damage of the endothelial lining, cell death, and activation of fibroblasts, promoting fibrosis and worsening cardiac function. This complex interplay of metabolic and molecular disturbances is central to the progression of DCM.[1]

Molecular and Cellular Basis

At the cellular level, DCM involves disturbances in calcium balance, impaired coordination between electrical signals and muscle contraction, and disrupted energy metabolism. Persistent high blood sugar reduces the activity of glucose transporter-4 (GLUT4), limiting glucose entry into heart muscle cells and shifting their energy source toward fatty acid oxidation.[3] This metabolic change contributes to lipid toxicity, mitochondrial damage, and increased vulnerability to injury caused by interrupted blood flow and reperfusion. These cellular dysfunctions collectively worsen heart muscle performance in diabetic individuals.[10]

Inflammation is a key player in the development of DCM. Activation of transcription factors such as NF-κB and AP-1 drives the production of proinflammatory cytokines, which in turn promote fibrosis in the heart muscle.[11] Moreover, disrupted nitric oxide signaling leads to endothelial dysfunction and decreases the heart muscle's flexibility, further impairing cardiac functions.

HISTORICAL PERSPECTIVE

Early Recognition (1972)

Diabetic cardiomyopathy was initially identified by Rubler and colleagues in 1972 when they examined autopsy findings from four diabetic patients who had heart failure but showed no evidence of coronary artery disease. This groundbreaking discovery challenged the then-common belief that heart failure in diabetes was solely due to coronary artery disease or high blood pressure. Their work established DCM as a unique clinical condition separate from other cardiovascular diseases.[12]

Evolution of Understanding

The understanding of diabetic heart disease advanced significantly after Lundbaek first proposed in 1954 that heart disease in diabetic patients could occur independently of hypertension and coronary artery disease.[13] Over the following decades, there was gradual refinement in the criteria used for diagnosis and deeper insights into the underlying mechanisms. Both type 1 and type 2 diabetes are now acknowledged as important contributors to this condition, highlighting its complex nature.[14]

Landmark Studies

Several important epidemiological studies have established the clinical importance of DCM. The Framingham Heart Study was among the first to show that diabetes itself is an independent risk factor for developing heart failure. This finding was further supported by the Strong Heart Study and the Cardiovascular Health Study, which reported that diabetic individuals face a 1.5–2 times higher risk of heart failure compared to those without diabetes.[14]

EPIDEMIOLOGY AND CURRENT BURDEN

Global Prevalence

Studies of general populations estimate that DCM occurs in about 1.1% of individuals overall, with approximately 17% of those with diabetes meeting diagnostic criteria for the condition. Among diabetic patients, around 54%

show diastolic dysfunction, while roughly 7% demonstrate systolic dysfunction. However, prevalence rates vary substantially based on the diagnostic standards used, ranging from about 12% with restrictive criteria to as much as 67% when more inclusive definitions are applied.[6]

Population-based Studies

The landmark Olmsted County study, which included 2,042 randomly selected residents aged 45 years and older, found that DCM affects about 1.1% of the community population. Importantly, diabetes was shown to increase the risk of left ventricular dysfunction by nearly twofold, diastolic dysfunction by 1.7 times, and systolic dysfunction by more than twofold after adjusting for age and sex. This study provided crucial population-based evidence linking diabetes to significant impairment in heart muscle function.[2]

Recent analyses combining data from multiple large studies—ARIC, CHS, and CRIC—examined over 10,208 participants without prior cardiovascular disease and confirmed that DCM poses a significant burden across various populations. The studies found that the 5-year incidence of heart failure among individuals diagnosed with DCM ranged between 8.4% and 12.8%, depending on the diagnostic criteria applied.[6]

Risk Factors and Demographics

Several important factors increase the risk of developing DCM, including the length of time a person has had diabetes, their level of blood sugar control, age, presence of hypertension, and kidney dysfunction. In patients with type 1 diabetes, each 1% rise in HbA1c is linked to a 30% higher risk of heart failure, while in those with type 2 diabetes, the risk increases by 8%. Modern predictive models also highlight other significant indicators such as systolic blood pressure, urinary albumin-to-creatinine ratio, size of the left atrium, and thickness of the left ventricular posterior wall.[15]

CLINICAL EVALUATION AND DIAGNOSIS

Diagnostic Criteria and Guidelines

Modern diagnostic strategies aim to detect structural and functional heart abnormalities in diabetic patients using a combination of assessment methods. A major challenge in the field is the lack of standardized diagnostic criteria.[15] Experts agree on the importance of developing unified approaches that integrate echocardiographic measurements, blood biomarkers, and advanced imaging techniques to more accurately identify and manage DCM.[15]

Echocardiographic Assessment

Echocardiography remains the primary tool for diagnosing DCM, with advanced techniques such as tissue Doppler imaging and strain rate imaging enabling early detection of subtle heart dysfunction. Important parameters include evaluating diastolic function through measures such as the E/e′ ratio, left atrial volume index, and tissue velocity assessments. Additionally, global longitudinal strain is a sensitive marker that can detect early systolic dysfunction often before any reduction in ejection fraction is apparent.[16]

Advanced echocardiographic methods, especially speckle tracking echocardiography (STE), are particularly valuable in identifying subtle myocardial dysfunction that might otherwise go undetected. Among the earliest changes observed is left ventricular diastolic dysfunction, which typically appears before any noticeable abnormalities in systolic function. STE provides sensitive measurements of myocardial strain, enabling early diagnosis of cardiac involvement in diabetic patients and potentially guiding timely therapeutic intervention.[15]

Advanced Imaging Modalities

Cardiac magnetic resonance imaging (CMR) offers advanced tissue characterization capabilities, allowing for precise detection of myocardial fibrosis using techniques such as late gadolinium enhancement and T1 mapping. Additionally, magnetic resonance spectroscopy provides valuable insights into myocardial metabolism, where alterations like reduced phosphocreatine to ATP ratios and increased triglyceride accumulation serve as early markers of DCM. These imaging methods offer a comprehensive, noninvasive approach to identifying early structural and metabolic changes in diabetic heart disease.[16]

Positron emission tomography (PET) allows detailed assessment of heart muscle metabolism, specifically measuring glucose and fatty acid utilization. This technique offers valuable mechanistic insights into the metabolic remodeling that characterizes DCM. PET and other advanced imaging modalities complement traditional echocardiography by providing a comprehensive evaluation of diabetic heart disease, particularly useful in research settings and complex clinical cases.[3]

BIOMARKERS AND LABORATORY TESTS

New biomarkers are showing great promise for the early detection and monitoring of DCM. Proteins such as galectin-3, growth differentiation factor-15 (GDF-15), and soluble suppression of tumorigenicity 2 (sST2) have been found to correlate with the early stages of DCM and provide valuable prognostic information. Additionally, long noncoding RNAs (lncRNAs) are emerging as novel biomarkers, offering insights not only for early diagnosis but also for understanding the underlying mechanisms of the disease.[15]

Traditional cardiac biomarkers such as brain natriuretic peptide (BNP) and NT-proBNP have shown limited effectiveness in detecting DCM during its early stages. However, increased levels of these markers are often seen in more advanced phases of the disease. Inflammatory markers, including C-reactive protein and interleukin-6, can indicate ongoing pathological processes in the heart but still require further research to confirm their usefulness in routine clinical practice.[17]

RECENT ADVANCES IN PATHOPHYSIOLOGY

Metabolic Dysregulation

Recent research has emphasized the critical role of metabolic reprogramming in the development of DCM. Chronic high blood sugar impairs glucose uptake and boosts gluconeogenesis, which leads to reduced expression of glucose transporters GLUT1 and GLUT4 in heart muscle cells. As a result, the heart relies more heavily on fatty acid oxidation, which contributes to lipid toxicity and mitochondrial damage.

The formation of AGEs is a crucial mechanism in the pathophysiology of DCM. AGEs lead to the cross-linking of extracellular matrix proteins, which promotes cardiac fibrosis. Furthermore, the buildup of lipid intermediates such as ceramide and diacylglycerol plays a significant role in damaging heart muscle cells, contributing to their dysfunction and death.[9]

Inflammatory Pathways

Inflammation is a vital factor in the progression of DCM. Persistent high blood sugar levels lead to an overproduction of reactive oxygen species, which in turn triggers inflammatory pathways. Important inflammatory agents such as tumor necrosis factor-α, interleukin-6, and C-reactive protein play significant roles in promoting changes in the heart muscle's structure and impairing its function.[17]

Nuclear factor-κB (NF-κB) and activator protein-1 (AP-1) are key transcription factors that regulate inflammatory responses in DCM. Recent studies have highlighted peroxisome proliferator-activated receptor beta/delta (PPARβ/δ) as a promising therapeutic target. Activating PPARβ/δ can inhibit proinflammatory transcription factors such as NF-κB and AP-1 and block the mitogen-activated protein kinase (MAPK) signaling pathways, potentially reducing inflammation and cardiac damage in DCM.[18]

Oxidative Stress and Fibrosis

Nuclear factor-κB (NF-κB) and activator protein-1 (AP-1) are essential transcription factors that control inflammatory processes in DCM. Recent research has identified peroxisome proliferator-activated receptor beta/delta (PPARβ/δ) as a potential target for therapy. By activating PPARβ/δ, it is possible to suppress proinflammatory factors such as NF-κB and AP-1, as well as inhibit MAPK signaling pathways, which may help decrease inflammation and protect the heart from damage in DCM.[9]

Myocardial fibrosis is a defining feature of DCM, characterized by excessive collagen buildup and cross-linking that stiffen the heart's ventricles, reducing their ability to expand and contract efficiently. The degree of fibrosis is closely linked to increased heart size and worsening heart function. Because of its significant impact, targeting fibrosis is considered a crucial approach for treating DCM.[13]

Novel Therapeutic Targets

New therapeutic targets under investigation for DCM include regulators of calcium balance, pathways involved in autophagy, and epigenetic factors. Promising candidates for drug development are proteins such as FoxO, endothelin-1, and calcium/calmodulin-dependent protein kinase II. Furthermore, stem cell therapy has shown encouraging results in preclinical studies, although its effectiveness in clinical settings has yet to be established.[16]

RECENT PIVOTAL CLINICAL TRIALS

SGLT2 Inhibitor Trials

SGLT2 inhibitors have shown impressive heart-protective effects in several major clinical trials. The *EMPA-REG OUTCOME* study found that empagliflozin lowered the risk of hospitalization for heart failure by 35% in patients with type 2 diabetes who were at cardiovascular risk.[19] Likewise, the *CANVAS program* investigating canagliflozin and the *DECLARE-TIMI 58 trial* evaluating dapagliflozin both reported significant and consistent reductions in heart failure-related events.[18]

The *DAPA-HF trial* marked a pivotal moment by showing that dapagliflozin significantly reduced the risk of cardiovascular death and hospitalizations for heart failure in patients with heart failure with reduced ejection fraction (HFrEF), regardless of whether they had diabetes.[20] The primary combined outcome occurred in 16.3% of patients treated with dapagliflozin compared to 21.2% in the placebo group, corresponding to a 26% risk reduction (hazard ratio 0.74, $p < 0.001$[21]). This trial established dapagliflozin as an important therapy for heart failure beyond its glucose-lowering effects.[22]

The *EMPEROR-Reduced trial* reinforced the cardiovascular benefits seen with SGLT2 inhibitors by demonstrating that empagliflozin similarly reduced cardiovascular death and hospitalizations for heart failure. Supporting these findings, meta-analyses that included nearly 47,000 patients from six major trials consistently showed that SGLT2 inhibitors reduce the risk of major adverse cardiovascular events by 10% (hazard ratio 0.90, 95% CI: 0.85–0.95) and lower heart failure hospitalizations by 32% (hazard ratio 0.68, 95% CI: 0.61–0.76).[23]

Glucagon-like Peptide-1 Receptor Agonist Studies

Glucagon-like peptide-1 receptor agonists have demonstrated meaningful cardiovascular benefits in diabetic patients at high risk for heart problems.[24] The *LEADER trial* showed that liraglutide reduced major adverse cardiovascular events by 13% over a period of 3.5 years in individuals with type 2 diabetes and elevated cardiovascular risk.[22] Notably, liraglutide also contributed to improvements in left ventricular function, partly by reducing systemic inflammation.[25]

The *HARMONY Outcomes trial* with albiglutide and the *SURPASS* series studying tirzepatide have reinforced the cardiovascular advantages of GLP-1 receptor agonists. Tirzepatide, which activates both GLP-1 and GIP receptors, has shown superior improvements in measures of heart function such as left ventricular strain and myocardial work index compared to traditional GLP-1 receptor agonists. These findings suggest enhanced cardiac benefits with this dual agonist approach.[26]

Meta-analyses have demonstrated that GLP-1 receptor agonists significantly lower the risk of major adverse cardiovascular events, all-cause death, cardiovascular death, and stroke. These cardiovascular benefits go beyond simply controlling blood sugar levels and include direct positive effects on the heart muscle. Specifically, GLP-1 receptor agonists improve left ventricular function and decrease arterial stiffness, enhancing overall cardiovascular health.[22]

Angiotensin-converting Enzyme Inhibitors/ Angiotensin Receptor Blockers Evidence

Inhibiting the renin-angiotensin system is a fundamental strategy in managing DCM, with differing impacts seen between ACE inhibitors and angiotensin receptor blockers (ARBs). Meta-analyses reveal that ACE inhibitors reduce cardiovascular events by 14% and lower cardiovascular mortality by 17% in hypertensive patients with diabetes. On the other hand, ARBs primarily help by decreasing heart failure rates by 30%, but they do not show a significant effect on mortality.[10]

Clinical studies strongly support using ACE inhibitors as the first-line treatment for DCM, with consistent evidence showing they help reduce mortality.[23] The enhanced benefits of ACE inhibitors compared to ARBs may be due to their ability to increase bradykinin levels, a mechanism unique to this drug class. Nonetheless, both ACE inhibitors and ARBs effectively lower the risk of heart failure in diabetic patients.[27]

Emerging Therapies

Emerging treatments under investigation for DCM include peroxisome proliferator-activated receptor (PPAR) agonists, sodium-hydrogen exchanger (NHE) inhibitors, and anti-inflammatory drugs.[28] The recent discovery of PPARβ/δ's protective effects presents promising new opportunities to prevent inflammation and fibrosis in the diabetic heart. Additionally, resveratrol has shown cardioprotective properties in preclinical studies, working through its anti-inflammatory and antioxidant actions.[29]

EVIDENCE-BASED TREATMENT STRATEGIES

Glucose Control Strategies

Maintaining optimal blood sugar control is essential for preventing and managing DCM. Metformin, widely used as the first-line treatment for type 2 diabetes, has demonstrated cardiovascular safety and may benefit patients with heart failure, although direct evidence specific to DCM is still limited. Long-acting insulin formulations such as glargine and degludec appear to have neutral or possibly positive effects on reducing hospitalizations for heart failure.[30]

SGLT2 inhibitors have emerged as a major breakthrough in treating DCM, offering significant cardiovascular benefits that go beyond their blood sugar-lowering effects. These drugs improve heart muscle metabolism, decrease left ventricular mass, and boost endothelial function through several mechanisms independent of glycemic control. Their multifaceted actions make SGLT2 inhibitors a cornerstone in the modern management of diabetic heart disease.[26]

Cardiovascular Medications

Effective cardiovascular risk reduction in DCM involves a multifaceted strategy targeting high blood pressure, abnormal lipid levels, and heart failure management. The 2024 ACC Expert Consensus highlights the importance of promptly initiating and optimizing guideline-directed medical therapies. Key treatments include ACE inhibitors or ARBs, β-blockers, mineralocorticoid receptor antagonists, and SGLT2 inhibitors to improve patient outcome.

Modern heart failure treatment now centers around the "four pillars" of therapy, which include SGLT2 inhibitors alongside traditional neurohormonal blockers such as ACE inhibitors, β-blockers, and mineralocorticoid receptor antagonists. Early initiation and rapid uptitration of these medications are crucial to achieving the greatest improvements in symptoms, lowering hospital admissions, and reducing mortality.[28]

Novel Therapeutic Approaches

New therapeutic approaches are focusing on key underlying mechanisms driving DCM. Activators of AMP-activated protein kinase (AMPK) show potential in protecting the heart by boosting autophagy and regulating metabolism. Additionally, anti-inflammatory treatments that specifically target certain cytokines or transcription factors offer promising strategies to reduce inflammation and cardiac damage.

Precision medicine approaches that integrate genomic, proteomic, and metabolomic data hold the potential to tailor treatments specifically for individual patients with DCM. Early developments using machine learning techniques show promise in improving risk prediction and optimizing therapy choices. However, these innovative methods still need thorough validation before they can be widely adopted in clinical practice.[1]

Lifestyle Interventions

Lifestyle changes such as regular aerobic exercise, maintaining a healthy weight, and quitting smoking are effective strategies for preventing DCM. Consistent blood sugar control achieved through these interventions lowers the risk of developing DCM and related cardiovascular diseases. However, there is limited specific evidence on the impact of lifestyle modifications in patients with established DCM, indicating an important area for further research.

KEY KNOWLEDGE GAPS

Diagnostic Standardization

The lack of universally accepted diagnostic criteria poses a significant challenge in both research and clinical management of DCM. Variability in how DCM is defined leads to wide differences in reported prevalence, making it difficult to compare findings across studies and to apply results in clinical practice. Establishing standardized diagnostic protocols that combine echocardiographic measurements, biomarker assessments, and advanced imaging techniques is a crucial priority to improve consistency and translation of research into patient care.

The absence of standardized echocardiographic phenotyping, even in well-established epidemiologic cohorts, creates obstacles for translating research into clinical practice. Variability in how heart failure subtypes and cardiometabolic factors are clinically characterized adds complexity, making it challenging to interpret study results consistently and apply them effectively to patient care.

Therapeutic Targets

Although significant progress has been made in unraveling the pathophysiology of DCM, many potential therapeutic targets lack thorough validation. The disease involves a complex interaction among metabolic, inflammatory, and fibrotic pathways, necessitating integrated treatment strategies that address multiple mechanisms at once. Emerging targets such as regulators of autophagy, epigenetic modifiers, and pathways controlling cell death warrant comprehensive investigation to assess their potential efficacy.

The involvement of molecular targets like PPAR-α in the development of DCM is not yet fully understood and requires more in-depth research. Furthermore, regenerative therapies, including stem cell-based treatments, show promise but still need rigorous clinical trials to establish their safety and effectiveness.

Biomarker Development

Current biomarkers do not provide adequate sensitivity and specificity for detecting DCM at early stages. Although new biomarkers such as galectin-3, sST2, and long non-coding RNAs show encouraging potential, they require extensive validation across diverse patient populations. Developing multi-biomarker panels that integrate metabolomic, proteomic, and genomic data is a promising avenue for improving early diagnosis and risk stratification.

Standardized protocols for the collection, processing, and interpretation of biomarkers are essential to facilitate their effective use in clinical practice. Moreover, the long-term value of biomarkers in tracking treatment responses and disease progression requires systematic study to establish their reliability and utility.

Clinical Trial Design

The varied presentations of DCM and the lack of standardized diagnostic criteria pose significant challenges for designing and interpreting clinical trials. Existing preclinical models often fail to capture the full complexity of human DCM, which hampers successful translation of findings. There is a critical need to develop more representative animal models and to design clinical trials that specifically target distinct DCM phenotypes.

The lack of large-scale cardiac clinical trials specifically focused on patients with DCM restricts the available evidence for targeted therapies. Future research should prioritize thoughtful patient selection, appropriate outcome measures, and sufficient trial duration to effectively evaluate interventions tailored to DCM.

FUTURE DIRECTIONS

Precision Medicine

Integrating multi-omics approaches—encompassing genomics, proteomics, and metabolomics—offers significant promise for personalized management of DCM. Identifying genetic factors and molecular signatures could facilitate precise risk stratification and enable targeted therapy tailored to individual patients. Additionally, applying machine learning to analyze these complex datasets and predict treatment responses represents a cutting-edge area of research.

Pharmacogenomic strategies have the potential to optimize drug selection and dosing by tailoring treatments based on each patient's unique genetic makeup. In parallel, creating personalized biomarker panels could allow for individualized monitoring and targeted interventions, enhancing the precision and effectiveness of managing DCM

Novel Drug Development

Emerging therapeutic targets such as PPARβ/δ agonists, autophagy modulators, and antifibrotic agents warrant thorough clinical investigation to determine their efficacy in DCM. Combining therapies that address multiple underlying disease pathways may offer synergistic effects, enhancing treatment outcomes. Furthermore, drug repurposing approaches hold promise for uncovering existing medications that could provide specific benefits for managing DCM.

Nanotechnology-based drug delivery systems offer the potential to improve targeted delivery of therapies directly to cardiac tissues, reducing systemic side effects. Coupling this with biomarker-guided therapy selection could further enhance treatment efficacy and safety by personalizing interventions based on patient-specific molecular profiles.

Artificial Intelligence Applications

Machine learning models that combine clinical information, imaging results, and biomarker data hold great promise for the early detection and risk stratification of DCM. Artificial intelligence (AI) tools for automated analysis of echocardiograms may enhance diagnostic accuracy and make advanced cardiac imaging more accessible. Additionally, deep learning techniques applied to large clinical datasets have the potential to uncover new therapeutic targets and predictive biomarkers.

The creation of clinical decision support systems that integrate AI-based risk assessment tools has the potential to significantly improve clinical care for DCM. These systems can assist healthcare providers in making more informed, personalized decisions. However, thorough validation of these tools across diverse patient populations and varied healthcare settings is essential before widespread adoption.

Preventive Strategies

Early identification of individuals at risk for DCM through systematic screening programs can facilitate timely preventive interventions. Developing risk prediction models that integrate both traditional and novel risk factors may help guide personalized preventive care. Additionally, lifestyle intervention programs tailored specifically for DCM prevention need comprehensive evaluation to determine their effectiveness.

Population-level strategies that address social determinants of health and improve access to healthcare could significantly reduce the burden of DCM within communities. Innovations within healthcare systems that facilitate early detection and timely intervention are also critical priorities to enhance outcomes.

CONCLUSIONS

Key Clinical Recommendations

- *Diagnostic approach:* Clinicians should remain vigilant for DCM in all patients with diabetes, especially those with poor glycemic control or a diabetes duration exceeding 10 years. A thorough cardiac evaluation is essential and should include echocardiography with tissue Doppler imaging to assess diastolic function. For patients suspected of having DCM but showing normal results on conventional echocardiography, advanced imaging techniques should be considered to improve diagnostic accuracy.
- *Therapeutic management:* SGLT2 inhibitors are considered first-line therapy for patients with DCM due to their well-established cardiovascular benefits that extend beyond glucose lowering. ACE inhibitors are preferred over ARBs because of their superior mortality reduction demonstrated in diabetic populations. Overall, comprehensive cardiovascular risk management using guideline-directed medical therapy remains the cornerstone of care for these patients.
- *Monitoring and follow-up:* For diabetic patients, regular cardiac evaluation every 1–2 years is recommended to facilitate early detection of DCM. Monitoring biomarkers can offer additional prognostic insights, although standardized protocols for their use are still needed. Educating patients about heart failure symptoms and emphasizing the importance of consistent medication adherence is also vital for effective management.

Practice Implications

Recognizing DCM as a distinct clinical condition should be integrated into standard diabetic care pathways. Healthcare systems need to adopt systematic screening programs for early detection of DCM, especially targeting high-risk groups. Multidisciplinary care teams—including cardiologists, endocrinologists, and heart failure specialists—play a crucial role in optimizing outcomes for these patients.

Newer antidiabetic medications, particularly SGLT2 inhibitors and GLP-1 receptor agonists, provide substantial cardiovascular benefits and should be prioritized in treatment algorithms for diabetic patients at cardiovascular risk. Although these drugs have higher upfront costs, cost-effectiveness analyses demonstrate that their use is justified by reductions in hospitalizations and improved clinical outcomes.

Research Priorities

Immediate priorities: The development of standardized diagnostic criteria and screening protocols is one of the most urgent research priorities in DCM. Systematic validation of novel biomarkers across diverse populations and healthcare environments is also critical to ensure their broad applicability. Additionally, clinical trials tailored specifically for DCM patients, employing standardized endpoints, are essential to generate robust evidence for targeted therapies.

Long-term Objectives

Mechanistic studies that clarify how metabolic, inflammatory, and fibrotic pathways interact in DCM are crucial for identifying new therapeutic targets. Incorporating multiomics data into precision medicine approaches could facilitate personalized treatment strategies tailored to individual patient profiles. Additionally, implementation research focused on healthcare delivery and population health interventions is essential to reduce the overall burden of DCM at the community level.

Innovation opportunities: Artificial intelligence applications for automated diagnosis and risk stratification in DCM show significant promise but still require thorough validation across diverse patient groups and clinical settings. Developing novel drugs that specifically target the underlying pathways of DCM is an important area of future research. Additionally, systematic evaluation of preventive interventions focusing on modifiable risk factors is needed, particularly in high-risk populations.

Diabetic cardiomyopathy is at a pivotal stage, marked by important progress in understanding its underlying mechanisms and expanding therapeutic options. However, major challenges persist in establishing standardized diagnostic criteria and developing targeted treatment strategies. Ongoing research to fill these gaps, alongside the implementation of evidence-based clinical practices, holds great promise for significantly improving outcomes for the millions affected by this condition.

REFERENCES

1. Hassooni FRH, Aljubori E, Abbas GMA, Dheyab AYD, Abdulatif MQA, Sadeq Sadeq MA, et al. Advances in diabetic cardiomyopathy: current and potential management strategies and emerging biomarkers. Ann Med Surg (Lond). 2025;87(1):224-33.
2. Dandamudi S, Slusser J, Mahoney DW, Redfield MM, Rodeheffer RJ, Chen HH. The Prevalence of Diabetic Cardiomyopathy. J Card Fail. 2014;20(5):304-9.
3. Miki T, Yuda S, Kouzu H, Miura T. Diabetic cardiomyopathy: pathophysiology and clinical features. Heart Fail Rev. 2013;18(2):149-66.
4. Radzioch E, Dąbek B, Balcerczyk-Lis M, Frąk W, Fularski P, Młynarska E, et al. Diabetic Cardiomyopathy—From Basics through Diagnosis to Treatment. Biomedicines. 2024; 12(4):765.
5. Zhao X, Liu S, Wang X, Chen Y, Pang P, Yang Q, et al. Diabetic cardiomyopathy: Clinical phenotype and practice. Front Endocrinol (Lausanne). 2022;13:1032268.
6. Segar MW, Khan MS, Patel KV, Butler J, Tang WHW, Vaduganathan M, et al. Prevalence and Prognostic Implications of Diabetes With Cardiomyopathy in Community-Dwelling Adults. J Am Coll Cardiol. 2021; 78(16):1587-98.
7. Gulsin GS, Athithan L, McCann GP. Diabetic cardiomyopathy: prevalence, determinants and potential treatments. Ther Adv Endocrinol Metab. 2019;10:2042018819834869.
8. Matsushita K, Harada K, Kohno T, Nakano H, Kitano D, Matsuda J, et al. Prevalence and clinical characteristics of diabetic cardiomyopathy in patients with acute heart failure. Nutr Metab Cardiovasc Dis. 2024;34(5):1325-33.
9. Huo JL, Feng Q, Pan S, Fu WJ, Liu Z, Liu Z. Diabetic cardiomyopathy: Early diagnostic biomarkers, pathogenetic mechanisms, and therapeutic interventions. Cell Death Discov. 2023;9:256.
10. Hao G, Wang Z, Guo R, Chen Z, Wang X, Zhang L, et al. Effects of ACEI/ARB in hypertensive patients with type 2 diabetes mellitus: a meta-analysis of randomized controlled studies. BMC Cardiovasc Disord. 2014;14:148.
11. Rizza V, Tondi L, Patti AM, Cecchi D, Lombardi M, Perone F, et al. Diabetic cardiomyopathy: pathophysiology, imaging assessment and therapeutical strategies. Int J Cardiol Cardiovasc Risk Prev. 2024;23:200338.
12. Levelt E, Gulsin G, Neubauer S, McCann GP. MECHANISMS IN ENDOCRINOLOGY: Diabetic cardiomyopathy: pathophysiology and potential metabolic interventions state of the art review. Eur J Endocrinol. 2018;178(4):R127-39.
13. Yilmaz S, Canpolat U, Aydogdu S, Abboud HE. Diabetic Cardiomyopathy; Summary of 41 Years. Korean Circ J. 2015;45(4):266-72.
14. Bellemare M, Bourcier L, Iglesies-Grau J, Boulet J, O'Meara E, Bouabdallaoui N. Mechanisms of diabetic cardiomyopathy: Focus on inflammation. Diabetes Obes Metab. 2025;27(5):2326-38.
15. Galis P, Bartosova L, Farkasova V, Bartekova M, Ferenczyova K, Rajtik T. Update on clinical and experimental management of diabetic cardiomyopathy: addressing current and future therapy. Front Endocrinol (Lausanne). 2024;15:1451100.
16. Monzo L, Kobayashi M, Ferreira JP, Lamiral Z, Delles C, Clark AL, et al. Echocardiographic and biomarker characteristics in diabetes, coronary artery disease or both: insights from HOMAGE trial. Cardiovasc Diabetol. 2025;24(1):111.
17. Kumric M, Ticinovic Kurir T, Borovac JA, Bozic J. Role of novel biomarkers in diabetic cardiomyopathy. World J Diabetes. 2021;12(6):685-705.
18. Yeung AM, Huang J, Pandey A, Hashim IA, Kerr D, Pop-Busui R, et al. Biomarkers for the Diagnosis of Heart Failure in People with Diabetes: A Consensus Report from Diabetes Technology Society. Prog Cardiovasc Dis. 2023;79:65-79.
19. Shou Y, Li X, Fang Q, Xie A, Zhang Y, Fu X, et al. Progress in the treatment of diabetic cardiomyopathy, a systematic review. Pharmacol Res Perspect. 2024;12(2):e1177.
20. Abdelrahman AH, Salama II, Salama SI, Elmosalami DM, Ibrahim MH, Hassan EM, et al. Role of some serum biomarkers in the early detection of diabetic cardiomyopathy. Future Sci OA. 2021;7(5):FSO682.
21. Huang K, Luo X, Liao B, Li G, Feng J. Insights into SGLT2 inhibitor treatment of diabetic cardiomyopathy: focus on the mechanisms. Cardiovasc Diabetol. 2023;22(1):86.
22. Andrikou E, Tsioufis C, Andrikou I, Leontsinis I, Tousoulis D, Papanas N. GLP-1 receptor agonists and cardiovascular outcome trials: An update. Hellenic J Cardiol. 2019; 60(6):347-51.
23. Iwane S, Nemoto W, Miyamoto T, Hayashi T, Tanaka M, Uchitani K, et al. Clinical and preclinical evidence that angiotensin-converting enzyme inhibitors and angiotensin receptor blockers prevent diabetic peripheral neuropathy. Sci Rep. 2024;14(1):1039.
24. Usman MS, Siddiqi TJ, Anker SD, Bakris GL, Bhatt DL, Filippatos G, et al. Effect of SGLT2 Inhibitors on Cardiovascular Outcomes Across Various Patient Populations. J Am Coll Cardiol. 2023;81(25):2377-87.

25. Moka MK, K SD, George M. Emerging clinical approaches in diabetic cardiomyopathy: insights from clinical trials and future directions. Acta Diabetol. 2025;62(1):1-10.
26. Hosseinpour A, Sood A, Kamalpour J, Zandi E, Pakmehr S, Hosseinpour H, et al. Glucagon-Like Peptide-1 Receptor Agonists and Major Adverse Cardiovascular Events in Patients With and Without Diabetes: A Meta-Analysis of Randomized-Controlled Trials. Clin Cardiol. 2024;47(7):e24314.
27. Singh B, Cusick AS, Goyal A, Patel P. ACE Inhibitors [Internet]. Treasure Island (FL): StatPearls Publishing; 2025.
28. McGuire DK, Shih WJ, Cosentino F, Charbonnel B, Cherney DZI, Dagogo-Jack S, et al. Association of SGLT2 Inhibitors With Cardiovascular and Kidney Outcomes in Patients With Type 2 Diabetes: A Meta-analysis. JAMA Cardiol. 2021;6(2):148-58.
29. Greene SJ, Butler J, Kosiborod MN. Chapter 3: Clinical Trials of Sodium-Glucose Co-Transporter-2 Inhibitors for Treatment of Heart Failure. Am J Med. 2024;137(2S):S25-34.
30. Zheng Z, Zong Y, Ma Y, Tian Y, Pang Y, Zhang C, et al. Glucagon-like peptide-1 receptor: mechanisms and advances in therapy. Signal Transduct Target Ther. 2024; 9(1):234.

Index

Page numbers followed by *b* refer to box, *f* refer to figure, *fc* refer to flowchart, and *t* refer to table.

A

B

C

I

J

K

L

M

N

O

Q

R

S

T